Nutrition and Exercise Concerns of Middle Age

Nutrition and Exercise Concerns of Middle Age

Edited by
Judy A. Driskell

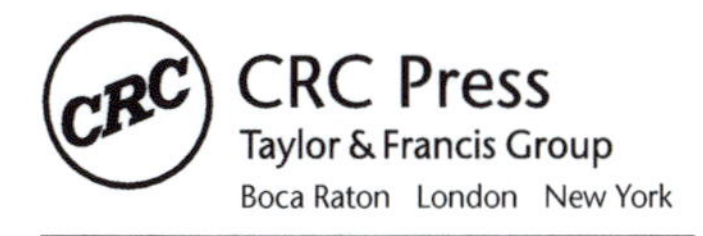

CRC Press is an imprint of the
Taylor & Francis Group, an **informa** business

CRC Press
Taylor & Francis Group
6000 Broken Sound Parkway NW, Suite 300
Boca Raton, FL 33487-2742

Printed in the United States of America on acid-free paper
10 9 8 7 6 5 4 3 2 1

International Standard Book Number-13: 978-1-4200-6601-2 (Hardcover)

Library of Congress Cataloging-in-Publication Data

Nutrition and exercise concerns of middle age / editor, Judy A. Driskell.
p. cm.
Includes bibliographical references and index.
ISBN 978-1-4200-6601-2 (alk. paper)
1. Middle-aged persons--Nutrition. 2. Exercise for middle-aged persons. I. Driskell, Judy A. (Judy Anne)

TX361.M47N88 2008
613.2'0844--dc22 2009001261

Visit the Taylor & Francis Web site at
http://www.taylorandfrancis.com

and the CRC Press Web site at
http://www.crcpress.com

This book is dedicated to the experts
who wrote the included chapters.

Contents

SECTION IV Minerals

SECTION V Fluids and Hydration

SECTION VI Other Commonly Consumed Substances

SECTION VII Recreational Activities

SECTION VIII Age-Related Disorders

Preface

The scientific and lay media extol the health benefits of good nutrition and physical activity. Most books that have been published about nutrition and physical activity have dealt with nutritional needs of young adults who exercise vigorously. At around 30 years of age or so, individuals start to become more concerned about having and maintaining good health and realizing the personal benefits of good nutrition and moderate-intensity physical activity. Some health professionals seem to believe that nutrition and physical activity information is the same for all people. What constitutes good nutrition and exercise habits is generally not interpreted for middle-aged individuals. Middle age is considered to be around 30 to 60 years of age. Middle-aged individuals most often are not involved in collegiate or professional sports but frequently do exercise on a regular basis as a form of recreation. Middle-aged adults are concerned about obtaining and maintaining good health and how they can reduce their risk of chronic diseases.

This volume includes a collection of chapters written by scientists from several academic disciplines who have expertise in an area of nutrition or kinesiology as it relates to exercise and sport. The introductory chapter on nutrition and exercise concerns of middle age is followed by chapters on the energy-yielding nutrients (carbohydrates, lipids, and proteins), three chapters on the vitamins (fat-soluble vitamins, vitamin C, and B-vitamins), three chapters on the minerals (major minerals, iron, and trace elements excluding iron). A chapter is included on fluids, electrolytes, and hydration. Chapters are included on the commonly consumed substances caffeine and tannins as well as herbal supplements. Two chapters describe resistance training and endurance training relating these to nutrient intakes, exercise recommendations, and overall health. The age-related chronic diseases cardiovascular disorders and cancer are discussed in relation to nutrition and exercise.

The book also includes appendices that list nutrient recommendations for middle-aged adults established by three major organizations: the Institute of Medicine, National Academy of Sciences for those living in the United States and Canada; the National Health and Medical Council (Australia and New Zealand Government for those living in Australia and New Zealand); and the World Health Organization. The daily values for vitamins and minerals are also listed.

Sports nutritionists, sports medicine and fitness professionals, researchers, coaches, trainers, physicians, dietitians, nurses, athletes, students, and the well-informed layperson will find this book to be informative and timely. It discusses "cutting edge" research on the topics of nutrition and exercise.

Judy A. Driskell, Ph.D., R.D.
Professor, University of Nebraska

The Editor

Judy Anne Driskell, Ph.D., R.D. is Professor of Nutritional Science and Dietetics at the University of Nebraska. She received her B.S. degree in Biology from the University of Southern Mississippi in Hattiesburg. Her M.S. and Ph.D. degrees were obtained from Purdue University. She has served in research and teaching positions at Auburn University, Florida State University, Virginia Polytechnic Institute and State University, and the University of Nebraska. She has also served as the Nutrition Scientist for the U.S. Department of Agriculture/Cooperative State Research Service and as a Professor of Nutrition and Food Science at Gadjah Mada and Bogor Universities in Indonesia.

Dr. Driskell is a member of numerous professional organizations including the American Society of Nutritional Sciences, the American College of Sports Medicine, the International Society of Sports Nutrition, the Institute of Food Technologists, and the American Dietetic Association. In 1993 she received the Professional Scientist Award of the Food Science and Human Nutrition Section of the Southern Association of Agricultural Scientists. In addition, she was the 1987 recipient of the Borden Award for Research in Applied Fundamental Knowledge of Human Nutrition. She is listed as an expert in B-Complex Vitamins by the Vitamin Nutrition Information Service.

Dr. Driskell co-edited the CRC book *Sports Nutrition: Minerals and Electrolytes* with Constance V. Kies. In addition, she authored the textbook *Sports Nutrition* and co-authored the advanced nutrition book *Nutrition: Chemistry and Biology*, both published by CRC. She co-edited *Sports Nutrition: Vitamins and Trace Elements, first and second editions*; *Macroelements, Water, and Electrolytes in Sports Nutrition; Energy-Yielding Macronutrients and Energy Metabolism in Sports Nutrition*; *Nutritional Applications in Exercise and Sport*; *Nutritional Assessment of Athletes*; *Nutritional Ergogenic Aids*; and *Sports Nutrition: Energy Metabolism and Exercise*; all with Ira Wolinsky. She also edited the book *Sports Nutrition: Fats and Proteins*, published by CRC Press. She has published more than 160 refereed research articles and 16 book chapters as well as several publications intended for lay audiences and has given numerous presentations to professional and lay groups. Her current research interests center around vitamin metabolism and requirements, including the interrelationships between exercise and water-soluble vitamin requirements.

Contributors

Farid E. Ahmed, Ph.D.
GEM Tox Consultants and Labs, Inc.
Greenville, North Carolina

Valerie A. Amend, B.S.
Department of Family and Consumer Sciences
Ball State University
Muncie, Indiana

Gayatri Borthakur, Ph.D.
Department of Kinesiology and Nutrition
University of Illinois at Chicago
Chicago, Illinois

J. Andrew Doyle, Ph.D.
Department of Kinesiology and Health
Georgia State University
Atlanta, Georgia

Judy A. Driskell, Ph.D., R.D.
Department of Nutrition and Health Sciences
University of Nebraska
Lincoln, Nebraska

Sarah J. Ehlers, M.S.
Department of Nutrition and Health Sciences
University of Nebraska
Lincoln, Nebraska

David W. Giraud, M.S.
Department of Nutrition and Health Sciences
University of Nebraska
Lincoln, Nebraska

Michael S. Green, Ph.D.
Department of Kinesiology and Health Promotion
Troy University
Troy, Alabama

Mark D. Haub, Ph.D.
Department of Human Nutrition
Kansas State University
Manhattan, Kansas

Emily M. Haymes, Ph.D.
Department of Nutrition, Food and Exercise Sciences
Florida State University
Tallahassee, Florida

Douglas S. Kalman, Ph.D., R.D., C.C.R.C., F.A.C.N.
Nutrition and Applied Clinical Research
Miami Research Associates
South Miami, Florida
and
Department of Dietetics and Nutrition
Florida International University

Jay Kandiah, Ph.D.
Department of Family and Consumer Sciences
Ball State University
Muncie, Indiana

Tait Lawrence, M.S., C.S.C.S.
Department of Nutrition, Food and Exercise Sciences
Florida State University
Tallahassee, Florida

Ji-Young Lee, Ph.D.
Department of Nutrition and Health Sciences
University of Nebraska
Lincoln, Nebraska

Yi Li, M.S.
Department of Biology
McMaster University
Hamilton, Ontario, Canada

George U. Liepa, Ph.D., F.A.C.N.
School of Health Sciences
Eastern Michigan University
Ypsilanti, Michigan

Henry C. Lukaski, Ph.D.
Grand Forks Human Nutrition Research Center
U.S. Department of Agriculture, Agricultural Research Service
Grand Forks, North Dakota

Stephen J. McGregor, Ph.D.
School of Health Promotion and Human Performance
Eastern Michigan University
Ypsilanti, Michigan

Susan Hazels Mitmesser, Ph.D.
Mead Johnson Nutrition
Evansville, Indiana

Robert J. Moffatt, Ph.D., M.P.H.
Department of Nutrition, Food and Exercise Sciences
Florida State University
Tallahassee, Florida

Forrest H. Nielsen, Ph.D.
Grand Forks Human Nutrition Research Center
U.S. Department of Agriculture, Agricultural Research Center
Grand Forks, North Dakota

Sandra D. Pernecky, M.S., R.D.
Department of Dietetics and Human Nutrition
Eastern Michigan University
Ypsilanti, Michigan

Steven J. Pernecky, Ph.D.
Department of Chemistry
Eastern Michigan University
Ypsilanti, Michigan

Heather E. Rasmussen, Ph.D., R.D.
Department of Nutrition and Health Sciences
University of Nebraska
Lincoln, Nebraska

Catherine G. Ratzin-Jackson, Ph.D.
Department of Kinesiology
Fresno State University
Fresno, California

Herb E. Schellhorn, Ph.D.
Department of Biology
McMaster University
Hamilton, Ontario, Canada

Angus G. Scrimgeour, Ph.D.
Military Nutrition Division
U.S. Army Research Institute for Environmental Medicine
Natick, Massachusetts

Shawn R. Simonson, Ed.D., C.S.C.S., A.C.S.M., H.F.S.
Department of Kinesiology
Boise State University
Boise, Idaho

Brian S. Snyder, M.S.
Department of Human Nutrition
Kansas State University
Manhattan, Kansas

Maria Stacewicz-Sapuntzakis, Ph.D.
Department of Kinesiology and Nutrition
University of Illinois at Chicago
Chicago, Illinois

Jidong Sun, Ph.D.
Perrigo Company
Holland, Michigan

Jacob M. Wilson, M.S., C.S.C.S.
Department of Nutrition, Food and Exercise Sciences
Florida State University
Tallahassee, Florida

Section I

Introduction

1 Introduction: *Nutrition and Exercise Concerns of Middle Age*

Judy A. Driskell

CONTENTS

I. INTRODUCTION

Middle-aged adults should have good nutritional and exercise habits. These habits influence their physical performance as well as their overall health. The American College of Sports Medicine, American Dietetic Association, and Dietitians of Canada issued a joint position statement on nutrition and athletic performance in 2000.[1–3] The key points of this joint position statement are given in Table 1.1. These key points summarize the current energy, nutrient, and fluid recommendations for physically active adults and competitive athletes. These recommendations would also apply to physically active middle-aged adults. This position statement is intended to provide guidance to health professionals working with physically active adults and is not intended for use with children or adolescents. It is currently being updated. The updated version, once it is available, can be accessed via the websites of these organizations.

According to the World Health Organization (WHO), about 30% of deaths in the world in 1999 were due to cardiovascular diseases, and this percentage is expected to increase.[4] One of the main objectives of the WHO's global strategy for the prevention and control of noncommunicable diseases is to reduce exposure in an integrated manner to the major risk factors of tobacco use, unhealthy diet, and physical inactivity. Unhealthy diets and physical inactivity are a problem to populations worldwide.

TABLE 1.1

Key Points of the Joint Position Statement of the American College of Sports Medicine, American Dietetic Association, and Dietitians of Canada on Nutrition and Athletic Performance

- During times of high-intensity training, adequate energy needs to be consumed to maintain body weight, maximize the training effects, and maintain health. Low-energy intakes can result in loss of muscle mass, menstrual dysfunction, loss or failure to gain body density, and increased risk of fatigue, injury, and illness.
- Body weight and composition can affect exercise performance but should not be used as the sole criterion for participation in sports; daily weigh-ins are discouraged. Optimal body-fat levels vary depending upon the sex, age, and heredity of the athlete, as well as the sport itself. Body-fat assessment techniques have inherent variability, thus limiting the precision with which they can be interpreted. If weight loss (fat loss) is desired, it should start early—before the competitive season—and involve a trained health and nutrition professional.
- Protein requirements are slightly increased in highly active people. Protein recommendations for endurance athletes are 1.2 to 1.4 g/kg body weight per day, whereas those for resistance and strength-trained athletes may be as high as 1.6 to 1.7 g/kg body weight per day. These recommended protein intakes can generally be met through diet alone, without the use of protein or amino acid supplements, if energy intake is adequate to maintain body weight.
- Fat intake should not be resisted, because there is no performance benefit in consuming a diet with less than 15% of energy from fat, compared with 20% to 25% of energy from fat. Fat is important in the diets of athletes as it provides energy, fat-soluble vitamins, and essential fatty acids. Additionally, there is no scientific basis on which to recommend high-fat diets to athletes.
- The athletes at greatest risk of micronutrient deficiencies are those who restrict energy intake or use severe weight-loss practices, eliminate one or more food groups from their diet, or consume high-carbohydrate diets with low micronutrient density. Athletes should strive to consume diets that provide at least the RDAs/DRIs for all micronutrients from food.
- Dehydration decreases exercise performance; thus, adequate fluid before, during, and after exercise is necessary for health and optimal performance. Athletes should drink enough fluid to balance their fluid losses. Two hours before exercise 400 to 600 mL (14 to 22 oz) of fluid should be consumed, and during exercise 150 to 350 mL (5 to 12 oz) of fluid should be consumed every 15 to 20 minutes depending on tolerance. After exercise the athlete should drink adequate fluids to replace sweat losses during exercise. The athlete needs to drink at least 450 to 675 mL (16 to 24 oz) of fluid for every pound (0.5 kg) of body weight lost during exercise.
- Before exercise, a meal or snack should provide sufficient fluid to maintain hydration, be relatively low in fat and fiber to facilitate gastric emptying and minimize gastrointestinal distress, be relatively high in carbohydrate to maximize maintenance of blood glucose, be moderate in protein, and be composed of foods familiar and well tolerated by the athlete.
- During exercise, the primary goals for nutrient consumption are to replace fluid losses and provide carbohydrate (approximately 30 to 60 g per hour) for the maintenance of blood glucose levels. These nutrition guidelines are especially important for endurance events lasting longer than an hour, when the athlete has not consumed adequate food or fluid before exercise, or if the athlete is exercising in an extreme environment (heat, cold, or altitude).

- After exercise, the dietary goal is to provide adequate energy and carbohydrates to replace muscle glycogen and to ensure rapid recovery. If an athlete is glycogen-depleted after exercise, a carbohydrate intake of 1.5 g/kg body weight during the first 30 minutes and again every 2 hours for 4 to 6 hours will be adequate to replace glycogen stores. Protein consumed after exercise will provide amino acids for the building and repair of muscle tissue. Therefore, athletes should consume a mixed meal providing carbohydrates, protein, and fat soon after a strenuous competition or training session.
- In general, no vitamin and mineral supplements should be required if an athlete is consuming adequate energy from a variety of foods to maintain body weight. Supplementation recommendations unrelated to exercise—such as folic acid in women of childbearing potential—should be followed. If an athlete is dieting, eliminating foods or food groups, is sick or recovering from injury, or has a specific micronutrient deficiency, a multivitamin/mineral supplement may be appropriate. No single nutrient supplements should be used without a specific medical or nutritional reason (e.g., iron supplements to reverse iron deficiency anemia).
- Athletes should be counseled regarding the use of ergogenic aids, which should be used with caution and only after careful evaluation of the product for safety, efficacy, potency, and legality.
- Vegetarian athletes may be at risk for low-energy, -protein, and micronutrient intakes because of high intakes of low-energy-dense foods and the elimination of meat and dairy from the diet. Consultation with a registered dietitian will help to avoid these nutrition problems.

Sources: American College of Sports Medicine, Joint position statement: nutrition and athletic performance, *Med. Sci. Sports Exerc.* 32, 2130–45, 2000.[1] Used with the permission of Wolters Kluwer Health.

RDAs = Recommended Dietary Allowances; DRIs = Dietary Reference Intakes.

II. DEFINITION OF MIDDLE AGE

Exactly what is middle age? Simply stated, middle age is the period of life between young adulthood and old age. The idea that midlife or middle age is a separate and distinct life stage is a cultural conception that originated in the 20th century.[5] The emergence of middle age as a life stage is linked to the increase in longevity and the decrease in fertility.[6] Little research has been conducted on the middle aged, especially with regard to nutrition and exercise.

Middle age is better defined by a pattern of characteristics as opposed to chronological age. Generally by middle age, adults are expected to have established a family of their own, have found a clear career direction, and have taken on responsibility with respect to their children, their aging parents, and sometimes their community.[7]

Many physiological changes occur during aging. Aging is a gradual process. Many of the physiological changes that usually occur in healthy individuals during middle age are given in Table 1.2. Good nutrition and exercise practices can moderate the effects of aging on the body's physiological functioning. Caloric restriction may slow some of the changes that occur in aging.[8] Conclusive evidence indicates that endurance and strength training generally slow some of the age-related changes.[8–11] The chapters in this book discuss how good nutrition and exercise practices are beneficial to the health status of individuals, particularly during middle age.

TABLE 1.2

Major Physiological Changes That Occur in Healthy Individuals during Middle Age

Brain weight declines around 10% from age 20 or 30 to age 90; however, intellectual performance tends to be maintained until at least age 80 in individuals who do not have neurologic disease.[10]

Lung function gradually declines after age 20.[10]

A decrease in height begins at around age 25 in men and 20 in women.[8]

Loss of muscle mass begins around age 30.[9]

The number and size of muscle fibers progressively decrease, beginning when individuals are in their 30s; this results in a decrease in skeletal muscle mass and lean body mass.[10]

A modest increase in the size of the heart occurs from age 20 to 80.[8]

Plasma endothelin-1 concentration, which is produced by vascular endothelial cells and has been implicated in regulation of vascular tonus and progression of atherosclerosis, was higher in healthy middle aged women (31–47 years) than in healthy young women (21–28 years).[11]

Intellectual abilities peak during the 30s and plateau through the 50s and 60s.[10]

Renal blood flow progressively decreases at age 30 to 40 years to age 80.[10]

Bone density begins to decrease between ages 40 and 50 in both genders, but most rapidly in women.[10]

The abilities to taste and smell start to gradually diminish when people are in their 50s.[9]

Adapted from: Masoro, E.J., *Challenges of Biological Aging*, Springer, New York, 1999;[8] Beers, M.H. and Jones, T.V., Eds., *The Merck Manual of Health & Aging*, Merck Research Laboratories, Whitehouse Station, NJ, 2005;[9] Beers, M.H. and Berkow, R., Eds., *The Merck Manual of Geriatrics, 3rd ed.*, Merck Research Laboratories, Whitehouse Station, NJ, 2006;[10] Maeda S. et al., Aerobic exercise training reduces plasma endothelin-1 concentration in older women, *J. Appl. Physiol.* 96, 336–41, 2003.[11]

Some researchers, governmental agencies, and others have utilized chronological age in designating the middle years of adulthood. These designations vary from 40 to 65 years,[12] 35 to 54 years,[13] 25 to 75 years,[14] 40 to 60 years,[15] and 31 to 50 years.[16] No consensus exists regarding the entry and exit points of middle age.

III. ENERGY BALANCE

Energy balance in individuals depends on their energy intakes as well as their energy outputs. The majority of the population in the United States consumes more food energy than they expend, primarily because they are sedentary. Data from the 2006 National Health Interview Survey indicates that 35% of adults 18 years of age and older in the United States were overweight (but not obese) and 26% were obese.[17] Sixty-two percent of adults included in the survey reported not participating in any type of vigorous leisure-time physical activity. This is also true in other developed countries, though in some developing countries, most of the population consumes too little food energy. In the United States, food energy is expressed as calories (properly referred to as kilocalories), while some other countries express food energy as kilojoules; one calorie is equal to 4.186 kilojoules[18] or 4.18 kilojoules.[19]

The three major components of energy expenditure are basal metabolism (though sometimes resting metabolism is utilized), thermic effect of food (previously known as specific dynamic action), and physical activity (also known as thermic effect of exercise and as energy expenditure of physical activity). All three of these components decrease as one ages, with a more rapid decline occurring around 40 years of age in men and 50 years of age in women.[20,21]

The Institute of Medicine, National Academy of Sciences, uses the term Estimated Energy Requirement (EER) which is the average dietary intake predicted to maintain energy balance in a healthy adult of a certain gender, age, weight, height, and level of physical activity that is consistent with good health.[18] The formula for calculating the EER for men 19 years of age and older is given below:

$$\text{EER} = 662 - (9.53 \text{ x age [y]}) + \text{PA x } (15.91 \text{ x weight [kg]} + 539.6 \text{ x height [m]})$$

The physical activity coefficient (PA) for men is 1.00 for those who are sedentary; 1.11, for low active; 1.25, for active; and 1.48, for very active. The formula for calculating the EER for women 19 years of age and older is given below:

$$\text{EER} = 354 - (6.91 \text{ x age [y]}) + \text{PA x } (9.36 \text{ x weight [kg]} + 726 \text{ x height [m]})$$

The PA for women is 1.00 for those who are sedentary; 1.12, low active; 1.27, active; and 1.45, very active.

Individuals who take 30 minutes of moderately intense activity (such as walking 2 miles in 30 minutes) or an equivalent amount of physical exertion in addition to activities involved in maintaining a sedentary lifestyle have a physical activity level (PAL) of about 1.5 and are classified as low active. PALs of ≥1.0–<1.4 are classified as sedentary, ≥1.4–<1.6 as low active, ≥1.6–<1.9 as active, and ≥1.9–<2.5 as very active.[18] Total energy expenditure (TEE) predictive equations were also developed by the Institute of Medicine (IOM), National Academy of Sciences[18] for use in estimating body weight maintenance in normal weight, overweight, and obese adults. The National Institutes of Health (NIH)[22] in the United States and the World Health Organization (WHO)[23] utilized body mass index (BMI as kg/m^2) in defining these body weight categories. BMIs <18.5 are considered underweight, 18.5 to 24.99 as healthy or desirable body weight, 25 to 29.99 as overweight, and ≥30 as obese. Total daily expenditures as calculated from TEE equations for normal weight, overweight, and obese men and women intended for use for those living in the United States and Canada[18] are given in Tables 1.3 and 1.4.

The group responsible for establishing the nutrient recommendations for Australia and New Zealand EERs of adults using predicted basal metabolic rate (BMR) multiplied by PAL, with PAL values varying from 1.2 to 2.2. PAL values of 1.75 and above are consistent with good health while values below 1.4 are incompatible with moving around freely or earning a living.[19] To determine maintenance or actual energy requirements (EERM), an individual's current body weight is utilized. In determining desirable estimated energy requirements (DEER), the current body weight is used

TABLE 1.3

Total Daily Energy Expenditure in Men 30 Years of Age as Calculated from Total Energy Expenditure (TEE) Equations for Normal-Weight, Overweight, and Obese Men[a] living in the United States and Canada

Height		TEE (kcal/d) for Body Mass Index (kg/m^2) of:			
m (in)	PAL[b]	18.5	25	30	40
1.5	sedentary	1,848	2,126	2,285	2,605
(59)	low active	2,010	2,312	2,491	2,849
	active	2,216	2,545	2,748	3,154
	very active	2,554	2,964	3,210	3,702
1.7	sedentary	2,144	2,453	2,659	3,069
(67)	low active	2,339	2,679	2,909	3,369
	active	2,586	2,961	3,222	3,743
	very active	2,993	3,469	3,785	4,417
1.9	sedentary	2,464	2,810	3,066	3,579
(75)	low active	2,694	3,078	3,365	3,939
	active	2,986	3,414	3,739	4,390
	very active	3,466	4,018	4,412	5,202

Adapted from: Institute of Medicine, National Academy of Sciences, *Dietary Reference Intakes for Energy, Carbohydrate, Fiber, Fat, Fatty Acids, Cholesterol, Protein, and Amino Acids*, National Academies Press, Washington, DC, 2002/2005.[18]

[a] For each year above 30, subtract 10 kcal/d from TEE.

[b] PAL = physical activity level. PAL = ≥1.0<1.4, sedentary; ≥1.4<1.6, low active; ≥1.6<1.9, active; ≥1.9<2.5, very active.

if it is within the healthy weight range (BMI between 18.5 and 24.99), but if the BMI is ≥25, the desirable body weight is determined by assuming a BMI of 22. The EER, in megajoules, using predicted BMR multiplied by PAL are intended for use by men and women living in Australia and New Zealand are given in Table 1.5. The estimated total energy recommendations of Australia and New Zealand for men and women approximate those of the United States and Canada, though slightly different terms are used and the recommendations are given in a different unit of measurement.

Energy expenditure is discussed in greater detail in chapters 14 and 15 of this book. Detailed information on energy balance is also available in references 18 and 19 of this chapter, several chapters in the books *Energy-Yielding Macronutrients and Energy Metabolism in Sports Nutrition*[24] and *Sports Nutrition: Energy Metabolism and Exercise*.[25] Additional research is needed on the influence of age as well as obesity on energy expenditure.

IV. NUTRIENT RECOMMENDATIONS

Water is the largest single constituent of the body. The IOM established an Adequate Intake (AI) for total water (from drinking water, beverages, and foods) based on the

TABLE 1.4

Total Daily Energy Expenditure in Women 30 Years of Age as Calculated from Total Energy Expenditure (TEE) Equations for Normal-Weight, Overweight, and Obese Women[a] Living in the United States and Canada

Height		TEE (kcal/d) for Body Mass Index (kg/m²) of:			
m (in)	PAL[b]	18.5	25	30	40
1.5	sedentary	1,625	1,771	1,894	2,139
(59)	low active	1,803	1,996	2,136	2,415
	active	2,025	2,205	2,360	2,672
	very active	2,291	2,493	2,671	3,027
1.7	sedentary	1,881	2,078	2,235	2,550
(67)	low active	2,090	2,345	2,525	2,884
	active	2,350	2,594	2,794	3,194
	very active	2,662	2,938	3,166	3,623
1.9	sedentary	2,151	2,406	2,603	2,993
(75)	low active	2,392	2,720	2,944	3,393
	active	2,693	3,011	3,261	3,760
	very active	3,053	3,414	3,699	4,270

Adapted from: Institute of Medicine, National Academy of Sciences, *Dietary Reference Intakes for Energy, Carbohydrate, Fiber, Fat, Fatty Acids, Cholesterol, Protein, and Amino Acids*, National Academies Press, Washington, DC, 2002/2005.[18]

[a] For each year above 30, subtract 7 kcal/d from TEE.

[b] PAL = physical activity level. PAL =≥ 1.0<1.4, sedentary; ≥1.4<1.6, low active; ≥1.6<1.9, active; ≥1.9<2.5, very active.

median total water intake from surveys performed in the United States. The AIs for water for men and women 31 to 70 years of age are 3.7 L total water daily (around 13 cups) and 2.7 L total water daily (around 9 cups), respectively.[26] Individuals who are physically active or exposed to hot temperatures require higher intakes of total water. A 2007 position stand of the American College of Sports Medicine (ACSM) indicates that, to avoid compromising physical performance,[27] during exercise individuals should drink enough fluids to prevent excessive (>2% body weight loss) dehydration and excessive changes in electrolyte balance. Some individuals sweat more than others. American athletes often achieve sweat rates of 0.5 to 2 L per hour. The hydration status of individuals can be monitored by utilizing urine measurements (specific gravity and osmolality) and body weight measurements. The ACSM recommends customized fluid replacement programs for individuals who exercise vigorously.[27] Such individuals should hydrate themselves before, during, and after exercise via fluid replacement.

In that scientific evidence suggests that individuals can consume moderate levels of the energy-yielding macronutrients carbohydrates, lipids (fats), and protein without risk of adverse health effects, increased risk may occur with chronic consumption of diets that are too high or too low in each of these macronutrients. Much of this

TABLE 1.5

Estimated Energy Requirements (MJ/d) of Men and Women using Predicted Basal Metabolic Rate (BMR) Multiplied by Physical Activity Level (PAL) for Men and Women Living in Australia and New Zealand

	BMI = 22[a]		Physical activity level (PAL)[b]			
Age (y)	Ht (m)	Wt (kg)	1.2	1.6	1.8	2.2
			MEN			
31–50	1.5	49.5	–	–	–	–
	1.7	63.6	8.0	10.7	12.1	14.8
	1.9	79.4	9.0	11.9	13.4	16.4
51–70	1.5	49.5	–	–	–	–
	1.7	63.6	7.3	9.8	11.1	13.6
	1.9	79.4	8.3	11.1	12.4	15.2
			WOMEN			
31–50	1.5	49.5	6.3	8.4	9.4	11.5
	1.7	63.6	6.8	9.1	10.3	12.5
	1.9	79.4	7.5	10.0	11.2	13.7
51–70	1.5	49.5	6.0	7.9	8.9	10.9
	1.7	63.6	6.5	8.7	9.8	12.0
	1.9	79.4	7.2	9.6	10.8	13.2

Adapted from: Australian National Health and Medical Research Council and New Zealand Ministry of Health, *Nutrient Reference Values for Australia and New Zealand*, Available at: http://www.nrv.gov.au.[19]

[a] A BMI of 22 is approximately the midpoint of the World Health Organization healthy weight range.

[b] PAL ranges from 1.2 (bed rest) to 2.2 (very active or heavy occupational work.

evidence is based on associations of high or low intakes of these macronutrients with risks of coronary heart disease, cancer, diabetes, and obesity. Hence, the IOM established Acceptable Macronutrient Distribution Ranges (AMDR) intended for use by healthy individuals in the United States and Canada. The AMDR is given as a range of intakes for a food energy source that is associated with reduced risk of chronic disease yet ensuring sufficient intakes of essential nutrients. The AMDRs for adults are as follows: carbohydrates, 45–65% of calories (not more than 25% of calories from added sugars); lipids, 20–35% of calories (0.6–1.2% of calories from α-linolenic acid and 5–10% of calories from linoleic acid); and protein, 10–35% of calories.[18] The Australian National Health and Medical Research Council in conjunction with the New Zealand Ministry of Health, while establishing Nutrient Reference Values in 2006 reviewed and discussed the AMDRs intended for use by United States and Canadian healthy populations but did not set any for use by their populations.[19]

The IOM[16] has established a set of reference nutrient intake values called Dietary Reference Intakes (DRIs) intended for use with the healthy populations in the United

TABLE 1.6

Categories of Dietary Reference Intakes

Estimated Average Requirement (EAR)	The daily intake value estimated to meet the nutrient requirement of 50% of the healthy individuals in a life stage/gender group.
Recommended Dietary Allowance (RDA)	The average daily dietary nutrient intake sufficient to meet the needs of 97–98% of healthy individuals in a life stage/gender group. The RDA is calculated from the EAR.
Adequate Intake (AI)	The daily nutrient intake or approximation of observed mean intakes by a group(s) of healthy individuals in a life stage/gender group. The daily nutrient intake calculated when scientific evidence is not available to calculate an EAR.
Tolerable Upper Intake Level (UL)	The highest daily nutrient intake that is likely to pose no risk of adverse health for almost all individuals in a life stage/gender group.

Adapted from: Institute of Medicine, National Academy of Sciences, *Dietary Reference Intakes for Calcium, Phosphorus, Magnesium, Vitamin D, and Fluoride*, National Academies Press, Washington, DC, 1997.[16]

States and Canada. The DRIs encompass the Estimated Average Requirements (EARs), Recommended Dietary Allowances (RDAs), Adequate Intakes (AIs), and Tolerable Upper Intake Levels (ULs). These terms are defined in Table 1.6. The RDAs and the AIs are the values intended for use in guiding individuals to achieve adequate nutrient intakes.[16,28] The uses of the DRIs for healthy individuals and groups as given by the IOM[16,28] are given in Table 1.7.

Healthy middle-age adults living in the United States and Canada should consume at least the RDA or AI for a nutrient but not more than the UL. The RDAs or AIs for the essential nutrients for individuals 31 to 70 years of age are given in Appendices A–C and the ULs are given in Appendices D and E.[16,18,26,29–31]

The group responsible for establishing the nutrient recommendations for Australia and New Zealand decided to adopt the approach of the United States/Canada DRIs but to vary some of the terminology.[19] Their Nutrient Reference Values included EARs, Recommended Dietary Intakes (RDIs; similar to the United States/Canadian Recommended Dietary Allowances or RDAs), AIs, and Upper Levels of Intake (ULs; similar to the Tolerable Upper Intake Levels or ULs of the United States and Canada). The RDIs, AIs, and ULs for healthy adults living in Australia and New Zealand are given in Appendices F–J. Many of the numerical values of the Australia/New Zealand Nutrient Reference Values are similar to those of the United States and Canada, though some are slightly different. Likely the small differences that exist in these recommendations are influenced by the fact that different experts served on the two groups that established the recommendations. Several other countries have

TABLE 1.7

Uses of the Dietary Reference Intakes in Evaluating Nutrient Intakes

Term	For an Individual	For a Group of Individuals
Estimated Average Requirement	Utilized in examining the probability that usual intake is inadequate.	Utilized in estimating the prevalence of inadequate intakes within the group.
Recommended Dietary Allowance	Usual intake at or higher than this level has a low probability of being inadequate.	Not utilized in evaluating intakes of groups.
Adequate Intake	Usual intake at or higher than this level has a low probability of being inadequate.	Mean usual intake or higher than this level implies a low prevalence of inadequate intakes. However, this assessment is made with less confidence when not based on mean intakes of healthy people.
Tolerable Upper Intake Level	Usual intake higher than this level may put the individual at risk of adverse effects from excessive intake of the nutrient.	Utilized in estimating the percentage of the population at potential risk of adverse effects from excessive intakes of the nutrient.

Adapted from: Institute of Medicine, *Dietary Reference Intakes: Applications in Dietary Assessment*, National Academies Press, Washington, DC, 2002/2005.[28]

established nutrient recommendations for their populations. The Recommended Nutrient Intakes of Vitamins and Minerals for adults established by the WHO[32] are given in Appendices K and L.

Some evidence exists that athletes and others who are vigorously active may benefit from the consumption of larger amounts of some of the vitamins and minerals than from the amounts recommended for the general public in the same lifestage (gender/age) groupings. The following suggestions come from the IOM:

Because of the functioning of niacin in the oxidation of fuel molecules at least a 10% adjustment should be be made to reflect differences in the average energy utilization and body sizes of individuals who exercise vigorously.[29]

Those spending much time training for active sports may require additional thiamin and those who are ordinarily physically active may require more riboflavin.[29]

Those who exercise vigorously may need more of the antioxidant nutrients vitamin A, carotenoids, vitamin E, and vitamin C.[30]

Potassium can be lost, primarily via sweat, during heat exposure and exercise; however, it is not known how much the intake should be increased to compensate for this loss.

Individuals who exercise strenuously in the heat on a daily basis can lose substantial amounts of sodium (along with chloride), but it has not been ascertained how much. The United States Army Research Institute of Environmental Medicine (USARIEM) estimated sodium and water losses at four levels of energy expenditure (1900, 2400, 2900, and 3600 kcal daily). This report estimated the daily sodium requirements at average day-time dry bulb temperatures varying from 59–104 °F to be as follows: 1900 kcal/d, ~1600–4020 mg sodium/d; 2400 kcal/d, ~2000–6200 mg sodium/d; 2900 kcal/d, ~2500–7500 mg sodium/d; and 3600 kcal/d, ~3020–9600 mg sodium/d. This USARIEM model is an empirical model that includes an equation to predict sweating rate during work.[26]

The vitamin and mineral needs of middle-aged individuals who exercise moderately or vigorously are discussed in more detail in Chapters 5–10.

The contents of specific nutrients in processed foods must be placed on the product label in the United States. Specific nutrient content information may also be provided for nonprocessed foods, but it is not mandatory. The term Daily Value is used in stating the nutrient content of processed foods and dietary supplements in the United States. The Daily Value is not the same as the RDA. However, the Daily Values were developed utilizing the 1968[33] and the 1974[34] RDAs. The Daily Values include Daily Reference Values (DRVs) and Reference Daily Intakes (RDIs). DRVs have been established for fat (meaning total fat), saturated fat, carbohydrates (including fiber), protein, cholesterol, sodium, and potassium. RDIs have been established for most of the vitamins and essential minerals. The Daily Values[35] for adults and children 4 or more years of age, based on a 2,000-calorie diet, are given in Appendix M.

V. DIETARY GUIDELINES

The Department of Health and Human Services (HHS) and the Department of Agriculture (USDA) have developed Dietary Guidelines for Americans[36] (Table 1.8). These guidelines are intended for use by healthy individuals 2 years of age and above. The Dietary Guidelines for Australian adults[37] are given in Table 1.9. The dietary guidelines for the United States and for Australia are rather similar, although those for the United States are more detailed. Both the United States and Australia update their dietary guidelines on a regular basis. Several other countries also have developed dietary guidelines for use by individuals living in their countries.

Some health organizations have also developed dietary guidelines and these are updated from time to time. For example, the American Heart Association Dietary Guidelines[38] are currently available online at http://www.americanheart.org/presenter.jhtml?identifier=4561. The World Cancer Research Fund in conjunction with the American Institute for Cancer Research[39] in 2007 made eight basic dietary recommendations expected to reduce the incidence of cancer and issued personal recommendations for each of the eight. These recommendations are given in Appendix N. The

TABLE 1.8

Dietary Guidelines for Americans, Key Recommendations

Adequate Nutrients Within Calorie Needs

- Consume a variety of nutrient-dense foods and beverages within and among the basis food groups while choosing foods that limit the intake of saturated and *trans* fats, cholesterol, added sugars, salt, and alcohol.
- Meet recommended intakes within energy needs by adopting a balanced eating pattern, such as the USDA Food Guide or the DASH Eating Plan.

Weight Management

- To maintain body weight in a healthy range, balance calories from foods and beverages with calories expended.
- To prevent gradual weight gain over time, make small decreases in food and beverage calories and increase physical activity.

Physical Activity

- Engage in regular physical activity and reduce sedentary activities to promote health, psychological well-being, and a healthy body weight.
  - To reduce the risk of chronic disease in adulthood: Engage in at least 30 minutes of moderate-intensity physical activity, above usual activity, at work or home on most days of the week.
  - For most people greater health benefits can be obtained by engaging in physical activity of more vigorous intensity or longer duration.
  - To help manage body weight and prevent gradual, unhealthy body weight gain in adulthood: Engage in approximately 60 minutes of moderate- to vigorous-intensity activity on most days of the week while not exceeding caloric intake requirements.
  - To sustain weight loss in adulthood: Participate in at least 60 to 90 minutes of daily moderate-intensity physical activity while not exceeding caloric intake requirements. Some people may need to consult with a healthcare provider before participating in this level of activity.
- Achieve physical fitness by including cardiovascular conditioning, stretching exercises for flexibility, and resistance exercises or calisthenics for muscle strength and endurance.

Food Groups To Encourage

- Consume a sufficient amount of fruits and vegetables while staying within energy needs. Two cups of fruit and 2 ½ cups of vegetables per day are recommended for a reference, 2,000-calorie intake, with higher or lower amounts depending on the calorie level.
- Choose a variety of fruits and vegetables each day. In particular, select from all five vegetable subgroups (dark green, orange, legumes, starchy vegetables, and other vegetables) several times a week.
- Consume 3 or more ounce-equivalents of whole-grain products per day, with the rest of the recommended grains coming from enriched or whole-grain products. In general, at least half the grains should come from whole grains.
- Consume 3 cups per day of fat-free or low-fat milk or equivalent milk products.

Fats

- Consume less than 10 percent of calories from saturated fatty acids and less than 300 mg/day of cholesterol, and keep *trans* fatty acid consumption as low as possible.
- Keep total fat intake between 20 and 35 percent of calories, with most fats coming from sources of polyunsaturated and monounsaturated fatty acids, such as fish, nuts, and vegetable oils.
- When selecting and preparing meat, poultry, dry beans, and milk or milk products, make choices that are lean, low-fat, or fat-free.
- Limit intake of fats and oils high in saturated and/or *trans* fatty acids, and choose products low in such fats and oils.

Carbohydrates

- Choose fiber-rich fruits, vegetables, and whole grains often.
- Choose and prepare foods and beverages with little added sugars or caloric sweeteners, such as amounts suggested by the USDA Food Guide and the DASH Eating Plan.
- Reduce the incidence of dental caries by practicing good oral hygiene and consuming sugar- and starch-containing foods and beverages less frequently.

Sodium and Potassium

- Consume less than 2,300 mg (approximately 1 teaspoon of salt) of sodium per day.
- Choose and prepare foods with little salt. At the same time consume potassium-rich foods, such as fruits and vegetables.

Alcoholic Beverages

- Those who choose to drink alcoholic beverages should do so sensibly and in moderation—defined as the consumption of up to one drink per day for women and up to two drinks per day for men.
- Alcoholic beverages should not be consumed by some individuals, including those who cannot restrict their alcohol intake, women of childbearing age who may become pregnant, pregnant and lactating women, children and adolescents, individuals taking medications that can interact with alcohol, and those with specific medical conditions.
- Alcoholic beverages should be avoided by individuals engaging in activities that require attention, skill, or coordination, such as driving or operating machinery.

Food Safety

- To avoid microbial foodborne illness:
  - Clean hands, food contact surfaces, and fruits and vegetables. Meat and poultry should not be washed or rinsed.
  - Separate raw, cooked, and ready-to-eat foods while shopping, preparing, or storing foods.
  - Cook foods to a safe temperature to kill microorganisms.

Taken from: U.S. Department of Health and Human Services and of Agriculture, Dietary Guidelines for Americans 2005. Available at http://www.health.gov/dietaryguidelines/dga2005/document/html/executivesummary.htm.[36]

TABLE 1.9

Dietary Guidelines for Australian Adults

Enjoy a wide variety of nutritious foods

- Eat plenty of vegetables, legumes and fruits
- Eat plenty of cereals (including breads, rice, pasta and noodles), preferably wholegrain
- Include lean meat, fish, poultry and/or alternatives
- Include milks, yoghurts, cheeses and/or alternatives. Reduced-fat varieties should be chosen where possible
- Drink plenty of water

and take care to

- Limit saturated fat and moderate total fat intake
- Choose foods low in salt
- Limit your alcohol intake if you choose to drink
- Consume only moderate amounts of sugars and foods containing added sugars

Prevent weight gain: be physically active and eat according to your energy needs

Care for your food: prepare and store it safely

Encourage and support breastfeeding

Taken from: National Health and Medical Research Council, Australian Government, Dietary Guidelines for all Australians, 2003. Available at http://www.nhmrc.gov.au/publications/synopses/dietsyn.htm.[3]

recommendations made by these health organizations are rather similar to those of the Dietary Guidelines for Americans[36] and the Dietary Guidelines for Australian adults.[37]

VI. FOOD GUIDANCE RECOMMENDATIONS

The USDA and HHS have developed a food guidance system known as MyPyramid.[40] MyPyramid is given in Figure 1.1 and can be viewed in more detail and utilized at http://www.MyPyramid.gov. The pyramid is intended for use by healthy individuals 2 years of age and above. The pyramid gives the amount of foods from the various food groups that one should consume (Figure 1.2). People can use the pyramid website in evaluating their diets and their physical activity. Some other countries have also developed food guidance systems for their populations.

VII. EXERCISE RECOMMENDATIONS

In June, 1998 the ACSM issued a position stand entitled "The Recommended Quantity and Quality of Exercise for Developing and Maintaining Cardiorespiratory and Muscular Fitness and Flexibility in Healthy Adults."[41] This position stand will likely be updated soon, and readers are encouraged to check the organization's website for the update. These recommendations are for healthy adults who are not athletes. These recommendations are summarized in Table 1.10. After seeking advice of

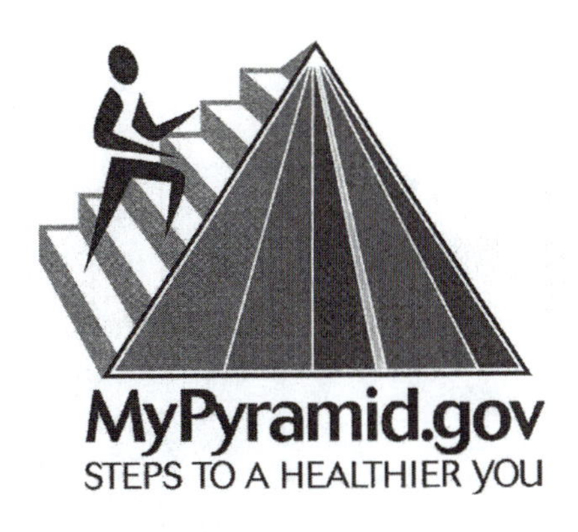

FIGURE 1.1 MyPyramid. (U.S. Department of Agriculture. Available at http://www.mypyramid.gov/.[40])

those invited to a workshop planned by the Food and Nutrition Board, IOM, and the Board on Population Health and Public Health Practice, the USDA and HHS considered developing a comprehensive set of physical activity guidelines for Americans.[42] These Physical Activity Guidelines for Americans[43] were recently released and the Key Guidelines for Physical Activity for Adults are given in Table 1.11.

VIII. CONCLUSIONS

Nutrition and exercise influence the physical performance of individuals of all ages, including middle-aged adults. Experts do not agree as to when middle age begins or ends. In this book, middle age is considered to be around 30 to 60 years of age.

Many individuals, particularly those living in developed countries, consume more food energy than they expend, primarily because they are sedentary. Individuals who exercise vigorously need to consume more food energy because they expend more energy. Maintaining energy balance is of great importance to athletes, as it has been shown to influence physical performance.

Athletes and nonathletes need to always be hydrated as this influences their physical performance as well as their health. Acceptable macronutrient distribution ranges have been established for the energy-yielding macronutrients carbohydrates, lipids (fats), and proteins. The recommended intakes of vitamins and minerals for individuals living in the United States and Canada,[16,26,29–31] in Australia and New Zealand,[19] and those given by the WHO[32] are detailed in Appendices A–L in the back of this book.

Dietary guidelines have been established for Americans[36] and for Australians,[37] as well as those living in several other countries. These guidelines are intended for use by both athletes and nonathletes.

Exercise recommendations, particularly those of the ACSM,[41] are given. Chapters 14 and 15 of this book discuss in detail the benefits of resistance and endurance training.

Little is known regarding the relationships among nutrition, exercise, and health during middle age. Additional research is needed on this topic, as the middle aged are a substantial portion of the population.

GRAINS Make half your grains whole	VEGETABLES Vary your veggies	FRUITS Focus on fruits	MILK Get your calcium-rich foods	MEAT & BEANS Go lean with protein
Eat at least 3 oz. of whole-grain cereals, breads, crackers, rice, or pasta every day 1 oz. is about 1 slice of bread, about 1 cup of breakfast cereal, or ½ cup of cooked rice, cereal, or pasta	Eat more dark-green veggies like broccoli, spinach, and other dark leafy greens Eat more orange vegetables like carrots and sweetpotatoes Eat more dry beans and peas like pinto beans, kidney beans, and lentils	Eat a variety of fruit Choose fresh, frozen, canned, or dried fruit Go easy on fruit juices	Go low-fat or fat-free when you choose milk, yogurt, and other milk products If you don't or can't consume milk, choose lactose-free products or other calcium sources such as fortified foods and beverages	Choose low-fat or lean meats and poultry Bake it, broil it, or grill it Vary your protein routine — choose more fish, beans, peas, nuts, and seeds

For a 2,000-calorie diet, you need the amounts below from each food group. To find the amounts that are right for you, go to MyPyramid.gov.

Eat 6 oz. every day	Eat 2½ cups every day	Eat 2 cups every day	Get 3 cups every day; for kids aged 2 to 8, it's 2	Eat 5½ oz. every day

Find your balance between food and physical activity

- Be sure to stay within your daily calorie needs.
- Be physically active for at least 30 minutes most days of the week.
- About 60 minutes a day of physical activity may be needed to prevent weight gain.
- For sustaining weight loss, at least 60 to 90 minutes a day of physical activity may be required.
- Children and teenagers should be physically active for 60 minutes every day or most days.

Know the limits on fats, sugars, and salt (sodium)

- Make most of your fat sources from fish, nuts, and vegetable oils.
- Limit solid fats like butter, stick, margarine, shortening, and lard, as well as foods that contain these
- Check the Nutrition Facts label to keep saturated fats, *trans* fats, and sodium low.
- Choose food and beverages low in added sugars. Added sugars contribute calories with few, if any, nutrients.

MyPyramid.gov
STEPS TO A HEALTHIER YOU

U.S. Department of Agriculture
Center for Nutrition Policy and Promotion
April 2005
CNPP-15

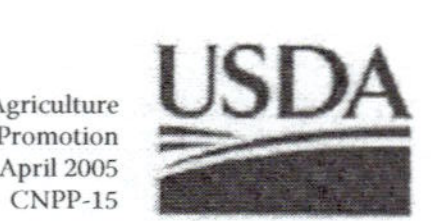

USDA is an equal opportunity provider and employer.

FIGURE 1.2 Food group comments for MyPyramid. (U.S. Department of Agriculture. Available at http://www.mypyramid.gov/.[40])

TABLE 1.10

The Recommended Quantity and Quality of Exercise for Developing and Maintaining Cardiorespiratory and Muscular Fitness, and Flexibility in Adults

For Cardiorespiratory Fitness and Body Composition

- Frequency of training:
  3 to 5 days weekly.
- Intensity of training:
  55 or 65 up to 90% of maximum heart rate or 40 or 50 up to 85% of maximum oxygen uptake reserve or maximum heart rate reserve. The lower percentages are for individuals who are sedentary.
- Duration of training:
  20 to 60 minutes of continuous or intermittent aerobic activity. The intermittent activity should be for 10 minutes or more time periods during the day. The 20 to 60 minutes is dependent on the activity's intensity.
- Mode of activity:
  Any activity that utilizes the large muscle groups and is maintained continuously.

For Muscular Strength and Endurance, Body Composition, and Flexibility

- Resistance training:
  One repetition of 8-10 exercises that trains the major muscle groups 2 to 3 days weekly. Additional repetitions may provide greater benefits.
- Flexibility training:
  Flexibility exercises sufficient to develop and maintain range of motion 2 to 3 days weekly.

Adapted from: Pollock, M.L., Gaesser, G.A., Butcher, J.D., Després, J.P., Dishman, R.K., Franklin, B.A. and Garber, C.E., The recommended quantity and quality of exercise for developing and maintaining cardiorespiratory and muscular fitness and flexibility in healthy adults: American College of Sports Medicine position stand, *Med. Sci. Sports Exerc.* 30, 975–91, 1998.[41]

REFERENCES

1. American College of Sports Medicine, Joint position statement: Nutrition and athletic performance, *Med. Sci. Sports Exerc.* 32, 2130–45, 2000.
2. American Dietetic Association, Joint position statement: Nutrition and athletic performance, *J. Am. Diet. Assoc.* 100, 1543–56, 2000.
3. Dietitians of Canada, Joint position statement: Nutrition and athletic performance, *Can. J. Diet. Prac. Res.* 61, 176–92, 2000.
4. World Health Organization, Diet, Physical Activity and Health: Report by the Secretariat, 55th World Health Assembly, Document WHA55/16, March 27, 2002.
5. Skolnick, A., *Embattled Paradise*, Basic, New York, 1991.
6. Moen P. and Wethington, E., Midlife development is a life course context, in *Life in the Middle*, Willis, S.L. and Reid, J.D., Eds., Academic Press, San Diego, CA, 1999, chap. 1.
7. Staudinger, U.M. and Bluck, S., A view on midlife development from life-span theory, in *Handbook of Midlife Development*, Lachman, M.E., Ed., John Wiley & Sons, New York, 2001, chap. 2.
8. Masoro, E.J., *Challenges of Biological Aging*, Springer, New York, 1999.

TABLE 1.11
Key Physical Activity Guidelines for Adults

All adults should avoid inactivity. Some physical activity is better than none, and adults who participate in any amount of physical activity gain some health benefits.

- For substantial health benefits, adults should do at least 150 minutes (2 hours and 30 minutes) a week of moderate-intensity, or 75 minutes (1 hour and 15 minutes) a week of vigorous-intensity aerobic physical activity, or an equivalent combination of moderate- and vigorous-intensity aerobic activity. Aerobic activity should be performed in episodes of at least 10 minutes, and preferably, it should be spread throughout the week.
- For additional and more extensive health benefits, adults should increase their aerobic physical activity to 300 minutes (5 hours) a week of moderate-intensity, or 150 minutes a week of vigorous-intensity aerobic physical activity, or an equivalent combination of moderate- and vigorous-intensity activity. Additional health benefits are gained by engaging in physical activity beyond this amount.
- Adults should also do muscle strengthening activities that are moderate- or high-intensity and involve all major muscle groups on 2 or more days a week, as these activities provide additional health benefits.
- All adults should avoid inactivity. Some physical activity is better than none, and adults who participate in any amount of physical activity gain some health benefits.

Adults should also do muscle strengthening activities that are moderate- or high-intensity and involve all major muscle groups on 2 or more days a week, as these activities provide additional health benefits.

Examples of Different Aerobic Physical Activities

Moderate Intensity

Walking briskly (3 miles per hour or faster, but not racewalking

Water aerobics

Bicycling slower than 10 miles per hour

Tennis (doubles)

Ballroom dancing

General gardening

Vigorous Intensity

Racewalking, jogging, or running

Swimming laps

Tennis (singles)

Aerobic dancing

Bicycling 10 miles per hour or faster

Jumping rope

Heavy gardening (continuous digging or hoeing, with heart rate increases)

Hiking uphill or with a heavy backpack.

Source: U.S. Department of Health and Human Services, 2008 Physical Activity Guidelines for Americans. Available at http://www.health.gov/paguidelines, accessed October 28, 2008.

9. Beers, M.H. and Jones, T.V., Eds., *The Merck Manual of Health & Aging*, Merck Research Laboratories, Whitehouse Station, NJ, 2005.
10. Beers, M.H. and Berkow, R., Eds., *The Merck Manual of Geriatrics, 3rd ed.*, Merck Research Laboratories, Whitehouse Station, NJ, 2006.
11. Maeda, S., Tanabe, T., Miyauchi, T., Otsuki, T., Sugawara, J., Iemitsu, M., et al., Aerobic exercise training reduces plasma endothelin-1 concentration in older women, *J. Appl. Physiol.* 95, 336–41, 2003.
12. Whitbourne, S.K., The physical aging process in midlife: Interactions with psychological and sociocultural factors, in *Handbook of Midlife Development*, Lackman, M.E., Ed., John Wiley & Sons, New York, 2001, chap. 4.
13. Middle Age. Wikipedia, http://en.wikipedia.org/wiki/Middle_age, accessed 08/06/2008.
14. Adams, R.L. Definition—When or What is Middle Age? http://www.middleage.org/definition.shtml, accessed 08/06/2008.
15. Middle Age. Britannica Encyclopedia Website, http://www.britannica.com/#search=tab~TOPICS%2Cterm~middle%20age, accessed 08/06/2008.
16. Institute of Medicine, National Academy of Sciences, *Dietary Reference Intakes for Calcium, Phosphorus, Magnesium, Vitamin D, and Fluoride*. National Academy Press, Washington, DC, 1997.
17. Pleis, J.R. and Lethbridge-Cejku, M., Summary Health Statistics for U.S. Adults: National Health Interview Survey, 2006. Vital Health Statistics Series 10, Number 235. Hyattsville, MD, National Center for Health Statistics, U.S. Department of Health and Human Services, 2007.
18. Institute of Medicine, National Academy of Sciences, *Dietary Reference Intakes for Energy, Carbohydrate, Fiber, Fat, Fatty Acids, Cholesterol, Protein, and Amino Acids*. National Academies Press, Washington, DC, 2002/2005.
19. Australian National Health and Medical Research Council and New Zealand Ministry of Health, Nutrient Reference Values for Australia and New Zealand. Available at http://www.nrv.gov.au, posted May, 2006, accessed 08/06/2008.
20. Poehlman, E.T., Energy expenditure and requirements in aging humans, *J. Nutr.* 122, 2057–65, 1992.
21. Poehlman, E.T., Regulation of energy expenditure in aging humans, *J. Am. Geriatr. Soc.* 41, 552–9, 1993.
22. National Heart, Lung, and Blood Institute and National Institute of Diabetes and Digestive and Kidney Diseases, *Clinical Guidelines on the Identification, Evaluation, and Treatment of Overweight and Obesity in Adults. The Evidence Report*, NIH Publication No. 98–4083, National Institutes of Health, Bethesda, MD, 1998.
23. World Health Organization, Obesity: Preventing and Managing the Global Epidemic. Report of a World Health Organization Consultation on Obesity, World Health Organization, Geneva, 1998.
24. Driskell, J.A., Wolinsky, I., Eds., *Energy-Yielding Macronutrients and Energy Metabolism in Sports Nutrition*, CRC Press LLC, Boca Raton, FL, 2000.
25. Wolinsky, I., Driskell, J.A., Eds., *Sports Nutrition: Energy Metabolism and Exercise*, Taylor and Francis, 2008.
26. Institute of Medicine, National Academy of Sciences, *Dietary Reference Intakes for Water, Potassium, Sodium, Chloride, and Sulfate*. National Academies Press, Washington, DC, 2005.
27. Sawka, M.N., Burke, L.M., Eichner, E.R., Maughan, R.J., Montain, S.J. and Stachenfeld, N.S., Exercise and fluid replacement: American College of Sports Medicine position stand, *Med. Sci. Sports Exer.* 39, 377–90, 2007.
28. Institute of Medicine, National Academy of Sciences, *Dietary Reference Intakes: Applications in Dietary Assessment*. National Academies Press, Washington, DC, 2000.

29. Institute of Medicine, National Academy of Sciences, *Dietary Reference Intakes for Thiamin, Riboflavin, Niacin, Vitamin B_6, Folate, Vitamin B_{12}, Pantothenic Acid, Biotin, and Choline*. National Academies Press, Washington, DC, 1998.
30. Institute of Medicine, National Academy of Sciences, *Dietary Reference Intakes for Vitamin C, Vitamin E, Selenium, and Carotenoids*. National Academies Press, Washington, DC, 2000.
31. Institute of Medicine, National Academy of Sciences, *Dietary Reference Intakes for Vitamin A, Vitamin K, Arsenic, Boron, Chromium, Copper, Iodine, Iron, Manganese, Molybdenum, Nickel, Silicon, Vanadium, and Zinc*. National Academies Press, Washington, DC, 2001.
32. World Health Organization and Food and Agriculture Organization of the United Nations, *Vitamin and Mineral Requirements in Human Nutrition, 2nd ed.*, World Health Organization, Geneva, 2004.
33. National Research Council, National Academy of Sciences, *Recommended Dietary Allowances, 7th rev. ed.*, Printing and Publishing Office of National Academy of Sciences, Washington, DC, 1968.
34. National Research Council, National Academy of Sciences, *Recommended Dietary Allowances, 8th rev. ed.*, Printing and Publishing Office of National Academy of Sciences, Washington, DC, 1974.
35. U.S. Food and Drug Administration, A Food Labeling Guide: Reference Values for Nutrition Labeling. Available at http://www.cfsan.fda.gov/~dms/flg–7a.html, editorial revisions June, 1999, accessed 08/06/2008.
36. U.S. Departments of Agriculture and of Health and Human Services, Dietary Guidelines for Americans, 2005. Available at http://www.health.gov/dietaryguidelines/dga2005/document, posted 2007, accessed 08/06/2008.
37. National Health and Medical Research Council of Australia, Dietary Guidelines for Australian Adults. Available at http://www.nhmrc.gov.au/publications/synopses/dietsyn.htm, posted 2003, accessed 1/25/08.
38. American Heart Association Dietary Guidelines, American Heart Association Dietary Guidelines. Available at http://www.americanheart.org/presenter.jhtml?identifier=4630, posted 2007, accessed 08/06/2008.
39. World Cancer Research Fund/American Institute for Cancer Research, *Food Nutrition, Physical Activity, and the Prevention of Cancer: A Global Perspective*, American Institute for Cancer Research, Washington, DC, 2007.
40. U.S. Departments of Agriculture and of Health and Human Services, MyPyramid. Available at http://www.mypyramid.gov, posted 2005, accessed 08/06/2008.
41. Pollock, M.L., Gaesser, G.A., Butcher, J.D., Després, J.P., Dishman, R.K., Franklin, B.A. and Garber, C.E., The recommended quantity and quality of exercise for developing and maintaining cardiorespiratory and muscular fitness and flexibility in healthy adults: American College of Sports Medicine position stand, *Med. Sci. Sports Exerc.* 30, 975–91, 1998.
42. Food and Nutrition Board, Institute of Medicine, *Adequacy of Evidence for Physical Activity Guidelines Development: Workshop Summary*, National Academies Press, Washington, DC, 2007.
43. U.S. Department of Health and Human Services, 2008 Physical Activity Guidelines for Americans. Available at http://www.health.gov/paguidelines, posted 10/7/2008, accessed 10/28/2008.

Section II

Energy-Yielding Nutrients

2 Carbohydrates

Michael S. Green and J. Andrew Doyle

CONTENTS

I. INTRODUCTION

Carbohydrates are the main source of energy during prolonged moderate- to high-intensity endurance exercise and repetitive, high-intensity activities that utilize the anaerobic energy systems. Sugars and starches consumed in the diet are stored within the body mostly in the form of glycogen, which can be rapidly mobilized as a source of energy during exercise. Carbohydrate stores in the body are limited, and are not able to indefinitely sustain moderate- to high-intensity exercise. Considerable research over the last 30 years has investigated dietary carbohydrate and methods of manipulating its intake at several key time points before, during, and after exercise. This chapter will present information regarding the metabolism of carbohydrate during exercise, as well as methods for manipulating carbohydrate consumption before, during, and after training or competition with the aim of enhancing performance and recovery.

II. CARBOHYDRATE METABOLISM

A. Dietary Sources of Carbohydrates

Carbohydrates, an economical and plentiful source of calories, can be found in varying amounts in a wide variety of foods. The basic diet should be consistent with the recommendations for chronic disease prevention and long-term health promotion. Such a diet is high in carbohydrate (>55% of total calories), low in fat (≤30% of total calories), and places a significant emphasis on a wide variety of foods.[1]

The various recommendations made in this chapter regarding carbohydrate intake can be satisfied via consumption of a wide range of carbohydrates, depending on personal and cultural preference. Although structure and consistency are important aspects of an athlete's daily routine, consumption of the same carbohydrate-containing foods day in and day out can lead to a reduction in the joy of eating. Incorporating traditional foods from different ethnic groups can be an excellent way of creating variety in an athlete's diet. For example, although most athletes are familiar with the fact that the main carbohydrate source in Italian food is pasta-based, it should be noted that Asian food is rice- and soybean-based, Mexican food is rice- and bean-based, and South American food is tuber-, bean-, and nut-based. Being largely composed of carbohydrates, food types such as these can be incorporated into the diet to promote varied and interesting carbohydrate consumption patterns. A selection of common sources of dietary carbohydrate can be found in Table 2.1.

B. Classification of Carbohydrates

Carbohydrates can be classified according to several criteria, including those based on the structure and number of sugar molecules, as well as the degree to which they induce a rise in blood glucose and insulin levels.

Monosaccharides contain only one sugar molecule and include glucose, fructose, and galactose. Disaccharides, which contain two sugar molecules, include sucrose, lactose, and maltose. Disaccharides can be distinguished from each other based on their specific monosaccharide building blocks, with sucrose made up of glucose and fructose, lactose made up of glucose and galactose, and maltose made of two glucose molecules.

Monosaccharides and disaccharides are collectively referred to as simple sugars or carbohydrates. Simple sugars, or food products containing large amounts of simple sugars, have often been referred to as "bad" carbohydrates, mostly as a method of describing the fact that they contain little additional nutritional value other than the provision of calories. Simple sugars are not inherently bad, but should certainly not make up the bulk of dietary carbohydrate intake. This may be especially true for sedentary or obese individuals, with studies suggesting that consumption of large amounts of rapidly absorbed sugars can predispose such individuals to chronic diseases such as type 2 diabetes.[2–4]

Polysaccharides, which include starch, fiber, and glycogen, contain many glucose units linked together and are referred to as complex carbohydrates. Maltodextrins, another type of polysaccharide, are glucose polymers containing no starch or fiber and are subsequently metabolized like simple sugars. Examples of simple and complex carbohydrates and their dietary sources can be found in Table 2.2.

TABLE 2.1

Common Sources of Dietary Carbohydrate

Food Group	Food	Serving Size	Carbohydrate (g)
Starches	Bagel	4" (71 g)	38
	Bread	1 slice (25 g)	14
	Cereal, sweet (Lucky Charms)	1 cup (35 g)	29
	Cereal, low sugar (Corn Flakes)	1 cup (28 g)	24
	Oatmeal, cooked	1 cup (234 g)	25
	Pasta, cooked	0.5 cup (70 g)	19
	Potato chips	1 ounce (28 g)	15
	Rice, cooked	0.5 cup (97 g)	22
Starchy vegetables	Corn, cooked	0.5 cup (75 g)	15
	Green peas, cooked	0.5 cup (75 g)	11
	Potatoes, mashed	0.75 cup (140 g)	25
Beans/legumes	Dried beans, cooked	0.5 cup (98 g)	20
	Lentils, cooked	0.5 cup (98 g)	20
Fruits	Apple, medium	3" (182 g)	25
	Banana, medium	7" (118 g)	27
	Orange	2.5" (141 g)	16
Vegetables	Broccoli, cooked	0.5 cup (78 g)	6
	Carrot	8" long (72 g)	6
	Tomato	2.5" (105 g)	5
Milk	Milk	1 cup (245 g)	12
	Chocolate milk	1 cup (245 g)	26
	Soy milk	1 cup (245 g)	18
	Yogurt, plain	1 cup (245 g)	17
	Yogurt, sweetened	1 cup (245 g)	26
Sugared beverages	Orange juice	0.5 cup (125 g)	13
	Sports beverage (6%)	1 cup (244 g)	14
	Soft drink	12 ounces (368 g)	40
Other foods	Pizza, cheese, thick crust	2 slices (142 g)	55
	Pizza, cheese, thin crust	2 slices (166 g)	46
	Cheese lasagna	1 cup (250 g)	45
	Chili with beans	1 cup (260 g)	22

TABLE 2.2

Classification of Carbohydrates

	Comments
Simple Carbohydrates	
Monosaccharides	
Glucose	Also known as dextrose; found in plant foods, fruits, honey
Fructose	Also known as fruit sugar; found in plant foods, fruits, honey
Galactose	Product of lactose digestion
Disaccharides	
Sucrose	Also known as white or table sugar; composed of glucose and fructose; used as a sweetener
Lactose	Composed of galactose and glucose; found in milk and dairy products
Maltose	Composed of two glucose molecules; product of starch digestion
Complex Carbohydrates	
Polysaccharides	
Amylopectin	Starch; found in plant foods and grains
Amylose	Starch; found in plant foods and grains
Carrageenan	Soluble fiber; found in the extract of seaweed and used as food thickener and stabilizer
Cellulose	Insoluble fiber; found in the bran layers of grains, seeds, edible skins, and peels
Corn Syrup	Hydrolyzed starch; found in processed foods
Dextrins	Starch; found in processed foods
Glycogen	Animal starch; found in meat, liver
Hemicellulose	Insoluble fiber; found in the bran layers of grains, seeds, edible skins, and peels
Inulin	Soluble fiber; found in Jerusalem artichokes
Invert Sugar	Hydrolyzed sucrose; found in processed foods
Lignin	Insoluble fiber; found in plant cell walls
Pectin	Soluble fiber; found in apples

C. Digestion and Absorption

Digestion of carbohydrates begins to a small degree in the mouth. Enzymes (salivary amylases) begin the process of digestion of complex carbohydrates by initiating the breakdown of starches. Chewing (mastication) is an important part of the digestive process, reducing foods to smaller-sized particles. Continuing this process of size reduction, mechanical action of the stomach increases both the rate of gastric emptying of food from the stomach into the small intestine and the surface area of the food particles made accessible to intestinal enzymes.

The majority of carbohydrate digestion and absorption occurs in the small intestine. After moving into the small intestine, the monosaccharides (glucose, fructose, and galactose) are absorbed directly into the blood via the capillaries within the intestinal villi. Glucose (and galactose) is absorbed via numerous sodium-dependent glucose transporters (SGLT-1), whereas fructose is absorbed via less numerous sodium-independent carriers. Disaccharides (sucrose, lactose, and maltose) are split into their constituent monosaccharides by specific disaccharidases, which are then absorbed directly into the blood. Complex carbohydrates are acted upon by pancreatic amylase and brush border enzymes, splitting polysaccharides to monosaccharides that are then absorbed as described above. The monosaccharides absorbed into the intestinal circulation are transported to the liver via the hepatic portal vein. Ultimately, glucose is the end point of carbohydrate digestion and absorption regardless of whether the original compound was a polysaccharide, disaccharide, or monosaccharide.

Not all of the carbohydrate content of foods consumed is digested and absorbed. Carbohydrate that is not absorbed may be related to the form of the food, the type of starch, or the amount of fiber present in the food. Undigested and unabsorbed carbohydrates go to the large intestine, where they are acted upon by colonic bacteria or excreted in the feces. Large amounts of indigestible carbohydrates, or excessive amounts of simple sugars consumed rapidly, may result in excessive gas production or gastrointestinal disturbances such as cramping and diarrhea. The fiber content of carbohydrate foods, which is largely indigestible by humans, plays an important role in maintaining appropriate gastric transit, may influence the eventual glycemic response to the foods consumed, and has important long-term health implications.

D. Glycemic Index

Consumption, digestion, and absorption of carbohydrates results in a postprandial increase in blood glucose, stimulation of insulin secretion by the pancreas, and subsequent increase in glucose uptake by various tissues in the body. The time course and magnitude of this glycemic response are highly variable with different foods, and do not follow the basic structural characterization of carbohydrates as simple or complex. For example, consumption of identical amounts of two simple sugars, the monosaccharides glucose and fructose, results in very different blood glucose responses. Glucose ingestion provokes a rapid, large increase in blood glucose, which in turn rapidly returns to baseline levels, whereas fructose consumption results in a much slower and lower glycemic response.

The concept of the Glycemic Index (GI) was developed to facilitate prediction of the glycemic response to a wide variety of foods.[5] The GI is a ranking based on the postprandial blood glucose response of a particular food compared with a reference food (glucose or white bread containing 50 g of carbohydrate). Test foods contain an identical amount of carbohydrate, and the blood glucose response is determined for several hours after consumption of the test food.[6] Specifically, the GI is a percentage of the area under the glucose response curve for a specific food compared with the area under the glucose response curve for the reference food.[7]

Extensive testing of foods has resulted in the publication of tables of glycemic indices for a wide variety of foods.[8] The GI of glucose (GI = 100) and fructose (GI = 19) clearly demonstrates the vast differences in glycemic response that can occur with the consumption of these two structurally similar monosaccharides. A GI of 19 indicates that fructose induces a blood glucose response that is 19% of that resulting from consumption of 50 g of glucose, and would therefore be described as having a significantly lower GI. The GI of sucrose is 68, which reflects the fact that sucrose consists of both glucose and fructose. The GI has become an important reference tool for prescribing appropriate diets for clinical populations that have a need for close regulation of blood glucose, such as people with diabetes. Athletes may also benefit from considering the GI of the carbohydrates they consume as well as their classification as simple or complex carbohydrates. There may be situations where an athlete would want to consume high-glycemic-index foods and provoke a large blood glucose and insulin response, such as when attempting to synthesize muscle glycogen quickly.[9] Conversely, there may be occasions when the athlete may want to consume lower-GI foods and avoid large increases in glucose and insulin, such as in the hours before an exercise bout.[10] As it relates to general health, consumption of low-GI foods may assist in preventing chronic diseases such as type 2 diabetes.[2,3] Figure 2.1 illustrates the GI for selected foods.

E. Carbohydrate Transportation and Storage

Increases in circulating glucose following carbohydrate consumption stimulate the pancreas to release insulin into the blood, where it functions to facilitate the uptake of glucose into various tissues. Glucose transport across cell membranes occurs via a process of facilitated diffusion, utilizing a family of glucose transporter carrier proteins (GLUT). The GLUT-4 isoform, normally located intracellularly, is translocated to the cell membrane when insulin binds to its receptor (or upon stimulation by muscular contractions), and is intimately related to the amount of glucose that can enter the cell. Upon entering the cell, glucose is subsequently metabolized for energy production or storage.

Although an important substrate for moderate- to high-intensity exercise, carbohydrate is stored in the body only in limited amounts. For each gram of carbohydrate metabolized there is the release of approximately 4 kilocalories (kcal) of available energy, compared with 9 kcal for each gram of fat oxidized. A small amount of glucose (5 g) circulates in the blood, but this amount cannot really be considered much of a "storage" form. The same can be said for free glucose existing within tissues and interstitial spaces.

Glycogen, the major store of carbohydrate, is found primarily in the liver and skeletal muscles. Other tissues, such as the kidneys and heart, only store small amounts of glycogen. For practical purposes, it is thus acceptable to consider the liver and skeletal muscles as the only areas of significant carbohydrate storage. Although various factors, including diet and training status, can affect the amount of glycogen stored in these tissues, useful estimates are that the liver contains 100 g of glycogen (~400 kcal) and skeletal muscle contains 400 g of glycogen (~1600 kcal).[11] Thus, skeletal muscle, by virtue of its significantly larger total mass, contains most of the glycogen stored in the body.

Glycogen is a large branched polymer that is composed of hundreds to thousands of glucose molecules. The branched structure allows for the convenient storage of relatively large amounts of rapidly accessible energy. Glycogen per se is not

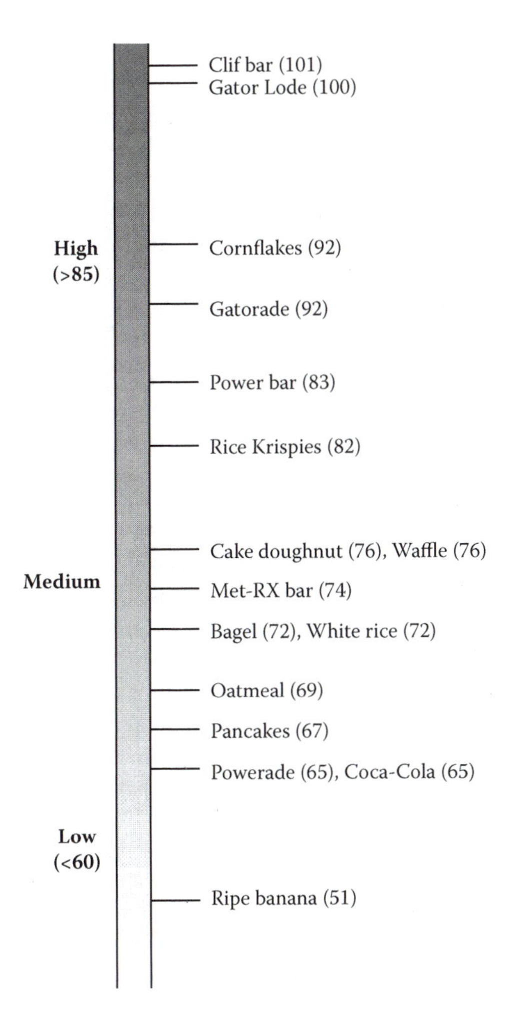

FIGURE 2.1 Glycemic index (GI) for selected foods. (Dunford, M., and Doyle, J.A. 2008. *Nutrition for Sports and Exercise*, p. 114. Belmont: Thomson Wadsworth. With permission).

consumed in appreciable amounts in the diet, since it is rapidly degraded in animal meat during cooking. Plants store glucose as starch, which is structurally rather similar to glycogen. Animals thus store glucose as glycogen, much like plants store glucose as starch.

Glycogen contained within the liver is utilized to maintain blood glucose levels in the postabsorptive state (i.e., between meals), whereas the glycogen contained within skeletal muscle is utilized directly by the muscle for its energy needs, particularly during moderate- to high-intensity exercise. The liver (and to a lesser extent the kidneys) is also capable of producing glucose from substrates such as fatty acids, amino acids, and lactate via the process of gluconeogenesis. Thus, in addition to that absorbed directly from the small intestine following a meal, blood glucose can be derived from the breakdown of stored liver glycogen or from glucose manufactured by the liver via gluconeogenesis. It is important to note that the process of gluconeogenesis can be a vital source of blood glucose during times of prolonged fasting or exercise when the liver's store of glycogen has been exhausted. It is the ability of the liver to maintain blood glucose via these pathways that allows individuals to last for several hours between meals without becoming hypoglycemic (low blood glucose levels). Of note is that the liver's glycogen stores can be depleted following 10–12 hours of fasting, which indicates that following a night's sleep the liver's glycogen levels can be almost totally exhausted.

Blood glucose derived from the liver can also enter the muscle and be utilized for energy. However, skeletal muscle lacks the enzyme glucose 6-phosphatase that allows glycogen to be degraded to free glucose and released into the blood. Thus, stored muscle glycogen is present primarily to satisfy the carbohydrate and energy requirements of the muscle cells themselves, with the task of maintaining blood glucose essentially left to the liver.

To put the total amount of skeletal muscle glycogen into perspective, an individual on a typical mixed diet (i.e., 50–60% of calories from carbohydrate or 4–5 g of carbohydrate consumed per kg of body weight) will typically possess 1–2 g of glycogen per 100 g of muscle. A trained individual on a high-carbohydrate diet (i.e., 70–80% of calories from carbohydrate or 8–10 g of carbohydrate consumed per kg of body weight) can often increase these muscle glycogen levels to values above 4 g per 100 g muscle. This ability to double the amount of stored muscle glycogen via dietary and training interventions was first shown by Scandinavian researchers in the 1960s,[12] and further refined by the work of Sherman and colleagues in the 1980s.[13] Muscle glycogen supercompensation will be further examined in the sections on carbohydrate manipulation that follow.

F. Carbohydrate Utilization During Exercise

Free fatty acids (derived from fat stored in adipose tissue) provide the majority of the energy during rest and low intensity exercise, with relatively small (but nevertheless necessary) contributions to the metabolic pathways made by carbohydrate. The brain, retina, and red blood cells are totally dependent on glucose for energy,[11] and tissues such as these thus have an absolute requirement for glucose whether during rest or exercise.

It is apparent that, during moderate- to high-intensity endurance exercise, carbohydrate, and in particular muscle glycogen, is a vital and major substrate contributing to the overall energy requirement of an individual.[14] Carbohydrates are used almost exclusively during maximal- and supramaximal-intensity exercise.

The physiological source of carbohydrate used during endurance performance can be conveniently partitioned between endogenous and exogenous sources. Endogenous carbohydrate can be thought of as that present in the body prior to any form of supplementation (e.g., liver and muscle glycogen, circulating blood glucose, and glucose derived via gluconeogenesis). As described earlier, the greatest amount of carbohydrate is stored in the form of muscle glycogen (300–400 g or 1,200–1,600 kcal). Glucose found in the blood totals approximately 5 g (20 kcal), while the liver contains about 75–100 g of glycogen (300–400 kcal).[11] The total body storage of carbohydrate is therefore approximately 1,500–2,000 kcal. Exogenous carbohydrate refers to that provided via ingested carbohydrate during or just prior to exercise and the role of this form of carbohydrate will be discussed in the section describing carbohydrate consumption during exercise.

The primary source of carbohydrate energy for physical exertion is muscle glycogen. As muscle glycogen is utilized, blood glucose enters the muscle to maintain the energy requirements of the active tissue. Consequently, the liver will release glucose to maintain blood glucose and prevent hypoglycemia. As blood glucose is used during exercise, it has to be replenished by liver glycogen stores (or via gluconeogenesis). Depletion of liver glycogen may lead to hypoglycemia. One hour of moderate-intensity exercise can reduce about half of the liver glycogen supply, whereas 15 or more hours of starvation (such as an overnight fast) can completely deplete liver glycogen. Although gluconeogenesis can be an important source of glucose during these times, it lacks the capacity to be able to fully maintain the flux of glucose. Hypoglycemia has been shown to impair the functioning of the central nervous system and is accompanied by feelings of dizziness, muscular weakness, and fatigue.

During exercise, glycogen breakdown is stimulated by both the increased free calcium present in the contracting muscle and the increase in circulating epinephrine (adrenaline). Glycogen use during exercise is dependent on several variables, including exercise intensity and duration, initial glycogen levels, and training status.

Exercise intensity has a significant effect on the source of substrate used for energy. Low-intensity exercise (20–30% of VO2max) places less emphasis on the use of muscle glycogen and allows for an increased utilization of free fatty acids as a substrate. As exercise intensity increases from low to moderate the relative amount of energy derived from carbohydrates (both blood glucose and muscle glycogen) increases. Energy derived from carbohydrate predominates above exercise intensities of 30–40% of VO2max in untrained individuals. Although blood glucose (derived itself from liver glycogen) and muscle glycogen both contribute increasingly as exercise intensity increases, it should be noted that at increasingly higher intensities the contribution of blood glucose is far outweighed by that of muscle glycogen.[14]

The shift toward an increased reliance on carbohydrate and a decreased reliance on fats as exercise intensity increases has been termed the crossover concept of substrate utilization.[15] It has been determined that as exercise intensity increases there is a gradual increase in the reliance on carbohydrate and a decreased reliance on fats. When graphed together this is illustrated as a crossover of the relative use of substrate, typically occurring at an exercise intensity of 30–40% of VO2max in untrained people. Further increases in exercise intensity up to maximum further diminish the use of fat as a substrate.

Supramaximal exercise results in the highest rates of glycogen utilization,[16] although these high rates cannot be maintained for extended periods due to the very high intensity of exercise. Thus, moderate- to high-intensity exercise (~75% VO2max) that can be maintained for longer periods not only results in relatively high rates of degradation but is also likely to result in large total amounts of glycogen degradation. Alternatively, supramaximal exercise performed repetitively with rest intervals (such as interval training) can also result in a combination of high rates and absolute amounts of glycogen depletion.

During prolonged exercise there is also a crossover phenomenon, although under these circumstances the crossover is to an increased reliance on fats as exercise proceeds. This is related to the decrease in glycogen levels present in the body of an individual exercising for prolonged periods, but is also caused as a result of a fatty acid–glucose cycle that operates to inhibit the use of glucose via glycolysis when fatty acids are being oxidized as a substrate. Even in the leanest individual, fatty acids offer an immense store of energy, but are able to sustain exercise only at rather low- to moderate-intensity levels when not supplemented with oxidation of adequate amounts of carbohydrate.

Utilization of carbohydrate during exercise is also influenced by its availability. An abundance of carbohydrate (whether endogenous or exogenous) will generally result in higher rates of carbohydrate oxidation during exercise. Individuals with higher amounts of muscle glycogen present in their muscles preceding an exercise bout will deplete their glycogen at a more rapid rate.[17] This may seem contradictory, since using glycogen more quickly should lead to more rapid glycogen depletion and fatigue. However, in concert with this elevated rate of glycogen use is the fact that performance is improved, thus allowing a more rapid completion of a fixed amount of exercise.

The training status of an individual can affect the degree to which he or she utilizes muscle glycogen during exercise. Trained, well fed individuals possess more glycogen in their muscles, so under some circumstances (such as during exercise intensities that surpass the ability of fat to provide energy) they will oxidize high amounts of the abundant muscle glycogen. However, compared with an unfit individual, an aerobically fit individual will utilize less total carbohydrate at the same absolute workload. Training induces adaptations (such as increased mitochondrial volume and number) that allow for a greater utilization of fats at a given exercise intensity. Thus, a trained individual will exhibit somewhat of a glycogen sparing effect when performing the same absolute-intensity exercise as an untrained person. The substrate "crossover" from fats to carbohydrate utilization occurs at higher relative and absolute exercise intensities in aerobically trained individuals.[15] This indicates that a trained individual will actually use less carbohydrate (and hence more fat) at a given submaximal workload than an untrained individual, an extremely beneficial adaptation since this will place less strain on the limited carbohydrate stores while allowing the plentiful fat stores to be utilized.

III. MANIPULATION OF CARBOHYDRATE INTAKE AND PHYSICAL PERFORMANCE

It should be apparent from the discussions above that carbohydrate is an important substrate used to provide energy during moderate- to high-intensity exercise. It is therefore not surprising that high carbohydrate intakes have been recommended for athletes to consume during training and competition. Research has clearly identified that fatigue typically coincides with the attainment of low muscle glycogen or blood glucose levels. Early research identified that subjects undergoing prolonged exercise were unable to maintain pace or were forced to stop when their muscle glycogen reached levels of ~5 g per kg of muscle (~30 mmol·kg^{-1}).[12,18] These are very low levels considering that well-trained, glycogen-supercompensated athletes may possess over 40 g of glycogen per kg of muscle (220 mmol·kg^{-1}) when they initiate such exercise. Thus, significant muscle glycogen depletion marks a serious inability to continue exercising at an appreciable or "competitive" intensity. This has obvious ramifications for competitive performance and the ability to tolerate repeated training bouts, and such early observations stimulated much of the research into carbohydrate manipulation.

A. Daily Training Diet

Carbohydrates should make up the bulk of total energy intake, primarily in the form of grain products, vegetables, and fruits. Individuals should further seek to limit total fat, saturated fat, and cholesterol in their diets. The recommended dietary allowance (RDA) for carbohydrate is 130 grams per day.[1] This amount should not really be viewed as a goal intake because it merely indicates the minimum amount of dietary carbohydrate necessary to provide adequate glucose for use by the brain. Athletes must further consider if the carbohydrate content of their diet is sufficient to support optimal performance in training and competition.

The carbohydrate content of the diet should be sufficient to maintain muscle glycogen stores during periods of intense training. Current recommendations for total carbohydrate intake for athletes is 5 to 10 g·kg^{-1} body weight daily,[19] although the volume and intensity of training play important roles in determining where in this range an individual falls.

During periods of heavy or increased training, many athletes may not consume adequate carbohydrate or calories to maintain muscle glycogen levels. Costill [20] showed that during a 3-day period of increased training while on a moderate-carbohydrate diet (43% of calories from carbohydrate) subjects were unable to maintain their glycogen levels. Indeed, glycogen progressively dropped during the study, and failed to return to baseline even after several days of recovery. Thus, a moderate carbohydrate diet providing ~5 g·kg^{-1}·day^{-1} does not seem to be adequate during heavy training. Kirwan [21] performed a similar study where attempts were made to match the carbohydrate expenditure of the athletes during a 5-day period of increased training. Even when carbohydrate intake was matched to estimated carbohydrate use (~8 g·kg^{-1}·day^{-1}), subjects continued to experience declines in their muscle glycogen levels over the training period (although not as large a decline as those consuming only ~4 g·kg^{-1}·day^{-1}). Despite this, subjects in both groups were able to adequately perform all training sessions, although perceived exertion was higher when on the low-carbohydrate regimen. For those athletes engaged in exhaustive training, it is therefore apparent that the diet may need to contain up to 10 g·kg^{-1}·day^{-1} to adequately replace the muscle glycogen they utilize during their daily training. Evidence for this was provided by Sherman,[22] who investigated the provision of 5 or 10 g·kg^{-1}·day^{-1} during 7 days of increased training. It was observed that muscle glycogen levels could be maintained with the high carbohydrate intake, but interestingly did not enhance daily training or high-intensity-exercise performance compared with the lower-carbohydrate group (who experienced declines in their muscle glycogen levels). The studies described above did not extend beyond a 7-day period, which may not allow enough time for the compromised muscle glycogen to exert an effect on the ability to train. Simonsen[23] showed that prolonged (4 weeks) supplementation of high amounts of carbohydrate can actually enhance the ability to continue hard training on consecutive days. Of note is that the subjects consuming 10 $g \cdot kg^{-1} \cdot day^{-1}$ were actually able to increase their glycogen levels throughout the intervention despite rather exhaustive daily training, and also exhibited larger improvements in mean power output during daily training. An interesting benefit of a high-carbohydrate diet is that it has also been shown to result in an enhanced maintenance of positive mood states during intensified training, a factor that may help promote motivation to continue participating in arduous training.[24]

A high-carbohydrate diet on a daily basis is therefore required to maintain or increase glycogen levels, and research suggests that this may promote the ability to perform more intense daily training. It may be difficult to consistently consume large amounts of carbohydrate as solid food, and athletes may want to consider using carbohydrate supplements, particularly in liquid form, to increase their intake. Liquid carbohydrate supplements have the added advantage of increasing fluid intake, thus helping the athlete maintain adequate hydration levels. People involved in activities or training of lesser intensity and duration do not need to consume as much carbohydrate, but should maintain their carbohydrate intake at 5–7 $g \cdot kg^{-1} \cdot day^{-1}$.

It is important to note that total energy intake must be sufficient in order to obtain the necessary amount of carbohydrate. If total caloric intake is too low, even a diet that is >70% carbohydrate (which is often recommended for athletic individuals) may yield an inadequate amount of carbohydrate. Carbohydrate consumption should therefore be considered on an absolute basis (i.e., number of grams for each kilogram of body weight) to ensure adequate intake. The example below illustrates this concept.

A 70-kg (154-lb) individual consuming a 2800 kcal diet and obtaining 70% of his or her calories from carbohydrate would consume 7.0 $g \cdot kg^{-1} \cdot day^{-1}$ and fall within the recommended range for carbohydrate intake based on body weight. However, this same person consuming 70% of calories from carbohydrate within a 1900 kcal diet would consume only 4.75 $g \cdot kg^{-1} \cdot day^{-1}$ and likely fall below the amount of carbohydrate necessary to sustain glycogen levels. In terms of percentages, both of these diets can be described as "high-carbohydrate" diets, but only the diet providing sufficient carbohydrate per kg of muscle would be considered acceptable. Conversely, 70-kg individuals consuming 5000 kcal per day will require only 50% of their calories (625 g total or 8.9 $g \cdot kg^{-1} \cdot day^{-1}$) to more than satisfy their carbohydrate need. It may therefore be more practical to assign carbohydrate intake based on body weight with the assumption that total calories are being supplied by this and other components of the diet. Under these circumstances, as long as the individual is weight stable and the remainder of the dietary intake is in line with nutritional guidelines for protein, fat, and other nutrients, it is probably safe to assume a diet is being consumed with sufficient total calories and carbohydrate to sustain glycogen levels and promote training adaptations.

B. Preparation for Prolonged Endurance Exercise and Competition

1. Carbohydrate Loading Protocols

Acute manipulation of exercise habits and carbohydrate content of the diet over short periods of time has been shown to result in supranormal levels of muscle glycogen, which in turn enhance carbohydrate oxidation and may improve endurance capacity in prolonged endurance activities such as cycling and running.[12,13] Such carbohydrate "loading" or "supercompensation" strategies have been shown to result in increased time to exhaustion during exercise at a fixed moderate-to-high intensity, but few studies have assessed the effect on more valid and reliable measures of endurance performance, such as actual competitive performance, time trials, time to perform a set amount of work, or use of protocols that more accurately mimic competitive events. Indeed, a recent well-designed study utilizing a reliable laboratory cycle protocol found no discernible effect of supercompensation on cycling performance.[25] However, the potential these strategies possess warrants serious consideration if only to help ensure that an optimal amount of glycogen is stored ahead of an important event.

Early studies showed a near doubling of muscle glycogen following the strategy referred to as the "classical" carbohydrate loading method.[12] However, this method possesses exercise and dietary demands that may be unacceptable to an athlete undergoing final preparations for an important event. The classical approach requires that muscle glycogen is depleted with prolonged, exhaustive exercise and is subsequently maintained in a suppressed state for three days with a virtually carbohydrate-free diet. Depleting exercise is performed again to further reduce glycogen stores, after which the athlete rests and consumes a carbohydrate-rich diet for the 3 days before the event. Although resulting in very high muscle glycogen stores, this method of carbohydrate loading may have other adverse physical and psychological effects that may not be advantageous for subsequent performance.

Although developed and refined over 25 years ago, many athletes are unaware of the so-called "modified" or "contemporary" carbohydrate loading method (see Figure 2.2).[13] In this method, athletes taper their training and follow a more realistic exercise preparation during the week before an important event. For the first

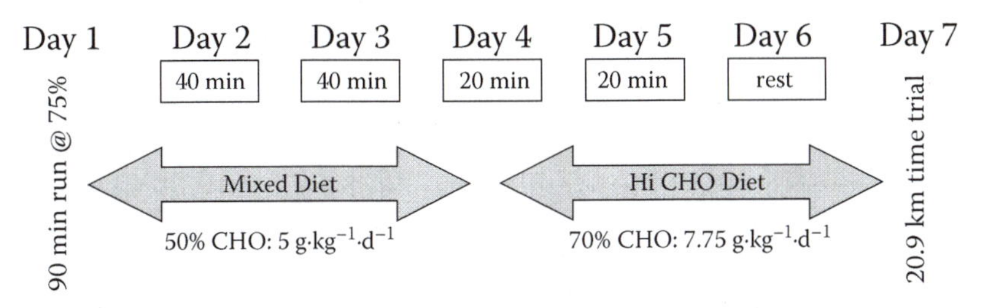

FIGURE 2.2 Modified carbohydrate loading protocol. (Adapted from Sherman, W.M., Costill, D.L., Fink, W.J., and Miller, J.M. 1981. *Int. J. Sports Med.*, 2, 114. With permission).

3 days of the week, when athletes are exercising for longer durations, the diet is manipulated to include a higher percentage of fat and protein and less carbohydrate (approximately 50% of total calories or ~5 $g \cdot kg^{-1} \cdot day^{-1}$). For many athletes, this may not necessitate much of a departure from their normal dietary routine, whereas those on already high carbohydrate diets may have to cut back their carbohydrate intake accordingly. The final 3 days before the event, when the athlete is exercising the least (i.e., tapering), the amount of carbohydrate in the diet is increased to 70% or more of total calories (i.e., ~8 $g \cdot kg^{-1} \cdot day^{-1}$), stimulating muscle glycogen storage. The amount of muscle glycogen synthesis following this modification is nearly as great as with the classical method, but the difficulties associated with exhaustive exercise and a period of very low carbohydrate intake are avoided. Although it usually requires a conscious effort to plan out the exercise and dietary modifications in this way, the procedure is not complicated and simply requires some attention to detail.

A few notes of caution should be observed regarding carbohydrate loading. Care should be taken to not become overzealous regarding carbohydrate consumption. Although a concerted effort is often required to consume 8–10 $g \cdot kg^{-1} \cdot day^{-1}$, possibly requiring supplementation with carbohydrate-containing liquids, the overriding principle of this procedure is a redistribution of calories from a mixed diet to one containing a greater amount of carbohydrate in concert with a tapered exercise program. Total daily caloric intake should remain relatively constant during the week, although it is an acceptable tendency to consume a slightly increased number of calories. It is also worth noting that each gram of stored glycogen is associated with several grams of water. As a result, weight gain and bloating can often occur, which can be of concern for athletes involved in events where they must support their own body weight (such as running).

Studies investigating the efficacy of one type of carbohydrate over the other have concluded that there is no advantage of either a predominately simple- or complex-carbohydrate diet in the 3-day high-carbohydrate period of the loading phase.[4,26]

2. Pre-Event Meal

The meal consumed prior to a training bout or competitive event may also be used to maximize carbohydrate stores. Fasting before prolonged endurance events results in diminished performance, so it is important to consume a meal in the hours before long-duration training sessions or competitive efforts.[27] The meal should provide adequate energy and carbohydrate to support the metabolic demands of the exercise, be consumed in adequate time before the onset of exercise to allow for gastric emptying, digestion, and absorption, and should also be palatable and acceptable to the athlete.

Carbohydrate meals of 1–2 $g \cdot kg^{-1}$ eaten 1 hour before exercise, or meals containing up to 4.5 $g \cdot kg^{-1}$ consumed 3–4 hours before exercise have been shown to improve endurance performance.[28,29] There appears to be a positive synergistic effect when pre-exercise meals are consumed in conjunction with carbohydrate intake during exercise.[30]

Meals high in carbohydrate, particularly high-glycemic foods, consumed in the hour or so before exercise result in high insulin and in decreasing blood glucose at the time exercise begins. It has been hypothesized that this glycemic response, coupled with the enhanced glucose uptake by exercising muscle, may result in a "rebound" hypoglycemia, inhibition of free fatty acid oxidation, and subsequent impairment of endurance exercise performance. This concern has led to recommendations to consume only low-GI foods prior to exercise.[10,31] However, most studies show that in the first 30–60 minutes of exercise, blood glucose does not decrease to the low levels at which symptoms of hypoglycemia are experienced, and very few studies have shown an impairment in subsequent performance. Blood glucose and insulin generally return to normally expected levels, and most studies show that carbohydrate consumption 1 hour before exercise improves performance, regardless of the GI.[32–34]

From a practical perspective, most athletes would not choose to eat within an hour of beginning a long exercise bout. The meal should be timed so that it is largely cleared from the gastrointestinal tract (typically 3–4 hours) before the onset of exercise to minimize the possibility of gastric upset. This additional time allows for the return of glucose and insulin toward baseline levels, and diminishes any lingering effects of the GI of the meal consumed.[35]

It is important for an athlete to consume a meal before prolonged exercise (especially following an overnight fast) in order to maximize endogenous carbohydrate stores. The meal should be largely composed of carbohydrate, and should consist of food the athlete is familiar with. This strategy should be employed consistently in training; new foods or meal patterns should not be implemented before important competitive events. The GI of the food is not as important as the familiarity, tolerance, and timing of the meal. For example, in the early morning hours before a marathon, it would be more practical for a runner to consume a familiar high-carbohydrate breakfast food such as oatmeal (GI = 69), rather than attempting to meet an unwarranted recommendation to consume a low-GI meal by consuming a bowlful of lentils (GI = 30).

C. Carbohydrate Consumption During Exercise

Prolonged moderate-intensity exercise will result in significant depletion of muscle glycogen stores. When the body's reserves of carbohydrate fall there is an inevitable reduction in exercise intensity, if not complete cessation from exercise. Concomitant with the decline in muscle glycogen there is an increasingly important role played by blood glucose in maintaining the necessary flux through glycolysis and the aerobic energy pathways. Although fats may also begin to contribute a larger role as exercise proceeds, the intensity–substrate relationship dictates that continued moderate- to high-intensity exercise requires a continued supply of carbohydrate. The supply of glucose is not unlimited, and its rate of production by the liver from gluconeogenic precursors, while profoundly increased, is not able to keep up with demand indefinitely. Resting and exercise blood glucose can usually be well maintained at 70–90 $mg{\cdot}dL^{-1}$ (3.9-5.0 $mmol{\cdot}L^{-1}$), but this can drop to 40–50 $mg{\cdot}dL^{-1}$ (2.2-2.8 $mmol{\cdot}L^{-1}$) during the most exhaustive and prolonged exercise. Although some athletes are able to tolerate hypoglycemia better than others, most athletes at this point will experience a significant decline in performance.

A large body of research provides evidence that consumption of carbohydrate during exercise maintains blood glucose levels and carbohydrate oxidation, and significantly improves both endurance capacity and performance.[36,37] Seminal research conducted in the 1980s by researchers such as David Costill, Edward Coyle, and Andrew Coggan laid the foundation for many of the current recommendations for carbohydrate supplementation during exercise.

Coyle[38] showed that trained cyclists were able to delay fatigue by 23 min (157 vs. 134 min) when consuming glucose solutions during exercise. This 17% increase in time to fatigue was achieved via provision of 1.0 $g \times kg^{-1}$ glucose (50% solution) at 20 min into exercise along with 0.25 $g \times kg^{-1}$ glucose (6% solution) at 60, 90, and 120 min into exercise, as opposed to provision of a non-caloric placebo. A follow-up study with the addition of muscle biopsies determined that supplementation with glucose during prolonged endurance exercise does not seem to spare muscle glycogen,[39] with the mechanism of performance enhancement likely being the ability to maintain high rates of carbohydrate oxidation late in exercise when muscle glycogen levels are low. Carbohydrate supplementation may also spare liver glycogen, which will assist with the maintenance of carbohydrate oxidation and blood glucose levels.[40,41]

Although carbohydrate consumption should occur at regular intervals throughout exercise in order to delay or avoid fatigue, consumption late in exercise can still be beneficial. A single large (3 $g \times kg^{-1}$ glucose in a 50% solution) carbohydrate feeding after 135 min of continuous cycling exercise halted the decline in blood glucose levels and allowed cyclists to exercise 21% longer compared with consumption of a non-caloric placebo.[42] In a related study, cyclists who exercised until fatigue and then rested for 20 min were able to exercise for an additional 26 min following consumption of 3 $g \times kg^{-1}$ glucose in a 50% solution, compared with only 10 min following consumption of a non-caloric placebo.[43]

Based on estimates of the maximum rate of glucose absorption from the small intestine, general recommendations are to consume 30 to 60 g of carbohydrate each hour during prolonged exercise. Although carbohydrate solutions of 20% or more are well tolerated by many individuals, the human gastrointestinal system's capacity to handle carbohydrate can certainly be exceeded. Higher nutrient densities generally hinder gastric emptying, and a significantly reduced rate of gastric emptying will cause less glucose to be presented to the small intestine and subsequently absorbed. Glucose remaining in the stomach waiting to pass into the small intestine is of no help in the provision of glucose to the blood. Indeed, severe GI distress may result from such situations. Research has ultimately shown that a 6–8% carbohydrate solution (typical of many commercially available sports beverages; see Table 2.3) presents itself as an adequate compromise between impaired gastric emptying and increased intestinal absorption. Thus, for every 100 milliliter (mL) of water, there should be 6–8 g of carbohydrate. To consume the recommended 60 g per hour, 1000 mL (1 liter) of a 6% solution would need to be consumed (or 750 mL of an 8% solution).

Due to factors related to the saturation of intestinal sodium-dependent glucose transporters (SGLT-1), as well as possible limitations exerted by the liver, it appears that oxidation of exogenous glucose peaks at 1.0–1.1 $g \cdot min^{-1}$ when provided in a beverage supplying 1.2 $g \cdot min^{-1}$ of glucose.[44,45] This rate of oxidation cannot be exceeded by supplying glucose in higher amounts (e.g. 2.4 $g \cdot min^{-1}$). Similar investigations

TABLE 2.3

Carbohydrate Content of Selected Sports Beverages, Gels, and Bars

	Serving Size	Energy (kcal)	Carbohydrate Content		
			Source	g	%
Beverage					
Accelerade	8 oz	80	Sucrose; maltodextrin; fructose	14	6
AllSport Body Quencher	8 oz	60	High fructose corn syrup (HFCS)	16	7
Gatorade Original	8 oz	50	Sucrose; glucose; fructose	14	6
Gatorade Endurance	8 oz	50	Sucrose; glucose; fructose	14	6
Gleukos Sports Fuel	8 oz	70	Glucose	17	7
Hydrade	8 oz	55	HFCS	10	4
POWERade	8 oz	64	HFCS; glucose polymers	17	7
Gels and Bars					
AccelGel	1 pack (32 g)	90	Maltodextrin; HFCS	20	—
Gu Energy Gel	1 pack (32 g)	100	Maltodextrin	25	—
Balance Bar	1 bar	200	HFCS; honey; high maltose corn syrup; sugar	23	—
Clif Bar	1 bar	240	Brown rice syrup; oats; cane juice; fig paste	46	—
Power Bar	1 bar	230	HFCS; fruit juice concentrate	20	—

utilizing fructose have demonstrated oxidation rates 20–25% lower (peaking at ~0.7 g·min^{-1}) than glucose, suggesting that the fructose intestinal transporter (GLUT-5) may act as a limiting factor, with the added possibility that conversion of fructose to glucose in the liver may also limit its oxidation.[45–47] The disaccharide sucrose (composed of equal amounts of glucose and fructose) also exhibits similar maximal oxidation rates (~1.0 g·min^{-1}) to glucose.[48]

An intriguing step is to combine mono- and disaccharides of various types in an attempt to overcome the apparent saturation limitation of their individual intestinal transport mechanisms. Building on the findings of the above studies and the apparent ceiling of exogenous carbohydrate oxidation that is reached at a glucose intake of 1.2 g·min^{-1}, the effects of various glucose, sucrose, and fructose combinations and amounts has continued to provide interesting findings. High peak oxidation rates of 1.7 g·min^{-1} have been found as a result of ingestion of a mixture providing 1.2 g·min^{-1} glucose, 0.6 g·min^{-1} sucrose, and 0.6 g·min^{-1} fructose (for a total of 2.4 g·min^{-1} of carbohydrate).[49] Of particular note, ingesting a total of 2.4 g·min^{-1} of carbohydrate in the form of 1.2 g·min^{-1} glucose and 1.2 g·min^{-1} fructose has resulted in some of the highest oxidation measurements to date, resulting in peak oxidation rates of 1.75 g·min^{-1}.[50]

Oxidation rates for exogenous carbohydrate have thus been shown to be highest when a prudent mixture of glucose and fructose (1.2 $g \cdot min^{-1}$ of each) are combined together in a beverage consumed during prolonged exercise. It also appears that a mixture of glucose (1.2 $g \cdot min^{-1}$), sucrose (0.6 $g \cdot min^{-1}$), and fructose (0.6 $g \cdot min^{-1}$) can provide similar oxidation maximums. Glucose consumed in isolation cannot sustain oxidation rates above 1.0 $g \cdot min^{-1}$, and does not need to be consumed in amounts higher than 1.2 $g \cdot min^{-1}$, which comes conveniently close to the recommended amount of 60 g of carbohydrate per hour typically recommended during prolonged endurance performance.

The studies discussed above provide a strong theoretical basis for enhancing endurance performance via supplementation with a mixture of specific mono- and/or disaccharides. The ability to utilize greater levels of exogenous carbohydrate, especially in the latter stages of an endurance event, would seem to hold great potential for maintaining high levels of endurance performance. Preliminary research has indicated that ingestion of glucose-fructose mixtures can improve endurance performance, with one study indicating that cycling time trial performance in conjunction with glucose-fructose ingestion was improved by 8% compared with ingestion of glucose only.[51] Further research is warranted to determine if higher carbohydrate oxidation rates indeed translate into improved endurance performance. A major factor to keep in mind is that these studies (and many of the studies regarding carbohydrate supplementation) have taken place using cyclists as subjects. Consuming the amount of fluid that these subjects typically consume may make the recommendations difficult to follow for runners who cannot conceivably consume as much liquid.

There is thus unequivocal support for the use of carbohydrate during prolonged (>2 h) continuous exercise. Although research findings are inconclusive, carbohydrate supplementation during continuous high-intensity exercise of less than 2 h (i.e., ~1 h) does appear to be beneficial.[52–54] This may be especially true if subjects are glycogen depleted prior to the exercise bout. Research looking at intermittent exercise also lends support for carbohydrate supplementation before and during repeated (6–8), short-duration (2–3 min), high-intensity (120–130% VO2max) exercise.[55] It is feasible that glycogen may actually be resynthesized during the rest periods that intermittent activities afford.

Consumption of other forms of carbohydrate (e.g., solid food) may be difficult or poorly tolerated during activities such as running. Other activities, such as cycling, may provide the opportunity for consumption of solid food with less discomfort. The few studies of solid food consumption during endurance exercise show improvements in performance compared with a placebo, but there is no evidence that solid or semi-solid carbohydrate consumption has any physiological or performance advantage over carbohydrate intake in liquid form.[56,57] Under some circumstances, such as during ultra endurance events, the consumption of solid food may enhance the feelings of satiety.

Athletes should maximize their glycogen stores prior to an event and, if the event is either intermittent or continuous and prolonged for over an hour, should certainly attempt to supplement with some form of carbohydrate if the nature of the activity permits. Carbohydrate should be consumed at regular intervals during exercise at a rate of no more than ~60 g per h in a 6–8 % solution. Ideally, delaying consumption of carbohydrate until late in exercise should be avoided, since blood glucose may have reached a precipitously low level that cannot be appreciably reversed. Attention should also be paid to the specific type of carbohydrate consumed, with solutions containing glucose, fructose, and/or sucrose offering the most potential. Typically, adequate carbohydrate consumption before and during exercise, as opposed to only before or only during, will help ensure the best endurance performance.[30] Carbohydrate consumption during exercise may be particularly beneficial to those who commence such activities in an already glycogen depleted state. Table 2.3 illustrates the carbohydrate content of several commercially available sports beverages, gels, and bars.

Recent research has also investigated the combined consumption of carbohydrate-protein beverages during prolonged exercise. Initial findings suggested that a carbohydrate sports drink containing additional calories from protein enhanced endurance performance above and beyond that of a drink containing only carbohydrate.[58–60] This remains a controversial area of research with several studies not supporting these findings,[61–63] although the degree of exercise-induced muscle injury that occurs during prolonged exercise may be attenuated.[61,62]

D. Carbohydrate Consumption During Recovery from Exercise

A significant proportion of the recovery from prolonged, moderate- to high-intensity exercise is the replacement of the body's stores of carbohydrate. Adequate glycogen replacement following exercise depends upon the provision of exogenous carbohydrate. In the event that carbohydrate is not consumed following exercise, the rate of muscle glycogen synthesis is rather low, and assumes a rate of 7-12 $mmol \cdot kg^{-1} dw \cdot h^{-1}$, with much higher rates (20–50 $mmol \cdot kg^{-1} dw \cdot h^{-1}$) occurring when carbohydrate is provided in the correct time frame and sufficient amounts.[64]

Carbohydrate intakes are typically expressed as grams of carbohydrate consumed per kilogram of body weight per hour ($g \cdot kg^{-1} \cdot h^{-1}$). Provided that sufficient carbohydrate is consumed, complete restoration of glycogen stores within 24 h has been shown.[65] Such a time frame is adequate for most individuals who do not regularly fully tax their glycogen stores, especially when combined with the fact that several meals will be consumed within this period. However, maximizing glycogen synthesis takes on greater importance for athletes who significantly deplete their glycogen stores on consecutive days of training or, as is very common, perform more than one training session per day.

There appears to be a rapid and a slow phase of glycogen synthesis following exercise-induced glycogen depletion.[66] An initial rapid period (30–60 min) is characterized by an insulin-independent translocation of glucose transporters (GLUT-4),[67] with a more extended period (up to 48 h) characterized by an insulin-dependent phase of glycogen synthesis at a slower rate.[68] Resynthesis of glycogen following exercise is thus heavily dependent on the timing and amount of carbohydrate consumed.

Withholding provision of carbohydrate results in significantly lower levels of muscle glycogen synthesis. Glycogen synthesis rates are 45% lower when post-exercise carbohydrate ingestion is delayed by 2 h.[64] A delay in administration reduces the amount of glucose that can enter the cell and subsequently be incorporated into glycogen. Thus, immediate (within 30 min of completion of exercise) consumption of carbohydrate is necessary to ensure adequate glycogen synthesis.

Provision of a sufficient amount of carbohydrate is important in order to maximize glycogen synthesis rates. The highest rates of glycogen synthesis are observed when carbohydrate is provided immediately after exercise and at frequent (every 15–30 min) intervals in amounts sufficient to provide 1.2 $g \cdot kg^{-1} \cdot h^{-1}$.[69] Providing this same hourly amount less frequently results in slower glycogen synthesis.[70] Supplying more than 1.2 $g \cdot kg^{-1} \cdot h^{-1}$ does not seem to result in higher glycogen synthesis rates.[71]

Research has also focused on the addition of amino acids or protein to the carbohydrate in attempts to further stimulate glycogen synthesis, perhaps by further elevating insulin levels or providing an additional gluconeogenic substrate. Increased glycogen synthesis rates have been observed when amino acids are added to moderate amounts of carbohydrate (0.8 $g \cdot kg^{-1} \cdot h^{-1}$).[69] Jentjens and colleagues[72] investigated the addition of amino acids to a drink containing 0.8 or 1.2 $g \cdot kg^{-1} \cdot h^{-1}$ carbohydrate and found that the addition of amino acids was beneficial only in the group receiving the lower amount of carbohydrate. Therefore, the presence of protein or amino acids in post-exercise supplements does not appear to be necessary as long as sufficient (1.2 $g \cdot kg^{-1} \cdot h^{-1}$) amounts of carbohydrate are present, although the addition of protein or amino acids may possibly assist with muscular growth and repair.[71]

Endurance-trained individuals possess significantly higher rates of glycogen synthesis. For example, one study determined that trained cyclists demonstrated glycogen synthesis rates over two times higher than untrained cyclists.[73] Muscle GLUT-4 content was also three times higher in the trained individuals. Further research has illustrated that just 10 weeks of training in previously untrained individuals resulted in significantly greater muscle glycogen synthesis rates and increased levels of GLUT-4.[74]

The magnitude of glycogen depletion plays a very important role in its subsequent synthesis. Glycogen inhibits its own formation, and it appears that the absolute amount of glycogen remaining in the muscle (and not the relative percentage that has been depleted) strongly controls the rate of glycogen synthesis.[75] Thus, it is the glycogen concentration remaining in the muscle that determines its subsequent rate of synthesis.

The type of prior exercise can affect the degree of subsequent glycogen synthesis. Activities that result in significant amounts of exercise-induced muscle injury (such as downhill running or prolonged exercise) have been shown to reduce glycogen synthesis rates by up to 25%, even when large amounts of carbohydrate are ingested.[76]

Consumption of CHO in the post-exercise period is therefore essential to ensure high rates of glycogen re-synthesis. Consumption of carbohydrate should commence immediately after exercise, and should be consumed at the rate of 1.2 $g \cdot kg^{-1} \cdot h^{-1}$ for 4–6 h in order to maintain maximum glycogen synthesis rates.

IV. CONSIDERATIONS FOR THE MIDDLE-AGED ATHLETE

The vast majority of research regarding carbohydrate manipulation and athletic performance has been conducted with young populations. A logical question is to ask whether the recommendations that have been set forth based on these studies are applicable to older populations. With respect to this, it is important to consider the age-related changes in lifestyle, body composition, resting energy expenditure, and training habits that may seriously curtail the energy and carbohydrate requirements of an aging individual.

Daily energy intake requirements for reasonably active (but non-athletic) individuals have been estimated to be 2400 and 3000 kcal for females and males, respectively.[1] Energy intake can also be expressed as a function of body weight, with the suggestion that 37–41 kcal should be consumed per day for each kg of body weight.[1] These energy requirements account for resting energy expenditure and typical activities of daily living, and must be scaled up (sometimes significantly so) to account for additional energy expended for exercise and larger amounts of daily physical activity. Thus, alterations in resting energy expenditure, amount of exercise, and amount of additional physical activity can significantly affect the amount of total calories and carbohydrate that should be consumed.

The energy requirements of an individual athlete of any age result from an interaction of the above mentioned factors. In general, an older athlete may have lower energy requirements than a younger athlete.[77] Possibly accounting for this is the observation that older athletes exhibit lower resting energy expenditures and training volumes.[78] It cannot always be ruled out that lower training volumes may be the causative factor accounting for the decline in resting energy expenditure, and not the independent effect of aging per se. Conversely, an older athlete will likely have an increased energy requirement in comparison with an age-matched sedentary person.[79] The fact remains that an aging athlete needs to take into account any reductions in training volume and general physical activity as it relates to carbohydrate (and caloric) intake. Adherence to guidelines designed for athletes performing more prolonged and intense physical activity may result in excessive caloric intake and subsequent weight gain in the progressively less-active individual, a point that is true regardless of age. Older athletes who maintain their training volume do not seem to exhibit a decline in resting energy expenditure or daily energy requirements.[78] Interestingly, when previously sedentary older subjects initiate endurance or resistance-training programs it has been noted that during the first few months the expected increase in dietary energy intake is absent, possibly as a result of a compensatory decrease in the amount of energy expenditure throughout the rest of the day.[79–81]

Skeletal muscle glycogen storage has been shown to be less in both sedentary and endurance trained older subjects when compared with sedentary or similarly trained younger individuals, and seems to be utilized at higher rates for a given sub-maximal intensity of exercise.[82] Reassuringly, following a period of endurance training, previously sedentary older individuals are able to increase the amount of glycogen that can be stored in the muscle, as well as the ability to replenish it after depleting exercise.[82] Although skeletal muscle glycogen stores still remain somewhat suppressed in comparison with younger individuals, endurance training does induce peripheral adaptations that promote the ability to synthesize glycogen at similar relative rates in an older individual.

Older individuals should consider their exercise and physical activity habits when determining their total caloric and carbohydrate intakes. Monitoring of body weight and feedback from training and competitive performance should be used as a guide in determining whether an adequate diet is being consumed. Decreased training loads should be met with a decrease in total caloric and carbohydrate intake toward the lower end of the ranges indicated in this chapter. Additionally, if training is to be performed with more prolonged recovery periods (such as every other day) less emphasis can be placed on the specific timing of carbohydrate intake and more placed on simply consuming an adequate amount throughout the day in the form of snacks and meals that conveniently conform to the individual's schedule.

V. RESEARCH NEEDS

The effect of carbohydrate consumption before, during, and after exercise has been heavily investigated over the last 30 years. It is reasonably well accepted that a diet high in carbohydrate promotes a favorable physiological environment that promotes repeated training and performance enhancement. Unequivocal evidence supports the use of carbohydrate during prolonged exercise, as well as the timely application of carbohydrate immediately following exercise to promote rapid restoration of glycogen.

Research is currently focusing on the effects of the interaction of carbohydrate with other nutrients, such as protein and amino acids, on the enhancement of athletic performance and promotion of exercise recovery and training adaptations. Mixtures of different mono- and disaccharides (such as glucose, fructose, and sucrose) also hold continued hope as ways of maximizing carbohydrate absorption and oxidation during exercise. Unfortunately, numerous methodological issues hinder the practical application of many of these research findings, and it is hoped that continued investigation will uncover the correct application of these various nutrients to further promote exercise performance. Although more studies should also be performed utilizing athletic older populations, there is no apparent reason that the vast majority of findings obtained using younger subjects cannot be successfully applied to aging athletes.

VI. CONCLUSIONS

Carbohydrates are present in a wide variety of foods and should make up the bulk (> 55–75%) of the diet in both active and inactive people. However, it is recommended that active individuals pay particular attention to their carbohydrate intake to ensure consumption of sufficient energy in the form of carbohydrate to maximize endogenous carbohydrate stores prior to exercise, as well as to promote adequate recovery from repeated exercise bouts. For this reason, carbohydrate intake prescribed based on body weight can be more useful than expressing it as a percentage of total calories.

Older individuals should take into consideration any alterations in their lifestyle and training habits that may impact the amount of carbohydrate they consume. Carbohydrate guidelines should be interpreted with these factors in mind, and adjusted up or down as necessary. Coordinating carbohydrate intake within a well balanced diet is important for the long-term health of all individuals.

TABLE 2.4

Summary of Carbohydrate Recommendations

Time Period	Carbohydrate Amount	Comments
Daily Training	7-10 $g \times kg^{-1} \times day^{-1}$	Amount depends upon duration and intensity of daily training; may need to supplement
Carbohydrate Loading	5 $g \times kg^{-1} \times day^{-1}$ for 3 days, then 8 + $g \times kg^{-1} \times day^{-1}$ for 3 days	For prolonged events (>2 h); depleting exercise bout followed by tapered training for 6 days
Pre-exercise Meal	1-2 $g \times kg^{-1}$ 1 to 2 h before, or up to 4-5 $g \times kg^{-1}$ 3 to 4 h before	Consume familiar foods; time meal before exercise to insure complete digestion
During Exercise	0.5-1.0 $g \times kg^{-1} \times hour^{-1}$	For prolonged events (>2 h); sports drinks up to 10% concentration; may consider mixed carbohydrate types (glucose and fructose)
After Exercise	0.75-1.5 $g \times kg^{-1} \times hour^{-1}$	Evaluate need for rapid replacement of muscle glycogen; small, frequent feedings beginning as soon as possible for 2-4 h; may consider addition of amino acids or protein

This chapter has presented various methods of manipulating carbohydrate consumption before, during, and after training or competition. Table 2.4 provides a concise summary of recommendations for carbohydrate consumption during the daily training and carbohydrate loading phases, as well for immediately before, during, and after exercise.

REFERENCES

1. Institute of Medicine, National Academy of Sciences, *Dietary Reference Intakes for Energy, Carbohydrate, Fiber, Fat, Fatty Acids, Cholesterol, Protein, and Amino Acids (Macronutrients)*. National Academies Press, Washington, DC, 2002.
2. Bell, S.J. and Sears, B., Low-glycemic-load diets: Impact on obesity and chronic diseases. *Crit. Rev. Food Sci. Nutr.* 43, 357–377, 2003.
3. Ludwig, D.S., The glycemic index: Physiological mechanisms relating to obesity, diabetes, and cardiovascular disease. *JAMA* 287, 2414–2423, 2002.
4. Roberts, K.M., Noble, E.G., Hayden, D.B., and Taylor, A.W., Simple and complex carbohydrate-rich diets and muscle glycogen content of marathon runners. *Eur. J. Appl. Physiol. Occup. Physiol.* 57, 70–74, 1988.
5. Jenkins, D.J., Wolever, T.M., Taylor, R.H., Barker, H., Fielden, H., Baldwin, J.M., et al., Glycemic index of foods: A physiological basis for carbohydrate exchange. *Am. J. Clin. Nutr.* 34, 362–366, 1981.
6. Wolever, T.M., Jenkins, D.J., Jenkins, A.L. and Josse, R.G., The glycemic index: Methodology and clinical implications. *Am. J. Clin. Nutr.* 54, 846–854, 1991.

7. Jenkins, D.J., Wolever, T.M., Jenkins, A.L., Josse, R.G. and Wong, G.S., The glycaemic response to carbohydrate foods. *Lancet* 2, 388–391, 1984.
8. Foster-Powell, K., Holt, S.H. and Brand-Miller, J.C., International table of glycemic index and glycemic load values: 2002. *Am. J. Clin. Nutr.* 76, 5–56, 2002.
9. Burke, L.M., Collier, G.R. and Hargreaves, M., Muscle glycogen storage after prolonged exercise: Effect of the glycemic index of carbohydrate feedings. *J. Appl. Physiol.* 75, 1019–1023, 1993.
10. Walton, P. and Rhodes, E.C., Glycaemic index and optimal performance. *Sports Med.* 23, 164–172, 1997.
11. Schils, M.E., Olson, J.A., Shike, M., and Ross, A.C., *Modern Nutrition in Health and Disease*. Williams and Wilkins, Baltimore, MD, 1999.
12. Bergstrom, J., Hermansen, L., Hultman, E., and Saltin, B., Diet, muscle glycogen and physical performance. *Acta Physiol. Scand* .7, 140–150, 1967.
13. Sherman, W.M., Costill, D.L., Fink, W.J., and Miller, J.M., Effect of exercise–diet manipulation on muscle glycogen and its subsequent utilization during performance. *Int. J. Sports Med.* 2, 114–118, 1981.
14. Romijn, J.A., Coyle, E.F., Sidossis, L.S., Gastaldelli, A., Horowitz, J.F., Endert, E., and Wolfe, R.R., Regulation of endogenous fat and carbohydrate metabolism in relation to exercise intensity and duration. *Am. J. Physiol.* 265, E380–E391, 1993.
15. Brooks, G.A. and Mercier, J., Balance of carbohydrate and lipid utilization during exercise: the “crossover” concept. *J. Appl. Physiol.* 76, 2253–2261, 1994.
16. Saltin, B. and Karlsson, J., Muscle glycogen utilization during work of different intensities, in *Muscle Metabolism during Exercise*, Pernow, B. and Saltin, B., Eds. Plenum Press, New York, 1971, p. 289–300.
17. Hargreaves, M., McConell, G., and Proietto, J., Influence of muscle glycogen on glycogenolysis and glucose uptake during exercise in humans. *J. Appl. Physiol.* 78, 288–292, 1995.
18. Karlsson, J. and Saltin, B., Diet, muscle glycogen, and endurance performance. *J. Appl. Physiol.* 31, 203–206, 1971.
19. Burke, L.M., Cox, G.R., Culmmings, N.K., and Desbrow, B., Guidelines for daily carbohydrate intake: Do athletes achieve them? *Sports Med.* 31, 267–299, 2001.
20. Costill, D.L., Bowers, R., Branam, G., and Sparks, K., Muscle glycogen utilization during prolonged exercise on successive days. *J. Appl. Physiol.* 31, 834–838, 1971.
21. Kirwan, J.P., Costill, D.L., Mitchell, J.B., Houmard, J.A., Flynn, M.G., Fink, W.J., and Beltz, J.D., Carbohydrate balance in competitive runners during successive days of intense training. *J. Appl. Physiol.* 65, 2601–2606, 1988.
22. Sherman, W.M., Doyle, J.A., Lamb, D.R., and Strauss, R.H., Dietary carbohydrate, muscle glycogen, and exercise performance during 7 d of training. *Am. J. Clin. Nutr.* 57: 27–31, 1993.
23. Simonsen, J.C., Sherman, W.M., Lamb, D.R., Dernbach, A.R., Doyle, J.A., and Strauss, R., Dietary carbohydrate, muscle glycogen, and power output during rowing training. *J. Appl. Physiol.* 70, 1500–1505, 1991.
24. Achten, J., Halson, S.L., Moseley, L., Rayson, M.P., Casey, A., and Jeukendrup, A.E., Higher dietary carbohydrate content during intensified running training results in better maintenance of performance and mood state. *J. Appl. Physiol.* 96, 1331–1340, 2004.
25. Burke, L.M., Hawley, J.A., Schabort, E.J., St Clair, G.A., Mujika, I., and Noakes, T.D., Carbohydrate loading failed to improve 100-km cycling performance in a placebo-controlled trial. *J. Appl. Physiol.* 88, 1284–1290, 2000.
26. Brewer, J., Williams, C., and Patton, A., The influence of high carbohydrate diets on endurance running performance. *Eur. J. Appl. Physiol. Occup. Physiol.* 57, 698–706, 1988.

27. Dohm, G.L., Beeker, R.T., Israel, R.G., and Tapscott, E.B., Metabolic responses to exercise after fasting. *J. Appl. Physiol.* 61, 1363–1368, 1986.
28. Sherman, W.M., Brodowicz, G., Wright, D.A., Allen, W.K., Simonsen, J., and Dernbach, A., Effects of 4 h preexercise carbohydrate feedings on cycling performance. *Med. Sci. Sports Exerc.* 21, 598–604, 1989.
29. Sherman, W.M., Peden, M.C., and Wright, D.A., Carbohydrate feedings 1 h before exercise improves cycling performance. *Am. J. Clin. Nutr.* 54, 866–870, 1991.
30. Wright, D.A., Sherman, W.M., and Dernbach, A.R., Carbohydrate feedings before, during, or in combination improve cycling endurance performance. *J. Appl. Physiol.* 71, 1082–1088, 1991.
31. Guezennec, C.Y., Oxidation rates, complex carbohydrates and exercise: Practical recommendations. *Sports Med.* 19, 365–372, 1995.
32. Febbraio, M.A., and Stewart, K.L. CHO feeding before prolonged exercise: Effect of glycemic index on muscle glycogenolysis and exercise performance. *J. Appl. Physiol.* 81, 1115–1120, 1996.
33. Horowitz, J.F. and Coyle, E.F., Metabolic responses to preexercise meals containing various carbohydrates and fat. *Am. J. Clin. Nutr.* 58, 235–241, 1993.
34. Thomas, D.E., Brotherhood, J.R., and Brand, J.C., Carbohydrate feeding before exercise: Effect of glycemic index. *Int. J. Sports Med.* 12, 180–186, 1991.
35. Coyle, E.F., Substrate utilization during exercise in active people. *Am. J. Clin. Nutr.* 61, 968S–979S, 1995.
36. Coggan, A.R. and Coyle, E.F., Carbohydrate ingestion during prolonged exercise: effects on metabolism and performance. *Exerc. Sport Sci. Rev.* 19, 1–40, 1991.
37. Jeukendrup, A.E., Carbohydrate intake during exercise and performance. *Nutr.* 20, 669–677, 2004.
38. Coyle, E.F., Hagberg, J.M., Hurley, B.F., Martin, W.H., Ehsani, A.A., and Holloszy, J.O., Carbohydrate feeding during prolonged strenuous exercise can delay fatigue. *J. Appl. Physiol.* 55, 230–235, 1983.
39. Coyle, E.F., Coggan, A.R., Hemmert, M.K., and Ivy, J.L., Muscle glycogen utilization during prolonged strenuous exercise when fed carbohydrate. *J. Appl. Physiol.* 61, 165–172, 1986.
40. Bosch, A.N., Dennis, S.C., and Noakes, T.D., Influence of carbohydrate ingestion on fuel substrate turnover and oxidation during prolonged exercise. *J. Appl. Physiol.* 76, 2364–2372, 1994.
41. McConell, G., Fabris, S., Proietto, J., and Hargreaves, M., Effect of carbohydrate ingestion on glucose kinetics during exercise. *J. Appl. Physiol.* 77, 1537–1541, 1994.
42. Coggan, A.R. and Coyle, E.F., Metabolism and performance following carbohydrate ingestion late in exercise. *Med. Sci. Sports Exerc.* 21, 59–65, 1989.
43. Coggan, A.R. and Coyle, E.F., Reversal of fatigue during prolonged exercise by carbohydrate infusion or ingestion. *J. Appl. Physiol.* 63, 2388–2395, 1987.
44. Jeukendrup, A.E., Mensink, M., Saris, W.H., and Wagenmakers, A.J., Exogenous glucose oxidation during exercise in endurance-trained and untrained subjects. *J. Appl. Physiol.* 82, 835–840, 1997.
45. Jeukendrup, A.E., and Jentjens, R., Oxidation of carbohydrate feedings during prolonged exercise: Current thoughts, guidelines and directions for future research. *Sports Med.* 29, 407–424, 2000.
46. Massicotte, D., Peronnet, F., Allah, C., Hillaire-Marcel, C., Ledoux, M., and Brisson, G., Metabolic response to [13C]glucose and [13C]fructose ingestion during exercise. *J. Appl. Physiol.* 61, 1180–1184, 1986.
47. Massicotte, D., Peronnet, F., Brisson, G., Bakkouch, K., and Hillaire-Marcel, C., Oxidation of a glucose polymer during exercise: Comparison with glucose and fructose. *J. Appl. Physiol.* 66, 179–183, 1989.

48. Wagenmakers, A.J., Brouns, F., Saris, W.H., and Halliday, D., Oxidation rates of orally ingested carbohydrates during prolonged exercise in men. *J. Appl. Physiol.* 75, 2774–2780, 1993.
49. Jentjens, R.L., Achten, J., and Jeukendrup, A.E., High oxidation rates from combined carbohydrates ingested during exercise. *Med. Sci. Sports Exerc.* 36, 1551–1558, 2004.
50. Jentjens, R.L. and Jeukendrup, A.E., High rates of exogenous carbohydrate oxidation from a mixture of glucose and fructose ingested during prolonged cycling exercise. *Br. J. Nutr.* 93, 485–492, 2005.
51. Currell, K. and Jeukendrup, A.E., Superior endurance performance with ingestion of multiple transportable carbohydrates. *Med. Sci. Sports Exerc.* 40, 275–281, 2008.
52. Below, P.R., Mora-Rodriguez, R., Gonzalez-Alonso, J., and Coyle, E.F., Fluid and carbohydrate ingestion independently improve performance during 1 h of intense exercise. *Med. Sci. Sports Exerc.* 27, 200–210, 1995.
53. Jeukendrup, A., Brouns, F., Wagenmakers, A.J., and Saris, W.H., Carbohydrate-electrolyte feedings improve 1 h time trial cycling performance. *Int. J. Sports Med.* 18, 125–129, 1997.
54. Davis, J.M., Jackson, D.A., Broadwell, M.S., Queary, J.L., and Lambert, C.L., Carbohydrate drinks delay fatigue during intermittent, high-intensity cycling in active men and women. *Int. J. Sport Nutr.* 7, 261–273, 1997.
55. Mason, W.L., McConell, G., and Hargreaves, M., Carbohydrate ingestion during exercise: Liquid vs solid feedings. *Med. Sci. Sports Exerc.* 25, 966–969, 1993.
56. Peters, H.P., van Schelven, W.F., Verstappen, P.A., de Boer, R.W., Bol, E., Erich, W.B., et al., Exercise performance as a function of semi-solid and liquid carbohydrate feedings during prolonged exercise. *Int. J. Sports Med.* 16, 105–113, 1995.
57. Ivy, J.L., Res, P.T., Sprague, R.C., and Widzer, M.O., Effect of a carbohydrate-protein supplement on endurance performance during exercise of varying intensity. *Int. J. Sport Nutr. Exerc. Metab.* 13, 382–395, 2003.
58. Saunders, M.J., Kane, M.D., and Todd, M.K., Effects of a carbohydrate-protein beverage on cycling endurance and muscle damage. *Med. Sci. Sports Exerc.* 36, 1233–1238, 2004.
59. Williams, M.B., Raven, P.B., Fogt, D.L., and Ivy, J.L., Effects of recovery beverages on glycogen restoration and endurance exercise performance. *J. Strength Cond. Res.* 17, 12–19, 2003.
60. Millard-Stafford, M., Warren, G.L., Thomas, L.M., Doyle, J.A., Snow, T., and Hitchcock, K., Recovery from run training: Efficacy of a carbohydrate-protein beverage? *Int. J. Sport Nutr. Exerc. Metab.* 15, 610–624, 2005.
61. Romano-Ely, B.C., Todd, M.K., Saunders, M.J., and Laurent, T.S., Effect of an isocaloric carbohydrate-protein-antioxidant drink on cycling performance. *Med. Sci. Sports Exerc.* 38, 1608–1616, 2006.
62. van Essen, M. and Gibala, M.J., Failure of protein to improve time trial performance when added to a sports drink. *Med. Sci. Sports Exerc.* 38, 1476–1483, 2006.
63. Ivy, J.L., Katz, A.L., Cutler, C.L., Sherman, W.M., and Coyle, E.F., Muscle glycogen synthesis after exercise: Effect of time of carbohydrate ingestion. *J. Appl. Physiol.* 64, 1480–1485, 1988.
64. Casey, A., Short, A.H., Hultman, E., and Greenhaff, P.L., Glycogen resynthesis in human muscle fibre types following exercise-induced glycogen depletion. *J. Physiol.* 483 (Pt 1), 265–271, 1995.
65. Garetto, L.P., Richter, E.A., Goodman, M.N., and Ruderman, N.B., Enhanced muscle glucose metabolism after exercise in the rat: The two phases. *Am. J. Physiol.* 246, E471–E475, 1984.

66. Maehlum, S., Hostmark, A.T., and Hermansen, L., Synthesis of muscle glycogen during recovery after prolonged severe exercise in diabetic and non-diabetic subjects. *Scand. J. Clin. Lab. Invest.* 37, 309–316, 1977.
67. Ivy, J.L., Muscle glycogen synthesis before and after exercise. *Sports Med.* 11, 6–19, 1991.
68. van Loon, L.J., Saris, W.H., Kruijshoop, M., and Wagenmakers, A.J., Maximizing postexercise muscle glycogen synthesis: Carbohydrate supplementation and the application of amino acid or protein hydrolysate mixtures. *Am. J. Clin. Nutr.* 72, 106–111, 2000.
69. Ivy, J.L., Lee, M.C., Brozinick, J.T., Jr., and Reed, M.J., Muscle glycogen storage after different amounts of carbohydrate ingestion. *J. Appl. Physiol.* 65, 2018–2023, 1988.
70. Jentjens, R., and Jeukendrup, A., Determinants of post-exercise glycogen synthesis during short-term recovery. *Sports Med.* 33, 117–144, 2003.
71. Jentjens, R.L., van Loon, L.J., Mann, C.H., Wagenmakers, A.J., and Jeukendrup, A.E., Addition of protein and amino acids to carbohydrates does not enhance postexercise muscle glycogen synthesis. *J. Appl. Physiol.* 91, 839–846, 2001.
72. Hickner, R.C., Fisher, J.S., Hansen, P.A., Racette, S.B., Mier, C.M., Turner, M.J., and Holloszy, J.O., Muscle glycogen accumulation after endurance exercise in trained and untrained individuals. *J. Appl. Physiol.* 83, 897–903, 1997.
73. Greiwe, J.S., Hickner, R.C., Hansen, P.A., Racette, S.B., Chen, M.M., and Holloszy, J.O., Effects of endurance exercise training on muscle glycogen accumulation in humans. *J. Appl. Physiol.* 87, 222–226, 1999.
74. Price, T.B., Laurent, D., Petersen, K.F., Rothman, D.L and Shulman, G.I., Glycogen loading alters muscle glycogen resynthesis after exercise. *J. Appl. Physiol.* 88, 698–704, 2000.
75. Doyle, J.A., Sherman, W.M., and Strauss, R.L., Effects of eccentric and concentric exercise on muscle glycogen replenishment. *J. Appl. Physiol.* 74, 1848–1855, 1993.
76. Reaburn, P., Nutrition and the ageing athlete, in *Clinical Sports Nutrition*, Burke, L. and Deakin, V., Eds. McGraw Hill, Melbourne, 2000, 602.
77. van Pelt, R.E., Dinneno, F.A., Seals, D.R., and Jones, P.P., Age-related decline in RMR in physically active men: Relation to exercise volume and energy intake. *Am. J. Physiol. Endocrinol. Metab.* 281, E633–E639, 2001.
78. Butterworth, D.E., Nieman, D.C., Perkins, R., Warren, B.J., and Dotson, R.G., Exercise training and nutrient intake in elderly women. *J. Am. Diet. Assoc.* 93, 653–657, 1993.
79. Campbell, W.W., Kruskall, L.J., and Evans, W.J., Lower body versus whole body resistive exercise training and energy requirements of older men and women. *Metabolism* 51, 989–997, 2002.
80. Keytel, L.R., Lambert, M.I., Johnson, J., Noakes, T.D., and Lambert, E.V., Free living energy expenditure in post menopausal women before and after exercise training. *Int. J. Sport Nutr. Exerc. Metab.* 11, 226–237, 2001.
81. Meredith, C.N., Frontera, W.R., Fisher, E.C., Hughes, V.A., Herland, J.C., Edwards, J., and Evans, W.J., Peripheral effects of endurance training in young and old subjects. *J. Appl. Physiol.* 66, 2844–2849, 1989.

3 Lipids

Sarah J. Ehlers, Heather E. Rasmussen, and Ji-Young Lee

CONTENTS

I. INTRODUCTION

Lipids are broadly defined as molecules that are soluble in organic solvents such as acetone, alcohols, chloroform, and ether. The word lipid comes from the Greek word *lipos*, meaning fat.[1] Lipids are a substantial component of the human diet, contributing approximately 100 to 150 g per day in a typical Western diet.[2,3] Lipids are commonly referred to as fats, and can originate from animal sources, existing in a solid state at room temperature, or from plant sources existing as liquid at room temperature.[4] Dietary lipids can be described as visible fats or invisible fats. Visible fats are those that the consumer can see, such as condiments such as butter, margarine, mayonnaise, or salad dressing. Invisible fats are those that are incorporated into the food product so the consumer can't necessarily see the fat itself. Examples of invisible fats are meats, baked goods, and fried foods.[5]

It is easy to understand why lipids are the primary source of energy both at rest and during low- to moderate-intensity physical exercise. Carbohydrate and protein each contain 4 kcal per g, while fats contain more than twice the energy, with 9 kcal per g.[2,5] Although certain lipids have a negative reputation for their role in obesity, inflammatory processes, atherosclerosis, carcinogenesis, and aging,[2] they are an important component of foods and a vital component of the human body. Food lipids enhance flavor, create unique texture, carry nutrients, and contribute to the feeling of satiety. In the body, lipids are a dense energy source, a critical component of cell membranes, a substrate for prostaglandin and leukotriene synthesis, and a carrier of fat-soluble vitamins. As our knowledge of lipids has evolved, it has become more apparent that not all lipids should be associated with negative health effects. The different structural characteristics of lipids determine their functionality and health effects, and certain lipids are now thought to play a positive role in human health. This chapter will serve to identify those characteristics and address the ways in which lipids are utilized in the body.

II. CLASSIFICATIONS AND STRUCTURES

A. Major Classes

Although some components of the major classes of lipids share similar structures or biological function, lipids are divided into three major classes: simple lipids, compound lipids, and derived lipids.

1. Simple Lipids

Simple lipids consist of free fatty acids, triglycerides, diglycerides, monoglycerides, and waxes. Triglycerides, the most common dietary lipid, consist of three fatty acids esterified to a glycerol backbone. Approximately 95% of lipids are consumed in the form of triglycerides, whereas monoglycerides and diglycerides, consisting of one and two fatty acids esterified to a glycerol backbone, respectively, exist in smaller amounts within the body.[2] Fatty acids that are not associated with a triglyceride, diglyceride, or monoglyceride molecule are considered free, or non-esterified, fatty acids. However, it is possible for these free fatty acids to be attached to proteins in the body, and only a fraction of a percentage of fatty acids are not bound to any other component in human plasma. Waxes are esters of long-chain fatty acids and alcohols. The alcohol component of a wax may be a sterol, such as cholesterol, or a non-sterol such as vitamin A.[6] In both plants and animals waxes are used as protective coatings.

2. Compound Lipids

The class of compound lipids includes phospholipids, glycolipids, and lipoproteins. As denoted in the name, phospholipids contain a phosphate group esterified to one or more fatty acids. The amphipathic nature of phospholipids is important in the formation of cell membrane, where phospholipids form a bilayer with the hydrophobic fatty acids facing the center, while the hydrophilic phosphate groups face outward toward the aqueous environment of the body. This structure allows for the transport of both water-soluble and fat-soluble nutrients. Phospholipids can be categorized as glycerophosphatides and sphingophosphatides, in which the building block of the molecule is a glycerol and sphingosine, respectively. A common glycerophosphatide is phosphatidylcholine, commonly known as lecithin, which is a very important cell membrane component. Sphingomyelins are an abundant example of sphingophosphatides. Sphingomyelins are also found in cell membranes, most notably in the myelin sheath of nerve tissue, and play a role in signal transduction.[6]

Glycolipids are made up of carbohydrate and fatty acid. They are classified as either cerebrosides or gangliosides. The carbohydrate portion of a cerebroside is a monosaccharide unit, generally either glucose or galactose, linked to a sphingosine and a fatty acid. Like sphingomyelins, cerebrosides are also an important component of neural tissue. Gangliosides are similar to cerebrosides in structure, except the carbohydrate moiety is an oligosaccharide. The more than 40 known gangliosides are involved in cell recognition and immune responses[7], and the ganglioside composition is a determinant of human blood types.[8,9]

Compound lipids may also include lipoproteins, as these particles contain lipids and proteins. Lipoproteins are the main transporter of lipids within the circulation, and depending on the ratio of lipid to protein, lipoproteins can be classified as chylomicrons, very-low-density lipoprotein (VLDL), low-density lipoprotein (LDL), and high-density lipoprotein (HDL). Lipoproteins can also be characterized by the composition of the lipids they carry, which can include triglycerides, phospholipids, free cholesterol, and cholesteryl esters.[6]

3. Derived Lipids

Derived lipids include sterols and alcohols left as a result of hydrolysis of simple or compound lipids that still retain properties of the lipids.[6] Sterols are a class of lipids that consist of a steroid and an alcohol. The most physiologically abundant sterol in humans is cholesterol, which is an integral part of the plasma membranes and a key determinant in the fluidity of the lipid bilayer. The amphipathic nature of cholesterol allows it to be an important structural component of cell membranes and the outer layer of plasma lipoproteins. Cholesterol is a precursor to corticosteroids, mineral corticoids, bile acids, vitamin D, and sex hormones such as testosterone, estrogen, and progesterone. Because excess free cholesterol is toxic in cells, it can be esterified to a fatty acid and becomes a neutral form of cholesterol termed cholesteryl ester. Cholesteryl esters can be stored in the lipid droplets of cells without cytotoxicity and therefore cholesterol esterification is increased when free cholesterol content in cells becomes excessive.

Whereas cholesterol is exclusively an animal sterol, more than 40 sterols have been identified in plants. Similar to cholesterol, plant sterols serve to maintain the structural integrity of a cell. The most abundant plant sterols are sitosterol, campesterol and stigmasterol, which differ from cholesterol by the presence of an extra methyl or ethyl group within the sterol side chain. This addition of the methyl or ethyl group on the sterol side chain results in poor intestinal absorption of plant sterols in humans,[10] with only 1.5 to 5.0% of sitosterol absorbed when typical amounts of sterols are consumed (240–320 mg).[2,11] Despite minimal amounts of plant sterol absorption into the blood stream, plant sterols function within the intestine as effective cholesterol-lowering agents.[12,13]

Because triglycerides are the primary source of energy-yielding dietary lipid, the remainder of the chapter will focus on the structures and characteristics of fatty acids and triglycerides rather than the compound lipids and lipid derivatives.

B. Fatty Acids

As a simple lipid, the fatty acid is often a basic unit of more complex lipid structures, namely triglycerides. Fatty acids consist of a methyl group (CH_3) and a carboxyl group (COOH) joined by a hydrocarbon chain. Properties of fatty acids depend upon carbon chain length, degree of saturation, and the position of the double bonds. Short chain fatty acids (2–8 carbons in length) and unsaturated fatty acids tend to be liquid oils at room temperature, whereas long chain (9–24 carbons in length) and saturated fatty acids exist as solid fats at room temperature. In unsaturated hydrocarbons, the fatty acid may have the exact same chemical composition, but the number of double bonds, or the position of the double bonds may differentiate how the molecule reacts in the body. Although a wide variety of fatty acids exist in nature, just four (palmitic, stearic, oleic, and linoleic acid) compose over 90% of the average American diet.[6]

1. Nomenclature

To describe the structure and characteristics of fatty acids, two common naming systems exist. Both utilize shorthand notation, with the number of carbon atoms listed first and the number of double bonds listed second after a colon, e.g., stearic acid (18:0) or oleic acid (18:1). This provides information on two of the three key characteristics of fatty acids (carbon chain length and number of double bonds) but provides no information on the position of the double bonds. The omega (ω) notation system provides the position of the first double bond as counted from the carboxyl end of the hydrocarbon chain. For example, oleic acid would be written as 18:1 ω-9, linoleic acid as 18:2 ω-6, and α-linolenic acid as 18:3 ω-3. Sometimes the Greek symbol ω is replaced with an n, and this same naming system can use both characters interchangeably. Although the omega system provides more information than just the chemical structure shorthand, it only provides the location of the first double bond. It can be assumed that the double bonds of a fatty acid in nature occur on every third carbon, so one can extrapolate the position of all double bonds from the omega notation. The second fatty acid notation system, the delta (Δ) notation system, provides the position of each double bond in the fatty acid. In this system, double bonds are also counted from the carboxyl end and the carbon atom at which the double bonds begin is listed in superscript behind the delta symbol. Therefore, linoleic acid is written as 18:2 $\Delta^{9,12}$, α-linolenic acid as 18:3 $\Delta^{9,12,15}$, and eicosapentaenoic acid (EPA) as 20:5 $\Delta^{5,8,11,14,17}$.[6]

2. Saturation

Saturated fatty acids are those that contain no double bonds in their hydrocarbon chain. The length of the carbon chains of saturated fatty acids varies from 4–24 carbon atoms. The most common saturated fatty acids found in nature are lauric acid (12:0), myristic acid (14:0), palmitic acid (16:0), and stearic acid (18:0), ranging in chain length from 12–18 carbons as indicated. Saturated fats mainly exist in a solid state at room temperature, with several exceptions such as coconut oil and palm kernel oil that are liquid at room temperature. Saturated fats can exist naturally, or can be produced by a processing method called hydrogenation, creating fully or partially saturated fatty acids from unsaturated fatty acids. This hydrogenation provides a more desirable structure and texture, longer shelf life, and stability during deep frying in a variety of manufactured food products and baked goods. However, health concerns have been raised over hydrogenation due to the by-production of *trans* fats during this process.[2] The *cis* and *trans* geometric isomers will be discussed in the next section.

Unsaturated fatty acids contain at least one carbon-carbon double bond in the hydrocarbon chain. Fatty acids containing only one double bond are called monounsaturated fatty acids (MUFA) and those with two or more double bonds are called polyunsaturated fatty acids (PUFA). Subfamilies of the PUFA include ω-3 and ω-6 fatty acids. A basic example of an ω-3 fatty acid in a Western diet is α-linolenic acid and a common ω-6 fatty acid is linoleic acid. The predominant ω-9 MUFA in the Western diet is oleic acid (18:1), with its single double bond located between the ninth and tenth carbons. Oleic acid and other ω-9 fatty acids are found in olive oil and some sunflower oils.[14]

3. Essential Fatty Acids

Two essential fatty acids have been identified, α-linolenic acid (ALA) and linoleic acid (LA), mentioned previously as ω-3 and ω-6 fatty acids, respectively. Plants, but not mammals, contain the desaturase enzymes needed to produce these fatty acids. Therefore, ω-3 and ω-6 fatty acids are considered essential fatty acids.[14,15] Once supplied in the diet, ALA and LA can be elongated in the body to 20-carbon molecules and desaturated to arachidonic acid (20:4), EPA (20:5)) and docosahexaenoic acid (DHA, 22:6) by a series of enzymes. In addition to ALA and LA, EPA and DHA can also be found naturally in food systems and are often used as supplements to promote health.[15] Through the cyclooxygenase (COX) enzyme system, arachidonic acid and EPA can be converted to eicosanoids.[14] Eicosanoids are an entire category of signaling molecules involved in inflammation. The four families of eicosanoids are prostaglandins, prostacyclins, thromboxanes, and leukotrienes.[14]

PUFA content of such oils can be as high as 75%, and daily intake averages between 12 and 20 grams per day.[14,15] Major sources of LA are plant seed oils and margarines made from corn, sunflower, and soybeans. High amounts of ALA are found in nuts, canola oil, and green leafy vegetables.[14,15] In a typical Western diet, the average ratio of LA to ALA is roughly 20:1 or higher.[15] Recommendations for a cardio-protective diet through PUFA consumption suggest the ratio of 4:1 or lower, containing at least 2 grams per day of ALA.[15] Oily fish such as salmon, herring, tuna, and mackerel are major sources of ω-3 EPA and DHA.

4. Geometric Isomers

Geometric isomers are molecules of same chemical composition but with different physical properties. In fatty acid geometric isomers, the physical structures differ around carbon-carbon double bonds. In a saturated hydrocarbon chain, the four available bonds of each carbon atom are shared between two other carbon atoms and two hydrogen atoms. In the case of unsaturation, the carbon-carbon double bond takes the place of one of the bonds to a hydrogen atom and causes a kink in the otherwise straight-chain molecule. Two forms of geometric isomers in fatty acids are called *cis* and *trans*, designated as such to describe the orientation of the hydrogen atoms around the double bond. In the *cis* configuration, both of the hydrogen atoms surrounding the carbon-carbon double bond are on the same side of the molecule. This causes a U-shaped kink in the chain. In the *trans* configuration the hydrogen atoms are on opposite sides of the double bond, resulting in a structure that is more straight and mimics that of a saturated fatty acid. Therefore, a *cis* bond retains the properties of an unsaturated fatty acid, but the same molecule containing a *trans* bond has different physical properties more closely related to those of a saturated fatty acid.

As mentioned previously, *trans* fats are often a result of the hydrogenation process, but they also exist naturally in foods. Common sources of industrially produced *trans* fats are products containing hydrogenated oils (margarines, fried foods, snack foods, baked goods) while natural sources are from animal products (meats, dairy products). Americans consume on average 2–3% of their total calories from *trans* fats produced during food processing, while only 0.5% of total calories come from naturally occurring *trans* fats.[16] Intake of *trans* fatty acids have been linked to negative alterations in plasma lipids, an increase in inflammation, and dysfunction of endothelial cells.[16] The health effects of *trans* fats will be discussed later.

C. Triglycerides

In addition to being the predominant form of dietary lipid, triglycerides are also the major form of lipid storage in the body. The basic structure of a triglyceride is a glycerol backbone esterified to three fatty acid chains. The glycerol molecule contains three hydroxyl groups, allowing ester bond formation with the carboxyl end of a free fatty acid. A triglyceride may be composed of three similar fatty acids, thus called a simple triglyceride, or different fatty acids, called a mixed triglyceride. It is the physical properties of the individual fatty acids that give the overall triglyceride its characteristics. The fatty acids may vary in chain length as well as saturation, so a triglyceride containing long chain or saturated fatty acids tends to be solid at room temperature while triglycerides containing short chain or unsaturated fatty acids are liquid at room temperature. A naming system has been developed to differentiate the position of each fatty acid based upon the carbon to which it is esterified. The carbons are labeled *sn*-1, *sn*-2, and *sn*-3. To be utilized for energy, the fatty acids from the triglyceride must be cleaved from the molecule by enzymes called lipases, to the free fatty acid form. Only the free fatty acids can be oxidized.[2,6]

III. LIPID INTAKE

A. Digestion

Because nearly all dietary lipids are in the form of triglycerides, they will be used as the primary example for discussion on digestion, absorption, and transport. The majority of triglyceride digestion occurs in the lumen of the small intestine, but also occurs partially in the stomach and mouth. Digestion of triglycerides is initiated in the mouth by the salivary enzyme lingual lipase, secreted from serous glands beneath the tongue, and continued in the stomach. Lingual lipase secretion is continuous at basal levels, but can be increased by neural stimulus, high dietary fat content, and sucking or swallowing motions.[6] It is responsible for 10–30% of triglyceride digestion.[1] Lingual lipase cleaves mainly fatty acids at the *sn*-3 position, and works most effectively on short chain (4–6 carbons) and medium chain (8–10 carbons) triglycerides, while long chain triglycerides (12–24 carbons) are mostly digested in the duodenum, the upper section of the small intestine. For lingual lipase to exert its effect on triglycerides, emulsification must take place by a combination of stomach contraction and acid milieu. The partially digested food, or chyme, containing the lipid emulsion exits the stomach and in the proximal small intestine, it is introduced to bile composed mostly of bile acids and salts that are synthesized from cholesterol. In the fasting state, bile acids are concentrated in the gallbladder, where they are stored until stimulated for secretion. Emulsification by bile is necessary to increase the surface of the lipid droplets for digestion.[3] Bile acids are suitable for emulsification because of their amphipathic properties, thus being able to dissolve the lipid particles into the body's aqueous environment. The bile acids orient so that their nonpolar end faces inward in the lipid droplet with their polar end facing the water phase.[6]

After food consumption, bile enters the duodenum in response to the hormone cholecystokinin (CCK).[15] CCK is a peptide hormone released in response to lipid or protein-rich chime emptied from the stomach into the duodenum. It is also responsible for an increase in satiety. Bicarbonate simultaneously secreted from the pancreas creates a favorable pH for emulsification and hydrolysis of triglycerides, and, in conjunction with bile, creates an optimal environment for pancreatic lipase. Hydrolysis of triglycerides by pancreatic lipase results in a mixture of monoglycerides, diglycerides and free fatty acids. Pancreatic lipase favors cleavage of fatty acids in the *sn*-1 and *sn*-3 position.[6] Only a small portion of triglycerides are completely hydrolyzed to glycerol and free fatty acids.

B. Absorption

Lipid absorption occurs in the duodenum and the jejunum sections of the small intestine with the aid of micelles. Micelles are small particles, roughly 5mm in diameter, whose size suits them well to travel to the villi of the intestinal mucosal membrane and fit into the spaces between the microvilli, an area known as the brush border. This aggregation of molecules is a colloidal system that allows for the solubility of the hydrophobic molecules by positioning the polar portions of bile salts, bile acids, and phospholipids outward. This outward polarity enables the micelle to penetrate the area surrounding the absorptive cells, called the unstirred water layer, allowing for absorption into the intestinal mucosal cells, or enterocytes. At the brush border, the micelle essentially fuses with the membrane so that the lipid contents can enter the enterocytes by several mechanisms, i.e., simple diffusion and facilitated diffusion and active transport involving membrane transporters. Once micelles deliver their lipid contents to the enterocytes, the bile acids can be reabsorbed in the ileum. Through a pathway known as entero-hepatic circulation, bile salts can travel from the intestine to the liver via portal blood to be used again in micelle formation. Roughly 94% of bile salts are recycled in this manner.[1] Bile salts are crucial to lipid absorption as described. In the presence of bile salts, absorption of fatty acids is 97%, whereas in their absence absorption is only 50%.[1]

Once in the enterocytes, long chain fatty acids are re-esterified into triglycerides in the endoplasmic reticulum. Medium chain and short chain fatty acids, as well as remaining glycerol molecules, can be directly shuttled into the portal blood and transported to the liver. As mentioned previously, very few fatty acids are truly "free" in plasma. Short chain fatty acids typically bind to albumin proteins for transport.

C. Transport

After absorption and reassembly of the long chain fatty acids, the resulting triglycerides are packaged into chylomicrons. The chylomicron, containing approximately 90% triglyceride, and 10% cholesterol, phospholipids and protein, is secreted into the lymphatic system by exocytosis.[6,17] After triglycerides in chylomicron are hydrolyzed by lipoprotein lipase (LPL), an extracellular enzyme that resides on the capillary walls, for energy use in tissues such as adipose tissue, and cardiac and skeletal muscle, the remaining lipoprotein particle, termed a chylomicron remnant, travels through the bloodstream to be taken into the liver by apolipoprotein E receptor-mediated endocytosis.[17]

D. Storage

1. Adipose Tissue

Fatty acids introduced to the tissues are either utilized for energy or stored for later use, depending on the energy state of the body. Adipose tissue is the main site of energy in the body, with roughly 95% of total body lipid's being stored as triglycerides in adipose tissue.[16] While only approximately 450 g of glycogen can be stored in the body at one time, a nearly unlimited capacity for fat storage exists. Adipose growth can occur in two ways: by increasing the number of adipocytes, called hyperplasia, or by increasing the size of adipocytes, called hypertrophy. A single adipocyte may contain more than 85% lipid by volume.[6] The total amount of fat stored depends on the individual and varies with body size and body composition. For non-obese males, average triglyceride storage ranges between 9 and 15 kg, translating into total energy storage of 80,000 to 140,000 kcal, which is equivalent to ~200 meals.[16] Females typically have a higher percentage of body fat than males. While trained athletes have less fat reserves than the average individual, ample amounts remain to provide energy in times of prolonged periods of insufficient energy intake. Not only in caloric deprivation, but in states of high energy expenditure, carbohydrate availability may be limited and utilization of fat stores may be warranted.

Several depots of adipose tissue exist in the body. Some are considered structural, such as fat pads of the hands, feet, and around the eyes, or as part of body cavities, such as visceral fat protecting vital organs. A major remaining depot is subcutaneous fat, the most visible depot of adipose.[18] In addition to total adiposity, it is also important how lipid is partitioned within the body. Increased adiposity may occur by lipid deposition in the subcutaneous abdominal region, in the liver, or intracellular accumulation, all of which have different health implications.

Triglycerides in the adipocytes are in continuous flux through the pathways of lipolysis and reesterification. When the body is in a fed energy state, the deposition of triglyceride is favored. In a fasting or post-absorptive energy state, lipolysis of fat is favored for free fatty acid oxidation to fuel the liver and kidney, as well as the heart and muscles at rest.[16] The lipolysis of fat tissue is regulated by the enzyme hormone-sensitive lipase (HSL). HSL is subject to control by insulin and catecholamines. Insulin regulates the uptake of glucose and free fatty acids or triglycerides from plasma and is a powerful inhibitor of lipolysis. Catecholamines function in response to the sympathetic nervous system, and different subtypes of these compounds can either stimulate or inhibit lipolysis.

In addition to being an energy store, adipose tissue is a biologically active tissue. It secretes a number of endocrine molecules, including leptin, adiponectin, visfatin, omentin, tumor necrosis factor-α, and resistin. These molecules collectively influence hunger physiology, energy balance, inflammation, fatty acid oxidation, and glucose and insulin sensitivity.[18]

2. Intramuscular Lipid

In addition to the fat storage in adipose tissue, a small amount of fat is present as lipid droplets within muscle tissues, known as intramyocellular triglyceride (IMCL) or intramuscular triglyceride (IMTG). The amount of energy stored in this capacity is difficult to quantify, as it is variable, transient, and not necessarily found in consistent concentrations within a single tissue or throughout the body. The amount of fat stored in muscle varies according to several factors, including energy state, fitness level, age, gender, and dietary fat intake. For example, IMTG levels can increase 50–100% after consumption of a high-fat meal, whereas consuming a high-carbohydrate meal can decrease IMTG stores by 10–30%.[3,16,18] This higher incorporation of IMTG with high-fat meals is partially explained by the inverse relationship between plasma insulin levels and the activity of LPL.[3] There are also several different methods for measuring IMTG, and analysis of a single tissue may get varied estimates depending on the method used. A very rough estimate of IMTG in an average human at rest is around 0.2 kg, or roughly 1850 kcal of stored energy.[16]

Cell staining experiments have shown IMTG to be present in droplets near the mitochondria of the muscle cells. This location supports the theory that IMTG is a buffer pool of energy utilized for oxidation, as the free fatty acids in plasma are unable to account for all energy expenditure during exercise. Studies have shown that muscles at rest will re-esterify plasma free fatty acids into IMTGs, but that during muscle contraction the free fatty acids are oxidized rather than being stored as IMTG.[19] In trained subjects, the IMTG droplets appear to be located close to the mitochondria, while in untrained subjects there does not seem to exist a similar pattern.[1] It has also been observed that the content of IMTG varies with fiber type of the muscle. Type I fibers, or the slow-oxidative endurance fibers, have been shown to contain three times as much IMTG than the Type II, or fast-oxidative fibers used for short and quick bursts of energy.[16] While it is generally accepted that IMTG is a useful source of energy in muscles at rest and during exercise, their relative contribution and mechanisms controlling their storage versus oxidation are not well understood. More about IMTG use as a fuel source for exercise will be discussed in the next section.

Interesting differences in the levels and implications of IMTG exist between trained athletes and untrained individuals. In endurance athletes, increased levels of IMTG correlate with increased insulin sensitivity. Conversely, in untrained individuals, increased IMTG correlate with decreased insulin sensitivity.[20] In untrained individuals, many studies have shown a relationship between high plasma free fatty acid levels and IMTG accretion with insulin resistance and type 2 diabetes. Increased plasma free fatty acid concentrations is characteristic of the obese and diabetic population, which in combination with a lower ability to oxidize plasma free fatty acids, may cause high IMTG accretion. However, this relationship is paradoxical with trained athletes. In this population, the increased IMTG accretion is more likely associated with their increased oxidative ability as well as a result of regular intense training causing cycles of high turnover in IMTG stores. Physical activity level is a major determinant of the rate of turnover in both muscle protein and IMTG.[16]

IV. LIPID METABOLISM IN PHYSICAL ACTIVITY

At times of adequate energy supply, lipogenesis, or the synthesis of lipids, is prevalent. In an energy deficient state, such as during exercise, there is an increase in lipolysis, or the hydrolysis of triglyceride stores, resulting in liberation of fatty acids to provide energy through β-oxidation. Fatty acids are released from adipocytes and are obtained from the plasma as albumin-bound long chain fatty acids or liberated from VLDL by LPL. The IMTG pool can also serve as a dynamic fuel source during physical activity. Because no blood transport is required, intramuscular fatty acids can be readily used for energy in exercising muscle.

During exercise, fat and carbohydrate metabolism are tightly coupled, both being controlled by nervous and hormonal mechanisms. Specific hormones increase during exercise, stimulating fat mobilization, transport, and oxidation.

At rest and during low-intensity exercise, total energy provision is primarily from fatty acids, whereas a majority of the energy is obtained from glycogen stores during intense short-term exercise. The proportion of each substrate utilized depends on factors such as the duration and intensity of exercise, the fitness level of the individual, gender, and age, as well as the composition of the meal prior to exercise.

A. Lipolysis and β-Oxidation

Triglycerides utilized for energy in muscle cells mainly come from adipose tissue of IMTG, but plasma triglycerides in VLDL may also be used. Triglycerides in adipose tissues are hydrolyzed to glycerol and three fatty acids, after which free fatty acids are released to circulation through fatty acid binding proteins and usually bound to albumin. Lipolysis of triglyceride in adipose and IMTG and is mediated by HSL, which is regulated by several different hormones and the sympathetic nervous system. HSL can be activated by epinephrine and norepinephrine, and inhibited by insulin. In addition to direct control of HSL, epinephrine and norepinephrine inhibit the release of insulin from the pancreas, resulting in an indirect decrease of insulin inhibition of HSL. Both epinephrine and insulin are controlled by blood glucose concentrations, as opposed to demand or availability of fatty acids.[16,21] Lipolysis can also be stimulated by exercise-induced catecholamine and its effect on β-adrenergic receptors.[16] Plasma triglyceride lipolysis is mediated by LPL on the endothelial lining of blood vessels and the fatty acids are free to be taken up first by the endothelial and then muscle cells. It is generally accepted that plasma triglycerides contribute as little as 3% of energy expended during exercise. However, LPL activity can be increased in response to high dietary fat intake and with higher levels of training, resulting in increased rates of fat oxidation.[1] While the fatty acids can be utilized in muscle tissue, the glycerol molecule is transported to the liver. The glycerol molecule is essentially useless to adipose and muscle tissues because they do not contain high enough concentrations of glycerokinase. Because glycerol diffuses from the cells back into plasma for transport to the liver, plasma glycerol concentrations can be used as an indicator of the rate of lipolysis.[1,6]

Once the fatty acids are hydrolyzed and released into the circulation, uptake into muscle cells are mediated by two transporters within the sarcolemma; plasma membrane fatty acid binding protein (FABPpm) and fatty acid transporter protein (FAT/CD36). The presence of these transporters is the limiting factor in fatty acid uptake into muscle cells. Fatty acid uptake can be increased during muscle contraction, a time of energy need, through increased FAT/CD36 in the sarcolemma. Once they have passed through the sarcolemma, fatty acids can be transported through the sarcoplasm to the mitochondria attached to a cytolasmic fatty acid binding protein. During this transport, the fatty acid may become activated before entering the mitochondria for β-oxidation. Activation is mediated by acyl-CoA synthetase and yields a fatty acyl-CoA complex, or activated fatty acid. Because this process involves hydrolysis of a pyrophosphate to prevent a reversal of the activation, the reaction uses two ATP molecules.[6,16]

The activated fatty acid is then ready to be transported into the mitochondria, and is mediated by two transporters: carnitine palmitoyl transferase I (CPT I) and carnitine palmitoyl transferase II (CPT II), which are located on the outer mitochondrial membrane and on the inner mitochondrial membrane, respectively. The carrier protein in this complex is carnitine, which is synthesized from lysine and methionine while also requiring vitamin C, vitamin B_6, niacin, and iron for synthesis.[5] At the outer mitochondrial membrane, the fatty acyl-CoA binds to CPT I and CoA is released, leaving a fatty acyl-carnitine complex that is then translocated across the outer membrane. Then CPT II transfers the molecule across the inner mitochondrial membrane and converts the molecule back to fatty acyl-CoA, where it is now in the matrix and available for β-oxidation. The carnitine molecules used for transport are able to diffuse back across the membrane, available again to shuttle across more activated fatty acids. CPT I is the rate-limiting factor in fatty acid uptake into the mitochondria for oxidation, and is inhibited by high glucose availability and malonyl-CoA.[21]

The process of β-oxidation is termed a cyclic degradative pathway. Regardless of the hydrocarbon chain length, each fatty acid cleavage results in one two-carbon unit of acetyl CoA. The degradation begins at the carboxyl end of the fatty acid, and the cycles continue until there are four carbon units left, which are then cleaved into two final acetyl CoA molecules. Acetyl CoA is sent to the Krebs cycle and $FADH_2$ and NADH, by-products of this cycle, shuttle through the electron transport chain to generate ATP. One cycle of β-oxidation produces 2 ATP by oxidative phosphorylation of $FADH_2$, 3 ATP by NADH, and each oxidized acetyl CoA molecule results in 12 ATP. Therefore, the energy produced from a fatty acid is dependent upon hydrocarbon chain length.

Fat oxidation is limited in many individuals, proving discouraging for those looking to lose weight or fat mass. Steps in the process that are likely to limit the ability of the body to burn fat are the ability to mobilize fatty acids from adipose or IMTG by LPL or HSL, transport by albumin to tissue, the transfer of fatty acids into muscle cells via FABPpm and FAT/CD36, and transport across the mitochondrial membrane by CPT 1 and II.[21] With so many potential limitations to utilizing fat, many products on the market claim to enhance fat as a preferred substrate for energy to aid in weight loss. Most of these claims are unjustified, but fat oxidation can be improved with exercise. Physical activity increases oxygen intake, number of mitochondria, the electron transport system, Kreb's cycle, LPL and carnitine for CPT I and II. Exercise also increases the ability of tissues to take up fatty acids and increases levels of IMTG.[21–23]

B. Energy Substrate Utilization During Exercise

The two primary sources of energy are fat and carbohydrate, whether that be as plasma fatty acids, IMTG, muscle glycogen, etc., whereas protein is a minor contributor. The primary substrate for oxidation during exercise depends on a variety of factors.[16] Fat is the primary fuel substrate during mild-intensity exercise, while carbohydrate is the primary energy source during high-intensity exercise. Absolute levels of fat oxidation will increase with duration and increased intensity; however, its relative contribution to total energy may be decreased.

The standard measure of intensity and fitness is the maximal oxygen uptake, or VO_{2max}, which measures the maximal amount of oxygen transported and utilized during a period of exercise. Intensities of exercise can be categorized as mild (25% VO_{2max}), moderate (65% VO_{2max}), or high (85% VO_{2max}).[5] At rest or during regular activities of daily living when VO_{2max} is low, fats provide 80–90% of energy while carbohydrates provide 5–18% and protein supplies around 2–5%.[6] Exercise for up to 2 hours at mild intensity will continue to utilize plasma free fatty acids and IMTG as the major fuel sources.[21]

At 25% VO_{2max}, the primary fuel source is plasma free fatty acids, but as intensity increases to 65% VO_{2max}, the primary fuel source is IMTG.[22] During moderate-intensity exercise, fat oxidation from both plasma free fatty acids and IMTG contributes 40–60% of energy expenditure.[16] If exercise occurs at a high enough intensity, there is a "crossover point" in substrate utilization when carbohydrate sources overtake fat sources as primary substrates. This crossover point between fat and carbohydrate utilization is a function of VO_{2max}, and optimal fat oxidation occurs around 62–63% VO_{2max}. A threshold of fat oxidation exists at high-intensity exercise levels over 75% VO_{2max}, where fat utilization, both relative and absolute, decreases to negligible amounts.[24,25] The cause of this effect is still debated; however, it is suggested that the limiting factors in fat utilization at high-intensity exercise are blood circulation to tissue, transport of fatty acids via albumin, and transport of fatty acids into the mitochondria.[21,23,25]

A greater proportion of fat is oxidized during mild-intensity activities carried out for extended periods of time, such as walking and swimming; however, a greater amount of total energy will be spent during higher-intensity exercises such as running.[5] Therefore, individuals should determine appropriate exercise activities based on their fitness level, physical capabilities, and overall goals of exercise. Individuals whose goal is to burn fat should maintain exercise around the 62–63% VO_{2max} if able.

V. IMPLICATIONS OF LIPIDS ON HEALTH

Despite being a necessary component of many foods and providing integral biochemical components within the body, lipids are often negatively implicated in a number of health conditions. Generally, these negative health effects can be linked to the overconsumption of all fats or specific fats such as saturated and *trans* fats.

A. *TRANS* FATS

The study of *trans* fatty acids and their health implications has been around for decades. However, in recent years, the issue of *trans* fats has become a highly political topic, and one that is frequently debated due to recent government intervention. Research has shown that *trans* fat intake is associated with increased plasma LDL cholesterol and decreased plasma HDL cholesterol,[19,23] and thus an increased risk of CHD complications such as myocardial infarction may exist.[26] Data from the Cardiovascular Health Study showed that high levels of plasma *trans* fatty acids were associated with an increased risk of cardiovascular heart disease (CHD) in both older men and women, with subjects in the upper quintile having a fourfold higher risk.[27] In addition, dietary *trans* fats and saturated fats increase CHD risk by increasing proinflammatory cytokines (interleukin 6), acute phase proteins (C-reactive protein), and adhesion molecules (E-selectin).[23] Negative health effects have been shown in subjects with dietary intakes of as little as 2–7 grams per day of *trans* fatty acids, equivalent to 1–3% total kcal in a 2000 kcal/day diet.[16] A meta-analysis of recent prospective studies on *trans* fats concluded that a near elimination of *trans* fats to levels below 0.5% total kcal/day could potentially result in a reduction of CHD events by 6–19%.[16] With an estimated 1.2 million deaths from CHD and myocardial infarction in the United States per year, that calculates to the possible prevention of 72,000–228,000 deaths from CHD.[16]

Because of recent research showing a relationship between dietary *trans* fatty acids and CHD and lack of evidence showing any beneficial effects of *trans* fats, governments are taking action. In March of 2003, Denmark began regulating the sale of *trans* fat-containing foods, thus limiting the supply and consumption of *trans* fats in the Danish people. In 2004, Denmark passed legislation to limit food content of *trans* fats to less than 2% of total fat content.[28] The Danish Nutrition Council determined that the near elimination of *trans* fats could be accomplished without detriment to taste, quality, price, or availability of food products.[21] In Canada, legislation was introduced in 2004 to limit *trans* fats. The bill called for all vegetable products and soft margarines to contain less than 2% *trans* fats, and all food products to contain less than 5% of total fat content from *trans* fats. However, any food containing less than 0.2 grams per serving may be labeled as zero *trans* fat. The Canadian Health Minister announced in 2007 that the industry would be allowed 2 years to comply with the recommendations of the Canadian Trans Fat Task Force.[21]

The United States Food and Drug Administration (FDA) mandated that all conventional foods and supplements must declare the *trans* fat content on their nutrition label, effective January 1, 2006.[21] By U.S. law, any product containing less than 0.5 grams of *trans* fat is allowed to declare zero grams of *trans* fat per serving.[16] A landmark, yet controversial, case against *trans* fats gained widespread media attention in New York in 2006. On December 5, 2006, the New York City Board of Health approved an amendment to the city's health code that would phase out the use of *trans* fats in restaurants and food service establishments in two stages. The first stage, completed on July 1, 2007, mandates limitation of *trans* fats to less than 0.5 grams per serving in all cooking oils, margarines, and shortenings. The second stage, completed on July 1, 2008, requires that all foods contain less than 0.5 grams per serving of *trans* fat.[28–30] The ban still faces opposition by the industries subject to the changes, critics opposing the emotionally charged wording of many of the publications regarding *trans* fats, as well as politicians and citizens opposing the level of government involvement. Despite the strong opposition, a trickle-down effect is already being seen in the United States and beyond. An ordinance similar to the legislation in New York City was submitted in 2006 to the Chicago city government.[29,30] To date, the initiative is still being debated. Another local ban on *trans* fats was approved in Philadelphia on February 8, 2007. Other areas successfully passing local bans to date are Albany County, New York; Brookline, Massachusetts; Montgomery County, Maryland; and King County, Washington. Some areas, however, are making the transition willingly. Restaurants in Tiburon, California; Westchester County, New York; and Boston, Massachusetts; have formed voluntary "trans fat-free zones" by meeting a mutual set of nutritional criteria. Even state legislatures are jumping on the bandwagon, as statewide bans are currently being considered in California, Connecticut, Georgia, Illinois, Michigan, Mississippi, New Jersey, Pennsylvania, Rhode Island, Tennessee, and Vermont. These statewide bans are also highly controversial, as demonstrated by initial rejection of such legislation in the Maryland State Senate and New Hampshire House of Representatives. The effects are even broadening outside of the United States, as Puerto Rico and parts of Australia are now also considering legislation against *trans* fats.[31]

There is no current guideline or official dietary recommendation for intake of *trans* fats. A general recommendation is to limit *trans* fat intake to as low as possible, however eliminating it completely from the diet is impossible, because the isomer exists naturally in several food products such as trace amounts in meat and dairy products.[6]

B. Obesity and Diabetes

Obesity, often resulting from chronic excess of dietary energy, is strongly linked to both increased inflammatory status and type 2 diabetes.[31] Visceral obesity, dyslipidemia, and insulin resistance are all conditions that, when occurring simultaneously, compose metabolic syndrome, increasing the risk for both diabetes and cardiovascular disease. Weight loss has been shown to increase insulin sensitivity.[23]

Obesity can be influenced by a variety of factors, including genetics, metabolism, environment, and socioeconomic status. Obesity is positively correlated to excess energy intake and low levels of physical activity. In addition, both the degree of total fat consumption and the type of fat consumed play a role in obesity. Dietary fat intake is a significant predictor of sustained weight gain and progression of type 2 diabetes in high-risk subjects.[32] Short-term studies suggest that very high intakes of fat (>35% of calories) may modify metabolism and potentially promote obesity.[33] Cross-cultural studies have also shown an increase in body mass index (BMI) in countries with higher intakes of fat.[23] In part, the dietary intake of both saturated and total fat is related to the risk of developing diabetes, primarily through its association with a higher BMI.[34] According to the National Institute of Health, obesity is defined as a BMI of 30.0 or greater.[35] An upward trend in overweight has occurred since 1980 and obesity prevalence doubled between 1980 and 2004 in adults as well as children.[36,37] Rates of obesity have increased every year since the 1976–1980 National Health and Nutrition Examination Survey (NHANES), except for the 2003–2004 vs. 2005–2006 NHANES data.[36] Although there was no statistically significant increase between these periods, obesity was still prevalent in more than one third of all adults—33.3% in men and 35.5% in women.[36] The age group of 40–59 years of age has the highest prevalence of obesity compared with younger (20–39 years old) or older age groups (60 years and older), with 40% and 41.1% obesity prevalence in men and women, respectively.[36] While no racial or ethnic disparities have been identified in men, non-Hispanic black and Mexican-American women have a higher prevalence of obesity than non-Hispanic white women.[36] Modest reductions in total fat intake are suggested to facilitate a decrease in caloric intake, leading to better weight control and potential improvement in metabolic syndrome.[38]

C. Coronary Heart Disease

Atherosclerosis, the underlying pathological process of CHD, is characterized by an accumulation of plaque and fatty material within the intima of the coronary arteries, cerebral arteries, iliac and femoral arteries, and the aorta. The atherosclerotic development in the coronary arteries leads to CHD and its manifestations. The deposition and buildup of cholesterol in the arteries, along with inflammation, create reduced blood flow to the heart and possible thrombosis, and is the principle cause of myocardial and cerebral infarction.

Of all cardiovascular diseases, CHD is the leading cause of death for both men and women in the United States, causing one in five deaths in the United States in 2004. It is predicted that 1.2 million Americans will have a new or recurrent coronary attack in 2008 and the estimated direct and indirect cost of CHD for 2008 is $156.4 billion.[32] After the age of 40, the lifetime risk of having CHD is 49% for men and 32% for women.[39] Risks for CHD include both modifiable and non-modifiable factors, including male gender, age, overweight or obesity, saturated-fat intake, and elevated plasma total and LDL cholesterol levels.

One of the major risk factors for CHD is dyslipidemia, including increases in plasma concentrations of total and LDL cholesterol, along with a decrease in HDL cholesterol concentration. A direct correlation exists between human deaths caused by CHD and plasma cholesterol concentrations.[26,40] In particular, a positive correlation between death from CHD and total cholesterol levels exceeding 200 mg/dl prompted the National Cholesterol Education Program (NCEP) to recommend serum cholesterol levels to remain at 200 mg/dL or lower for the general population.[41] Two thirds of CHD-related mortality occurs in individuals who had plasma total cholesterol concentrations higher than 200 mg/dl when they were young adults.[18] Between the years of 1999–2002, 17% of adults age 20 and over possessed high serum cholesterol levels of 240 mg/dl or higher in the Unites States.[37] Elevated plasma LDL cholesterol has been shown to play a major role in the formation of atherosclerotic plaque, making it a common target for prevention strategies.[18] According to the 2006 American Heart Association Statistical Update, approximately 40% of individuals in the United States have plasma LDL cholesterol concentrations greater than 130 mg/dl, above the recommendation for individuals with a moderate (2+ risk factors and 10–year risk of developing CHD of < 10%) or moderately high risk (2+ risk factors and 10-year risk of developing CHD of 10% to 20%).[18] The risk of CHD falls as concentrations of plasma HDL cholesterol increase, especially to levels >40 mg/dl.

Contrary to previous beliefs, altering the amount of cholesterol ingested has only a minor effect on total plasma cholesterol concentration in most people. A study performed on more than 80,000 female nurses found that increasing cholesterol intake by 200 mg for every 1000 calories in the diet did not appreciably increase the risk for heart disease.[18] Because the body is well equipped with compensatory mechanisms to maintain cholesterol homeostasis, if a decrease in dietary cholesterol intake occurs, cholesterol biosynthesis increases, almost fully compensating for the decrease in cholesterol intake; in contrast, when the body has excess cholesterol, cholesterol biosynthesis decreases with a concomitant increase in cholesterol excretion pathways through biliary cholesterol and bile acids.

Plasma cholesterol concentrations are more subject to regulation by dietary fat than dietary cholesterol is. Contradicting evidence exists regarding the relationship between the quantity of fat intake and CHD. As previously noted, short-term studies indicate that very high intakes of fat (>35% of calories) may have the ability to modify metabolism and potentially promote obesity.[42] The Women's Health Initiative Dietary Modification Trial, a long term dietary intervention study on approximately 49,000 women, was designed to investigate the effect of dietary intervention on the risk of cancer and CHD. The 8.1 year follow-up showed trends toward greater reductions in CHD risk; i.e., reduction in LDL cholesterol levels in individuals consuming lower intakes of saturated fat (2.9% decrease by year 6), but found nearly identical rates of heart attacks, strokes, and other forms of cardiovascular disease.[43] Findings from the study are similar to both the Nurses' Health Study and the Health Professionals Follow-up Study, indicating no link between the overall percentage of calories from fat and several health outcomes including cancer, heart disease, and weight gain.

A majority of saturated fatty acids appear to have a negative effect on plasma cholesterol profiles, i.e., increases in LDL cholesterol levels and LDL:HDL ratio and a decrease in HDL cholesterol levels, which can enhance the risk of CHD. Hypercholesterolemic effects of saturated fatty acids are attributed, in part, to their abilities to alter the secretion of bile acids, to decrease the removal of LDL from circulation, and to enhance LDL formation. Therefore, recent clinical trials replacing saturated fatty acids with monounsaturated fatty acids showed an improvement in plasma lipid profiles, as well as beneficial effects on insulin sensitivity.[18,44,45] Decreasing saturated fat intake from 12% to 8% has shown to decrease plasma LDL cholesterol by 5–7 mg/dl, based upon equations from Hegsted et al.[46] and Mensink and Katan.[39] While most saturated fatty acids such as lauric (12:0), myristic (14:0), and palmitic (16:0) acids are all considered hypercholesterolemic, researchers have shown that stearic acid (18:0) actually has a neutral or mild hypocholesterolemic effect on plasma total and LDL cholesterol concentrations.[44,47–50] In addition, 18:0 was as effective as 18:1 in lowering plasma cholesterol levels when it replaced 16:0 in the diet.[51]

The intake of other fatty acids has been linked to cardiovascular health. Omega-3 fatty acid intake has been linked to a decrease in plasma triglycerides and has been recommended for consumption in the National Cholesterol Education Program (NCEP) adult treatment panel III guidelines.[41] Increasing fish consumption has been shown to have a direct, dose-dependent relationship to reduced CHD-related mortality.[52] Consumption of long-chain ω-3 fatty acids such as EPA and DHA, were found to be significantly reduced in patients experiencing CHD events.[53]

D. Cancer

Varying evidence exists in regard to the effect of total fat consumption on the risk of various cancers. A report of the NCEP indicates that the percentage of total fat in the diet, independent of caloric intake, has not been documented to be related to cancer risk in the general population.[35] However, diets high in fat are often correlated with those high in calories, potentially contributing to obesity and overweight, a risk factor linked to the incidence of multiple cancers such as cancer of the pancreas, kidney, colon and esophagus.[54]

The Women's Health Initiative Dietary Modification Trial involving approximately 49,000 subjects showed that those exposed to dietary intervention that included a 8.1% lower fat intake than the control group developed colon cancer at the same rate as the control.[55] As with colon cancer, the study showed similar rates of breast cancer risk in women eating a low-fat diet (8.1% decrease from control) and in the control group without diet modification. The Nurses' Health Study also reported no association between total fat intake or specific types of fat and breast cancer risk.[56] In contrast, a higher risk of prostate cancer progression has been seen in men with a high fat intake, with fat of animal origin correlating to the highest risk of prostate cancer.[57,58] A literature search on dietary fat and breast cancer risk involving published articles from January 1990 through December 2003 found a positive association between increased total and saturated fat intake and the development of breast cancer.[51] The review acknowledges that not all epidemiological studies provided a strong positive association between dietary fat and breast cancer risk, but a moderate association does exist.[51,58,59]

Additional research has shown a correlation between saturated fat intake and cancer risk. A recent prospective cohort study performed by the European Prospective Investigation into Cancer project found no association between breast cancer and saturated fat intake measured by food-frequency questionnaire, but when using a food diary, a daily intake of 35 g of saturated fat doubles the risk of breast cancer in comparison with women who had a daily intake of 10 g or less.[60] A greater intake of saturated fat intake may increase the risk of esophageal adenocarcinoma and distal stomach cancer.[61] In addition, a meta-analysis of the association between dietary fat intake and breast cancer found significant summary relative risks for saturated fat.[51] In contrast, a recent review of prospective epidemiologic studies have found no consistent, statistically significant association between diet and breast cancer except for alcohol consumption, overweight, and weight gain.[62]

While both fat and saturated fat have been implicated in the risk of various cancers, both have not conclusively been positively correlated with cancer risk amongst all cancers. However, some evidence reveals a positive association between fat intake and certain cancers, and it is recommended to reduce total and saturated fat intake to decrease cancer risk.

VI. LIPID SUPPLEMENTS

A. Omega-3 Fatty Acids

As mentioned, ω-3 fatty acids are polyunsaturated fatty acids that are considered an essential nutrient. The intake of ω-3 fatty acids has been shown to have beneficial effects in inflammatory diseases including CHD and certain cancers. While the intake of seed oils has been investigated for its health benefits, much of the focus has been on the intake of ω-3 fatty acid found in fish oils. In 2002, the Institute of Medicine of the National Academies set an Adequate Intake (AI) for α-linolenic acid as 1.6 g/d for men and 1.1 g/day for women aged 19–50 years, and up to 10% of the AI for α-linolenic acid may be provided by EPA and DHA. At the same time, an accepted macronutrient distribution range was set for ω-3 fatty acids at 0.6–1.2% of energy.[63] For the general population, the American Heart Association recommends consuming two servings of oily fish per week, while also including dietary oils and foods rich in α-linolenic acid to obtain appropriate amounts of ω-3 fatty acids. To obtain these recommendations and increase ω-3 intake, fish oil supplements have been marketed. The soft-gel fish oil supplements are rich in the ω-3 DHA and EPA. The ω-3 fatty acids have been shown to be anti-inflammatory, anti-thrombotic, anti-arrhythmic, hypolipidemic, and anti-vasodilatry.[64] ω-6 fatty acids, however, are shown to be prothrombotic and proaggretory.[64] Because of the high ratio of ω-6 to ω-3 fatty acids typically seen in the Western diet, fish oil supplements are used to counteract the ω-6 intake and lower the ratio to levels closer to 4:1.[14]

Athero-protective effects of ω-3 fatty acid intake have been extensively investigated. Results of clinical trials have revealed that daily administration of low doses of ω-3 fatty acids reduces the risk of CHD outcomes, including heart attack.[46,65] Another study found that increasing intake of ω-3 and ω-9 fatty acids while decreasing intake of ω-6 fatty acids reduced the occurrence of fatal and nonfatal CHD complications.[39,66] Several studies have also been performed using fish oil supplements specifically, resulting in a reduction in plasma inflammatory markers and CHD risk factors.[15,67,68] It is thought that ω-3 fatty acids alter the inflammation response stimulated in atherosclerosis by inhibiting the signal transduction of nuclear factor κB (NF-κB), which is a transcription factor to increase the expression of pro-inflammatory molecules such as tumor necrosis factor-α (TNF-α) and interleukin-1β (IL-1β).[15] Another mechanism by which ω-3 fatty acids affect inflammation is the inhibition of eicosanoid production. As mentioned, arachidonic acid (ω-6) and EPA (ω-3) can be converted to eicosanoids through the COX enzyme system upon release from a cell membrane.[14] Eicosanoids are an entire category of signaling molecules involved in inflammation including prostaglandins, prostacyclins, thromboxanes, and leukotrienes.[14] A main difference among the subseries of eicosanoids is that the ω-6 derived prostaglandins and thromboxanes are more inflammatory, vasoconstrictive, and thrombotic than the ω-3 derived eicosanoids.[15,69,70] Therefore, a higher amount of dietary ω-3 consumption will result in increased production of the lesser inflammatory eicosanoids.[69] Additionally, ω-3 fatty acids may lower blood pressure and plasma triglycerides, decrease inflammation, improve endothelial function, and increase plaque stability, all of which could reduce the risk of CHD.[51,71–73]

Much research has been conducted to find possible beneficial effects of ω-3 fatty acids on various cancers, as epidemiological studies suggest a lower incidence of certain cancers in individuals with high ω-3 consumption.[51,74–77] Relationships have been studied between ω-3 intake and incidence of cancer in the aerodigestive tract (oral cavity, pharynx, esophagus, or larynx), stomach, colorectum, bladder, pancreas, lungs, ovaries, breast, prostate, and skin.[51] However, a systematic review of cohort studies on each of the above cancers revealed no overall significant effect of ω-3 fatty acids on cancer.[51] Out of 65 individual studies evaluated, only 10 produced significant results for breast cancer (4), colorectal cancer (1), lung cancer (2), and skin cancer (1).[51]

Although there has been a vast amount of research on the benefits of ω-3 or fish oil supplementation, little has been documented on the negative effects. One major drawback of all polyunsaturated fatty acids (PUFA) is their high susceptibility to oxidation due to the presence of unsaturated carbon bonds. Lipid oxidation of PUFA may occur preconsumption while in the food system, or postconsumption within the body, both with negative effects on health.[78–80] Oily fish and their oils have been shown to contain varying levels of toxic compounds such as methylmercury, dioxins, and polychlorinated biphenyls.[81] While not generally a concern at doses of normal dietary intake, harmful levels of these toxic compounds could be reached with long-term use of supplements.[81]

B. Conjugated Linoleic Acid

As indicated by its name, conjugated linoleic acid (CLA) is a form of linoleic acid. The term conjugated describes the bond structure in which two double bonds are separated by a single carbon–carbon bond instead of a methylene group.[81,82] CLA is actually a family of positional and geometric isomers, including the major isomers *cis*-9,*trans*-11 and *trans*-10,*cis*-12.[83] CLA is formed by the fermentative bacteria *Butyrvibrio fibrisolvens* in the stomach of ruminant animals, such as cows, sheep and goats.[84] It can be found in the products of these animals (milk, cheese, meat) in quantities ranging from 3–7 mg per gram of fat.[85] Estimated intake of CLA of an average diet is around 150–200 mg/day,[86,87] and for a diet high in fat-containing animal products the estimate is upwards of 650 mg/day.[88] Few plant sources of CLA exist, and can be found in pomegranate seed oil, bitter gourd oil, tung seed oil, catalpa seed oil, pot marigold seed oil, and several seaweeds.[88–90] CLA can also be commercially prepared through alkaline isomerization of linoleic acid or through utilizing bateria.[89] Several CLA supplements are available on the market, most of which are marketed for weight loss at dosage intakes of 3-4 g/day.[81]

Interest originated in CLA because of its potential beneficial effects on cancer. It has been suggested that CLA has anti-carcinogenic activity in liver cancer[91] and in colorectal cancer,[92] but the majority of research has been performed on breast cancer. Currently, there is inconclusive evidence regarding the effect of CLA on breast cancer. A significant positive relationship was seen between low plasma concentrations of CLA and incidence of breast cancer in postmenopausal women.[93] In addition, studies have shown anti-tumor and anti-cancer effects of CLA on breast cancer cells.[94] However, this evidence has been challenged by recent studies showing that CLA treatment at 0.5% of the diet can actually stimulate or accelerate tumor development in a rat breast cancer model, and that CLA supplementation of 1–2% of the diet in mice induced inflammation and fibrosis of mammary tissue.[15] Research analyzing the CLA content of breast adipose tissue in patients with breast cancer versus patients with benign breast tumor found that there was a significantly higher content of CLA in the breast tissue of cancer patients.[14] Because of conflicting research and the suggestion of such adverse effects, it cannot be recommended at this time that CLA supplements be used for treatment or prevention of breast cancer. The mechanism of the possible anti-cancer action is not fully understood, but research points to induction of apoptosis, decreased cancer cell growth, and modulation of cytokine production.[95,96]

Perhaps the best-known benefit of CLA is weight and fat mass loss. In mice, 6 weeks of treatment with 1% CLA in a low-fat diet resulted in a 10% decrease in body weight and a 70% decrease in body fat in CLA treatment groups compared with control.[97] In an obese mouse model, it was shown that treatment with 1% CLA in the diet for 6 weeks reduced white adipose tissue of the abdomen and lowered plasma and liver triglycerides. It was speculated that these changes were mediated by increased β-oxidation along with decreased hepatic fatty acid synthesis. This theory is supported by evidence that treatment of 1% CLA for a period of 6 weeks in rats increased expression of CPT-1 in the liver and adipose tissue, discussed earlier as the limiting factor in fatty acid uptake into the mitochondria for oxidation.[98] Despite positive results in animal studies, there have been variable and inconclusive results in human studies. Supplementation of 4.2 g/day of CLA for 12 weeks in healthy adults significantly reduced body fat compared with a control without CLA supplementation.[99] Also, middle-aged men with metabolic syndrome were supplemented with 4.2 g/day of CLA for 4 weeks; a significant reduction in waist circumference was seen.[100] Research also showed a dose of 3.4 g/day for 3 months caused a significant decrease in body fat in obese or overweight subjects.[101] Contrary to these findings, several studies found no significant effect on body weight, fat mass, or free fat mass using CLA doses ranging from 1.4–6 g/day for up to 64 days.[100,102,103] A meta-analysis of human clinical trials found no significant effect of CLA supplementation on weight loss or loss of fat.[81] One potential explanation for this discrepancy between animal and human trials may lie in the dosage requirements. Per body weight, CLA doses used in rodent and other animal studies are much higher than those given in human studies. One estimate shows comparable doses of CLA given to rats would translate to a dosage of 130 g/day for a human.[81]

Supplementation with CLA has also been implicated in reducing the area of aortic fatty streaks in atherosclerosis, normalizing glucose sensitivity and tolerance in impaired models at levels similar to pharmacological agents.[100] However, some studies have reported that CLA supplementation may also cause fatty liver and spleen,[17,104] increase insulin resistance,[105] decrease endothelial function,[106] and increase lipid peroxidation.[105,106] One possibility for negative outcomes may relate to the *trans* fat content, as both natural sources and CLA supplements contain a mixture of both *cis* and *trans* isomers. Because of inconclusive evidence regarding benefits, multiple reports of adverse effects, and questionable preparation and composition of CLA supplements, their use is cautioned at this time.

D. Medium-Chain Triglycerides

As mentioned in the discussion on lipid digestion, the metabolism of fatty acids differs depending on chain length. Of specific interest in this section are the medium-chain triglycerides (MCT), with a designated fatty acid chain length of 8–10 carbons. Natural sources of these triglycerides are coconut oil and palm kernel oil, and MCT can also be commercially synthesized and purified from those two oils as starting materials.[1] Because of their smaller size and higher polarity, MCT are more water-soluble than long-chain triglycerides (LCT) and can pass more quickly through the stomach. Importantly, once MCT are absorbed and hydrolyzed in the small intestine, they go directly into the portal blood system, whereas LCT need to be transported through the lymph system.[107,108] MCT are thought to bypass re-esterification within the cell and can be quickly taken up by the mitochondria independent of carnitine transporters for oxidation, thus suggesting a role as a quick energy source.[109,110]

MCT have been studied since the 1980s as a supplement to enhance exercise performance, especially in endurance sports. Supporters of this theory claim MCT intake results in increased plasma free fatty acids, as they are transported through portal blood rather than lymph, and may be used for oxidation during exercise while sparing muscle glycogen.[109] In a study of cyclists, Lambert et al. reported that intake of MCT resulted in improved performance over the control group in a timed trial.[111] However, Misell et al. found no significant effect of MCT intake on endurance or energy metabolism in male runners.[112] Other studies have shown that MCT supplementation prior to exercise does not affect the rate of fat oxidation or muscle glycogen stores.[113–115] One study reported that in male runners, supplementation with MCT in 30-gram doses twice a day for 14 days increased plasma total cholesterol, LDL cholesterol, and triglycerides compared with a control group supplemented with an equal amount of long-chain triglycerides.[116] Therefore, any potential benefits of MCT may be outweighed by the negative impact on blood lipid profiles.

More recently, focus on MCT has shifted to the use of MCT supplements for the reduction of body fat mass. Suggested theories of action include increased fat oxidation, decreased hepatic fatty acid synthesis, and increased effect on satiety. Overweight subjects in Japan given 10 g/day of MCT for 12 weeks exhibited significant reductions in body weight, body fat, abdominal subcutaneous fat, and waist and hip circumferences compared to a group given LCT.[117] Total energy expenditure was shown to be significantly higher in both normal weight and obese subjects following a meal containing MCT compared to LCT.[107,117,118] In contrast, overweight men given mixed MCT/LCT supplement had a short term increase in fat oxidation, but there were no changes in body weight or fat mass throughout the 6 week study.[119] Therefore, more research is required to understand the effect of MCT supplementation on body fat mass.

Although MCT supplement usage is not fully supported, it is recommended that doses do not exceed 30 grams/day due to incidence of gastrointestinal discomfort and diarrhea.[120] Research on the efficacy of MCT supplementation in exercise as well as for prevention of obesity appears inconclusive at this time. Due to possible adverse effects such as a negative impact on blood lipid profile and gastrointestinal discomfort, MCT use is not supported. There is also a near absence of studies on the long-term effects of MCT supplementation. It has been suggested that consumption of a diet low in fat is a more effective weight loss plan than supplementation with MCT.[121]

D. L-Carnitine

While not a lipid itself, L-carnitine has been touted as playing an important role in fat metabolism and supplementation is utilized by athletes to enhance exercise performance. L-carnitine, the predominant stereoisomer of carnitine in nature, is an amine that can be taken through the diet or be produced endogenously in the human body. Major dietary sources of L-carnitine are meat and dairy products, yet it can be synthesized in the liver and kidney from the amino acids lysine and methionine.[122] Because of dietary and endogenous sources, deficiencies in L-carnitine are rarely seen in humans, with the exception of strict vegetarians.[123] Most L-carnitine in the body, around 98%, is found in skeletal muscle and heart tissue.[1] It can be found in other tissues in varying quantities, but estimates of skeletal muscle content are 4000 μmol/kg, while concentrations in the plasma are as low as 60 μmol/L.[124] If plasma concentrations surpass the estimated range of 60–100 μmol/L, excess is eliminated through urine.[125,126] Proposed benefits of L-carnitine are increased fat oxidation, increased VO_{2max}, modulation of utilization of fuel substrates, and increased skeletal muscle carnitine pools.[124,127,128]

Because L-carnitine is required for long chain fatty acid oxidation, functioning as the precursor molecule to carnitine palmitoyl transferase I and II, some believe that L-carnitine supplementation will lead to increased fat oxidation. Karlic et al. reported that rats supplemented with L-carnitine increased the expression and activity of hepatic CPT I and CPT II.[129] In addition, it is thought that if fat oxidation is increased, glucose oxidation is theoretically decreased and therefore muscle glycogen stores are spared and the onset of exercise-induced fatigue can be delayed.[130] L-carnitine supplementation caused an increased rate of fat oxidation with a subsequent decrease rate of glucose oxidation in rats, but further evidence is lacking.[131] In addition, while studies have shown that carnitine content of skeletal muscle tissue may be increased with supplementation in animal models such as rats[132,133] and horses[134], the level of supplementation used in these studies are not likely to be obtained in humans, and therefore, changes in metabolism may not be seen.[135] In support of this, two studies administering L-carnitine at lower levels have reported that L-carnitine supplementation does not alter carnitine content of skeletal muscle tissue in humans.[136,137] In addition, analyses of various human studies looking at the relationship between L-carnitine and exercise have reported no effect of L-carnitine on fat oxidation, VO_{2max}, or overall exercise performance.[127,128]

Most studies that did find positive effects of L-carnitine supplementation have been performed in animals or trained athletes during exercise, but there are no apparent benefits for untrained individuals.[107,138] At this point, current research does not support substantial enough benefit in L-carnitine intake to warrant supplementation, as most claims tend to be based on theory rather than data.[127] Bioavailability of L-carnitine supplements given orally are only around 5–15% of the ingested amount, and large supplement doses have resulted in large L-carnitine recoveries in the urine.[107,126] In addition, inaccurate labeling of L-carnitine supplements' content may contribute to its nonsignificant effects. Chosing a random sample from a variety of marketed L-carnitine supplements found that the actual content of L-carnitine was merely half of what was declared on the label.[139] Although L-carnitine supplementation has inconclusive effects, it has been deemed a safe supplement up to 2000 mg/day on a short-term basis; however, long-term safety or efficacy have not been established.[140]

VII. DIETARY RECOMMENDATIONS

In 2005, the U.S. Department of Heath and Human Services (HSS) and the Department of Agriculture (USDA) released new dietary guidelines for Americans. The new guidelines recommend total fat intake to remain between 20–35% of total calories with less than 10% calories from saturated fat, to limit intake of *trans* fat to as low as possible, and to consume most fats from sources of polyunsaturated and monounsaturated fatty acids. In addition, consumption of less than 300 mg/day of cholesterol is recommended.

The range of 20–35% calories from fat was selected because consumption over 35% is associated with increased saturated fat intake and excessive caloric intake, while less than 20% is associated with a risk of inadequate intake of fat-soluble vitamins and essential fatty acids as well as unfavorable effects on plasma HDL cholesterol concentration. Very few Americans consume less than 20% calories from fat, so it is of greater concern to keep consumption under the recommended 35%. *Trans* fats tend to increase plasma LDL cholesterol level to nearly the same extent as saturated fat but saturated fats increase plasma HDL cholesterol while *trans* fats do not.[141] The American Heart Association diet and lifestyle recommendations, revised in 2006, include restricting saturated fat to less than 7% of total calories, and *trans* fat to less than 1%.[142] In 1999–2000, Americans in all age groups consumed a daily mean percentage of calories from saturated fat of 11.2%, while men and women ages 20–74 consumed average cholesterol intakes of 341mg and 242mg, respectively.[143] Although variable, *trans* fat intake was estimated to be approximately 2.7% of total calories.[142] Recommendations for saturated fat, *trans* fat, and cholesterol are related to decreasing the risk of elevated levels of plasma LDL cholesterol associated with CHD.[144] Goal plasma LDL cholesterol level for an individual with zero or one risk factor are less than 160 mg/dL and for those with two or more risk factors are less than 130 mg/dL. Individuals with CHD, LDL goal levels are less than 100 mg/dL.[144]

The additional recommendation of consuming most fats from sources containing polyunsaturated and monounsaturated fatty acids is twofold. First, consumption of two servings of fish per week high in EPA and DHA is associated with a reduced risk of CHD.[145,146] Second, consumption of these products often means replacement of sources of saturated and *trans* fats.[142] The three most common sources of saturated fat to the American diet are cheese, beef, and milk.[144] However, choices at the grocery store can help to greatly reduce the consumption of saturated fat from these sources by selecting lean, low-fat, or fat-free products. Other ways to replace saturated fats while also reducing cholesterol is to use vegetable-based meat alternatives, and[142] with meats, remember that choice of cooking method also has a large impact on fat content. Roasting, baking, or broiling meat will keep fat content lower than frying, as will removal of the skin from poultry before cooking.[144] It becomes increasingly important to make wise decisions regarding diet and exercise in the older adult population, especially because of the prevalence of CHD, obesity, and type 2 diabetes. Although the variety of recommendations and the task of making positive changes may be daunting, even small changes in plasma lipid profiles through dietary and lifestyle factors can produce considerable benefit regarding disease risk. An additional resource for determining dietary recommendations based upon age, gender, height, weight, and physical activity level can be found at www.mypyramid.gov as a service of the USDA.[146]

VII. CONCLUSIONS

Fat metabolism can be altered by energy status and exercise training. Certain activities may be better suited for utilizing fat as the primary fuel source during exercise. The effects of total fats, saturated fats, and cholesterol on health and disease have been well documented. While increased amounts of total fat and saturated fat in the diet have largely shown to be detrimental to personal health, such as an increased risk of CHD, some contradicting evidence exists concerning its impact on certain diseases, such as various cancers. Although the use of many lipid supplements cannot be supported based on current research, some, such as fish oil, may possibly provide advantageous effects.

The recommended intakes of total fat, saturated fat, and cholesterol have been established, by both the federal government HSS and USDA as well as the American Heart Association. Further research is warranted before definitive recommendations are made concerning the intake of total fat, saturated fat, and *trans* fats specific to the older adult population.

REFERENCES

1. Jeukendrup, A.E. and Gleeson, M., *Sport nutrition and introduction to energy production and performance,* Human Kinetics, Champaign, IL, 2004, chap. 1, 2 ,6, 10.
2. Driskell, J.A., *Sports Nutrition*, CRC Press, Boca Raton, FL, 2007, chap. 2.
3. Mu, H. and Porsgaard, T., The metabolism of structured triacylglycerols. *Prog. Lipid Res.* 44, 430–48, 2005.
4. Driskell, J.A., *Sports Nutrition*. CRC Press, Boca Raton, 2000, chap. 5.
5. Manore, M. and Thompson, J., *Sport Nutrition for Health and Performance*. Human Kinetics, Champaign, IL, 2000, chap. 3.
6. Gropper, S.A.S., Groff, J.L., and Smith, J.L., *Advanced Nutrition and Human Metabolism,* 4th ed, Thomson Wadsworth, Belmont, CA, 2005, chap. 2, 6, 8.
7. Potapenko, M., Shurin, G.V., and de Leon, J., Gangliosides as immunomodulators. *Adv. Exp. Med. Biol.* 601, 195–203, 2007.
8. Clausen, H. and Hakomori, S., ABH and related histo-blood group antigens; immunochemical differences in carrier isotypes and their distribution. *Vox Sang.* 56, 1–20, 1989.
9. Watkins, W.M., Biochemistry and Genetics of the ABO, Lewis, and P blood group systems. *Adv. Hum. Genet.* 10, 1–85, 1980.
10. Subbiah, M.T. and Kuksis, A., Differences in metabolism of cholesterol and sitosterol following intravenous injection in rats. *Biochim. Biophys. Acta* 306, 95–105, 1973.
11. Kritchevsky, D., Phytosterols. *Adv. Exp. Med. Biol.* 427, 235–43, 1997.
12. Pollak, O.J., Reduction of blood cholesterol in man. *Circulation* 7, 702–06, 1953.
13. Pollak, O.J. and Kritchevsky, D., Sitosterol. *Monogr Atheroscler.* 10, 1–219, 1981.
14. De Lorgeril, M., Essential polyunsaturated fatty acids, inflammation, atherosclerosis and cardiovascular diseases. *Subcell. Biochem.* 42, 283–97, 2007.
15. Calder, P.C., Polyunsaturated fatty acids and inflammation. *Biochem. Soc. Trans.* 33, 423–27, 2005.

16. De Lorgeril, M. and Salen, P., Alpha-linolenic acid and coronary heart disease. *Nutr. Metab Cardiovasc. Dis.* 14, 162–69, 2004.
17. Lapointe, A., Couillard, C., and Lemieux, S., Effects of dietary factors on oxidation of low-density lipoprotein particles. *J. Nutr. Biochem.* 17, 645–58, 2006.
18. Mozaffarian, D., Katan, M.B., Ascherio, A., Stampfer, M.J., and Willett, W.C., Trans fatty acids and cardiovascular disease. *N. Engl. J. Med.* 354, 1601–13, 2006.
19. Sacchetti, M., Saltin, B., Osada, T., and van Hall, G., Intramuscular fatty acid metabolism in contracting and non-contracting human skeletal muscle. *J. Physiol* 540, 387–95, 2002.
20. Salter, A.M. and Brindley, D.N., The biochemistry of lipoproteins. *J. Inherit. Metab Dis.* 11 Suppl 1, 4–17, 1988.
21. Large, V., Peroni, O., Letexier, D., Ray, H., and Beylot, M., Metabolism of lipids in human white adipocyte. *Diabetes Metab* 30, 294–309, 2004.
22. Rosen, E.D. and Spiegelman, B.M., Adipocytes as regulators of energy balance and glucose homeostasis. *Nature* 444, 847–53, 2006.
23. van Loon, L.J., Use of intramuscular triacylglycerol as a substrate source during exercise in humans. *J. Appl. Physiol* 97, 1170–87, 2004.
24. Johnson, N.A., Stannard, S.R., Mehalski, K., Trenell, M.I., Sachinwalla, T., Thompson, C.H. and Thompson, M.W., Intramyocellular triacylglycerol in prolonged cycling with high- and low-carbohydrate availability. *J. Appl. Physiol* 94, 1365–72, 2003.
25. Starling, R.D., Trappe, T.A., Parcell, A.C., Kerr, C.G., Fink, W.J., and Costill, D.L., Effects of diet on muscle triglyceride and endurance performance. *J. Appl. Physiol.* 82, 1185–89, 1997.
26. Ascherio, A., Hennekens, C.H., Buring, J.E., Master, C., Stampfer, M.J., and Willett, W.C., Trans-fatty acids intake and risk of myocardial infarction. *Circulation* 89, 94–101, 1994.
27. Thamer, C., Machann, J., Bachmann, O., Haap, M., Dahl, D., Wietek, B., et al., Intramyocellular lipids: Anthropometric determinants and relationships with maximal aerobic capacity and insulin sensitivity. *J. Clin. Endocrinol. Metab* 88, 1785–91, 2003.
28. Wolfe, R.R., Metabolic interactions between glucose and fatty acids in humans. *Am. J. Clin. Nutr.* 67, 519S–26S, 1998.
29. Berning, J.R. and Steen, S.N., *Nutrition for Sport and Exercise*, 2nd ed., Aspen Publishers, Gaithersburg, MD, 1998, chap. 4.
30. Jeukendrup, A.E., Saris, W.H., and Wagenmakers, A.J., Fat metabolism during exercise: A review–part II: Regulation of metabolism and the effects of training. *Int. J. Sports Med.* 19, 293–302, 1998.
31. Saltin, B. and Astrand, P.O., Free fatty acids and exercise. *Am. J. Clin. Nutr.* 57, 752S–7S, 1993.
32. Hodgetts, V., Coppack, S.W., Frayn, K.N., and Hockaday, T.D., Factors controlling fat mobilization from human subcutaneous adipose tissue during exercise. *J. Appl. Physiol* 71, 445–51, 1991.
33. Romijn, J.A., Coyle, E.F., Sidossis, L.S., Gastaldelli, A., Horowitz, J.F., Endert, E. and Wolfe, R.R., Regulation of endogenous fat and carbohydrate metabolism in relation to exercise intensity and duration. *Am. J. Physiol.* 265, E380–E391, 1993.
34. Achten, J., Gleeson, M., and Jeukendrup, A.E., Determination of the exercise intensity that elicits maximal fat oxidation. *Med. Sci. Sports Exerc.* 34, 92–97, 2002.
35. Ogden, C.L., Carroll, M.D., McDowell, M.A. and Flegal, K.M., Obesity among adults in the United States–no statistically significant changes since 2003–2004. 2007. http://www.cdc.gov/nchs/pressroom/07newsreleases/obesity.htm. Accessed 08/12/2008.

36. Achten, J., Venables, M.C., and Jeukendrup, A.E., Fat oxidation rates are higher during running compared with cycling over a wide range of intensities. *Metabolism* 52, 747–52, 2003.
37. Coyle, E.F., Jeukendrup, A.E., Wagenmakers, A.J., and Saris, W.H., Fatty acid oxidation is directly regulated by carbohydrate metabolism during exercise. *Am. J. Physiol.* 273, E268–E275, 1997.
38. Sidossis, L.S., Gastaldelli, A., Klein, S., and Wolfe, R.R., Regulation of plasma fatty acid oxidation during low- and high-intensity exercise. *Am. J. Physiol* 272, E1065–E1070, 1997.
39. Mensink, R.P. and Katan, M.B., Effect of dietary trans fatty acids on high-density and low-density lipoprotein cholesterol levels in healthy subjects. *N. Engl. J. Med.* 323, 439–45, 1990.
40. Zock, P.L. and Katan, M.B., Hydrogenation alternatives: Effects of trans fatty acids and stearic acid versus linoleic acid on serum lipids and lipoproteins in humans. *J. Lipid Res.* 33, 399–410, 1992.
41. Lemaitre, R.N., King, I.B., Mozaffarian, D., Sotoodehnia, N., Rea, T.D., Kuller, L.H., et al., Plasma phospholipid trans fatty acids, fatal ischemic heart disease, and sudden cardiac death in older adults: The cardiovascular health study. *Circulation* 114, 209–15, 2006.
42. Stender, S., Dyerberg, J., Bysted, A., Leth, T., and Astrup, A., A trans world journey. *Atheroscler. Suppl.* 7, 47–52, 2006.
43. Astrup, A., The trans fatty acid story in Denmark. *Atheroscler. Suppl.* 7, 43–46, 2006.
44. Ban Trans Fats. www.bantransfats.com. Accessed 08/12/2008.
45. United States Department of Health and Human Services, HHS to require food labels to include trans fat contentsImproved labels will help consumers choose heart-healthy foods. www.hhs.gov/news/press/2003pres/20030709.html. Accessed 08/12/2008.
46. Hegsted, D.M., Ausman, L.M., Johnson, J.A., and Dallal, G.E., Dietary fat and serum lipids: An evaluation of the experimental data. *Am. J Clin Nutr.* 57, 875–83, 1993.
47. Browning, L.M. and Jebb, S.A., Nutritional influences on inflammation and type 2 diabetes risk. *Diabetes Technol. Ther.* 8, 45–54, 2006.
48. Lindstrom, J., Peltonen, M., Eriksson, J.G., Louheranta, A., Fogelholm, M., Uusitupa, M. and Tuomilehto, J., High-fibre, low-fat diet predicts long-term weight loss and decreased type 2 diabetes risk: The Finnish Diabetes Prevention Study. *Diabetologia* 49, 912–20, 2006.
49. Lueck, T.J. and Severson, K., New York bans most trans fats in restaurants. *New York Times*, 2006.
50. Potteiger, J.A., Jacobsen, D.J., Donnelly, J.E., and Hill, J.O., Glucose and insulin responses following 16 months of exercise training in overweight adults: The Midwest Exercise Trial. *Metabolism* 52, 1175–81, 2003.
51. Third report of the National Cholesterol Education Program (NCEP) Expert panel on detection, evaluation, and treatment of high blood cholesterol in adults (Adult Treatment Panel III) final report. *Circulation* 106, 3143–421, 2002.
52. Bray, G.A. and Popkin, B.M., Dietary fat intake does affect obesity! *Am. J. Clin. Nutr.* 68, 1157–73, 1998.
53. van Dam, R.M., Willett, W.C., Rimm, E.B., Stampfer, M.J., and Hu, F.B., Dietary fat and meat intake in relation to risk of type 2 diabetes in men. *Diabetes Care* 25, 417–24, 2002.
54. Grundy, S.M., Abate, N., and Chandalia, M., Diet composition and the metabolic syndrome: What is the optimal fat intake? *Am. J. Med.* 113, 25–29, 2002.

55. Rosamond, W., Flegal, K., Furie, K., Go, A., Greenlund, K., and Haase, N., et al. Heart Disease and Stroke Statistics 2008 Update. A report from the American Heart Association Statistics Committee and Stroke Statistics Subcommittee. *Circulation*, 2007.
56. Thom, T., Haase, N., Rosamond, W., Howard, V.J., Rumsfeld, J., and Manolio, T., et al., Heart Disease and Stroke Statistics–2006 Update: A report from the American Heart Association Statistics Committee and Stroke Statistics Subcommittee. *Circulation* 113, e85–151, 2006.
57. Kjelsberg, M.O., Cutler, J.A., and Dolecek, T.A., Brief description of the Multiple Risk Factor Intervention Trial. *Am. J. Clin. Nutr.* 65, 191S–5S, 1997.
58. Stamler, J., Daviglus, M.L., Garside, D.B., Dyer, A.R., Greenland, P., and Neaton, J.D., Relationship of baseline serum cholesterol levels in 3 large cohorts of younger men to long-term coronary, cardiovascular, and all-cause mortality and to longevity. *JAMA* 284, 311–18, 2000.
59. Grundy, S.M., Primary prevention of coronary heart disease: Selection of patients for aggressive cholesterol management. *Am. J. Med.* 107, 2S–6S, 1999.
60. Grundy, S.M., Cleeman, J.I., Merz, C.N., Brewer, H.B., Jr., Clark, L.T., and Hunninghake, D.B., et al., Implications of recent clinical trials for the National Cholesterol Education Program Adult Treatment Panel III guidelines. *Circulation* 110, 227–39, 2004.
61. Hu, F.B., Stampfer, M.J., Rimm, E.B., Manson, J.E., Ascherio, A., and Colditz, G.A.,et al., A prospective study of egg consumption and risk of cardiovascular disease in men and women. *JAMA* 281, 1387–94, 1999.
62. Howard, B.V., Van Horn, L., Hsia, J., Manson, J.E., Stefanick, M.L., and Wassertheil–Smoller, et al., Low–Fat Dietary Pattern and Risk of Cardiovascular Disease: The Women's Health Initiative Randomized Controlled Dietary Modification Trial. *JAMA* 295, 655–66, 2006.
63. Lovejoy, J.C., Smith, S.R., Champagne, C.M., Most, M.M., Lefevre, M., and Delany, J.P., et al., Effects of diets enriched in saturated (palmitic), monounsaturated (oleic), or trans (elaidic) fatty acids on insulin sensitivity and substrate oxidation in healthy adults. *Diabetes Care* 25, 1283–88, 2002.
64. Perez-Jimenez, F., Lopez-Miranda, J., Pinillos, M.D., Gomez, P., Paz-Rojas, E., and Montilla, P., et al., A Mediterranean and a high-carbohydrate diet improve glucose metabolism in healthy young persons. *Diabetologia* 44, 2038–43, 2001.
65. Vessby, B., Unsitupa, M., Hermansen, K., Riccardi, G., Rivellese, A.A., and Tapsell, et al., Substituting dietary saturated for monounsaturated fat impairs insulin sensitivity in healthy men and women: The KANWU Study. *Diabetologia* 44, 312–19, 2001.
66. Ahrens, E.H., Jr., Insull, W., Jr., Blomstrand, R., Hirsch, J., Tsaltas, T.T., and Peterson, M.L., The influence of dietary fats on serum-lipid levels in man. *Lancet* 272, 943–53, 1957.
67. Hegsted, D.M., McGandy, R.B., Myers, M.L., and Stare, F.J., Quantitative effects of dietary fat on serum cholesterol in man. *Am. J. Clin. Nutr.* 17, 281–95, 1965.
68. Keys, A., Effects of different dietary fats on plasma-lipid levels. *Lancet* 17, 318–19, 1965.
69. Grundy, S.M. and Mok, H.Y., Determination of cholesterol absorption in man by intestinal perfusion. *J. Lipid Res.* 18, 263–71, 1977.
70. Grundy, S.M., Influence of stearic acid on cholesterol metabolism relative to other long-chain fatty acids. *Am. J. Clin. Nutr.* 60, 986S–90S, 1994.
71. Bonanome, A. and Grundy, S.M., Effect of dietary stearic acid on plasma cholesterol and lipoprotein levels. *N. Engl. J. Med.* 318, 1244–48, 1988.

72. Hassel, C.A., Mensing, E.A., and Gallaher, D.D., Dietary stearic acid reduces plasma and hepatic cholesterol concentrations without increasing bile acid excretion in cholesterol-fed hamsters. *J. Nutr.* 127, 1148–55, 1997.
73. He, K., Song, Y., Daviglus, M.L., Liu, K., Van Horn, L., Dyer, A.R., and Greenland, P., Accumulated evidence on fish consumption and coronary heart disease mortality: A meta-analysis of cohort studies. *Circulation* 109, 2705–11, 2004.
74. Beresford, S.A., Johnson, K.C., Ritenbaugh, C., Lasser, N.L., Snetselaar, L.G., and Black, H.R., et al., Low-fat dietary pattern and risk of colorectal cancer: the Women's Health Initiative Randomized Controlled Dietary Modification Trial. *JAMA* 295, 643–54, 2006.
75. Harris, W.S., Poston, W.C. and Haddock, C.K., Tissue n-3 and n-6 fatty acids and risk for coronary heart disease events. *Atherosclerosis* 193, 1–10, 2007.
76. Lagergren, J., Controversies surrounding body mass, reflux, and risk of oesophageal adenocarcinoma. *Lancet Oncol.* 7, 347–49, 2006.
77. Morita, T., Tabata, S., Mineshita, M., Mizoue, T., Moore, M.A., and Kono, S., The metabolic syndrome is associated with increased risk of colorectal adenoma development: the Self-Defense Forces Health Study. *Asian Pac. J. Cancer Prev.* 6, 485–89, 2005.
78. Holmes, M.D., Hunter, D.J., Colditz, G.A., Stampfer, M.J., Hankinson, S.E., and Speizer, F.E., et al., Association of dietary intake of fat and fatty acids with risk of breast cancer. *JAMA* 281, 914–20, 1999.
79. Optenberg, S.A., Thompson, I.M., Friedrichs, P., Wojcik, B., Stein, C.R., and Kramer, B., Race, treatment, and long-term survival from prostate cancer in an equal-access medical care delivery system. *JAMA* 274, 1599–605, 1995.
80. Whittemore, A.S., Kolonel, L.N., Wu, A.H., John, E.M., Gallagher, and R.P., et al., Prostate cancer in relation to diet, physical activity, and body size in blacks, whites, and Asians in the United States and Canada. *J. Natl. Cancer Inst.* 87, 652–61, 1995.
81. Binukumar, B. and Mathew, A., Dietary fat and risk of breast cancer. *World J. Surg. Oncol.* 3, 45, 2005.
82. Prentice, R.L., Caan, B., Chlebowski, R.T., Patterson, R., Kuller, L.H., and Ockene, J.K., et al., Low–Fat Dietary Pattern and Risk of Invasive Breast Cancer: The Women's Health Initiative Randomized Controlled Dietary Modification Trial. *JAMA* 295, 629–42, 2006.
83. Gonzalez, C.A., The European Prospective Investigation into Cancer and Nutrition (EPIC). *Public Health Nutr.* 9, 124–26, 2006.
84. Chen, H., Tucker, K.L., Graubard, B.I., Heineman, E.F., Markin, R.S., Potischman, N.A., Russell, R.M., Weisenburger, D.D. and Ward, M.H., Nutrient intakes and adenocarcinoma of the esophagus and distal stomach. *Nutr. Cancer* 42, 33–40, 2002.
85. Boyd, N.F., Stone, J., Vogt, K.N., Connelly, B.S., Martin, L.J. and Minkin, S., Dietary fat and breast cancer risk revisited: A meta-analysis of the published literature. *Br. J. Cancer* 89, 1672–85, 2003.
86. Michels, K.B., Mohllajee, A.P., Roset-Bahmanyar, E., Beehler, G.P. and Moysich, K.B., Diet and breast cancer: A review of the prospective observational studies. *Cancer* 109, 2712–49, 2007.
87. Trumbo, P., Schlicker, S., Yates, A.A., and Poos, M., Dietary reference intakes for energy, carbohydrate, fiber, fat, fatty acids, cholesterol, protein and amino acids. *J Am. Diet Assoc.* 102, 1621–30, 2002.
88. Simopoulos, A.P., Omega-3 fatty acids and athletics. *Curr. Sports Med. Rep.* 6, 230–36, 2007.
89. Burr, M.L., Fehily, A.M., Gilbert, J.F., Rogers, S., Holliday, R.M., and Sweetnam, et al., Effects of changes in fat, fish, and fibre intakes on death and myocardial reinfarction: Diet and reinfarction trial (DART). *Lancet* 2, 757–61, 1989.

90. Dietary supplementation with n-3 polyunsaturated fatty acids and vitamin E after myocardial infarction: Results of the GISSI-Prevenzione trial. *Lancet* 354, 447–55, 1999.
91. De Lorgeril, M., Renaud, S., Mamelle, N., Salen, P., Martin, J.L., and Monjaud, I., et al., Mediterranean alpha-linolenic acid-rich diet in secondary prevention of coronary heart disease. *Lancet* 343, 1454–59, 1994.
92. De Lorgeril, M., Salen, P., Martin, J.L., Monjaud, I., Delaye, J. and Mamelle, N., Mediterranean diet, traditional risk factors, and the rate of cardiovascular complications after myocardial infarction: Final report of the Lyon Diet Heart Study. *Circulation* 99, 779–85, 1999.
93. Zhao, G., Etherton, T.D., Martin, K.R., West, S.G., Gillies, P.J., and Kris-Etherton, P.M., Dietary alpha-linolenic acid reduces inflammatory and lipid cardiovascular risk factors in hypercholesterolemic men and women. *J. Nutr.* 134, 2991–97, 2004.
94. Zhao, G., Etherton, T.D., Martin, K.R., Gillies, P.J., West, S.G., and Kris-Etherton, P.M., Dietary alpha-linolenic acid inhibits proinflammatory cytokine production by peripheral blood mononuclear cells in hypercholesterolemic subjects. *Am. J. Clin. Nutr.* 85, 385–91, 2007.
95. Bhatnagar, D. and Durrington, P.N., Omega-3 fatty acids: Their role in the prevention and treatment of atherosclerosis related risk factors and complications. *Int. J. Clin. Pract.* 57, 305–14, 2003.
96. Din, J.N., Newby, D.E. and Flapan, A.D., Omega 3 fatty acids and cardiovascular disease–fishing for a natural treatment. *BMJ* 328, 30–35, 2004.
97. Geelen, A., Brouwer, I.A., Zock, P.L., and Katan, M.B., Antiarrhythmic effects of n-3 fatty acids: Evidence from human studies. *Curr. Opin. Lipidol.* 15, 25–30, 2004.
98. Thies, F., Garry, J.M., Yaqoob, P., Rerkasem, K., Williams, J., and Shearman, C.P., et al., Association of n-3 polyunsaturated fatty acids with stability of atherosclerotic plaques: A randomised controlled trial. *Lancet* 361, 477–85, 2003.
99. Kato, I., Akhmedkhanov, A., Koenig, K., Toniolo, P.G., Shore, R.E., and Riboli, E., Prospective study of diet and female colorectal cancer: The New York University Women's Health Study. *Nutr. Cancer* 28, 276–81, 1997.
100. MacLean, C.H., Newberry, S.J., Mojica, W.A., Khanna, P., Issa, A.M., and Suttorp, M.J., et al., Effects of omega-3 fatty acids on cancer risk: A systematic review. *JAMA* 295, 403–15, 2006.
101. Schuurman, A.G., van den Brandt, P.A., Dorant, E., Brants, H.A., and Goldbohm, R.A., Association of energy and fat intake with prostate carcinoma risk: Results from The Netherlands Cohort Study. *Cancer* 86, 1019–27, 1999.
102. Takezaki, T., Inoue, M., Kataoka, H., Ikeda, S., Yoshida, M., and Ohashi, Y., et al., Diet and lung cancer risk from a 14-year population-based prospective study in Japan: With special reference to fish consumption. *Nutr. Cancer* 45, 160–67, 2003.
103. Voorrips, L.E., Brants, H.A., Kardinaal, A.F., Hiddink, G.J., van den Brandt, P.A., and Goldbohm, R.A., Intake of conjugated linoleic acid, fat, and other fatty acids in relation to postmenopausal breast cancer: The Netherlands Cohort Study on Diet and Cancer. *Am. J. Clin. Nutr.* 76, 873–82, 2002.
104. Staprans, I., Pan, X.M., Rapp, J.H., and Feingold, K.R., The role of dietary oxidized cholesterol and oxidized fatty acids in the development of atherosclerosis. *Mol. Nutr. Food Res.* 49, 1075–82, 2005.
105. Kanner, J., Dietary advanced lipid oxidation endproducts are risk factors to human health. *Mol. Nutr. Food Res.* 51, 1094–101, 2007.
106. Hooper, L., Thompson, R.L., Harrison, R.A., Summerbell, C.D., Ness, A.R., and Moore, H.J., et al., Risks and benefits of omega 3 fats for mortality, cardiovascular disease, and cancer: systematic review. *BMJ* 332, 752–60, 2006.

107. Larsen, T.M., Toubro, S., and Astrup, A., Efficacy and safety of dietary supplements containing CLA for the treatment of obesity: Evidence from animal and human studies. *J. Lipid Res.* 44, 2234–41, 2003.
108. Taylor, C.G. and Zahradka, P., Dietary conjugated linoleic acid and insulin sensitivity and resistance in rodent models. *Am. J. Clin. Nutr.* 79, 1164S–8S, 2004.
109. Kepler, C.R., Hirons, K.P., McNeill, J.J., and Tove, S.B., Intermediates and products of the biohydrogenation of linoleic acid by *Butyrinvibrio fibrisolvens. J. Biol. Chem.* 241, 1350–54, 1966.
110. O'Shea, M., Bassaganya-Riera, J., and Mohede, I.C., Immunomodulatory properties of conjugated linoleic acid. *Am. J. Clin. Nutr.* 79, 1199S–206S, 2004.
111. Lin, H., Boylston, T.D., Chang, M.J., Luedecke, L.O., and Shultz, T.D., Survey of the conjugated linoleic acid contents of dairy products. *J. Dairy Sci.* 78, 2358–65, 1995.
112. Jiang, J., Wolk, A., and Vessby, B., Relation between the intake of milk fat and the occurrence of conjugated linoleic acid in human adipose tissue. *Am. J. Clin. Nutr.* 70, 21–27, 1999.
113. Kohno, H., Suzuki, R., Noguchi, R., Hosokawa, M., Miyashita, K., and Tanaka, T., Dietary conjugated linolenic acid inhibits azoxymethane-induced colonic aberrant crypt foci in rats. *Jpn. J. Cancer Res.* 93, 133–42, 2002.
114. Park, Y., McGuire, M.K., Behr, R., McGuire, M.A., Evans, M.A., and Shultz, T.D., High-fat dairy product consumption increases delta 9c,11t-18:2 (rumenic acid) and total lipid concentrations of human milk. *Lipids* 34, 543–49, 1999.
115. Ritzenthaler, K.L., McGuire, M.K., Falen, R., Shultz, T.D., Dasgupta, N., and McGuire, M.A., Estimation of conjugated linoleic acid intake by written dietary assessment methodologies underestimates actual intake evaluated by food duplicate methodology. *J. Nutr.* 131, 1548–54, 2001.
116. Suzuki, R., Noguchi, R., Ota, T., Abe, M., Miyashita, K., and Kawada, T., Cytotoxic effect of conjugated trienoic fatty acids on mouse tumor and human monocytic leukemia cells. *Lipids* 36, 477–82, 2001.
117. Nagao, K. and Yanagita, T., Conjugated fatty acids in food and their health benefits. *J. Biosci. Bioeng.* 100, 152–57, 2005.
118. Yamasaki, M., Nishida, E., Nou, S., Tachibana, H., and Yamada, K., Cytotoxity of the trans10,cis12 isomer of conjugated linoleic acid on rat hepatoma and its modulation by other fatty acids, tocopherol, and tocotrienol. *In Vitro Cell Dev. Biol. Anim.* 41, 239–44, 2005.
119. Roynette, C.E., Rudkowska, I., Nakhasi, D.K., and Jones, P.J., Structured medium and long chain triglycerides show short-term increases in fat oxidation, but no changes in adiposity in men. *Nutr. Metab Cardiovasc. Dis.* 2007.
120. Larsson, S.C., Bergkvist, L. and Wolk, A., High-fat dairy food and conjugated linoleic acid intakes in relation to colorectal cancer incidence in the Swedish Mammography Cohort. *Am. J. Clin. Nutr.* 82, 894–900, 2005.
121. Aro, A., Mannisto, S., Salminen, I., Ovaskainen, M.L., Kataja, V., and Uusitupa, M., Inverse association between dietary and serum conjugated linoleic acid and risk of breast cancer in postmenopausal women. *Nutr. Cancer* 38, 151–57, 2000.
122. Fite, A., Goua, M., Wahle, K.W., Schofield, A.C., Hutcheon, A.W., and Heys, S.D., Potentiation of the anti-tumour effect of docetaxel by conjugated linoleic acids (CLAs) in breast cancer cells in vitro. *Prostaglandins Leukot. Essent. Fatty Acids* 77, 87–96, 2007.
123. Ip, M.M., McGee, S.O., Masso-Welch, P.A., Ip, C., Meng, X., Ou, L., and Shoemaker, S.F., The t10,c12 isomer of conjugated linoleic acid stimulates mammary tumorigenesis in transgenic mice over-expressing erbB2 in the mammary epithelium. *Carcinogenesis* 28, 1269–76, 2007.

124. Russell, J.S., McGee, S.O., Ip, M.M., Kuhlmann, D., and Masso-Welch, P.A., Conjugated linoleic acid induces mast cell recruitment during mouse mammary gland stromal remodeling. *J. Nutr.* 137, 1200–07, 2007.
125. Belury, M.A., Inhibition of carcinogenesis by conjugated linoleic acid: Potential mechanisms of action. *J. Nutr.* 132, 2995–98, 2002.
126. Chajes, V., Lavillonniere, F., Maillard, V., Giraudeau, B., Jourdan, M.L., Sebedio, J.L., and Bougnoux, P., Conjugated linoleic acid content in breast adipose tissue of breast cancer patients and the risk of metastasis. *Nutr. Cancer* 45, 17–23, 2003.
127. Belury, M.A., Dietary conjugated linoleic acid in health: Physiological effects and mechanisms of action. *Ann. Rev. Nutr.* 22, 505–31, 2002.
128. Cimini, A., Cristiano, L., Colafarina, S., Benedetti, E., Di Loreto, S., and Festuccia, C., et al., PPARgamma-dependent effects of conjugated linoleic acid on the human glioblastoma cell line (ADF). *Int. J. Cancer* 117, 923–33, 2005.
129. West, D.B., Delany, J.P., Camet, P.M., Blohm, F., Truett, A.A., and Scimeca, J., Effects of conjugated linoleic acid on body fat and energy metabolism in the mouse. *Am. J. Physiol.* 275, R667–R672, 1998.
130. Martin, J.C., Gregoire, S., Siess, M.H., Genty, M., Chardigny, J.M., and Berdeaux, O., et al., Effects of conjugated linoleic acid isomers on lipid-metabolizing enzymes in male rats. *Lipids* 35, 91–98, 2000.
131. Smedman, A. and Vessby, B., Conjugated linoleic acid supplementation in humans–Metabolic effects. *Lipids* 36, 773–81, 2001.
132. Riserus, U., Berglund, L., and Vessby, B., Conjugated linoleic acid (CLA) reduced abdominal adipose tissue in obese middle-aged men with signs of the metabolic syndrome: A randomised controlled trial. *Int. J. Obes. Relat. Metab. Disord.* 25, 1129–35, 2001.
133. Blankson, H., Stakkestad, J.A., Fagertun, H., Thom, E., Wadstein, J., and Gudmundsen, O., Conjugated linoleic acid reduces body fat mass in overweight and obese humans. *J. Nutr.* 130, 2943–48, 2000.
134. Rivero, J.L., Sporleder, H.P., Quiroz-Rothe, E., Vervuert, I., Coenen, M., and Harmeyer, J., Oral L-carnitine combined with training promotes changes in skeletal muscle. *Equine Vet. J. Suppl* , 269–74, 2002.
135. Benito, P., Nelson, G.J., Kelley, D.S., Bartolini, G., Schmidt, P.C., and Simon, V., The effect of conjugated linoleic acid on plasma lipoproteins and tissue fatty acid composition in humans. *Lipids* 36, 229–36, 2001.
136. Kamphuis, M.M., Lejeune, M.P., Saris, W.H., and Westerterp-Plantenga, M.S., The effect of conjugated linoleic acid supplementation after weight loss on body weight regain, body composition, and resting metabolic rate in overweight subjects. *Int. J. Obes. Relat. Metab. Disord.* 27, 840–47, 2003.
137. Kreider, R.B., Ferreira, M.P., Greenwood, M., Wilson, M., and Almada, A.L., Effects of conjugated linoleic acid supplementation during resistance training on body composition, bone density, strength, and selected hematological markers. *J. Strength. Cond. Res.* 16, 325–34, 2002.
138. Mougios, V., Matsakas, A., Petridou, A., Ring, S., Sagredos, A., and Melissopoulou, A., et al., Effect of supplementation with conjugated linoleic acid on human serum lipids and body fat. *J. Nutr. Biochem.* 12, 585–94, 2001.
139. Houseknecht, K.L., Vanden Heuvel, J.P., Moya-Camarena, S.Y., Portocarrero, C.P., Peck, L.W., Nickel, K.P., and Belury, M.A., Dietary conjugated linoleic acid normalizes impaired glucose tolerance in the Zucker diabetic fatty fa/fa rat. *Biochem. Biophys. Res. Commun.* 244, 678–82, 1998.
140. Delany, J.P., Blohm, F., Truett, A.A., Scimeca, J.A., and West, D.B., Conjugated linoleic acid rapidly reduces body fat content in mice without affecting energy intake. *Am. J. Physiol.* 276, R1172–R1179, 1999.

141. Tsuboyama-Kasaoka, N., Takahashi, M., Tanemura, K., Kim, H.J., Tange, T., Okuyama, H., and Kasai, M., et al., Conjugated linoleic acid supplementation reduces adipose tissue by apoptosis and develops lipodystrophy in mice. *Diabetes* 49, 1534–42, 2000.
142. Riserus, U., Vessby, B., Arnlov, J., and Basu, S., Effects of cis-9, trans-11 conjugated linoleic acid supplementation on insulin sensitivity, lipid peroxidation, and proinflammatory markers in obese men. *Am. J. Clin. Nutr.* 80, 279–83, 2004.
143. Taylor, J.S., Williams, S.R., Rhys, R., James, P., and Frenneaux, M.P., Conjugated linoleic acid impairs endothelial function. *Arterioscler. Thromb. Vasc. Biol.* 26, 307–12, 2006.
144. Riserus, U., Vessby, B., Arner, P., and Zethelius, B., Supplementation with trans10cis12-conjugated linoleic acid induces hyperproinsulinaemia in obese men: Close association with impaired insulin sensitivity. *Diabetologia* 47, 1016–19, 2004.
145. Babayan, V.K., Medium chain triglycerides and structured lipids. *Lipids* 22, 417–20, 1987.
146. Bach, A.C. and Babayan, V.K., Medium-chain triglycerides: An update. *Am. J. Clin. Nutr.* 36, 950–62, 1982.

4 Proteins

Brian S. Snyder and Mark D. Haub

CONTENTS

I. INTRODUCTION

Aging is associated with many changes in body composition, including the reduction of bone density and lean body mass with a concomitant increase in fat mass. These changes can often have negative impacts on overall health and functional capacity. The loss of bone density may lead to osteopenia and osteoporosis, while the loss of lean body mass may lead to sarcopenia.

Sarcopenia is the degenerative loss of skeletal muscle mass and strength, beginning as early as age 30 and accelerating with advancing age.[50,51] The exact causes of sarcopenia are unknown but are thought to be related to decreasing hormones, reduced physical activity, and inadequate nutrition. Advancing sarcopenia is associated with increased risk of falls and fractures, decreased ability to complete activities of daily living, and decreased metabolic health.[1] Dietary protein and exercise strategies outlined in this chapter may be effective strategies to reduce or delay the onset of sarcopenia.

The decrease of lean body mass with aging is associated with decreased metabolic health and caloric needs.[1] The conditions allowing the accumulation of a large amount of body fat, namely sedentary behavior and excess energy intakes, are associated with Type 2 diabetes, cardiovascular disease, and other metabolic conditions. While these conditions are less prevalent in middle age, the nutritional and exercise habits of middle-aged adults can help to delay or prevent their occurrence later in life. This chapter will review the importance of dietary protein in aiding the prevention of these conditions and attempt to decipher what is an adequate protein intake and what may be an "optimal" protein intake for middle-aged adults.

II. ESTABLISHED PROTEIN REQUIREMENTS

A. The Importance of Protein in the Diet

Dietary proteins, composed of individual amino acids, are found in many food sources. These amino acids are the building blocks of many structural and functional components within the human body. Proteins are the major component of skeletal muscle and also make up other structures including enzymes, collagen, membrane carriers, and some hormones. Amino acids can also be metabolized for energy, and some can be converted to glucose or fat.

Amino acids contain an amino nitrogen group that is the essential portion of amino acids. Humans consume proteins daily to replace nitrogen that is excreted in the form of urea and other nitrogen-containing molecules. We are not able to store protein per se, and will metabolize skeletal muscle to obtain nitrogen in the absence of dietary protein intake. Amino acids are categorized into three subgroups, namely essential amino acids, conditionally essential amino acids, and non-essential or dispensable amino acids (Table 4.1). Protein sources containing all eight of the essential amino acids are needed to support normal growth and protein synthesis. Most protein sources contain a mixture of all three types of amino acids. The essential amino acids can be metabolized into the other subgroups of amino acids but cannot be produced themselves in humans. The conditionally essential amino acids are rate limiting for protein synthesis under some conditions. The dispensable amino acids can typically be synthesized in the body from other amino acids.

The ingestion of proteins containing all of the essential amino acids results in an increase in total body and muscle protein synthesis.[2–5] In healthy sedentary young adults, assuming protein and total energy intake are adequate, these small

TABLE 4.1
Essential, Conditionally Essential, and Nonessential Amino Acids

Essential Amino Acids	Conditionally Essential Amino acids	Nonessential Amino Acids
*^Leucine	Arginine	Alanine
*Isoleucine	Cystine	Asparagine
*Valine	Glutamine	Citruline
Lysine	Histadine	Glutamic acid
Methionine	Proline	Glycine
Phenylalanine	Taurine	Serine
Threonine	Tyrosine	
Tryptophan		

* Branched Chain Amino Acids (BCAAs); ^ Important Amino Acid Signal for protein synthesis.

increases in protein synthesis in response to a meal counteract protein breakdown during the postabsorptive and overnight periods result in nitrogen and protein balance. (Figure 4.1).[6]

B. Nitrogen Balance

Assessing dietary protein needs is very important for determining protein requirements, which affect the overall health and growth of all individuals. Nitrogen balance is the most commonly used method to asses the protein needs of an individual or population. Nitrogen or protein balance is the relationship between the intake of dietary proteins and the recycling of body nitrogen with all of the nitrogen excreted. Nitrogen is lost in feces, urine, sweat, hair, and skin on a daily basis.

There are inherent problems with the nitrogen balance method when protein intakes are high or inadequate. When consuming a very high-protein diet, nitrogen balance studies trend toward positive nitrogen balance.[7–9] The positive nitrogen balance experienced while consuming a high-protein diet (2.3–3.0 g/kg/day) has been shown to continue for the duration of studies lasting up to 50 days.[9] However, the amount of protein accretion that would be taking place at this level of positive nitrogen balance would lead to great gains of muscle mass over time. It is well known that increased protein intake without sufficient resistance training does not result in an increase in skeletal muscle mass. The potential site of this additional nitrogen deposition is not known but is thought to increase the urea pool. Additionally, nitrogen losses with a high protein intake may have been underestimated.

Inadequate and suboptimal dietary protein intakes may not be apparent using the nitrogen balance method. It is important to distinguish between adaptation and accommodation to lower protein intakes to assess the negative impact such a protein intake may have on overall health. An adaptation to a low protein intake is an appropriate response to an adequate, yet lower than optimal protein intake. The result is a

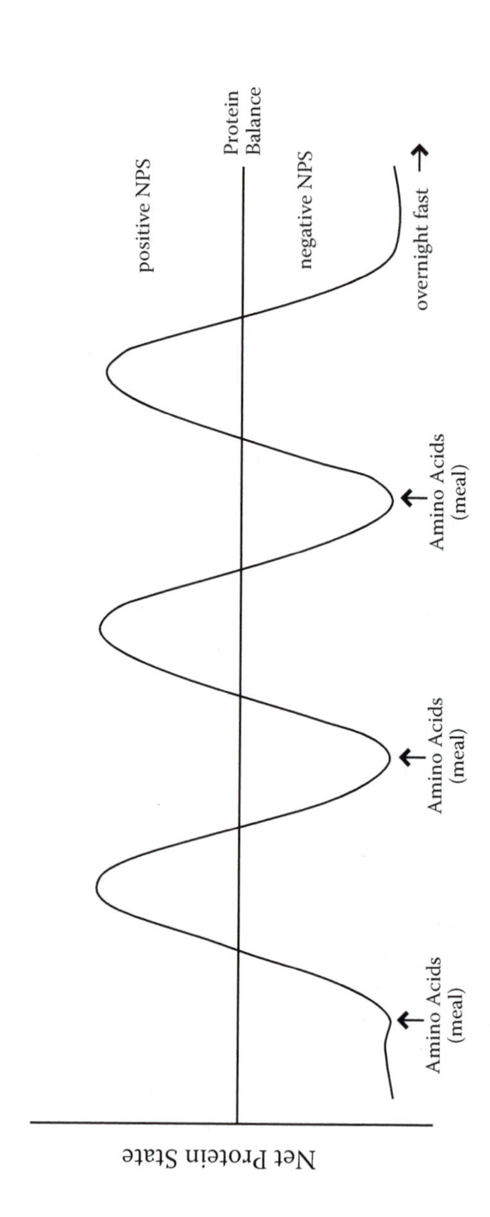

FIGURE 4.1 Adapted from Phillips et al [1]. Repeated daily protein containing meals result in nitrogen storage (positive NPS) which balances nitrogen losses (negative NPS). The overall result is nitrogen balance with no loss or gain of lean tissue. (Net Protein State = (NPS) nitrogen balance)

new steady state of nitrogen excretion without a compromise or loss of strength and physiological function. An accommodation is a survival response resulting in a new lower steady state of nitrogen excretion, but accompanying a decrease in strength or physiological function. The adaptations to low protein intakes will likely lead to muscle loss and impaired metabolic functioning.

C. RDA for Protein for Middle-Aged Adults

Based on the most recent meta-analysis by Rand et al.,[10] the recommended dietary allowance (RDA) for adults for protein remains set at 0.8 grams of protein per kilogram of body weight (0.8 g/kg/d).[11] This level of dietary protein intake is intended to meet the needs of almost all healthy people (97.5%) independent of age and physical activity. Ingesting 0.8 g/kg/d of quality protein should cover daily nitrogen losses with a built-in margin of error. This value was established largely based on nitrogen balance data and did not consider muscle mass, metabolic outcomes, nor physical capacity as end points in the meta-analysis. Additionally, there is very little data concerning older adults' protein needs and even less regarding protein needs specifically in middle age. The protein recommendations for older adults have been based on an extrapolation from nitrogen balance studies in younger adults and the few studies that measured nitrogen balance in older adults.[12] Some studies contest that the current RDA is adequate for middle-aged and older adults[13,14] because these individuals are able to adapt to a wide range of protein intakes. While the RDA value may be adequate to prevent deficiencies in many age groups based on nitrogen balance, that amount may be inadequate for maximizing metabolism, muscle mass, and functional capacity, especially in adults as they age. A dietary protein intake of 0.8 g/kg/d may be sufficient to keep an adult in nitrogen balance from a clinical standpoint, while still resulting in muscle loss over time, and ultimately leading to sarcopenia. Individuals can accommodate a suboptimal dietary protein intake by reducing nitrogen excretion and, if necessary, metabolizing muscle proteins.

A study conducted by Campbell et al[12] examined the effects of consuming 0.8 g/kg/d for 14 weeks in a tightly controlled setting. The healthy elderly men who participated in this study had a decrease in nitrogen excretion over the 14 weeks as well as a loss of mid-thigh muscle area assessed by CT scans even though they were consuming a weight-maintenance diet. These data illustrate that the protein intake in these subjects resulted in an accommodation to an inadequate protein intake to maintain skeletal muscle mass. If these subjects were to continue this level of dietary protein intake for a long period of time, they would most likely end up sarcopenic. Even in cases of extreme starvation, individuals may be able to maintain nitrogen balance until shortly before death by greatly reducing nitrogen excretion via recycling of endogenous nitrogen.[1] These examples illustrate some of the problems with relying on nitrogen balance as the sole method for establishing dietary protein needs.

Establishing an adequate or even optimal RDA for protein is important to middle-aged and older adults because up to 30% of older adults consume the RDA or less each day.[15] Inadequate dietary protein intake over an extended period of time leads to a decrease in total body protein turnover and increased loss of muscle mass in older adults.[16,17] Additionally, the nutritional habits of middle-aged adults are likely to influence their habits as they reach older adulthood.

While the dietary energy needs of older adults are less than those of young adults,[18] decreased portions and total energy will potentially decrease protein intake if protein intake is considered a percentage of total caloric intakes. To apply this concept to most consumers, it might be easiest to establish an absolute amount (g/d) instead of the traditional weight-relevant amount (g/kg/d), as many consumers likely do not even know how to calculate their needs.

III. PROTEIN METABOLISM

The source, timing, and composition of dietary protein all can have a significant impact on how they are handled by the body and will ultimately affect protein metabolism. To optimize the body's usage of protein, the following factors should be considered.

A. Protein Source

Not all protein sources were created equal. Both the quality and quantity of dietary protein can affect nitrogen balance and lean body mass. Dietary protein comes from two primary sources, animals and vegetables or plants. Animal protein in the human diet is typically derived from the muscles of these animals, their eggs, organs, or milk products. Vegetable and plant sources of protein are typically missing one or more of the essential amino acids and must be consumed in conjunction with another vegetable or animal protein source to make a complete protein able to support protein synthesis. The exception is soy protein, which contains all of the essential amino acids. However, it has been shown that soy proteins are less digestible on a nitrogen basis[19] and tend to produce more urea compared with casein intake, indicating an increased oxidation of soy proteins and reduced availability of its amino acids for protein synthesis.[20] Animal protein sources typically contain all of the essential amino acids and contain a higher concentration of the branched chain amino acid leucine. The essential amino acids must be included in the diet so that protein synthesis can be completed. The absence of even one essential amino acid will result in a protein deficiency by stopping the synthesis of any proteins that require that amino acid.

B. Protein Digestion and Absorption

The amount of time that a protein spends in the stomach is dependent on a number of variables including the type and form of protein consumed, the meal's fat content, fiber content, and total weight. Proteins are passed into the small intestine and absorbed throughout its entire length. The splanchnic tissues, which have first access to amino acids, have a relatively high demand for amino acids. The appearance of amino acids in peripheral circulation is dependent on splanchnic handling of a protein meal and can impact muscle protein synthesis.[21,22] Splanchnic and liver metabolism account for the majority of whole body protein metabolism at rest even though there is a greater amount of skeletal muscle mass.[23] The splanchnic zone acts as a buffer to amino acid ingestion to keep the level of circulating urea and free amino acids in check to prevent hyperaminoacidemia.[24] Thus, the amino acid content of a protein meal will affect the availability of amino acids for protein synthesis. The splanchnic tissues of older adults have an increased extraction of leucine compared with young adults[25], and there are differing opinions on the potential impact on total body and muscle protein synthesis with aging.

The speed with which the amino acids from a protein meal enter into systemic circulation will affect the concentration of the free amino acid pool as well as the duration of elevated amino acids. Both the peak and duration of elevated amino acids in the free amino acid pool greatly affect protein synthesis.[4,5,26]

Dietary fat has an interesting and confusing role in protein metabolism. The addition of sucrose to milk proteins increases whole body nitrogen retention mostly in splanchnic regions, and adding fat to milk proteins resulted in greatest nitrogen deposition in peripheral tissues.[27] Additionally, whole milk resulted in greater post-exercise protein synthesis in young adults than isocaloric skim milk.[28] More research is needed to determine the effects of fat on protein metabolism.

C. Anabolic Response to Protein

In healthy adults, muscle protein synthesis is the main determinant of net protein balance primarily due to the overall mass of skeletal muscle.[6,29] Studies have shown that total body protein synthesis[2,3] and muscle protein synthesis[4,5] are increased in response to amino acid provision at rest without provision of other macronutrients. Providing amino acids alone elevates plasma amino acids and stimulates muscle protein synthesis depending on dose, profile of the amino acids provided, means of delivery (bolus, pulse, or constant infusion), and the age and hormonal profile of the subject.[29] The increase in protein synthesis is transient, typically lasting about 2h during the postprandial state. Protein synthesis will typically fall after about 2h even if circulation amino acid levels remain elevated via an amino acid infusion.[5,29] However, ingestion of additional protein after 1h can re-stimulate protein synthesis.[30]

Approximately 80% of the effect of feeding amino acids on muscle protein synthesis is attributed to the amino acid content of the meal or infusion.[31–34] Studies have shown that ingestion of the essential amino acids alone are sufficient to elevate muscle protein synthesis.[29,35–38] Ingestion of nonessential amino acids alone does not have an effect on muscle nor total body protein synthesis.[29,39] While there is no direct effect of nonessential amino acids, consuming a diet devoid of these amino acids is not advised at this time.

Providing a single stimulatory amino acid such as valene, leucine, phenylalanine, or threonine results in an initial anabolic response that is transient, as all other amino acids in the intracellular pool fall.[39–41] Leucine has recently been discovered as the key regulatory amino acid.[42,43] The importance of adequate leucine intake will be discussed later in Section III E.

Some data suggest there may be an upper concentration of circulating amino acids above which additional amino acids have no supplementary effect. The muscle system may become saturated at approximately 2.5-fold normal circulating levels of amino acids.[34] A study by Bohe et al.[4] shows that the increase in muscle protein synthesis rises almost linearly until the plasma essential amino acids rise to 80% of basal. After this point, the system begins to saturate as the line flattens out. There is speculation that there may be some sort of signal that the "muscle is full," similar to that of a muscle full of glycogen.

The amount of protein synthesis caused by the amino acid meal is dose dependent, with greater doses causing a greater response to the saturation point.[4,44] The oral essential amino acid dose, which is thought to saturate the system is between 8 g[45] and 15 g[1] of essential amino acids at a given meal to maximally stimulate protein synthesis. These values have been shown to be effective in both the young and elderly. For example, 10 g of essential amino acids is approximately equal to 25 g of whole protein from lean meat, milk, or eggs. Studies have illustrated that repeated doses of amino acids are able to repeatedly stimulate protein synthesis.[30] Taken together, the intake of 25 g of quality protein per meal, spread out over five meals, could potentially result in maximal protein synthesis for sedentary adults. This level of dietary protein intake (125 g per day) is equal 1.8 g/kg/d for a 70-kg man, which is more than double the RDA of 0.8 g/kg/d.

D. Anabolic Response in Aging

In the healthy sedentary young individual, ingestion of dietary protein results in increased protein synthesis, which replaces proteins lost during the post-absorptive state, yielding a net protein balance. Muscle loss takes place when skeletal muscle breakdown is greater than skeletal muscle protein synthesis, leading to a net negative balance over a period of time. Muscle protein breakdown has been shown to remain relatively unchanged with advancing age in the post-absorptive state in healthy individuals.[46–48] Thus, it appears that the amount of muscle "lost" does not change with advancing age. However, it has been shown that older adults have a blunted increase in muscle protein synthesis in response to available dietary amino acids if the leucine concentration is not increased sufficiently.[49] Aging adults who do not consume enough leucine or essential amino acids per protein meal will theoretically not be replacing the protein lost during the post-absorptive state and may not maximize protein accretion (Figure 4.2).

E. The Importance of Leucine Rich Foods

Leucine is the primary amino acid regulator that "turns on" protein synthesis in the cells by signaling that quality protein is available for protein synthesis.[42,43] Aging tends to blunt muscle anabolic responses to a small dose (7 g) of essential amino acids as compared with younger adults.[49] Another study from the same authors recently illustrated that a high dose of leucine (2.79 g) in a mixture of essential amino acids can rebound the diminished anabolic muscle response of older adults to a level similar to that of young adults.[52] Paddon-Jones et al. confirmed these results in a study that reported that the isocaloric ingestion of essential amino acids containing 2.79 grams of leucine increased muscle protein synthesis to a greater extent than a whey protein supplement containing 1.75 grams of leucine.[53] While longer

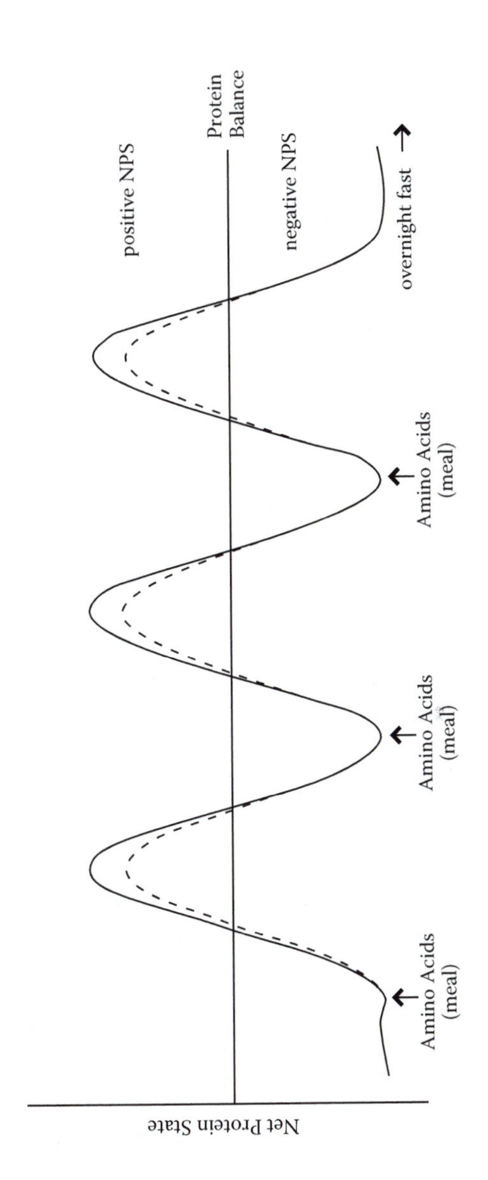

FIGURE 4.2 Adapted from [6]. Older adults have a blunted response to a protein meal (dashed line) compared to young adults (solid line) while protein breakdown does not change. This results in an overall negative net protein state, leading to the loss of lean tissue. Increasing the leucine content of each meal may rebound their protein response so that they respond similarly to young adults.

interventions are needed, one can speculate that higher repeated doses of leucine in conjunction with the other essential amino acids may be able to aide in maintaining skeletal muscle mass throughout adulthood.

A potential strategy to combat age-associated muscle loss is adding leucine to a protein-containing meal to maximize the anabolic response. A recent study by Rieu et al.[54] illustrated that the addition of leucine to a casein-containing meal increased the fractional synthesis rate compared with a control. A study by Koopman et al.[55] examined the effects of carbohydrate (C), carbohydrate plus protein (C+P), and carbohydrate plus protein plus added leucine (C+P+L) supplementation on post-exercise muscle protein synthesis. Relevant to this discussion, the greatest net protein balance occurred in the leucine-supplemented group (C+P+L). Another study from this group illustrated that the co-ingestion of protein, leucine and carbohydrates increased muscle protein synthesis similarly in young and older men.[56] However, supplementation in the elderly may not always produce the desired results, as they tend to compensate (decrease) their total energy intake to account for the supplement.[57]

F. Leucine and Insulin Interaction

The interaction between amino acids and insulin in stimulating protein synthesis is not fully understood. If insulin secretion is blocked artificially, (concentrations ≥5μU/mL) leucine is no longer able to stimulate protein synthesis.[43,58] Hence, the effect of leucine is linked to insulin action. Under normal conditions, leucine intake alone produces a slight transient increase in insulin concentration.[43] Only a small amount of insulin is needed to facilitate the increases in protein synthesis by leucine. Increased insulin concentration does not seem to augment protein synthesis, but does aid protein accretion by decreasing protein breakdown.[58]

High physiological levels of amino acids can also induce insulin resistance in humans.[59] Specifically, the increased availability of amino acids is thought to impair the ability of insulin to reduce glucose production and the ability of the muscle to take up glucose. Increased insulin resistance can accelerate muscle loss[60] and ultimately result in Type 2 diabetes. Prolonged increased fat, glucose, and total calorie intake can induce insulin resistance as well. This partially explains why increased energy intake (regardless of source of macronutrient) has been implicated in obesity and its associated co-morbidities. To confound the issue, individuals with Type 2 diabetes who supplemented daily with amino acids tended to have improved glycemic control and decreased HbA1c levels.[61] The etiology of Type 2 diabetes from a dietary intake standpoint is still under investigation.

While carbohydrate ingestion in combination with protein has been shown to enhance net protein balance in young adults,[62,63] the opposite has been observed in older adults.[46] The addition of carbohydrates to a protein meal in healthy older nondiabetic individuals actually blunted the anabolic response, resulting in a less positive net protein state.[46,64] It has been suggested that muscle protein synthesis in the elderly is at least somewhat resistant to the anabolic action of insulin even when glucose metabolism is not apparently altered.[65] Thus, the anabolic response to mixed meals (carbohydrates and protein) seems reduced in older adults.

It has been suggested that very low carbohydrate intake with higher protein intake could enhance the muscle mass of older adults. Increasing protein intake to 35% of total caloric intake and decreasing carbohydrate intake to approximately 5% increases fractional synthesis rate, which is positively associated with strength; thereby maintaining muscle mass in healthy young adults.[66] In that study, muscle protein synthesis was increased and muscle tissue loss was not observed in those consuming a low-carbohydrate diet while in energy balance. The insulin level of the individuals remained low, which may be beneficial for older adults. Longitudinal clinical trials in middle-aged and older adults are needed to determine if this strategy is realistic, beneficial, and healthy.

G. Pattern of Protein Ingestion

Both total daily intake and the amount of amino acids ingested per meal can affect retention of skeletal muscle mass. Two examples of patterns of protein intake would be ingesting up to 80% of dietary protein in one meal (pulse method) or distributing dietary protein throughout the day (spread method). Increasing the daily protein intake in elderly women from 0.75 to 1.05 g/kg/d increased nitrogen retention regardless of ingestion patterns. However, consuming 80% of the dietary protein intake at one meal (pulse method) resulted in greater lean mass and nitrogen retention, as shown by nitrogen balance and fat-free mass analysis. Some of the subjects in the spread feeding groups lost fat-free mass during the trial, with the pulse-feeding group maintaining fat-free mass.[67] The increased amount of amino acids exposed the aged muscle to greater leucine content, which likely enhanced muscle protein synthesis. Increasing the protein content of each meal may benefit fat-free body mass retention even further. The spread group was consuming up to 22 grams of protein spread over four meals. The pulse group ingested approximately 56 grams of protein at the noon meal.

Middle-aged and older adults who are consuming near or below the current RDA for protein would likely see benefits from adopting a strategic protein eating pattern. First, if they choose not to increase protein intake, they should ingest at least 25 grams of quality protein in two separate meals to ensure adequate leucine content. They may benefit further from ingesting all 56 grams (RDA for protein for a 70-kg individual) at one midday meal using the data from Arnal et al.[67] However, a theoretically better method would be to increase protein intake so that each of five meals contains at least 25 g of high-quality protein to theoretically maximize protein synthesis throughout the day.

IV. PROTEIN AND EXERCISE

A. Protein and Exercise Response

The amount of muscle mass of a healthy young to middle-aged person remains relatively unchanged, assuming adequate diet and level of physical activity (in the absence of either exercise or a muscle wasting condition). An acute bout of resistance exercise has a relatively large positive effect on the rate of muscle protein synthesis and protein breakdown.[68–71] This effect is dependent on many factors, including intensity, duration, mode of exercise, muscles stressed during the exercise bout, age of the individual, training status, and nutritional status of the individual both before and after the exercise bout. The increase in muscle protein synthesis can last up to 36–48h after the exercise bout.[68,70,71] While the increase in muscle protein breakdown is of less magnitude than the synthesis, muscle is still lost in the absence of adequate protein and total energy intake.[35,68,70–74] The combination of adequate total energy and protein intake with sufficient resistance training leads to muscle-mass accretion over time. Additionally, training status affects the amount of increase in muscle protein synthesis an individual experiences in response to a training bout.[6,70,71,74–76]

B. Protein Needs and Exercise

Dr. Peter Lemon has conducted numerous studies and literature reviews regarding the protein needs of athletes,[77–91] with many of these studies suggesting that amino acid oxidation increases with exercise. This led to the notion that athletes have greater protein needs than the general sedentary population.[89] The typical endpoint of these studies was the nitrogen balance of the subjects without accounting for athletic performance or strength.[8] However, using isotopic tracers, it has been shown that leucine oxidation increases with exercise,[8,87,92] potentially through its increased use as a fuel source in the exercising muscle. For protein needs to ultimately increase, greater amino acid oxidation during exercise cannot be compensated for after the exercise bout by the metabolic systems. However, some studies have shown that, while exercise increases amino acid (leucine) oxidation, 24 h leucine balance was the same between a moderate and high protein intake.[93,94]

There is evidence that training may actually increase protein efficiency. Studies have shown that endurance exercise makes protein metabolism more efficient, but some researchers feel that the exercise intensities and volume of exercise in these studies was not sufficient to induce the increased protein needs.[8] Two studies by Phillips et al.[71,76] have shown that training actually decreases protein needs for maintenance of body mass.

A key point is maintenance of body mass versus accretion of lean body mass. A positive nitrogen state must be achieved to attain an accretion of lean body mass. A study by Burke,[8,95] compared weightlifters fed either 1.2 or 2.1 g/kg/d. The group with the higher protein intake gained more lean mass. A study by Lemon et al.[90] examined the effects of either a supplement containing 2.62 g protein/kg or an isocaloric supplement containing 1.35 g protein/kg. The subjects also resistance trained for 1.5 h/d, 6 d/wk for 1 month. The results of the study indicated that while protein needs are increased, extra protein does not have an additive effect on muscle mass or strength gains over the 1 month period. The suggested intake posed by Lemon were that strength or speed athletes consume 1.2–1.7 g protein/kg/d and endurance athletes consume 1.2–1.4 g protein/kg/d.[79] Overall, it would appear that athletes could benefit from moderate increases in dietary protein, assuming this increase does not compromise performance via a suboptimal carbohydrate or energy intake.

C. Timing of Protein Intake with Exercise

The timing of protein ingestion in relation to a resistance exercise bout is an important determinant of the amount of muscle protein that can be attained, especially in older adults. In young adults, it appears that attaining a positive net protein state is possible by ingesting protein up to 3 h after the exercise bout.[37] However, older muscle appears to need an adequate protein dose immediately after exercise to elicit an increase in muscle protein accretion.[96] The results of this study suggest that aging muscle responds differently from its younger counterpart to amino acid provision. Studies are needed to test the suggested higher dose of essential amino acids (10 g) with mixed meals administered up to 3 h after resistance exercise in older adults.

V. ENERGY BALANCE

A. Protein and Energy State

Energy balance plays a crucial role in the maintenance of lean body mass. A negative energy state results in the loss of body mass while a positive energy state promotes mass gain. Whether body mass loss comes from fat tissue or lean tissue is highly dependent on dietary protein intake and mode of exercise.

B. Positive Energy State

Evidence suggests that total energy intake is more important for nitrogen balance than total dietary protein intake.[8] It is possible to gain lean body mass on a relatively low protein intake as long as total energy intake is sufficiently greater than energy expenditure.[8] Whether a lower protein intake, in light of excess total energy intake, is simply an adequate approach or the optimal approach is still under debate.

C. Negative Energy State

While a healthy lifestyle including exercise and healthy diet are critical for healthy living, many adults are concerned and sometimes obsessed with what their scale says they weigh. A negative energy state is critical for the loss of body mass. Ideally, most, if not all, of the intentional loss of body mass should come from fat mass while preserving lean body mass (especially organs and skeletal muscle). Evidence is mounting that a higher-protein diet in combination with resistive exercise is the best method to lose body fat while preserving metabolically active skeletal muscle.[8,97–100] The maintenance of skeletal muscle mass with weight loss is important due to the maintenance of basal metabolic rate. Approximately every 10 kg difference in lean body mass translates to a 100 kcal/d difference in total caloric need.[1] Additionally, muscle protein synthesis requires energy, and resistance exercise and higher protein intakes increase muscle protein synthesis.[65] Another variable pertinent to this discussion is the thermic effect of food,[101] which tends to decrease when consuming less energy to reduce weight (unless energy expenditure increases enough). Thus, the combination of these factors can aid in weight loss and maintenance of lean mass.

A study conducted by Layman et al.[100] examined the effects of diet alone or diet and exercise on body composition while consuming a hypocaloric diet. The four groups of middle-aged women (BMI of 33; n = 12) consumed the hypocaloric diet for 4 months. The higher-protein (102 g/kg/d) with exercise group did not "lose" any lean body mass, while body fat decreased by approximately 9 kg.[100] Additionally, both higher-protein groups decreased dietary fat intake during the feeding period from baseline. While the other groups decreased body fat, they also "lost" lean tissue. In another study, Demling et al.[102] examined the effects of casein or whey on body composition and strength measures during 12 weeks of hypocaloric, high-protein diets with resistance training in overweight police officers. Both the whey and casein groups decreased weight and gained lean mass while on a hypocaloric diet. A study by Piatti et al.[103] suggests that a high-protein, hypoenergetic diet improves insulin sensitivity while conserving lean tissue. Conversely, the higher-carbohydrate diet decreased insulin sensitivity and did not spare lean body mass.

Middle-aged overweight—and sometimes obese—individuals tend to have greater lean mass due to the added "weight training" they are obligated to do on a daily basis. They may be able to use this lean tissue to their advantage during weight loss when consuming higher-protein diets. While in a negative energy state (e.g., a hypocaloric diet), protein needs increase, especially in the elderly.[15] The current RDA for protein is seemingly inadequate for maintaining muscle mass during greater energy deficits, as more protein tends to be metabolized for energy.

D. Bed Rest and Trauma

As we age, we are more likely to suffer from illnesses and injuries that result in hospital stays that may last for extended periods. Injury, illness, surgery, and trauma increase protein oxidation. Consuming the current RDA for protein in these situations often leads to a negative nitrogen state and loss of skeletal muscle mass. Even higher protein intakes are often not sufficient to stave off muscle loss during some extended periods of bed rest or recovery from severe trauma. Thus, it is important to increase or maintain skeletal muscle mass during middle age to ensure that adequate amounts are available during or following medically stressful situations such as trauma and extended bed rest. In fact, individuals with the lowest protein mass have the lowest survivorship during recovery from burns and cancer.[1] Additionally, falls resulting in a bone fracture can be catastrophic for those with low skeletal muscle mass, as they are least likely to walk again.[1]

Nonetheless, muscle mass and strength can be improved by increased availability of essential amino acids, as was observed in younger people confined to bed rest. [104] A study by Paddon-Jones[105] illustrated that the group consuming excess nitrogen in the form of essential amino acids during 28 days of bed rest maintained more muscle mass than the group not consuming this extra nitrogen.

VI. CONCERNS

A. Renal Function

Almost any time the topic of increased protein intake is raised, the concern will turn to renal function with the increased nitrogen metabolism. In a Department of Health report from 1991, it was stated that there is no conclusive evidence for harmful effects of excess dietary protein intake in healthy people.[13] In fact, there appears to be no evidence that higher protein intakes initiate renal disease.[106] However, patients with preexisting renal disease may experience further renal deterioration due to increased intraglomerular pressure and glomerular filtration rate. This increase in glomerular filtration is often a concern regarding aging, but has not been shown to be detrimental.[107] However, individuals with Type 2 diabetes and hypertension may not want to increase their protein intake too dramatically due to already increased kidney stress.[106]

B. Bone Density

Another unsupported concern with higher protein intakes is bone loss leading to osteoporosis. While increased dietary protein intake can increase calcium excretion, the higher phosphorous content of these higher-protein foods can decrease urinary calcium.[13] The detrimental effects of increased protein intake on calcium do not appear to manifest until very high protein intakes.[108] Recent studies have, in fact, demonstrated the opposite—increased protein intakes are not detrimental to bone health and can actually benefit bone health during weight loss.[109–111]

C. Personal Barriers to Higher Protein Intakes

Optimal and even adequate protein intakes for middle-aged and older adults may be more difficult because of the cost of nutrient-dense and healthy foods and preconceived notions regarding saturated fat and cholesterol. While animal proteins have a high biological value and contain a large proportion of essential amino acids and leucine, they are more expensive than many lower-protein and convenience foods, which often contain increased amounts of refined carbohydrates or high fat (e.g., pastries, chips, cookies, etc.). Additionally, as adults age, their ability to chew and swallow some foods may be reduced. Outside of dysphagia therapy, a potential solution using whole foods would be increased milk or egg consumption as a means to obtain quality nonmeat proteins. It is often recommended that proteins for all adults should come primarily from high-quality lower fat sources of protein. Some examples include lean meats (including beef), chicken breasts, egg whites with some yolk, fish, milk, and whey. These high-quality protein sources tend to be low in fat and have a high proportion of leucine and other essential amino acids. They often have less total fat than some highly processed carbohydrates and fried foods.

VI. CONCLUSIONS

Dietary protein intake among middle-aged adults will likely affect an amount of lean tissue mass in older adulthood. The current RDA for protein has been shown to be inadequate to maintain skeletal muscle mass in aging adults and may not be sufficient to prevent sarcopenia. There is ample evidence that an increased dietary protein intake could benefit skeletal muscle mass and the metabolic health of middle-aged and older adults. An absolute protein intake of 125 g of quality lean protein spread over four or five meals appears to be a potential strategy to help reduce age-associated muscle loss. Higher protein intakes are also important while in a negative-energy state on a weight-reducing diet, having been shown to help maintain lean body mass, especially when combined with resistance training. Reduction of simple carbohydrates seems to improve overall body composition and retention of lean mass in middle-aged and older adults. While there needs to be more research regarding separating carbohydrate intake from protein intake, it may be beneficial to the overall rate of protein synthesis in older adults. Overall, in healthy middle-aged and older adults, there are no established reasons that a modest increase in dietary protein intake should be avoided, yet there is clear evidence that this type of dietary change can be beneficial.

REFERENCES

1. Wolfe, R.R., The underappreciated role of muscle in health and disease, *Am. J. Clin. Nutr.* 84, 475–82, 2006.
2. Boirie, Y., Dangin, M., Gachon, P., Vasson, M.P., Maubois, J.L., and Beaufrere, B., Slow and fast dietary proteins differently modulate postprandial protein accretion, *Proc. Natl. Acad. Sci. USA.* 94, 14930–5, 1997.
3. Dangin, M., Boirie, Y., Garcia-Rodenas, C., Gachon, P., Fauquant, J., and Callier, P., et al., The digestion rate of protein is an independent regulating factor of postprandial protein retention, *Am. J. Physiol. Endocrinol. Metab.* 280, E340–8, 2001.
4. Bohe, J., Low, A., Wolfe, R.R., and Rennie, M.J., Human muscle protein synthesis is modulated by extracellular, not intramuscular amino acid availability: A dose–response study, *J. Physiol.*. 552, 315–24, 2003.
5. Bohe, J., Low, J.F., Wolfe, R.R., and Rennie, M.J., Latency and duration of stimulation of human muscle protein synthesis during continuous infusion of amino acids, *J. Physiol.* 532, 575–9, 2001.
6. Phillips, S.M., Hartman, J.W., and Wilkinson, S.B., Dietary protein to support anabolism with resistance exercise in young men, *J. Am. Coll. Nutr.* 24, 134S–9S, 2005.
7. Price, G.M., Halliday, D., Pacy, P.J., Quevedo, M.R., and Millward, D.J., Nitrogen homeostasis in man: Influence of protein intake on the amplitude of diurnal cycling of body nitrogen, *Clin. Sci. (Lond.).* 86, 91–102, 1994.
8. Tipton, K.D. and Wolfe, R.R., Protein and amino acids for athletes, *J. Sports Sci.* 22, 65–79, 2004.
9. Tome, D. and Bos, C., Dietary protein and nitrogen utilization, *J. Nutr.* 130, 1868S–73S, 2000.
10. Rand, W.M., Pellett, P.L., and Young, V.R., Meta-analysis of nitrogen balance studies for estimating protein requirements in healthy adults, *Am. J. Clin. Nutr.* 77, 109–127, 2003.

11. Institute of Medicine, *Dietary Reference Intakes for Energy, Carbohydrate, Fiber, Fat, Fatty Acids, Cholesterol, Protein, and Amino Acids,* National Academies Press, Washington, DC, 2005, pp. 589–768.
12. Campbell, W.W., Trappe, T.A., Wolfe, R.R., and Evans, W.J., The recommended dietary allowance for protein may not be adequate for older people to maintain skeletal muscle, *J. Gerontol. A Biol. Sc.i Med. Sci.* 56, M373–80, 2001.
13. Millward, D.J., Optimal intakes of protein in the human diet, *Proc. Nutr. Soc.* 58, 403–13, 1999.
14. Munro, H.N., Suter, P.M., and Russell, R.M., Nutritional requirements of the elderly, *Annu. Rev. Nutr.* 7, 23–49, 1987.
15. Evans, W.J., Protein nutrition, exercise and aging, *J. Am. Coll. Nutr.* 23, 601S–9S, 2004.
16. Castaneda, C., Charnley, J.M., Evans, W.J., and Crim, M.C., Elderly women accommodate to a low-protein diet with losses of body cell mass, muscle function, and immune response, *Am. J. Clin. Nutr.* 62, 30–9, 1995.
17. Castaneda, C., Dolnikowski, G.G., Dallal, G.E., Evans, W.J., and Crim, M.C., Protein turnover and energy metabolism of elderly women fed a low-protein diet, *Am. J. Clin. Nutr.* 62, 40–8, 1995.
18. Roberts, S.B., Young, V.R., Fuss, P., Heyman, M.B., Fiatarone, M., and Dallal, G.E., et al., What are the dietary energy needs of elderly adults? *Int. J. Obes. Relat. Metab. Disord.* 16, 969–76, 1992.
19. Bos, C., Metges, C.C., Gaudichon, C., Petzke, K.J., Pueyo, M.E., and Morens, C., et al., Postprandial kinetics of dietary amino acids are the main determinant of their metabolism after soy or milk protein ingestion in humans, *J. Nutr.* 133, 1308–15, 2003.
20. Luiking, Y.C., Deutz, N.E., Jakel, M., and Soeters, P.B., Casein and soy protein meals differentially affect whole-body and splanchnic protein metabolism in healthy humans, *J. Nutr.* 135, 1080–7, 2005.
21. Fouillet, H., Gaudichon, C., Bos, C., Mariotti, F., and Tome, D., Contribution of plasma proteins to splanchnic and total anabolic utilization of dietary nitrogen in humans, *Am. J. Physiol. Endocrinol. Metab.* 285, E88–97, 2003.
22. Mariotti, F., Huneau, J.F., Mahe, S., and Tome, D., Protein metabolism and the gut, *Curr. Opin. Clin. Nutr. Metab. Care* 3:45–50, 2000.
23. Waterlow, J.C., Whole-body protein turnover in humans–Past, present, and future, *Annu. Rev. Nutr.* 15:,57–92, 1995.
24. Morens, C., Bos, C., Pueyo, M.E., Benamouzig, R., Gausseres, N., and Luengo, C., et al., Increasing habitual protein intake accentuates differences in postprandial dietary nitrogen utilization between protein sources in humans, *J. Nutr.* 133, 2733–40, 2003.
25. Volpi, E., Mittendorfer, B., Wolf, S.E., and Wolfe, R.R., Oral amino acids stimulate muscle protein anabolism in the elderly despite higher first-pass splanchnic extraction, *Am. J. Physiol.* 277, E513–520, 1999.
26. Bohe, J. and Rennie, M.J., Muscle protein metabolism during hemodialysis, *J. Ren. Nutr.* 16, 3–16, 2006.
27. Fouillet, H., Gaudichon, C., Mariotti, F., Bos, C., Huneau, J.F., and Tome, D., Energy nutrients modulate the splanchnic sequestration of dietary nitrogen in humans: A compartmental analysis, *Am. J. Physiol. Endocrinol. Metab.* 281, E248–60, 2001.
28. Elliot, T.A., Cree, M.G., Sanford, A.P., Wolfe, R.R., and Tipton, K.D., Milk ingestion stimulates net muscle protein synthesis following resistance exercise, *Med. Sci. Sports Exerc.* 38, 667–74, 2006.
29. Wolfe, R.R., Regulation of muscle protein by amino acids, *J. Nutr.* 132, 3219S–24S, 2002.

30. Miller, S.L., Tipton, K.D., Chinkes, D.L., Wolf, S.E., and Wolfe, R.R., Independent and combined effects of amino acids and glucose after resistance exercise, *Med. Sci. Sports Exerc.* 35, 449–55, 2003.
31. Bennet, W.M., Connacher, A.A., Scrimgeour, C.M., Jung, R.T., and Rennie, M.J., Euglycemic hyperinsulinemia augments amino acid uptake by human leg tissues during hyperaminoacidemia, *Am. J. Physiol.* 259, E185–94, 1990.
32. Bennet, W.M., Connacher, A.A., Scrimgeour, C.M., and Rennie, M.J., The effect of amino acid infusion on leg protein turnover assessed by L–[15N]phenylalanine and L–[1–13C]leucine exchange, *Eur. J. Clin. Invest.* 20, 41–50, 1990.
33. Cheng, K.N., Dworzak, F., Ford, G.C., Rennie, M.J., and Halliday, D., Direct determination of leucine metabolism and protein breakdown in humans using L–[1–13C, 15N]–leucine and the forearm model, *Eur. J. Clin. Invest.* 15, 349–54, 1985.
34. Rennie, M.J., Bohe, J., and Wolfe, R.R., Latency, duration and dose response relationships of amino acid effects on human muscle protein synthesis, *J. Nutr.* 132, 3225S–7S, 2002.
35. Tipton, K.D., Ferrando, A.A., Phillips, S.M., Doyle, D., Jr., and Wolfe, R.R., Postexercise net protein synthesis in human muscle from orally administered amino acids, *Am. J. Physiol.* 276, E628–34, 1999.
36. Borsheim, E., Tipton, K.D., Wolf, S.E., and Wolfe, R.R., Essential amino acids and muscle protein recovery from resistance exercise, *Am. J. Physiol. Endocrinol. Metab.* 283, E648–57, 2002.
37. Rasmussen, B.B., Tipton, K.D., Miller, S.L., Wolf, S.E., and Wolfe, R.R., An oral essential amino acid-carbohydrate supplement enhances muscle protein anabolism after resistance exercise, *J. Appl. Physiol.* 88, 386–92, 2000.
38. Tipton, K.D., Gurkin, B.E., Matin, S., and Wolfe, R.R., Nonessential amino acids are not necessary to stimulate net muscle protein synthesis in healthy volunteers, *J. Nutr. Biochem.* 10, 89–95, 1999.
39. Smith, K., Reynolds, N., Downie, S., Patel, A., and Rennie, M.J., Effects of flooding amino acids on incorporation of labeled amino acids into human muscle protein, *Am. J. Physiol.* 275, E73–8, 1998.
40. Alvestrand, A., Hagenfeldt, L., Merli, M., Oureshi, A., and Eriksson, L.S., Influence of leucine infusion on intracellular amino acids in humans, *Eur. J. Clin. Invest.* 20, 293–8, 1990.
41. Smith, K., Barua, J.M., Watt, P.W., Scrimgeour, C.M., and Rennie, M.J., Flooding with L-[1-13C]leucine stimulates human muscle protein incorporation of continuously infused L-[1-13C]valine, *Am. J. Physiol.* 262, E372–6, 1992.
42. Kimball, S.R. and Jefferson, L.S., Regulation of protein synthesis by branched-chain amino acids, *Curr. Opin. Clin. Nut.r Metab. Care* 4, 39–43, 2001.
43. Kimball, S.R. and Jefferson, L.S., Signaling pathways and molecular mechanisms through which branched-chain amino acids mediate translational control of protein synthesis, *J. Nutr.* 136, 227S–31S, 2006.
44. Paddon-Jones, D., Sheffield-Moore, M., Zhang, X.J., Volpi, E., Wolf, S.E., and Aarsland, A., et al., Amino acid ingestion improves muscle protein synthesis in the young and elderly, *Am. J. Physiol. Endocrinol. Metab.* 286, E321–8, 2004.
45. Cuthbertson, D., Smith, K., Babraj, J., Leese, G., Waddell, T., and Atherton, P., et al., Anabolic signaling deficits underlie amino acid resistance of wasting, aging muscle, *FASEB J.* 19, 422–4, 2005.
46. Volpi, E., Mittendorfer, B., Rasmussen, B.B.. and Wolfe, R.R., The response of muscle protein anabolism to combined hyperaminoacidemia and glucose-induced hyperinsulinemia is impaired in the elderly, *J. Clin. Endocrinol. Metab.* 85, 4481–90, 2000.

47. Volpi, E., Sheffield-Moore, M., Rasmussen, B.B., and Wolfe, R.R., Basal muscle amino acid kinetics and protein synthesis in healthy young and older men, *JAMA* 286, 1206–12, 2001.
48. Yarasheski, K.E., Zachwieja, J.J., and Bier, D.M., Acute effects of resistance exercise on muscle protein synthesis rate in young and elderly men and women, *Am. J. Physiol.* 265, E210–4, 1993.
49. Katsanos, C.S., Kobayashi, H., Sheffield-Moore, M., Aarsland, A., and Wolfe, R.R., Aging is associated with diminished accretion of muscle proteins after the ingestion of a small bolus of essential amino acids, *Am. J. Clin. Nutr.* 82, 1065–73, 2005.
50. Metter, E.J., Lynch, N., Conwit, R., Lindle, R., Tobin, J., and Hurley, B., Muscle quality and age: Cross-sectional and longitudinal comparisons, *J. Gerontol. A Biol. Sci. Med. Sci.* 54, B207–8, 1999.
51. Dreyer, H.C. and Volpi, E., Role of protein and amino acids in the pathophysiology and treatment of sarcopenia, *J. Am. Coll. Nutr.* 24, 140S–5S, 2005.
52. Katsanos, C.S., Kobayashi, H., Sheffield-Moore, M., Aarsland, A. and Wolfe, R.R., A high proportion of leucine is required for optimal stimulation of the rate of muscle protein synthesis by essential amino acids in the elderly, *Am. J. Physiol. Endocrinol. Metab.* 291, E381–7, 2006.
53. Paddon-Jones, D., Sheffield-Moore, M., Katsanos, C.S., Zhang, X.J. and Wolfe, R.R., Differential stimulation of muscle protein synthesis in elderly humans following isocaloric ingestion of amino acids or whey protein, *Exp. Gerontol.* 41, 215–9, 2006.
54. Rieu, I., Balage, M., Sornet, C., Giraudet, C., Pujos, E., and Grizard, J., et al., Leucine supplementation improves muscle protein synthesis in elderly men independently of hyperaminoacidaemia, *J. Physiol.* 575, 305–15, 2006.
55. Koopman, R., Wagenmakers, A.J., Manders, R.J., Zorenc, A.H., Senden, J.M., and Gorselink, M., et al., Combined ingestion of protein and free leucine with carbohydrate increases postexercise muscle protein synthesis in vivo in male subjects, *Am. J. Physiol. Endocrinol. Metab.* 288, E645–53, 2005.
56. Koopman, R., Verdijk, L., Manders, R.J., Gijsen, A.P., Gorselink, M., Pijpers, E., Wagenmakers, A.J. and van Loon, L.J., Co-ingestion of protein and leucine stimulates muscle protein synthesis rates to the same extent in young and elderly lean men, *Am. J. Clin. Nutr.* 84,623–32, 2006.
57. Timmerman, K.L. and Volpi, E., Amino acid metabolism and regulatory effects in aging, *Curr. Opin. Clin. Nut.r Metab. Care* 11, 45–9, 2008.
58. Rennie, M.J., Bohe, J., Smith, K., Wackerhage, H. and Greenhaff, P., Branched-chain amino acids as fuels and anabolic signals in human muscle, *J. Nutr.* 136, 264S–8S, 2006.
59. Krebs, M., Krssak, M., Bernroider, E., Anderwald, C., Brehm, A., and Meyerspeer, M., et al., Mechanism of amino acid-induced skeletal muscle insulin resistance in humans, *Diabetes* 51, 599–605, 2002.
60. Wang, X., Hu, Z., Hu, J., Du, J., and Mitch, W.E., Insulin resistance accelerates muscle protein degradation: Activation of the ubiquitin-proteasome pathway by defects in muscle cell signaling, *Endocrinology* 147, 4160–8, 2006.
61. Solerte, S.B., Gazzaruso, C., Schifino, N., Locatelli, E., Destro, T., and Ceresini, G., et al., Metabolic effects of orally administered amino acid mixture in elderly subjects with poorly controlled type 2 diabetes mellitus, *Am. J. Cardiol.* 93, 23A–9A, 2004.
62. Borsheim, E., Cree, M.G., Tipton, K.D., Elliott, T.A., Aarsland, A., and Wolfe, R.R., Effect of carbohydrate intake on net muscle protein synthesis during recovery from resistance exercise. *J Appl Physiol.* 96:674–678, 2004.
63. Borsheim, E., Aarsland, A., and Wolfe, R.R. Effect of an amino acid, protein, and carbohydrate mixture on net muscle protein balance after resistance exercise, *Int. J. Sport Nut. Exer.c Metab.* 14, 255–71, 2004.

64. Guillet, C., Prod'homme, M., Balage, M., Gachon, P., Giraudet, C., and Morin, L., et al., Impaired anabolic response of muscle protein synthesis is associated with S6K1 dysregulation in elderly humans, *FASEB J.* 18, 1586–7, 2004.
65. Fujita, S. and Volpi, E., Amino acids and muscle loss with aging, *J. Nutr.* 136, 277S–280S, 2006.
66. Harber, M.P., Schenk, S., Barkan, A.L., and Horowitz, J.F., Effects of dietary carbohydrate restriction with high protein intake on protein metabolism and the somatotropic axis, *J. Clin. Endocrinol. Metab.* 90:, 175–81, 2005.
67. Arnal, M.A., Mosoni, L., Boirie, Y., Houlier, M.L., Morin, L., and Verdier, E., et al., Protein pulse feeding improves protein retention in elderly women, *Am. J. Clin. Nutr.* 69, 1202–8, 1999.
68. Biolo, G., Maggi, S.P., Williams, B.D., Tipton, K.D., and Wolfe, R.R., Increased rates of muscle protein turnover and amino acid transport after resistance exercise in humans, *Am. .J Physiol.* 268, E514–20, 1995.
69. Chesley, A., MacDougall, J.D., Tarnopolsky, M.A., Atkinson, S.A., and Smith, K., Changes in human muscle protein synthesis after resistance exercise, *J. Appl. Physiol.* 73, 1383–8, 1992.
70. Phillips, S.M., Tipton, K.D., Aarsland, A., Wolf, S.E., and Wolfe, R.R., Mixed muscle protein synthesis and breakdown after resistance exercise in humans, *Am. J. Physiol.* 273, E99–107, 1997.
71. Phillips, S.M., Tipton, K.D., Ferrando, A.A., and Wolfe, R.R., Resistance training reduces the acute exercise-induced increase in muscle protein turnover, *Am. J. Physiol.* 276, E118–24, 1999.
72. Biolo, G., Tipton, K.D., Klein, S., and Wolfe, R.R., An abundant supply of amino acids enhances the metabolic effect of exercise on muscle protein, *Am. J. Physiol.* 273, E122–9, 1997.
73. Trappe, T.A., Raue, U., and Tesch, P.A., Human soleus muscle protein synthesis following resistance exercise, *Acta Physiol. Scand.* 182, 189–96, 2004.
74. Wolfe, R.R. Skeletal muscle protein metabolism and resistance exercise. *J Nutr.* 136:525S–528S, 2006.
75. Kim, P.L., Staron, R.S. and Phillips, S.M., Fasted-state skeletal muscle protein synthesis after resistance exercise is altered with training, *J. Physiol.* 568, 283–290, 2005.
76. Phillips, S.M., Parise, G., Roy, B.D., Tipton, K.D., Wolfe, R.R., and Tamopolsky, M.A., Resistance-training-induced adaptations in skeletal muscle protein turnover in the fed state, *Can. J. Physiol. Pharmacol.* 80, 1045–53, 2002.
77. Lemon, P.W, Beyond the zone: Protein needs of active individuals, *J. Am. Coll. Nutr.* 19, 513S–21S, 2000.
78. Lemon, P.W., Do athletes need more dietary protein and amino acids? *Int. J. Sport Nutr.* 5 Suppl, S39–61, 1995.
79. Lemon, P.W., Effect of exercise on protein requirements, *J. Sports Sci.* 9, Spec No:53–70, 1991.
80. Lemon, P.W., Effects of exercise on dietary protein requirements, *Int. J. Sport Nutr.* 8, 426–47, 1998.
81. Lemon, P.W., Is increased dietary protein necessary or beneficial for individuals with a physically active lifestyle? *Nutr. Rev.* 54, S169–75, 1996.
82. Lemon, P.W., Protein and amino acid needs of the strength athlete, *Int. J. Sport Nutr.* 1, 127–45, 1991.
83. Lemon, P.W., Protein and exercise: Update 1987, *Med. Sci. Sports Exerc.* 19, S179–90, 1987.
84. Lemon, P.W., Protein requirements of soccer, *J. Sports Sci.* 12, Spec No. S17–22, 1994.

85. Lemon, P.W., Benevenga, N.J., Mullin, J.P. and Nagle, F.J., Effect of daily exercise and food intake on leucine oxidation, *Biochem. Med.* 33, 67–76, 1985.
86. Lemon, P.W., Berardi, J.M., and Noreen, E.E., The role of protein and amino acid supplements in the athlete's diet: Does type or timing of ingestion matter? *Curr. Sports Med. Rep.* 1, 214–21, 2002.
87. Lemon, P.W., Dolny, D.G., and Yarasheski, K.E., Moderate physical activity can increase dietary protein needs, *Can. J. Appl. Physiol.* 22, 494–503, 1997.
88. Lemon, P.W. and Nagle, F.J., Effects of exercise on protein and amino acid metabolism, *Med. Sci. Sports Exerc.* 13, 141–9, 1981.
89. Lemon, P.W. and Proctor, D.N., Protein intake and athletic performance, *Sports Med.* 12, 313–25, 1991.
90. Lemon, P.W., Tarnopolsky, M.A., MacDougall, J.D., and Atkinson, S.A., Protein requirements and muscle mass/strength changes during intensive training in novice bodybuilders, *J. Appl. Physiol.* 73, 767–75, 1992.
91. Lemon, P.W., Yarasheski, K.E. and Dolny, D.G., The importance of protein for athletes, *Sports Med.* 1, 474–84, 1984.
92. Tarnopolsky, M.A., Atkinson, S.A., MacDougall, J.D., Senor, B.B., Lemon, P.W., and Schwarcz, H., Whole body leucine metabolism during and after resistance exercise in fed humans, *Med. Sci. Sports Exerc.* 23, 326–33, 1991.
93. el-Khoury, A.E., Forslund, A., Olsson, R., Branth, S., Sjodin, A., and Andersson, A., et al., Moderate exercise at energy balance does not affect 24-h leucine oxidation or nitrogen retention in healthy men, *Am. J. Physiol.* 273, E394–407, 1997.
94. Forslund, A.H., Hambraeus, L., Olsson, R.M., El-Khoury, A.E., Yu, Y.M., and Young, V.R., The 24-h whole body leucine and urea kinetics at normal and high protein intakes with exercise in healthy adults, *Am. J. Physiol.* 275, E310–20, 1998.
95. Burke, D.G., Chilibeck, P.D., Davidson, K.S., Candow, D.G., Farthing, J., and Smith-Palmer, T., The effect of whey protein supplementation with and without creatine monohydrate combined with resistance training on lean tissue mass and muscle strength, *Int. J. Sport Nutr. Exerc. Metab.* 11, 349–64, 2001.
96. Esmarck, B., Andersen, J.L., Olsen, S., Richter, E.A., Mizuno, M., and Kjaer, M., Timing of postexercise protein intake is important for muscle hypertrophy with resistance training in elderly humans, *J. Physiol.* 535, 301–11, 2001.
97. Layman, D.K., Protein quantity and quality at levels above the RDA improves adult weight loss, *J. Am. Coll. Nutr.* 23, 631S–6S, 2004.
98. Layman, D.K. and Baum, J.I., Dietary protein impact on glycemic control during weight loss, *J. Nutr.* 134, 968S–73S, 2004.
99. Layman, D.K., Boileau, R.A., Erickson, D.J., Painter, J.E., Shiue, H., Sather, C., and Christou, D.D., A reduced ratio of dietary carbohydrate to protein improves body composition and blood lipid profiles during weight loss in adult women, *J. Nutr.* 133, 411–7, 2003.
100. Layman, D.K., Evans, E., Baum, J.I., Seyler, J., Erickson, D.J., and Boileau, R.A., Dietary protein and exercise have additive effects on body composition during weight loss in adult women, *J. Nutr.* 135, 1903–10, 2005.
101. Smith, E.M., Finn, S.G., Tee, A.R., Browne, G.J., and Proud, C.G., The tuberous sclerosis protein TSC2 is not required for the regulation of the mammalian target of rapamycin by amino acids and certain cellular stresses, *J. Biol. Chem.* 280, 18717–27, 2005.
102. Demling, R.H. and DeSanti, L., Effect of a hypocaloric diet, increased protein intake and resistance training on lean mass gains and fat mass loss in overweight police officers. *Ann Nutr. Metab.* 44, 21–9, 2000.
103. Piatti, P.M., Monti, F., Fermo, I., Baruffaldi, L., Nasser, R., and Santambrogio, G., et al., Hypocaloric high-protein diet improves glucose oxidation and spares lean body mass: comparison to hypocaloric high-carbohydrate diet, *Metabolism* 43, 1481–7, 1994.

104. Paddon-Jones, D., Sheffield-Moore, M., Urban, R.J., Sanford, A.P., Aarsland, A., Wolfe, R.R., and Ferrando, A.A., Essential amino acid and carbohydrate supplementation ameliorates muscle protein loss in humans during 28 days bedrest, *J. Clin. Endocrinol. Metab.* 89, 4351–8, 2004.
105. Paddon-Jones, D., Sheffield-Moore, M., Creson, D.L., Sanford, A.P., Wolf, S.E., Wolfe, R.R., and Ferrando, A.A., Hypercortisolemia alters muscle protein anabolism following ingestion of essential amino acids, *Am. J. Physiol. Endocrinol. Metab.* 284, E946–53, 2003.
106. Walser, M., Hill, S., and Ward, L., Progression of chronic renal failure on substituting a ketoacid supplement for an amino acid supplement, *J. Am. So.c Nephrol.* 2, 1178–85, 1992.
107. Brenner, B.M., Meyer, T.W., and Hostetter, T.H., Dietary protein intake and the progressive nature of kidney disease: The role of hemodynamically mediated glomerular injury in the pathogenesis of progressive glomerular sclerosis in aging, renal ablation, and intrinsic renal disease, *N. Engl. J. Med.* 307, 652–9, 1982.
108. Orwoll, E.S., Weigel, R.M., Oviatt, S.K., Meier, D.E., and McClung, M.R., Serum protein concentrations and bone mineral content in aging normal men, *Am. J. Clin. Nutr.* 46, 614–21, 1987.
109. Bowen, J., Noakes, M., and Clifton, P.M., Effect of calcium and dairy foods in high protein, energy-restricted diets on weight loss and metabolic parameters in overweight adults, *Int. J. Obes. (Lond.)* 29, 957–65, 2005.
110. Bowen, J., Noakes, M., and Clifton, P.M., A high dairy protein, high–calcium diet minimizes bone turnover in overweight adults during weight loss, *J. Nutr.* 134, 568–73, 2004.
111. Pannemans, D.L., Schaafsma, G., and Westerterp, K.R., Calcium excretion, apparent calcium absorption and calcium balance in young and elderly subjects: Influence of protein intake, *Br. J. Nutr.* 77, 721–9, 1997.

Section III

Vitamins

5 Fat-Soluble Vitamins

Maria Stacewicz-Sapuntzakis
and Gayatri Borthakur

CONTENTS

I. INTRODUCTION

The preceding chapters discussed macronutrients (carbohydrates, lipids, and proteins), which provide energy and substrates for constant rebuilding of the middle-aged body, as required by an active lifestyle. Humans also need many micronutrients in their diet, and an adequate supply of vitamins and minerals may be of crucial importance in affluent Western societies, where the abundance of high-calorie food causes a high prevalence of obesity and various health problems of middle age.[1] The diet of 30–60 year-old-people should not be energy-dense, but rich in micronutrients and fiber, which is optimal for our species. Humans evolved as hunters-gatherers, omnivores consuming meat, seafood, and plants (various fruits, vegetables, seeds, and nuts). With the introduction of agriculture, only about 12,000 years ago, starchy grains and tubers became the basis of the human diet, with a corresponding decline in the health of human populations.[2] Progressive developments in nutrition and medicine identified many important micronutrients and their role in maintaining health. Among them, the fat-soluble vitamins are distinguished by physical properties associated with low polarity, absorption requiring the presence of fat, specific transport modes, accumulation in the liver, adipose, and certain other tissues. While adequate intake of fat-soluble vitamins is undoubtedly necessary over the life span, the body can store enough of these micronutrients to prevent deficiency during long periods of low intake. On the other hand, excessive intake of vitamins A and D may result in dangerous toxicity.

All fat-soluble vitamins can be derived from terpenes, hydrocarbon compounds constructed of 5-carbon isoprene units. The only vitamin completely synthesized by the human body is vitamin D, from squalene, a triterpene intermediate in the cholesterol pathway. Vitamin A is derived from carotenoid plant pigments, a special class of tetraterpenes. Other fat-soluble vitamins (E, K) are produced only by plants and bacteria.

Despite certain similarities in chemical structure and physical properties, fat-soluble vitamins all have very different functions, which will be described in this chapter. Vitamin A is necessary for vision, growth, regeneration and reproduction; vitamin D maintains bone health through the regulation of calcium balance; vitamin E is the most important antioxidant, protecting lipids in cell structures and circulation; while vitamin K is required for normal blood clotting. All these vitamins are also implicated in prevention of chronic diseases, such as cancer and cardiovascular problems, which tend to develop in middle age, causing premature morbidity and mortality.

II. VITAMIN A

In animals, including humans, vitamin A is derived from ingested carotenoids, which possess at least one β-ionone ring. Carotenoid oxygenases, variously expressed by different human tissues, may produce vitamin A from carotenoid precursors, by central cleavage or eccentric splitting of long C_{40} molecules.[3] The resulting vitamin A aldehyde (retinal) contains one β-ionone ring and a tetraene side chain (C_{20}). Other forms of vitamin A include retinoic acid (from irreversible oxidation of the aldehyde), retinol, (product of reversible reduction) and retinyl esters of various long-chain fatty acids (Figure 5.1). Therefore, the dietary sources of vitamin A include provitamin A carotenoids (β-carotene, α-carotene, β-cryptoxanthin) and retinyl esters.[4] The former are found in many deeply colored fruits and vegetables, the latter in foods of animal origin, mainly dairy products, egg yolks and organ meats, like liver and kidney (Table 5.1). The bioavailability of vitamin A from plant sources is very limited and depends on the food matrix, presence of dietary fat, efficiency of absorption and conversion.[5,6] Recently introduced conversion factors state that β-carotene in plant food is converted only in a 12:1 ratio, and other provitamin A carotenoids in a 24:1 ratio. An updated vitamin A activity database uses the new term retinol activity equivalents (1 μg RAE = 2 μg retinol, or 12 μg β-carotene, or 24 μg other provitamin A carotenoids).[4] The new conversion factors decrease the share of plant-derived food in total vitamin A intake and explain the relatively low vitamin A status of strict vegetarians. However, supplemental β-carotene in oil or gelatin beadlets is so efficiently absorbed that its conversion factor is 2:1 (1 RAE = 2 μg supplemental β-carotene). Animal sources contain easily absorbed retinyl esters, which are also added to fortified foods (breakfast cereals, margarine, reduced-fat dairy products, egg substitute) and supplements. Unfortunately, the pharmaceutical industry still lists the content of vitamin A in International Units (1 IU = 0.3 μg retinol, or 0.6 μg β-carotene), adding together the contributions from retinyl esters (acetate or palmitate) and β-carotene, which is often included in multivitamins.

The absorption of carotenoids from plant sources requires breaking down cell walls, a difficult feat for humans who cannot digest cellulose. Various food preparation techniques (mashing, cooking, and the addition of fat) help to release carotenoids from the food matrix.[7,8] The released fraction may be incorporated into mixed

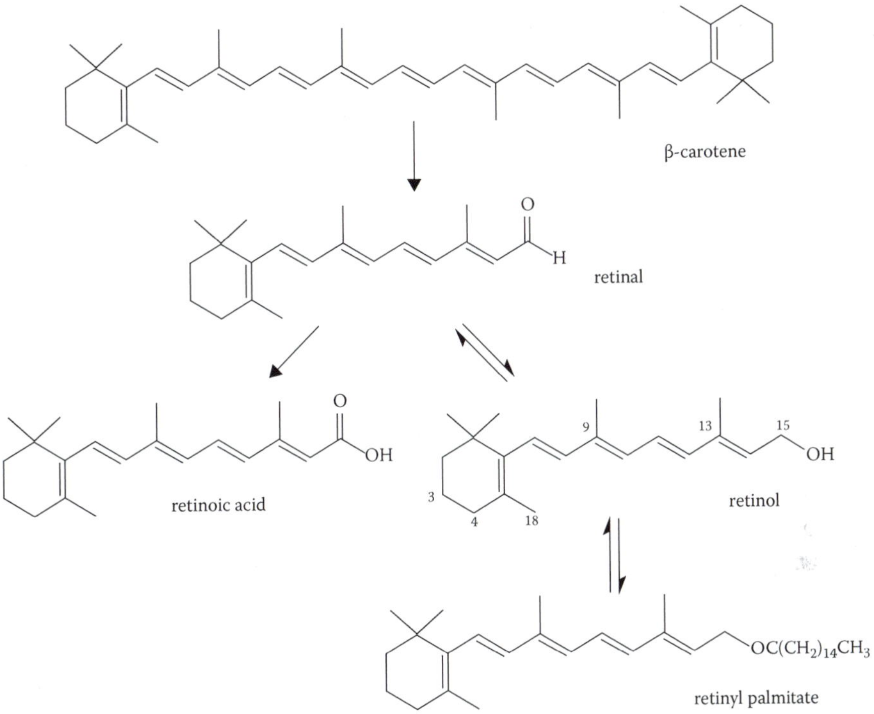

β-carotene

retinal

retinoic acid

retinol

retinyl palmitate

FIGURE 5.1 Structures of vitamin A and β-carotene.

micelles formed in the duodenum and small intestine when fat stimulates the secretion of bile, and then absorbed by enterocytes. Retinyl esters, together with triglycerides, undergo very efficient hydrolysis by pancreatic enzymes[9] and are easily absorbed by intestinal mucosa. Provitamin A carotenoids are partially converted to retinal by central cleavage carotenase (15,15'-oxygenase), and the resulting retinal is immediately reduced to retinol. The newly formed and the absorbed retinol are reestrified by fatty acids and transported in chylomicrons to the liver. The chylomicrons also carry the absorbed carotenoids, which were not directly converted to vitamin A, or are not its precursors. In the liver, hepatic cells hydrolyze retinyl esters and the resulting retinol is sent into plasma as a complex with retinol-binding protein and transthyretin. The liver maintains the level of circulating retinol at steady state by storing the excess in stellate cells as retinyl esters. All tissue cells contain cellular retinol-binding protein (CRBP) and retinoic acid-binding proteins (CRABP) in cytoplasm, as well as specific nuclear retinoid receptors (RAR and RXR), because of the retinoic acid role in regulation of gene expression.

The best known function of vitamin A is producing the visual impulse in the retina when 11-*cis*-retinal absorbs an incoming photon.[10] The rods, photoreceptors of the eye, contain the photosensitive pigment rhodopsin, a specific protein that forms a complex only with the *cis* configuration of retinal. The light isomerizes retinal to the all-*trans* form, which disengages from opsin and is immediately reduced to retinol.

TABLE 5.1

Food Sources of Vitamin A

Food, standard amount	Weight (g)	µg RAE
Fruits and nuts:		
Apricots, dry, 10 halves	35	63
Cantaloupe, cubes, 1 cup	160	270
Mango, raw, 1 cup	165	63
Papaya, raw, 1 cup	140	77
Tangerines, canned, 1 cup	252	2. 2
Peanut butter, smooth style, 1 tbsp	16	1. 4
Brazil nuts, 1 oz	28	1. 6
Vegetable oils:		
Sunflower oil, 1 tbsp	13. 6	5. 6
Cottonseed oil, 1 tbsp	13. 6	4. 8
Safflower oil, 1 tbsp	13. 6	4. 6
Canola oil, 1 tbsp	13. 6	2. 4
Peanut oil, 1 tbsp	13. 6	2. 1
Corn oil, 1 tbsp	13. 6	1. 9
Olive oil, 1 tbsp	13. 6	1. 9
Other fruits and vegetables:		
Turnip greens, cooked, 1/2 cup	82	2. 2
Spinach, cooked, ½ cup	85	1. 9
Tomato puree, canned, ½ cup	125	2. 5
Tomato sauce, canned, ½ cup	123	1. 7
Avocado, raw, 1 oz	28	0.75
Carrot juice, canned, 1 cup	236	2. 7
Seafood:		
Sardines, in oil, drained, 3 oz	85	1. 7
Blue crab, cooked, 3 oz	85	1. 6
Herring, pickled, 3 oz	85	1. 5
Breakfast cereal:		
Wheat germ, toasted, 2 tbsp	14	2. 3
Fortified ready-to-eat cereals, 1 cup	Varies by type of cereal	1. 6–13. 5

Adapted from: USDA National Nutrient Database for Standard Reference, Release 20. Agricultural Research Service. 2007. Nutrient Data Laboratory Home Page, http://www.ars.usda.gov/ba/bhnrc/ndl.

Retinal pigment epithelium of the eye contains a local pool of retinyl esters and enzymes, which convert all-*trans*-retinol to 11-*cis* retinol and oxidize it back to 11-*cis* retinal in the visual cycle of reactions. Vitamin A deficiency causes impaired dark adaptation, progressing to night blindness, a reversible condition cured by increased intake of retinol in supplements or animal products. Total irreversible blindness may result from the destruction of the cornea due to progressive xerophthalmia, which is caused by hyperkeratinization of epithelial tissues, including conjunctiva of the eye, skin, respiratory, and urogenital tracts. Retinoic acid, an oxidized form of vitamin A, is required for the proper differentiation and proliferation of cells, not only in epithelial tissues, but also in production of various classes of white blood cells, for normal immune function. The early symptoms of vitamin A deficiency include impaired dark adaptation, follicular hyperkeratosis and skin dryness, loss of appetite, and susceptibility to infection.

The estimated average requirement (EAR) for vitamin A is set at 500 μg/day for adult women, and 625 μg/day for adult men, based on average body weight and designed to maintain minimal acceptable liver reserves.[4] The recommended dietary allowance (RDA) exceeds EAR by 40%, since it is designed to supply the needs of 98% of targeted population, reaching 700 μg for adult women and 900 μg for adult men per day. At present, there is little vitamin A deficiency in the United States, especially in middle-aged people who have usually accumulated ample liver reserves. The evaluation of vitamin A intake among middle-aged subjects of the Third National Health and Nutrition Examination Survey (NHANES III, 1988–1994) found that the average total from food exceeded EAR, and more than 25% of adults consumed well above the RDA. Adult supplement users ingested on average additional 1300 μg RAE/day. Since these data were published, the use of supplements in the United States increased considerably at all socioeconomic levels among middle-aged adults.[11] The tolerable upper level (UL) of vitamin A intake is set at 3000 μg of retinol/ day, and includes only preformed vitamin A from animal sources and supplements, because large amounts of dietary provitamin A carotenoids do not cause the toxic effects of hypervitaminosis A. The UL may be reached and exceeded by some supplement users, especially males whose diet is also rich in animal products. In fact, about 5% of supplement users consumed more than the UL of vitamin A from supplements alone, and more than 1% of men 31–50 years old ingested such amounts just from food.

Long-term high intake of preformed vitamin A may cause serious adverse effects even at much lower doses of 1500 μg/day, which were associated with decreased bone mineral density (BMD) and increased risk of hip fractures in older men and women.[12] This amount may be contained in the pills of 25% supplement users, and in the food of more than 1% of middle-aged adults. Chronic toxicity, associated with doses larger than 30,000 μg/day causes liver abnormalities, joint and bone pain, redness and desquamation of skin, loss of hair, headache, irritability, and appetite loss. Acute poisoning increases cerebrospinal fluid pressure, causing severe headache, disorientation, blurred vision, vomiting, and loss of coordination. It may even be fatal.[13,14]

Vitamin A status cannot be assessed from intake but can be judged from a vitamin A profile of serum or plasma. High-performance liquid chromatography

(HPLC) after extraction of the fat-soluble vitamins with organic solvents allows the separation of retinol and individual retinyl esters.[15] The latter should not appear in the plasma of fasting subjects; their presence indicates recent intake of preformed vitamin A, a chronic excessive consumption with possible liver overload, or liver damage. Deficient vitamin A status is declared when plasma retinol falls below 0.7 μmol/L (20 μg/dL); marginal status includes the levels between 0.7 and 1.05 μmol/L (20–30 μg/dL) and indicates low liver stores.[16] Thenormal range in adults is regulated within 1.1–2.8 μmol/L (30–80 μg/dL). Higher levels are associated with increased bone fragility and indicate excessive intake of preformed vitamin A more reliably than dietary assessments. According to NHANES III (1988–1994) more than 10% of middle-aged men had too high serum retinol concentrations (above 2.8 μmol/L), and the same was found for women over 50 years of age.[17] The data show that only 5% of middle-age men were under 1.4 μmol/L, and 5% of women were below 1.15 μmol/L. The prevalence of high vitamin A intake increases with age and is confirmed by high serum levels of older people, precisely when their risk of osteoporosis is increased due to menopause and other age-related factors. Unfortunately, the assessment of fat-soluble vitamins in serum is not commonly utilized to ascertain nutritional status of middle-aged adults, and only the overt symptoms of deficiency or toxicity may alert medical personnel and dietitians to the necessity of drastic changes of diet or supplementation regime. In such cases, the liver stores of vitamin A may be checked directly in biopsy samples, or by indirect methods of isotope dilution, relative-dose response or modified-dose response.[18] The indirect methods measure vitamin A (stable isotope-labeled, retinol, or dehydroretinol, respectively) in blood samples after an oral dose administration.

The available studies indicate that the physical performance of middle-aged adults does not require increased doses of preformed vitamin A from food or supplements.[19] Even very strenuous exercise did not decrease plasma retinol levels in cyclists (170-km mountain stage).[20] After running a half-marathon, trained athletes had a significant 18% increase of plasma retinol, while their plasma volume decreased by only 6%.[21] It is possible that bouts of strenuous exercise may mobilize vitamin A from the liver and adipose tissue into circulation. However, long-term strenuous training may decrease plasma retinol, as observed in volunteers from the U. S. Marine Corps after 24 days in a cold environment.[22] Average loss of body weight in these volunteers was 5 kg, and their plasma retinol decreased significantly, from 1.7 to 1.4 μmol/L. Another group in the same study was taking antioxidant supplements (24 mg β-carotene/day, vitamin C and E, selenium, catechin, but not retinyl esters) and did not experience any change in plasma retinol. These results indicate increased utilization of vitamin A in conditions of sustained heavy physical labor, which may even be advantageous for healthy adults with large liver stores.

To prevent high accumulation of vitamin A and excessive liver stores, healthy middle-aged adults should limit their intake of preformed vitamin A from animal products and supplements, not to exceed EAR. Instead, carotenoid-rich foods, mainly fruits and vegetables, should be consumed in larger quantities because provitamin A carotenoids do not cause hypervitaminosis A, due to their limited absorption and low rate of conversion, regulated by the vitamin A status of the subject. High intakes may cause carotenemia, a harmless condition characterized by yellow color of plasma, skin and ovaries.[23] Low dietary intakes of provitamin A carotenoids are associated with higher risk of developing oesophageal and lung cancer.[24] Carotenoids are efficient antioxidants, and may prevent lipid peroxidation, thus decreasing oxidative stress and oxidative damage in inflammatory diseases. They increase tolerance of sunlight, protecting the skin against sunburn[25] and the eyes from developing cataracts and macular degeneration.[26] However, high-dose (15 mg/day and above) supplements of β-carotene are not advisable for smokers and alcohol drinkers, because large doses were found to increase the risk of lung and colorectal cancer in such subjects.[27,28] It is difficult to find multivitamin supplements without vitamin A activity, but some contain only β-carotene (100% of total vitamin A content) in a standard amount of 5000 IU, which corresponds to 3 mg β-carotene. That amount does not seem excessive, as it is easily available from food alone and about 25% of middle-aged Americans already consume as much in their diet. The optimal intake of provitamin A carotenoids may be as high as 6 mg/day for healthy, physically active adults,[29] which would provide most of their vitamin A needs and have other beneficial effects of decreased oxidative stress, enhanced immunity, and photoprotection for the eyes and skin.

III. VITAMIN D

The two major nutritional forms of vitamin D are cholecalciferol (vitamin D_3) generated in the skin of animals, and ergocalciferol (vitamin D_2) derived from yeasts, fungi, and microalgae. The precursor of vitamin D_3, 7-dehydrocholesterol, is a derivative of cholesterol produced in the liver and stored in the skin. Upon exposure to sunlight, 7-dehydrocholesterol in skin is converted to vitamin D_3. Therefore, vitamin D can be classified as both a vitamin and a steroid hormone. A substrate for vitamin D_2, the yeast sterol ergosterol, is converted to ergocalciferol by commercial irradiation with UVB rays. The synthesis and structures of vitamin D_2 and vitamin D_3 are presented in Figure 5.2. Until recently, the two vitamin D forms were considered equivalent, and vitamin D_2 has been used in most of the prescription formulations in North America. Either D_2 or D_3 were incorporated in multivitamins. However, a majority of the pharmaceutical companies have started to reformulate their supplements using vitamin D_3, because it has been demonstrated to be more potent than vitamin D_2 in raising and sustaining serum levels of circulatory vitamin D metabolite, 25-hydroxyvitamin D [25(OH)D], in both humans and nonhuman primates.[30–32] The equivalency of vitamin D_2 and D_3 is still a controversial issue. A recent report claims that D_2 is as effective as D_3 in maintaining both 25(OH)D and 1,25-dihydroxyvitamin D [1,25$(OH)_2$D] levels and bone health.[33]

Vitamin D_3 is present in only a few food sources such as egg yolks, fatty fish, fish liver oils, milk, and milk products (Table 5.2), while vitamin D_2 may occur only in wild mushrooms growing in sunlight.[34] Although sufficient skin exposure to sunlight can provide the required amount of the vitamin, many factors such as season, time of day, geographical location, heavy cloud cover, smog, clothing, and use of sunscreen can affect this natural synthesis of vitamin D_3. During the winter months (November through March) at latitudes above 37°, UVB rays do not reach the Earth, therefore vitamin D synthesis is minimal. Melanin pigment in the skin is the natural

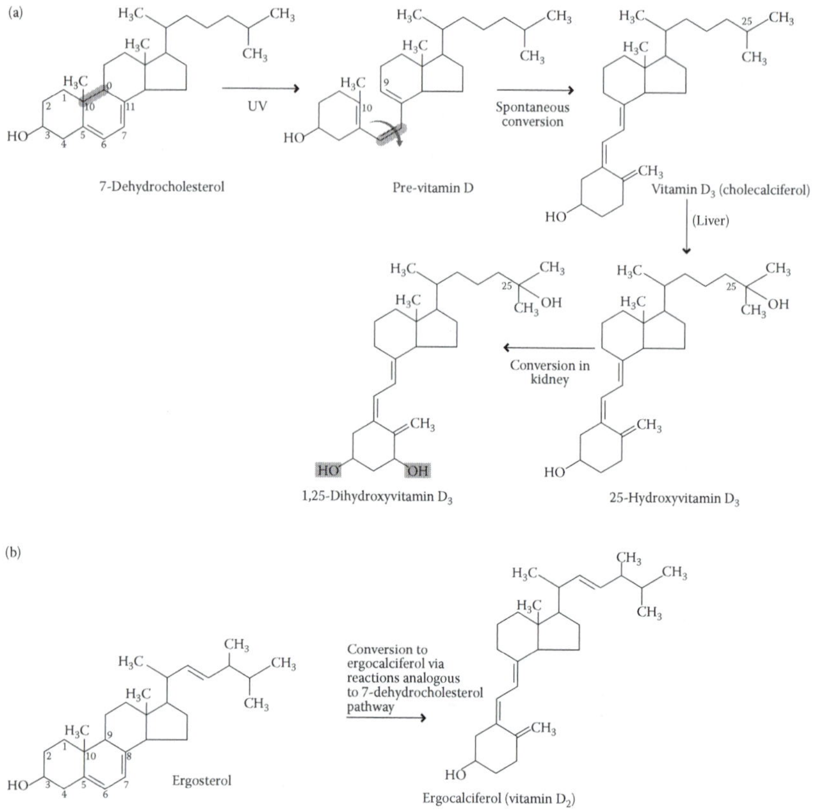

FIGURE 5.2 Structures and synthesis of two major forms of vitamin D.

sunscreen that can reduce vitamin D_3 synthesis by more than 90%, which makes many African American people with very dark skin chronically deficient in vitamin D. Aging is another important factor that significantly reduces natural synthesis of vitamin D. A 70-year-old person has only 25% of a young individual's efficiency to produce vitamin D naturally in the skin. People who do not get adequate sunlight for natural synthesis of vitamin D need to increase intake of vitamin D-rich or -fortified foods. Milk is the major food most commonly fortified with vitamin D due to its rich content of calcium and phosphorus, and fortification with vitamin D helps their absorption. Milk supply in the United States is fortified with 10 μg of vitamin D per quart, which is equivalent to 400 IU. One IU of vitamin D is defined as the activity of 0.025 μg of vitamin D_3, or 0.005 μg of 25(OH)D.[35] One cup of vitamin D-fortified milk supplies half of the adequate intake (AI) for adults between the ages of 30 and 50, or one fourth of the AI for adults between the ages of 51 and 70. Different foods are selected in other countries for vitamin D fortification. For example, margarine is fortified in Great Britain (1300–1600 IU/lb) and Germany (135 IU/lb), but not in the United States. Food manufacturers also add vitamin D to other products, such as infant formula, flour, ready-to-eat breakfast cereals, and bread.

TABLE 5.2

Food Sources of Vitamin D

Food, standard amount	Weight (g/mL)	Vitamin D per serving (IU)	Vitamin D per serving (μg)
Quaker Nutrition for Women Instant oatmeal, 1 packet	45	150	3. 8
General Mills, Cheerios, Yogurt Burst, 3/4 cup to 1 cup	30–50	60–100	1. 5-2. 5
Orange juice fortified, 8 oz.	236	94	2. 4
Soymilk, fortified, 8 oz.	236	100	2. 5
Milk, nonfat, reduced fat, and whole, vitamin D fortified, 8 oz.	236	94-123	2. 3-3. 1
Margarine, fortified, 1 tbsp	15	60	1. 5
Egg, 1 whole, fried	58	21	0.5
Egg, dried, 3. 5 oz.	100	188	4. 7
Cheese, Swiss, 1 oz.	28	12	0.3
Tuna fish, canned, 3 oz.	85	200	5
Cod liver oil, 1 tablespoon	15	1,360	34
Mackerel, canned, 3 oz.	85	214	5. 4
Mackerel, raw, 3. 5 oz.	99	357	8. 9
Sardines, canned, 3 oz.	85	231	5. 8
Sardines, canned in tomato sauce, 3 oz.	85	408	10.2
Pink salmon, canned, 3 oz.	85	530	13

Adapted from: USDA National Nutrient Database for Standard Reference, Release 20.

Insufficient cutaneous synthesis of vitamin D_3 to maintain adequate plasma concentration of 25(OH)D necessitates regular consumption of vitamin D-fortified foods or supplements. Pediatric multivitamin supplements usually contain 200–400 IU, and adult multivitamin supplements provide 400–1000 IU (10–25 μg) of vitamin D. Vitamin D is also combined with calcium, or present in fish oil supplements. The dose varies from 100–400 IU in calcium supplements, while fish oil supplements contain 135-400 IU of vitamin D.

Skin-synthesized vitamin D binds to vitamin D binding protein (DBP) in blood, also known as α-2-globulin, for its transport in the circulation. Ingested vitamin D (both D_2 and D_3) is solubilized within mixed micelles and incorporated into chylomicrons in the intestine. During transport in the lymphatic circulation, a major portion of vitamin D is released from the chylomicrons and taken up by the liver. Vitamin D binds to the DBP within the hepatocytes. The protein-bound vitamin D is released into the circulation for transport to the target tissues. Vitamin D, either formed in the skin or absorbed from dietary sources, is converted to its biologically active form, calcitriol [1,25$(OH)_2$D], in a two-step, hormonally controlled process. First, in the liver, it is hydroxylated in C-25 position to form the major circulatory metabolite

25(OH)D, or calcidiol. Serum levels of calcidiol reflect the amount of vitamin D produced in the skin or obtained from dietary sources. Most of the 25(OH)D is bound to DBP and enters the circulation for transport to the kidneys for a second hydroxylation in the renal tubule cells, where 25(OH)D is hydroxylated in C-1 position to form $1,25(OH)_2D$. Although kidneys are the primary site for calcitriol formation, a substantial amount is also formed in extrarenal tissues, such as placenta and brain. Calcitriol is released into the circulation and delivered to target cells, where it binds to the nuclear vitamin D receptor (VDR). The conversion of calcidiol to calcitriol is tightly controlled by parathyroid hormone (PTH), which activates 1-α-hydroxylase in the kidney and stimulates formation of $1,25(OH)_2D$. Low serum levels of phosphate also induce production of this key renal enzyme.

The major function of vitamin D is the mineralization of the skeleton. Both bone-forming cells (osteoblasts) and bone resorption cells (osteoclasts) are activated by vitamin D. Enhanced absorption of dietary calcium and phosphorus are essential for bone mineralization that is regulated by the vitamin D endocrine system, involving an interaction between calcitriol and parathyroid hormone. Calcitriol binds to the receptors in the nuclei of intestinal cells and stimulates production of calcium-binding protein, calbindin, which enhances the calcium uptake by intestinal cells. Calcium is then transported in the circulation to maintain the serum calcium level. Phosphorus absorption is also stimulated by calcitriol via increased activity of the enzyme alkaline phosphatase. Low serum calcium levels, induced by vitamin D deficiency, stimulate the parathyroid hormone, which activates the renal enzyme 1-α-hydroxylase to produce an increased amount of calcitriol. This results in bone resorption, as increased osteoclastic activity releases calcium from bones in order to maintain its normal serum level. Thus, the vitamin D endocrine system enhances the mobilization of calcium and phosphorus from bone and reabsorption of calcium in the kidney. Apart from bone mineralization, vitamin D is also essential for muscle contraction, transmission of nerve impulse, and other cellular functions, such as cell proliferation and differentiation.

Vitamin D deficiency is no longer considered just a common old-age health concern, but an epidemic in all age groups, including prepubertal children, adolescents, young and middle-aged adults. Osteoporosis and osteomalacia are the most common vitamin D deficiency symptoms in adults. Osteoporosis is a common metabolic bone disease characterized by poor bone mass and increased susceptibility to fractures. Initiated by long-term vitamin D deficiency combined with poor calcium status, it is the leading cause of bone fractures among the middle-aged and elderly population. According to the NIH Osteoporosis and Related Bone Diseases overview,[36] one in two women and one in four men over the age of 50 will suffer from an osteoporosis-related bone fracture in his or her lifetime, which may even result in death. About 20% of hip-fracture patients, aged 50 years and above, die within 1 year of incidence.[37] Osteoporosis-induced fractures affect four times more postmenopausal women than men of similar age, because a lack of estrogen after menopause facilitates bone mineral loss. Endocrine-related osteoporosis commonly occurs in postmenopausal women and castrated men, or it can be age related, occurring in both men and women after 60 years of age. Dietary vitamin D supplementation with or without calcium can lower the risk of bone fractures,[38] however, it is suggested that baseline vitamin D status and calcium intake may be important to produce a significant response to any supplementation.[39]

Osteomalacia, or adult rickets, is associated with bone aches and pains due to poor mineralization of the bone collagen matrix. It is common in women who are culturally prevented from exposing their skin to sunlight, and also in women who are continuously bearing and nursing children during their active reproductive years. Obesity is also highly associated with lower serum levels of 25(OH)D and higher incidence rate of bone fractures. Vitamin D deficiency significantly reduces dietary absorption of calcium (by 85–90%) and phosphorus (by 40%), resulting in poor bone health and reduced muscle strength in all age groups.[40] Vitamin D deficiency together with low calcium status produce a loss of skeletal bone mass at a rate of 0.25–0.5% per year in both young and middle-aged adults. Another serious vitamin D deficiency disorder is hypocalcaemia tetany, characterized by muscular weakness and convulsions due to insufficient supply of calcium to the nerves and muscles. It is also a major risk factor for increased frequency of falls and fractures.

Suboptimal serum vitamin D levels are prevalent among populations from around the world, including the industrialized nations in North America, Europe, and Australia. In Norway, middle-aged women (44–59 years) had decreased levels of serum 25(OH)D in the winter months.[41] Their vitamin D status was significantly associated with both the exposure to UVB radiation and vitamin D intake. NHANES III indicated a high prevalence of vitamin D deficiency, ranging from mild to severe, among women and the minority sections of 15,000 U.S. adult participants. Hispanic and African American men and women had significantly lower levels of serum vitamin D than white men and women.[42] Several studies indicate that suboptimal levels of vitamin D are widely prevalent among osteoporotic patients, especially postmenopausal women.[43]

Osteoporosis and bone fractures are associated with serum 25(OH)D concentrations below 75 nmol/L (30 ng/mL). A serum level of 25(OH)D below 50 nmol/L (20 ng/mL) is defined as vitamin D deficiency, associated with secondary hyperparathyroidism, increased bone resorption, decreased intestinal calcium absorption and BMD, increased risk of osteoporosis and bone fractures, and decreased leg function.[44] Serum levels of 25(OH)D between 52.5 and 72.5 nmol/L (21–29 ng/mL) are classified as vitamin D insufficiency.[45] Suggested safe levels of serum vitamin D are 80–100 nmol/L (32-40 ng/mL) for maximum calcium absorption and normal bone health. A regular consumption of 1000 IU of vitamin D_3 per day, or 50,000 IU every 2 weeks can maintain these levels, in total absence of cutaneous synthesis of vitamin D.[40]

The determination of individual vitamin D status requires an accurate measurement of plasma levels. A direct assay of the two common forms of vitamin D (D_2 and D_3) in plasma is not easy or practical due to their hydrophobic nature and very short half-life (24 h). Among vitamin D metabolites, 25(OH)D (major circulatory metabolite) and 1,25(OH)$_2$D (physiologically active metabolite) are the most significant for determination of vitamin D status. However, measurements of 1,25(OH)$_2$D are not very accurate since its plasma half-life is short (4–6 hours) and its levels are maintained tightly by the PTH stimulation of renal 1-α-hydroxylase enzyme to synthesize more calcitriol. Only during severe deficiency condition, when the substrate level is very low, is 1,25$(OH)_2$D depleted. Therefore, plasma level of DBP bound 25(OH)D is considered the most reliable biomarker,[46] since only 0.02–0.05% of it remains free in the circulation.[47] It has a long plasma half-life (2–3 weeks),[45] which permits the most accurate estimate of vitamin D status.

Unfortunately, the results reported by different laboratories for the same serum samples may differ widely due to variations in the methodologies and poor quality control. Some methods, like competitive protein binding with DBP and radioimmunoassay (RIA), overestimated the total 25(OH)D levels by recognizing other vitamin D metabolites.[45] Another RIA assay was found to have 100% specificity toward 25$(OH)D_3$ while it was only 75% specific for 25$(OH)D_2$. HPLC is the preferred assay method for vitamin D, because it separates and measures both forms of vitamin D. However, most clinicians and epidemiologists are interested in standardization of a simple method measuring total level of serum calcidiol [25$(OH)D_2$ plus 25$(OH)D_3$] to determine vitamin D status.[45,46]

Several studies found that the consumption of vitamin D in the United States is rather low in the adult population, ranging from 3.5 μg to 5 μg/day. The Food and Nutrition Board of Institute of Medicine recommended an AI of 200 IU (5 μg) per day for all adults 19–50 years old, and 400 IU (10 μg) per day for everyone 50–70 years old.[35] However, recent evidence indicates that, to maintain serum 25(OH)D level in the optimal range of >30 ng/mL (80 nmol/L), AI should be increased to 800–1000 IU (20–25 μg) per day when there is inadequate exposure to sunlight. A meta-analysis of primary prevention trials found that oral supplementation of vitamin D_3 at 700–800 IU per day, or 100,000 IU every 4 months, with or without calcium supplementation, could achieve serum 25(OH)D levels of 74 nmol/L and reduce significantly both hip and nonvertebral fracture risk.[48] A similar study concluded that an intake of 2.5 mg (100,000 IU) every 4 months could be recommended as a safe supplementary program to reduce the occurrence of osteoporotic fractures. A placebo-controlled longitudinal study on postmenopausal African American women reported that 50 μg (2000 IU) or more of vitamin D_3 supplementation per day could raise the serum vitamin D level to 50–75 nmol/L.[49] Recently, a risk assessment for oral consumption of vitamin D, conducted on all well designed human clinical trials, suggested that the current UL of 2000 IU (50 μg) per day[35] may be safely increased 5-fold, up to 10,000 IU (250 μg) per day for adults.[50]

However, vitamin D is very toxic in excessive dosages, potentially causing abnormal levels of calcium in the blood (hypercalcemia), which are associated with serious damaging effects such as calcification of soft tissues, including the heart, lungs, and kidneys. Hypercalcemia is manifested by early symptoms of decreased appetite, nausea, and weight loss, and if not treated, may result in death. Symptoms of vitamin D toxicity include headaches, weakness, constipation, excessive thirst and urination. Therefore, it is recommended that dietary intake should not exceed 250 μg (10,000 IU) per day.[50] Overexposure to sunlight does not cause hypervitaminosis, because continuous UV irradiation destroys excessive vitamin D_3 in the skin.[51]

Recently, questionnaire assessment of sunlight exposure is given much consideration. However, many factors can affect accuracy in quantifying cutaneous synthesis of vitamin D, such as wide variation in self-reports of personal sunlight exposure (use of sunscreen, clothing, amount of time under sunlight), and environmental UV exposure (season, cloud cover, time of the day, latitude).[52] Although a few reports indicate a low but statistically significant correlation between UV exposure and serum 25(OH)D,[53,54] the questionnaire method still lacks reliability and needs further standardization before it can be used to quantify vitamin D synthesized from sunlight exposure.[52]

Epidemiological studies suggest that high doses of vitamin D could prevent or eliminate several autoimmune diseases, such as rheumatoid arthritis, inflammatory bowel disease, and multiple sclerosis. Vitamin D is associated with better control of diabetes[51] and implicated in the prevention of other chronic diseases, such as cancer and cardiovascular diseases. High vitamin D intake is associated with a significant reduction in total mortality from any cause. A meta-analysis conducted on 18 previously published studies reported an increased risk of death from cancer, heart disease, and diabetes due to vitamin D deficiency. Individuals taking vitamin D supplements had a 7% lower risk of death than those who did not use any supplements.[55] People with high serum 25(OH)D levels had systolic and diastolic blood pressure 3.0 and 1.6 mm Hg lower, respectively, than people with levels below 40 nmol/L (16 ng/L).[56] An analysis of data from participants in the Framingham Offspring Study reported that individuals with serum levels of 25(OH)D below 15 ng/mL (<37.5 nmol/L) had a 62% higher risk of developing cardiovascular disease.[57] Even higher odds were found in the Health Professionals Follow-up Study, where men had more than twice the risk of heart attack at this low serum 25(OH)D level, compared with those above 30 ng/mL (>75 nmol/L).[58]

Observational studies report an inverse association between suboptimal vitamin D status and risk of cancer. A randomized placebo-controlled 4-year trial conducted in Nebraska reported that high intake of vitamin D reduced the rate of cancer incidence.[59] The subjects in the study were white women, 55 years of age and older, divided into three groups. One group received 1400–1500 mg of calcium supplements and 1100 IU of vitamin D_3, the second group received only calcium supplements, and the third group received a placebo. The group receiving vitamin D_3 supplements had a 60% reduction in cancer risk, while there were no statistically significant differences between the groups taking placebo and calcium supplements alone. The antiproliferative effect of calcitriol has been shown in *in vitro* studies of colon cancer cells.[60] The important role played by functional VDR in cancer prevention is indicated by recent animal studies. VDR null mice showed an increased rate of tumor growth in the mammary gland, epidermal, and lymphoid tissues, compared with the wild type mice, when carcinogenesis was induced by dimethylbenzanthracene (DMBA).[61] Similarly, topical application of DMBA on the skin of VDR and RXR null animals resulted in a higher incidence rate of skin cancer, compared with wild type animals.[62]

Prostate cancer is the leading cause of cancer death among men and its incidence rate is particularly high among African Americans, who are chronically deficient in vitamin D, and also in men living in high latitudes. The regulatory role of calcitriol in normal growth and differentiation of prostate cells was indicated by several *in vitro* and *in vivo* studies. Recently, population-based case control studies among middle-aged men reported a close association between polymorphisms in VDR genes and prostate cancer risk.[63,64]

A nested case-control study in Japan investigated the association between plasma 25(OH)D and risk of colorectal cancer. Low plasma vitamin D levels were associated with increased risk of rectal cancer in both men (OR 4.6; 95% CI 1.0–20) and women (OR 2.7; 95% CI 0.94–7.6).[65] Similar inverse associations between serum vitamin D and colorectal cancer mortality were observed in a prospective follow-up study based on the NHANES III survey in the United States. Serum vitamin D levels over 80 nmol/L, compared with levels below 50 nmol/L, were associated with a 72% reduction in the cancer mortality risk ($p<0.02$).[66] It was postulated that in North America a 50% reduction in colon cancer incidence would require an average intake of 2000 IU vitamin D per day. [67,68] Similar analysis of pooled data from observational studies indicates that a 50% reduction in breast cancer incidence may be achieved with 3500–4000 IU (75–100 μg) vitamin D per day, or 2000 IU (50 μg) vitamin D per day combined with moderate sun exposure.[69]

Even in healthy people, aging is associated with loss of muscle mass and bone density, but a regular exercise program combined with adequate intake of dietary calcium and vitamin D may prevent or slow down the process of bone loss. It is possible to increase bone density in middle age by following a varied program of exercise, including aerobics, high-impact sport activities, weight lifting, and resistance exercises. In Germany, a long-term exercise program was investigated to determine its effect on coronary heart disease, osteoporotic risk factors, and physical fitness parameters in postmenopausal women.[70] Both control and experimental groups were given calcium and vitamin D supplements, but only the experimental group exercised for 50 months. Maximum isometric strength and bone density significantly decreased in the control group, while both parameters were significantly increased in the experimental group. The results demonstrated that multipurpose high-intensity exercise programs are beneficial for postmenopausal women and therefore may be recommended as an alternative to hormone replacement therapy. However, another study reported that active non-athletic women, maintaining low- to moderate-intensity physical activity, had higher BMD than either sedentary or athletic women who had high-intensity training for competitive events.[71] Cycling, vigorous exercise, or sports were associated with higher levels of plasma 25(OH)D in most active women, while in men a similar but statistically insignificant trend was observed.[72] Vitamin D intake was low (2.1 μg/day) in older master athletes resulting in low serum levels of 25(OH)D.[73] However, even younger women may be at risk of bone fractures due to reduced BMD when strenuous exercising is not accompanied by optimal diet containing sufficient energy, vitamin D, and calcium. The female athletic triad (eating disorders, amenorrhea/oligomenorrhea, and decreased BMD) is receiving much attention, since the incidence of stress related fractures is increasing with the growing number of women in active sports programs.[74] A diet insufficient to meet the high calorie demand of a specific exercise training program results in a negative energy balance that stimulates the hypothalamus and reduces estrogen levels. A complex neuroendocrine adaptive condition is established, resulting in malfunction in the reproductive system. Low estrogen levels are further associated with reduced BMD and increase the risk of bone fractures.

IV. VITAMIN E

Vitamin E compounds are synthesized by plants and possess a chromanol ring with a 16-carbon side chain, which is saturated in tocopherols and unsaturated (3 double bonds) in tocotrienols. The number and position of methyl groups on the chromanol ring distinguish α, β, γ, δ forms of tocopherols and tocotrienols (Figure 5.3). Tocopherols contain three chiral centers in their side chain, of which the first, at the junction of the chromanol ring and side chain, is the most important for their function in the human body. The natural chiral form of α-tocopherol (*RRR*) is preferentially recognized by the α-tocopherol transfer protein (α-TTP) in the liver, which maintains a steady plasma level of this vitamin.[75,76] Synthetic α-tocopherol is a racemic mixture of eight stereoisomers (all-*rac*-α-tocopherol), four of them possessing vitamin E activity. Therefore, synthetic vitamin E is only half as effective as the natural form for meeting the human vitamin E requirement.[77]

There is a lot of confusion regarding the units of vitamin E activity. Traditionally, they were expressed in IUs based on the rat fetal resorption assay and defined as 1 mg of all-*rac*-α-tocopheryl acetate. This terminology is still used in labeling vitamin supplements. Vitamin E activity in food is often reported in nutrient databases and research literature as α-tocopherol equivalents (α-TE), also based on the activity of various tocopherols and tocotrienols in rat fetal resorption assay. Such reporting does not distinguish the proportion of various tocopherols and tocotrienols in diet and tends to overestimate intake by 20%, on average. Thus it is advisable to measure and report separately the actual content of each vitamin E compound.[77] At present, only four stereoisomeric forms of α-tocopherol (*RRR, RSR, RRS, RSS*) are considered to fulfill the vitamin E requirement. Therefore, the labels on supplements and fortified foods have to be carefully assessed and recalculated according to their content of synthetic or natural α-tocopherol, and total dietary estimates from unfortified food expressed in α-TE should be multiplied by a factor of 0.8.

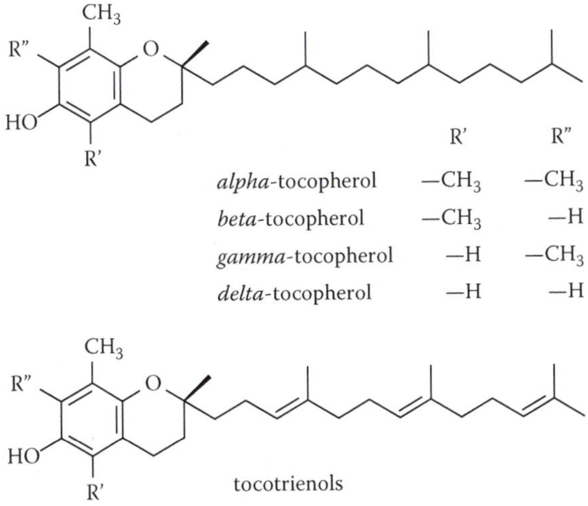

	R'	R"
alpha-tocopherol	$-CH_3$	$-CH_3$
beta-tocopherol	$-CH_3$	$-H$
gamma-tocopherol	$-H$	$-CH_3$
delta-tocopherol	$-H$	$-H$

tocotrienols

FIGURE 5.3 Structures of different forms of vitamin E.

The major sources of vitamin E in diet are seeds and nuts, as well as vegetable oils,[76] because vitamin E compounds protect the plant fats stored for the benefit of seedling development from oxidation (rancidity).[78] Green tissues of plants and some fruits (avocado, olives, tomato) also contain considerable amounts of α-tocopherol. Table 5.3 lists some of the most important foods that provide vitamin E.

TABLE 5.3

Food Sources of Vitamin E

Food, standard amount	Weight (g)	α-Tocopherol (mg)
Seeds and nuts:		
Sunflower seeds, dry roasted, 1 oz	28	7. 4
Almonds, 1 oz	28	7. 3
Hazelnuts, 1 oz	28	4. 3
Mixed nuts, dry roasted, 1oz	28	3. 1
Peanuts, 1 oz	28	2. 2
Peanut butter, smooth style, 1 tbsp	16	1. 4
Brazil nuts, 1 oz	28	1. 6
Wheat germ, toasted, 2 tbsp	14	2. 3
Vegetable oils:		
Sunflower oil, 1 tbsp	13. 6	5. 6
Cottonseed oil, 1 tbsp	13. 6	4. 8
Safflower oil, 1 tbsp	13. 6	4. 6
Canola oil, 1 tbsp	13. 6	2. 4
Peanut oil, 1 tbsp	13. 6	2. 1
Corn oil, 1 tbsp	13. 6	1. 9
Olive oil, 1 tbsp	13. 6	1. 9
Other fruit and vegetable foods:		
Turnip greens, cooked, 1/2 cup	82	2. 2
Spinach, cooked, ½ cup	85	1. 9
Tomato puree, canned, ½ cup	125	2. 5
Tomato sauce, canned, ½ cup	123	1. 7
Avocado, raw, 1 oz	28	0.75
Carrot juice, canned, 1 cup	236	2. 7
Seafood:		
Sardines, in oil, drained, 3 oz	85	1. 7
Blue crab, cooked, 3 oz	85	1. 6
Herring, pickled, 3 oz	85	1. 5
Fortified ready-to-eat cereals, 1 cup	Varies by type of cereal	1. 6–13. 5

Adapted from: USDA National Nutrient Database for Standard Reference, Release 20.

Vitamin E absorption requires the formation of micelles in the intestinal lumen, which is dependent on bile secretion.[77] Chylomicrons carry the newly absorbed tocopherols from the enterocytes to the liver, where a specific transfer protein (α-TTP) preferentially binds to 2R-α-tocopherol stereoisomers and regulates their resecretion to plasma and distribution to circulating lipoproteins. Other tocopherols and tocotrienols are not resecreted by the liver and quickly disappear from plasma, although they are absorbed in the intestine at a similar rate. Unlike vitamin A, tocopherols do not accumulate in tissues to produce toxic levels, and excess vitamin E is excreted in bile, while the metabolites are found in both urine and bile. Non-α-tocopherols are metabolized in preference to α-tocopherol; their concentrations and half-life in plasma are much lower.

The main function of α-tocopherol is that of a potent antioxidant, peroxyl radical scavenger that protects long-chain polyunsaturated fatty acids in cell membranes and in plasma lipoproteins from excessive oxidation.[79] In the absence of vitamin E, organic peroxyl radicals propagate in the chain reaction of lipid peroxidation. Tocopheryl radical usually breaks this propagation by forming nonreactive products, or it may be reduced back to vitamin E by water-soluble antioxidants, vitamin C, glutathione, or ubiquinols. The other important effect of vitamin E is the inhibition of platelet aggregation, mediated by the protein kinase C pathway, which may be independent of the antioxidant activity.[80] Tocopherols may also possess anti-inflammatory properties because they inhibit responses of activated macrophages *in vitro*.[81] These studies made vitamin E a promising candidate for prevention of chronic diseases, particularly cancer and cardiovascular disease, which are etiologically connected with oxidative stress.

In humans, severe vitamin E deficiency occurs very rarely, and only as a result of fat malabsorption, malnutrition, or genetic defect in α-TTP.[77] The symptoms are related to degeneration of sensory neurons and include slow development of ataxia, neuropathy, retinopathy, and muscular abnormalities. Experimental animals are much more sensitive to vitamin E deficiency and fail to produce offspring (rats),[82] or die within a few days when vitamin C is also withdrawn (guinea pigs).[83]

The human requirement for vitamin E was recently set at 12 mg of α-tocopherol per day for all adult men and women (except in pregnancy and lactation).[77] Therefore, the RDA for vitamin E, defined as at 120% of EAR to cover the needs of nearly all individuals, is 15 mg α-tocopherol per day. Estimates of dietary vitamin E intake in the U.S. population fall short of this goal; only 10% of middle-aged men and 5% of women were reporting dietary intake at or above RDA (NHANES III, 1988–94). More recent survey reports from 2004 indicate that 30–60 year-old-men consume on average 8.2 mg, and women only 6.4 mg α-tocopherol per day from food alone.[84] However, the dietary intake reporting is very unreliable in the case of vitamin E, because amounts of vegetable oil in diet are commonly underestimated, as is total energy intake, i.e., amount of food consumed. Many people take vitamin E supplements containing very significant doses, from 12 to 500 mg/day. Considering both dietary and supplemental vitamin E intake, more than 25% of middle-aged adults are well above the RDA.[77]

The assessment of vitamin E status in humans is based on plasma levels of α-tocopherol, which usually range from 14 to 36 μmol/L (600–1500 μg/dL). The plasma concentrations below 14 μmol/L (600 μg/dL) are considered too low, because they are accompanied by increased fragility of erythrocytes.[85] The test involves the rise in hydrogen peroxide-induced hemolysis *in vitro* above the normal 12%. According to this cut-off point, fewer than 1% of the middle-aged U.S. population exhibited such low serum vitamin E concentrations in NHANES III (1988–1994), but close to 10% had levels above 36 μmol/L (1500 μg/dL).[77] The UL for any form of supplementary α-tocopherol (including racemic formulations) was set at 1000 mg for all adults. Higher doses may cause hemorrhagic effects, especially in people deficient in vitamin K or undergoing anticoagulant therapy. It should be mentioned that in a Finnish placebo-controlled trial of male smokers consuming only 50 mg of all-rac-α-tocopherol per day for 6 years, there was a significant 50% increase in mortality from hemorrhagic stroke.[86] A meta-analysis of randomized prevention trials on antioxidant supplements revealed a small but significant increase in all-cause mortality with vitamin E supplementation (RR = 1.04; 95% CI 1.01-1.07) in a total of 55 studies. In 31 of them vitamin E was tested in combination with other antioxidants.[87] Vitamin E supplements had no effect for the prevention of cardiovascular disease in another meta-analysis of seven large vitamin E trials, in doses ranging from 50 to 800 IU.[88] More disturbing are the results of a large study (VITAL = VITamins And Lifestyle) in Washington state, where intake of supplemental vitamin E was associated with a small but significant increase in the risk of lung cancer. Among smokers, the incidence of lung cancer increased by 11% for every 100 mg vitamin E per day, while the whole population experienced 5% increase.[89] Despite this evidence, some researchers still advocate vitamin E supplementation at 15–100 IU/day[90,91] to maintain optimal concentrations of serum α-tocopherol at 13–14 mg/L (30–33 μmol/L), because they do not believe that such serum levels are possible to achieve by diet alone. High dietary intake of vitamin E from food and high serum α-tocopherol have been consistently correlated with decreased incidence of chronic diseases and all-cause mortality, especially in older adults.[91,92]

The main difference between supplementary and dietary vitamin E is the presence of various tocopherols and tocotrienols in food, while supplements usually contain only α-tocopherol. Some plant oils in seeds and nuts are rich in γ-tocopherol, an intermediate in the α-tocopherol pathway,[93,94] particularly soybean, corn, sesame, and peanut oil, which are widely used in the U.S. food supply. Olive oil and sunflower oil, which are more popular in Europe, contain mostly α-tocopherol. As a consequence, γ-tocopherol is much higher in the serum of Americans than Europeans, while the levels of α-tocopherol are comparable.[93] High intakes of supplementary α-tocopherol suppress serum γ-tocopherol,[95] possibly due to competition during incorporation of tocopherols in circulating lipids. *In vitro* studies show higher activity of γ-tocopherol in detoxification of reactive nitrogen species (peroxynitrite, NO_2, and NO).[96] Tocotrienols were reported to reduce oxidative damage to DNA in 37- to 78-year-old subjects supplemented with vitamin E extract from palm oil containing tocotrienols and α-tocopherol in a ratio of 74:26 for 6 months.[97] Some producers have started to include a mixture of tocopherols and tocotrienols in their "natural" supplements. However, tocotrienols are usually very minor forms of vitamin E in plant foods and their levels in plasma are very minute, not likely to exert significant effects.

Exercise greatly increases consumption of oxygen and production of free radicals in skeletal muscles and heart.[98] The resulting oxidative stress is particularly pronounced in untrained subjects,[99] beginning exercisers, intermittent exercisers ("weekend warriors"),[100] and in very strenuous endurance exercise conditions.[101] Training may improve body antioxidant defenses by stimulating the expression and activity of endogenous antioxidant enzymes (superoxide dismutases, glutathione peroxidase, catalase) and production of endogenous antioxidants (glutathione, uric acid, ubiquinone).[98] Exogenous antioxidants, such as vitamin E, vitamin C, or carotenoids, are mobilized during exercise and degraded at an increased rate. Although it may seem that exercise studies are a perfect model of vitamin E antioxidant effects, the abundant literature on this topic is rife with controversial results.

Relatively few studies measured the vitamin E status of exercising subjects, being more interested in assessing parameters of oxidative stress and athletic performance.[102] Most studies found transient increase of plasma α-tocopherol during exercise, especially endurance exercise such as cycling competition[20] or marathon running.[101] The participants of the annual McDonald Forest Ultramarathon Race (Corvallis, Oregon) were studied in a series of experiments related to oxidative stress and its possible alleviation by antioxidant supplementation. The subjects were mostly middle-aged men and women, recreationally trained, not professional athletes, and the trail of 50 km (32 miles) was rugged, with considerable change of elevation. In the first experiment, 11 subjects were given deuterium-labeled vitamin E on the evening before the race in order to study the kinetics of α-tocopherol during intense endurance exercise.[101] The experiment was repeated 1 month later with the same subjects at rest. Average total plasma α-tocopherol increased significantly during the race (from 30.1 to 33.9 μmol/L) and dropped below baseline level by 24 hr after the race (to 25.7 μmol/L). Labeled vitamin E disappeared faster during the race than at rest. The study also measured plasma F_2-isoprostanes as an indicator of lipid peroxidation, arising from free radical-induced oxidation of arachidonic acid. The plasma levels of F_2-isoprostanes nearly doubled during the race, but did not change during the rest period, suggesting that extreme endurance exercise increases lipid peroxidation and utilization of vitamin E.

In the second experiment,[103] 12 marathon runners received antioxidant supplements (300 mg vitamin E and 1000 mg vitamin C) daily for 6 weeks before the race, while 10 subjects received a placebo. The average plasma α-tocopherol increased in treated subjects from 28 to 45 μmol/L. DNA damage was evaluated in leukocytes by comet assay, showing a transient 10% increase mid-race followed by rapid decrease below baseline values post-race. The greatest decrease was observed in the supplemented women 1 day after the marathon. The marked decrease in DNA damage following exercise supports the inverse dose–response association between physical activity and cancer risk in a meta-analysis of 48 colon/colorectal cancer studies and 41 breast cancer studies.[104] Overall, antioxidant supplementation did not enhance the performance of marathon runners and did not decrease muscle damage, inflammation markers, fatigue, or recovery.[105,106] However, the runners in the Oregon studies had optimal plasma concentrations of plasma α-tocopherol before supplementation. Another study of seven healthy men (27–45 years old), competing in the half-marathon, indicated significant increase in erythrocyte susceptibility to peroxidation *in vitro* persisting for 4 days after the run.[21] It correlated with a decrease in their plasma tocopherol concentrations, which were low even before the race (16.8 μmol/L, decreased to 14.9 μmol/L at 48 hr post-race). Paradoxically, the erythrocyte tocopherols increased during this time, but it did not prevent the enhanced erythrocyte glutathione oxidation.

Trained ultraendurance athletes may have better antioxidant defenses at rest due to training response of antioxidant enzymes (catalase, glutathione peroxidase), but they are still under considerable oxidative stress during competitions. Half- and full-Ironmen athletes had a significant increase in plasma malondialdehyde (MDA, the commonly used marker of lipid peroxidation) and a decrease in erythrocyte antioxidant enzymes as a result of participation in triathlon events.[107] However, after competition, the users of antioxidant supplements among these athletes had significantly more elevated plasma MDA than nonusers. An interesting study compared middle-aged (36 ± 9 years old) alumni of the varsity rugby team with young players (21.5 ± 3.2 years old).[100] The alumni played rugby only once per week ("weekend warriors") and otherwise did not exercise, while young players participated in training regimen at least three times per week for 2.5 hr each time. The older group had higher lipid peroxidation markers (MDA and conjugated dienes in LDL and VLDL) at rest than young men, and the MDA levels were much more elevated after one game. Not surprisingly, a single session of resistance exercise produces significant oxidative damage in untrained subjects, as shown by a study of seven young male volunteers.[101] Their urinary excretion of F_2-isoprostanes increased significantly after exercise, despite the adaptive increase in the antioxidant capacity of blood (erythrocyte reduced glutathione, plasma uric acid) and muscle (uric acid, glutathione reductase, and glutathione-S-transferase).

Very few studies support the notion that antioxidant supplements may enhance aerobic performance in addition to the training effect. A study of 15 male amateur athletes assigned them to placebo or antioxidant supplement treatment (500 mg vitamin E and 30 mg β-carotene per day during 3-month training, plus 1 g vitamin C per day for the last 15 days).[108] A maximal exercise test on a cycle ergometer was performed by all men before and after the training period. Both groups significantly improved their maximal oxygen uptake (VO_{2max}), and maximal workload, but the efficiency was better in the supplemented group (lower maximal blood lactate). The antioxidant enzymes of leukocytes were more responsive to supplementation than those of erythrocytes.[109]

The discrepant results of different studies stem from variations in exercise regimens, nutritional status and fitness of subjects, and the methodologies employed to evaluate parameters of oxidative stress, fatigue, and recovery.[100] It is also difficult to evaluate the effect of supplemental doses of vitamin E because most studies involved multiple, possibly interacting, antioxidants.

V. VITAMIN K

The basic structure of vitamin K possesses a methylated naphthoquinone ring with a hydrophobic side chain of varying length and saturation at the 3-position (Figure 5.4). There are three major types of vitamin K:

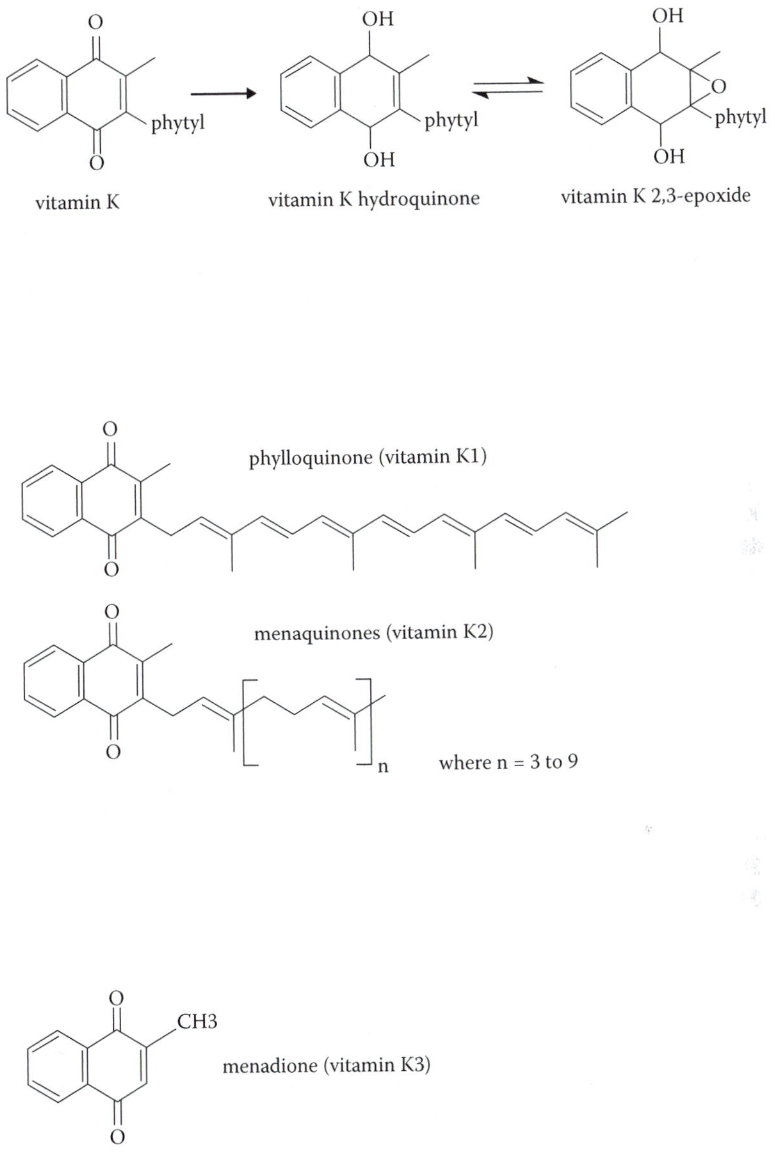

vitamin K → vitamin K hydroquinone ⇌ vitamin K 2,3-epoxide

phylloquinone (vitamin K1)

menaquinones (vitamin K2)

where n = 3 to 9

menadione (vitamin K3)

FIGURE 5.4 Structures of different forms of vitamin K.

1. Phylloquinone (vitamin K1) is obtained primarily from plant sources. It is a component of chloroplasts in plants and contains four isoprenoid residues, one of which is unsaturated. Phylloquinone is partially converted to dihydrophylloquinone during hydrogenation of vegetable oils.[110]
2. Menaquinones (vitamin K2 series) are synthesized by bacteria and designated as MK-n, where n refers to the number of isoprenoid units, all unsaturated. Long-chain menaquinones, such as MK-6 to MK-10, are the

most common vitamin K2 members synthesized by bacteria, while MK-4 can also be formed from phylloquinone in animals. Phylloquinone can be converted to menadione via cleavage of the side chain by the gut flora, which is then absorbed and converted to MK-4 in the target tissues by realkylation. There is also a possibility that the conversion of phylloquinone to MK-4 may occur in animal tissues without bacterial participation.[111,112] However, animals cannot form the napthoquinone ring, so it must be obtained from dietary sources. Plants and bacteria can synthesize the ring, so they are the primary source of this vitamin for animals.

3. Menadione, or vitamin K3, does not possess any side chain and it has been synthesized to be used as a vitamin K supplement for humans and animals. However, synthetic menadione may cause liver damage[113] and hemolytic anemia. It can also oxidize intracellular glutathione, the body's natural antioxidant, resulting in oxidative damage to cell membranes and mitochondrial dysfunction.[114,115] This form of synthetic vitamin K is therefore no longer used as a supplement for humans.

About 90% of dietary vitamin K is in the form of phylloquinone. The dietary sources of phylloquinone are green leafy vegetables, such as spinach, broccoli, cabbage, but also fruits and plant oils (Table 5.4). Menaquinones, which constitute about 10% of total vitamin K consumption, are derived from bacterial synthesis and are present in liver, egg yolk, milk, butter, and especially in fermented foods such as cheeses and natto (fermented soybean product) (Table 5.5).[116]

Although a considerable amount of menaquinone MK-10 is produced in the colon by bacterial microflora, the bacterial synthesis of menaquinones is not adequate to maintain normal blood clotting function in the absence of dietary phylloquinone.[117] This may be due to poor absorption of menaquinone in the colon. The bioavailability of vitamin K from different food sources may affect its blood levels. Only 10–20% of phylloquinone from green vegetables is absorbed, while the absorption rate is much higher for menaquinones from natto.[116,117] Due to its availability from a wide range of foods, dietary deficiency of vitamin K is rare, except in conditions associated with fat malabsorption. Vitamin K absorption is impaired in patients with extrahepatic biliary obstruction and pancreatic disorders. Use of laxatives in the form of mineral oils also reduces the rate of vitamin K absorption. Once absorbed in the intestinal cells, dietary phylloquinone and menaquinones are taken up by chylomicrons in the circulation and distributed among the different types of lipoproteins to be cleared in the liver. Hepatic cell uptake of vitamin K is mediated by apo-E receptors, which also influence the plasma level of phylloquinone.

Different tissues have distinct distribution of vitamin K forms. The level of phylloquinone, but not MK-4, in tissues is affected by a vitamin K deficient diet. Animal studies with germ-free rats and *in vitro* studies with mammalian cell lines showed that maintaining MK-4 level was not dependent on bacterial synthesis of this vitamer, suggesting an effective conversion of phylloquinone to MK-4 *in vivo*.[112,118] Since its discovery in early 1930s, vitamin K has been known for its participation in hemostasis mechanism, which comprises a highly regulated network of proteins that maintains

TABLE 5.4

Food Sources of Phylloquinone (vitamin K1)

Food, standard amount	Weight (g)	Phylloquinone (μg)
Kale, cooked, 1 cup	130	1062.1
Spinach, cooked, 1 cup	180	888.5
Onions, spring, 1 cup	100	207.0
Parsley, raw, 10 sprigs	10	164.0
Spinach, raw, 1 cup	30	144.9
Lettuce, romaine, raw, 1 cup	56	57.4
Broccoli, cooked, 1 cup	156	220.0
Plum, dried, stewed, 1 cup	248	64.7
Cabbage, raw, 1 cup	70	53.2
Beans, snap, canned, 1 cup	135	52.5
Cucumber, raw, 1 large	301	49.4
Peas, green, cooked, 1 cup	160	38.4
Blueberries, frozen, 1 cup	230	40.7
Cauliflower, frozen, cooked, 1 cup	180	21.4
Carrots, cooked, 1 cup	156	21.4
Canola oil, 1 tbsp	14	10.0
Soybean oil, 1 tbsp	14	27.0
Margarine, vegetable oil spread, 1 tbsp	14	14.5
Natto, 1 cup	175	60.7

Adapted from USDA National Nutrient Database for Standard Reference, Release 20, and Schurgers and Vermeer, 2000.[116]

regular blood flow. Vitamin K is one of the cofactors in the synthesis and activation of these proteins that mediate both coagulation and anticoagulation function.

The quinone form of dietary vitamin K is reduced in the tissues to hydroquinone, which serves as the cofactor for the γ-carboxylation of vitamin K dependent (VKD) proteins. Activation occurs through vitamin K-mediated γ-carboxylation of glutamic acid, resulting in γ-carboxyglutamyl (Gla) residues. The Gla proteins serve as chelating sites for calcium ions and therefore play an important role in membrane–protein interaction and hemostasis. Among the coagulation factors, factor II, VII, IX, and X are VKD proteins. They act as proenzymes and trigger the complex coagulation cascade upon binding to the cell membrane tissue factor during injury. This result in the formation of a stable platelet-fibrin clots and prevents blood loss. VKD proteins also actively participate in bone metabolism.

Vitamin K has been associated with several nonhemorrhagic disorders, such as osteoporosis, osteoarthritis, and vascular calcification. Osteocalcin, secreted by osteoblasts, and matrix Gla protein (MGP) found in bone and other tissues, such as cartilage and blood vessel walls, are two vitamin K-dependent proteins associated with these

TABLE 5.5

Food Sources of Menaquinones (Vitamin K2)

Food	Menaquinone type	Amount (µg/100g)
Goose liver	MK-4	369
Egg yolk	MK-4	31.4
Hard cheese	MK-8	16.9
	MK-9	51.1
Soft cheese	MK-8	11.4
	MK-9	39.6
Curd cheese	MK-8	5.1
	MK-9	18.7
Natto	MK-5	7.5
	MK-6	13.8
	MK-7	998
	MK-8	84.1

Adapted from Schurgers and Vermeer, 2000.[116]

disorders. Another VKD protein, activated protein C, regulates inflammatory responses by inhibition of the NF-κB pathway of inflammation,[119] and allergic responses by preventing leukocyte chemotaxis.[120] Impairment of the γ-carboxylation process leads to the synthesis of proteins induced by vitamin K absence or antagonism (PIVKA), which can be used as specific and sensitive biomarkers for detecting vitamin K deficiency.

Vitamin K deficiency may occur due to poor dietary intake, severe cholestasis (impaired bile flow from the liver) and impaired menaquinone (vitamin K2) production by intestinal bacteria due to treatment with broad-spectrum antibiotics, especially when fat malabsorption is present. In cases of severe coagulopathy due to impaired hepatic synthesis of coagulation factors, intravenous vitamin K1 can be given to prevent deficiency. The symptoms of vitamin K deficiency include prolonged blood clotting time resulting in hemorrhage, easy bruising, nosebleeds, bleeding gums, loss of blood in stool or urine, and heavy menstrual flow. Although vitamin K deficiency is rare in adults, it may occur in patients using anticoagulant drugs that function as vitamin K antagonists, and in cases of severe liver disease. Due to an efficient vitamin K recycling mechanism in mammals, the vitamin K requirement in healthy people is very small.[121] The AI level of vitamin K for adult men is 120 µg per day, and for women 90 µg per day.[117] According to the current USDA report, average daily intake of vitamin K is 99 µg for men and 87 µg for women.[122] This amount can be easily obtained by consumption of a half cup of cooked broccoli (Table 5.4). Phylloquinone or menaquinones do not cause toxic symptoms even at high doses, and therefore UL for vitamin K has not been established.[117]

Plasma phylloquinone concentration is associated with recent dietary intake of vitamin K.[123] In the adult population of Great Britain, average plasma levels were 1.13 nmol /L in men and 0.81 nmol/L in women, with seasonal variation affecting only women in this study.[124] Data obtained from the Framingham Offspring Study indicated that the average plasma concentration of phylloquinone in the United States was 0.99 nmol/L in men and 0.94 nmol/L in women.[125] Assessing prothrombin clotting time to determine vitamin K status is a classical method, but measuring the ratio of active prothrombin to total prothrombin is considered a more sensitive indicator of vitamin K status.[126] Another biological marker that links vitamin K with bone health is the percent of undercarboxylated osteocalcin (%ucOC) in serum.[127] Low dietary intake and reduced plasma phylloquinone level are highly associated with increased serum %ucOC.[125,128,129] The prevalence of high circulating ucOC among the healthy population indicates that vitamin K deficiency is a more common health concern than predicted from intake data.[121] With increased consumption of both dietary and supplementary phylloquinone, the serum %ucOC can be significantly reduced.[128]

Since osteocalcin, a VKD protein, can be measured in serum, much interest has been given to the role of vitamin K in maintaining bone health. Vitamin K activates osteocalcin by γ-carboxylation and the carboxylated osteocalcin participates in maintaining the bone mass by adequate mineralization. Inside the bone matrix, the calcium is anchored by activated osteocalcin and therefore vitamin K deficiency, which lowers the ratio of carboxylated to uncarboxylated osteocalcin, can adversely affect bone mineralization. Increased concentration of serum ucOC and reduced concentration of vitamin K have been associated with increased risk for hip fracture. To investigate this hypothesis, a prospective study was conducted by analyzing diet and reported hip fracture incidence of middle-aged women (38 to 63 years of age) participating in the Nurse's Health Study. Results suggest that poor vitamin K status may increase the risk of hip fracture in women.[130] Similar association of low dietary vitamin K intake with bone fracture risk has been reported by several other investigations.[131–133] Most of the clinical intervention trials used very high pharmacological doses of MK-4 and phylloquinone to reduce bone mineral loss and fracture risk in healthy premenopausal, postmenopausal, and osteoporotic subjects.[134,135] However, MK-7 can be used with similar beneficial effect on BMD at much lower nutritional doses due to its higher bioavailability, longer half-life, and extra-hepatic tissue distribution. It was found to be more potent than phylloquinone in maintaining a stable and higher serum level of vitamin K and in activating VKD proteins.[136] Epidemiological studies indicate that consumption of dietary menaquinone MK-7 significantly promotes cardiovascular and bone health and reduces risk of bone fracture.

The role of dietary vitamin K intake in preventing cardiovascular diseases needs further study because the observational data are inconclusive. High intake of phylloquinone may be a marker for a heart-healthy diet, rich in green vegetables.[137] However, the Framingham Offspring Study reported that both serum levels and dietary intake of phylloquinone were inversely correlated to inflammatory markers.[138] Increased postmenopausal bone loss and progressive arterial calcification with reduced elasticity are associated with poor vitamin K status[121,139] and also with anticoagulant treatment. High doses of K1 or MK-4 reduced arterial calcification in warfarin-treated rats.[140] *In vitro* cell culture from normal and varicose veins identified overexpression and incomplete carboxylation of matrix Gla-protein (MPG, a VDK protein) as a cause of increased smooth muscle cell proliferation and calcification of extracellular matrix.[141] These processes were enhanced by warfarin and reversed by vitamin K.

Adequate intake of vitamin K for physically active adults is very important to prevent excessive bruising and bleeding. Although it has not been established that deficiency of vitamin K promotes osteoporosis, supplementation may improve BMD and prevent bone loss, especially in female athletes. Due to strenuous exercise programs, female athletes may suffer from hypoestrogenism and amenorrhoea, resulting in osteoporosis. In a small study of eight elite athletes—20–44-year-old female long distance runners—four were amenorrhoeic for more than a year, and four were using oral contraceptives.[142] All had extremely low circulating sex hormones, in the range of prepubertal girls or postmenopausal women. The low calcium-binding capacity of circulating osteocalcin in amenorrheic runners was indicative of low vitamin K status, despite their self-reported ample intake of green vegetables and dairy products. Supplementation of vitamin K at a dose of 10 mg/day for 1 month increased calcium binding capacity of osteocalcin in all subjects and produced a 15–20% increase in bone formation with a 25% decrease in bone resorption markers of amenorrheic runners.

VI. INTERACTIONS OF FAT-SOLUBLE VITAMINS

The best known interaction is that of vitamin E and vitamin C (a water-soluble vitamin), the two main dietary antioxidants, which were shown *in vitro* to complement each other and prevent oxidation of cellular components. Vitamin C may regenerate α-tocopherol from tocopheryl radical, and also quench reactive oxygen species, sparing vitamin E in the process.[143] A human study of 30 healthy middle-aged adults investigated this interaction by supplementing the subjects with 73.5 mg vitamin E or 500 mg vitamin C per day for 6 weeks in a crossover double-blind experiment.[144] Supplementation with vitamin C increased plasma concentration of both vitamins C and E, when the latter was normalized to lipid concentration. Supplementation with α-tocopherol increased plasma levels of vitamin C and decreased γ-tocopherol. Half the subjects showed a significant increase in plasma α-tocopherol, but others had only a slight increase. Lipid-normalized values were increased by 30%, on average. Both vitamins caused a significant decrease in total plasma cholesterol and triglycerides, but increased blood glutathione peroxidase activity and partial thromboplastin time.

These results obtained in healthy nonsmoking subjects support the synergistic interaction of vitamins E and C, with respect to antioxidant status, antithrombotic tendency, and improvement in lipid profile. Even more convincing were studies of cigarette smokers, who are exposed to incessant oxidative assault of reactive oxygen and nitrogen species in the smoke and increased inflammatory responses. Deuterium-labeled vitamin E administration (150 mg/day for 6 days) indicated a faster disappearance rate of α-tocopherol in smokers, when compared with nonsmokers.[145] Since the rates of α-tocopherol disappearance were inversely correlated with plasma vitamin C in smokers, the second experiment involved supplementation with 1000 mg vitamin C or placebo for 2 weeks, followed by a single dose of deuterated α-tocopherol and γ-tocopherol (50 mg each).[146] Vitamin C supplementation decreased the disappearance rates of both tocopherols to normal levels of nonsmokers, but it did not reduce higher plasma lipid peroxidation in smokers (F_2-isoprostanes), or change the rate of tocopherol metabolism through the cytochrome P-450 system. These results indicate that vitamin C directly recycles vitamin E or spares it from oxidants, and both antioxidant vitamins act synergistically *in vivo*.

Vitamin E seems to protect hepatic stores of vitamin A, help in absorption, and alleviate toxicity.[147] In terms of growth and survival, early experiments on chicks show that severe vitamin A toxicity can be reversed by simultaneous administration of large doses of vitamin E. When well nourished rats were given a diet deficient in both vitamins, they showed signs of vitamin A deficiency sooner than on a vitamin E-sufficient diet, which spared hepatic stores of vitamin A. For ethical reasons, such trials cannot be performed on humans, although a study in India reported that single high doses of vitamin A to prevent deficiency in children were absorbed at a higher rate when vitamin E was simultaneously administered.[148]

The interaction of vitamins A and D is more plausible, because both VDR and RAR bind as heterodimers with the RXR to hormone response elements in DNA. *In vitro* experiments indicate a complex interaction resulting in co-activation or antagonist repression of gene transcription.[149] Through the interaction with nuclear receptors, both vitamins interact in cell proliferation and differentiation processes, so important in regeneration of tissues and cancer prevention. However, the epidemiological evidence points to opposite effects of vitamins A and D in maintaining BMD, with high plasma retinol associated with increased incidence of osteoporosis and bone fractures, while sufficiently high 25(OH)D is essential for bone health through its effects on calcium homeostasis. Vitamin K is also involved in adequate mineralization of bone matrix and collagen formation, at the same time preventing excessive calcification of blood vessels and enhancing their elastic properties. Matrix Gla-protein (MPG), synthesized in cartilage and arterial vessel walls, is an inhibitor of calcification, but requires vitamin D for its gene expressions and vitamin K for its biological activity.[139] MPG promoter contains a vitamin D response element, and vitamin D binding enhances the synthesis of this protein. Vitamin K is a cofactor in carboxylation of glutamate residues in MPGs, essential for its calcification inhibition function.

Hypothetically, the similarity of vitamin E and vitamin K structures may allow them to bind to the same site of pregnane xenobiotic receptor (PXR).[150] Dimerization of PXR with RXR allows in turn binding to the PXR response element and regulation of various xenobiotic enzymes, which metabolize a great variety of endogenous and exogenous compounds. This competition may explain opposite effects of vitamin E and K in blood clotting mechanism, where vitamin K promotes coagulation and vitamin E decreases platelet aggregation and acts as antithrombotic agent. Therefore, vitamin E may interfere with vitamin K activation of clotting factors and protect from heart attack or stroke due to thromboembolism, as well as decrease the tendency to form varicose veins. However, in healthy people, 12 weeks of supplementation with 681 mg *RRR*-α-tocopherol caused a marked increase in undercarboxylated prothrombin (PIVKA-II), but not in undercarboxylated osteocalcin.[151] Thus, the supplementation with a large dose of vitamin E caused abnormally high undercarboxylation of prothrombin despite normal plasma levels of vitamin K. In susceptible individuals, particularly on anticoagulant therapies, it could promote bleeding and bruising and even increase the risk of hemorrhagic stroke.

VII. RECOMMENDATIONS AND CONCLUSIONS

Adequate levels of fat-soluble vitamins in circulation and target tissues are required for optimal health at every stage of the life cycle. The middle-age years, 30 to 60, are of particular importance, because this is the most productive period in terms of work capacity and raising a family, both of utmost importance in maintaining human society. It is also the time of life when inactive life style, poor diet, and harmful habits (smoking, alcohol abuse) may result in the development of chronic diseases in old age. This chapter attempts to emphasize the role of fat-soluble vitamins in prevention of chronic diseases and in the maintenance of healthy physical activity throughout middle age and into later years. Most of the research studies on fat-soluble vitamins in the past were conducted on infants, children, healthy young people, old people, or special disease populations, which is understandable from the viewpoint of medical and nutritional practitioners, who are most concerned with the proper growth and development of the young and improving the health and longevity of old and sick persons. Professional athletes were also subjects of many studies, providing insight into the requirements of more extreme demands on the human body than are usually encountered by average people. In addition, researchers are far from agreement on many aspects of fat-soluble vitamin nutrition, including optimal intake levels and the use of supplements. However, the available data suggest that it is possible to give cautious recommendations for middle-aged adults who are concerned about their health and physical fitness.

The rising prevalence of obesity and the association of cardiovascular disease with high plasma cholesterol and triglycerides instilled fear of dietary fat in a sizable segment of the middle-aged population. However, it is necessary to ingest some fat (20–35% energy)[152,153] with every meal to ensure the absorption of fat-soluble vitamins, especially those from green leaves, fruits, and vegetables (vitamin E, K, provitamin A carotenoids), which contain little fat. Monounsaturated olive oil, the mainstay fat of the healthy Mediterranean diet, and other vegetable oils are the main source of vitamin E, while fish oils contain vitamin D.

Middle-age diets should contain a wide variety of foods, including plant and animal sources, to provide the best balance of fat-soluble vitamins and other nutrients. The American Dietetic Association recommends no additional vitamin and mineral supplements if adults, including athletes, obtain their optimum dietary energy intake from such a variety.[153] The complex interactions among vitamins indicate that an imbalance in their relative proportions may impair health and result in development of chronic diseases. Low intakes of vitamins D and K may be aggravated by excessive intake of preformed vitamin A, resulting in early osteopenia and osteoporosis in middle-aged subjects.

Dietary vitamin A is the only fat-soluble vitamin that has to be limited in middle-aged adults, who usually have accumulated large liver stores. The intake should not exceed the EAR, unless low status is confirmed by biochemical assessment. It is quite possible to exceed the RDA, and even the UL of vitamin A with food alone, by ingesting large portions of liver, liver products, and other organ meats, and certainly by the use of supplements containing vitamin A. There are no precautions for the dietary intake of provitamin A or other carotenoids, but excessive supplements of β-carotene were associated with increasing the risk of cancer, especially in smokers and drinkers of alcohol.

It is difficult to exceed recommendations for dietary vitamin D, because it is present in very few foods; therefore, the deficiency is quite common in all age groups of Western societies, especially among dark-skinnned people living far away from the equator. Sedentary work and lifestyle, embraced by a high proportion of middle-aged people, prevents them from cutaneous synthesis of adequate amounts of vitamin D, and obesity further decreases the availability of the vitamin, which is stored in adipose tissue.[154] Outdoor physical activity in warm weather is the best remedy for this situation, because even 15 min/d of sun exposure will increase circulating vitamin D to acceptable levels. The highest, but not excessive, levels of plasma 25(OH)D were registered in lifeguards,[45] but even a short vacation in Mexico raised it in an obese woman.[154] Many researchers advocate supplements of vitamin D far in excess of the RDA, which they consider inadequate. It is troublesome that the new recommendations are so close to the former UL for vitamin D, which may result in many cases of abuse, particularly in small-bodied individuals, who are most concerned about the risk for osteoporosis. On the other hand, most postmenopausal women should probably take 400–1000 IU of vitamin D along with the daily calcium supplement to prevent accelerated loss of BMD, osteoporosis, and risk of fractures. In the future, an improved and widespread testing of vitamin D status by measuring 25(OH)D in blood could accurately indicate the need and the necessary dose of supplementary vitamin D in middle-aged adults.

Vitamin E is also generally not overabundant in the diet and many people consume much less than the RDA, although there is probably much underreporting of vegetable fat in foods. Some researchers are in favor of very high supplements of vitamin E to prevent oxidative stress and cardiovascular disease, while others discourage such supplementation for the general population and cite a lack of protection in vulnerable subjects. It is probably safe to use a supplement of RDA value, but adequate amounts of dietary fat and vitamin C must also be consumed to ensure optimal absorption and utilization of vitamin E.

The vitamin K supply in green vegetables and fermented foods is quite adequate to fulfill the needs of healthy adults and no additional supplements are usually necessary. However, very high doses of supplemental vitamin E may cause a serious imbalance in the blood clotting mechanism, antagonizing vitamin K function and promoting hemorrhaging stroke. These interactions of vitamins require further research, but in the meantime, the best advice for active middle-aged people is to rely on a high-quality diet to meet their nutritional needs, maintain perfect weight for their height, exercise, and avoid smoking. It is practically impossible to provide sensible advice to heavy smokers, because the combination of unusually heavy oxidative stress, inflammation, and tar carcinogens with intensive exercise or vitamin therapy may result in unexpected outcomes of higher risk for cancer, cardiovascular, and other chronic diseases.

REFERENCES

1. Cordain, L., Eaton, S. B., Sebastian, A., Mann, N., Lindeberg, S., Watkins, B. A., et al., Origins and evolution of the Western diet: Health implications for the 21st century, *Am. J. Clin. Nutr.* 81, 341–54, 2005.
2. Eaton, S. B. and Konner, M., Paleolithic nutrition. A consideration of its nature and current implications, *N. Engl. J. Med.* 312, 283–9, 1985.
3. Krinsky, N. I., Wang, X. D., Tang, G., and Russell, R. M., Mechanism of carotenoid cleavage to retinoids, *Ann. NY Acad. Sci.* 691, 167–76, 1993.
4. Food and Nutrition Board, Institute of Medicine, Vitamin A, in *Dietary Reference Intakes for Vitamin A, Vitamin K, Arsenic, Boron, Chromium, Copper, Iodine, Iron, Manganese, Molybdenum, Nickel, Silicon, Vanadium and Zinc,* National Academy Press, Washington, D. C., 2001, pp. 82–161.
5. van Lieshout, M., West, C. E., Muhilal, P. D., Wang. Y., Xu, X., van Breemen, R.B., et al., Bioefficacy of β–carotene dissolved in oil studied in children in Indonesia, *Am. J. Clin. Nutr.* 73, 949–58, 2001.
6. West, C. E., Eilander, A., and van Lieshout, M., Consequences of revised estimates of carotenoid bioefficacy for the dietary control of vitamin A deficiency in developing countries, *J. Nutr.* 132, 2920S–6S, 2002.
7. Furr, H. C. and Clark, R. M., Intestinal absorption and tissue distribution of carotenoids, *J. Nutr. Biochem.* 8, 364–77, 1997.
8. Stahl, W. and Sies, H., Uptake of lycopene and its geometrical isomers is greater from heat-processed than from unprocessed tomato juice in humans, *J. Nutr.* 122, 2161–6, 1992.
9. Harrison, E. H., Mechanisms of digestion and absorption of dietary vitamin A, *Ann. Rev. Nutr.* 25, 87–103, 2005.
10. Saari, J. C., Retinoids in photosensitive systems, in *The Retinoids: Biology, Chemistry and Medicine*, 2nd ed., Sporn, M. B., Roberts, A. B., and Goodman, D. S., Eds. Raven Press, New York, 1994, pp. 351–85.
11. Archer, S. L., Stamler, J., Moag-Stahlberg, A., Van Horn, L., Garside, D., Chan, Q., et al., Association of dietary supplement use with specific micronutrient intakes among middle-aged American men and women: The INTERMAP Study, *J. Am. Med. Assoc.* 105, 1106–14, 2005.
12. Michaelsson, K., Lithell, H., Vessby, B., and Melhus, H., Serum retinol levels and the risk of fracture, *N. Eng. J. Med.* 348, 287–94, 2003.
13. Gerber, A., Raab, A. P., and Sobel, A. E., Vitamin A poisoning in adults with description of a case, *Am. J. Med.* 16, 729–45, 1954.
14. Shearman, D. J. C., Vitamin A and Sir Douglas Mawson, *Br. J. Med.* Vol. 1 (6108), 283–85, 1978.
15. Stacewicz-Sapuntzakis, M., Bowen, P. E., Kikendall, J. W., and Burgess, M., Simultaneous determination of serum retinol and various carotenoids: their distribution in middle-aged men and women, *J. Micronutr. Anal.* 3, 27–45, 1987.
16. Underwood, B. A., Hypovitaminosis A: International programmatic issues, *J. Nutr.* 124, 1467S–72S, 1994.
17. Ballew, C., Bowmen, B. A., Sowell, A. L., and Gillespie, C., Serum retinol distribution in residents of the United States: Third National Health and Nutrition Examination Survey, 1988–1994, *Am. J. Clin. Nutr.* 73, 586–93, 2001.
18. Olson, J. A., Recommmended dietary intakes (RDI) of vitamin A in humans. *Am. J. Clin. Nutr.* 45, 704–16, 1987.
19. Stacewicz-Sapuntzakis, M. and Borthakur, G., Vitamin A, in *Sports Nutrition*, 2nd ed., Driskell, J. A. and Wolinsky, I., Eds., CRC Press, Boca Raton, 2006, pp. 163–74.

20. Aguilo, A., Tauler, P., Pilar, G. M., Villa, G., Cordova, A., Tur, J. A., and Pons, A., Effect of exercise intensity and training on antioxidants and cholesterol profile in cyclists, *J. Nutr. Biochem.* 14, 319–25, 2003.
21. Duthie, G. G., Robertson, J. D., Maugham, R. J., and Morrice, P. C., Blood antioxidant status and erythrocyte lipid peroxidation following distance running, *Arch. Biochem. Biophys.* 282, 78–83, 1990.
22. Schmidt, M. C., Askew, E. W., Roberts, D. E., Prior, R. L., Ensign, W. Y., and Hesslink, R. E., Oxidative stress in humans training in a cold, moderate altitude environment and their response to a phytochemical antioxidant supplement, *Wilderness Environ. Med.* 13, 94–105, 2002.
23. Leung, A. K. C., Carotenemia, *Adv. Pediatr.* 34, 223–48, 1987.
24. World Cancer Research Fund / American Institute for Cancer Research, Food, nutrition, physical activity and the prevention of cancer: A global perspective, AICR, Washington DC, 2007, pp. 102–103.
25. Köpcke, W. and Krutmann, J., Protection from sunburn with β-carotene–a meta-analysis, *Photochem. Photobiol.* 84, 284–88, 2008.
26. Hammond, B. R. Jr., Wooten, B. R., and Curran-Celentano, J., Carotenoids in the retina and lens: Possible acute and chronic effects on human visual performance, *Arch. Biochem. Biophys.* 385, 41–6, 2001.
27. Omenn, G. S., Chemoprevention of lung cancer: The rise and demise of beta-carotene, *Ann. Rev. Public Health* 19, 73–99, 1998.
28. Baron, J. A., Cole, B. F., Mott, L., Haile, R., Grau, M., Church, T. R., et al., Neoplastic and antineoplastic effects of beta-carotene on colorectal adenoma recurrence: Results of a randomized trial, *J. Natl. Cancer Inst.* 95, 717–22, 2003.
29. Stacewicz-Sapuntzakis, M., and Diwadkar-Navsariwala, V., Carotenoids, in *Nutritional Ergogenic Aids*, Wolinsky, I. and Driskell, J. A. Eds., CRC Press, Boca Raton, 2004, pp. 325–53.
30. Marx, S. J., Jones, G., Weinstein, R. S., Chrousos, G. P., and Renquist, D. M., Differences in mineral metabolism among nonhuman primates receiving diets with only vitamin D_3 or only vitamin D_2, *J. Clin. Endocrinol. Metab.* 69, 1282–9, 1989.
31. Armas, L. A., Hollis, B. W., and Heaney, R. P., Vitamin D_2 is much less effective than vitamin D_3 in humans, *J. Clin. Endocrinol. Metab.* 89, 5387–91, 2004.
32. Mastaglia, S. R., Mautalen, C. A., Parisi, M. S., and Oliveri, B., Vitamin D_2 dose required to rapidly increase 25(OH)D levels in osteoporotic women, *Eur. J. Clin. Nutr.* 60, 681–7, 2006.
33. Holick, M. F., Biancuzzo, R. M., Chen, T. C., Klein, E. K., Young, A., Bibuld, D., et al., Vitamin D_2 is as effective as vitamin D_3 in maintaining circulating concentrations of 25-hydroxyvitamin D, *J. Clin. Endocrinol. Metab.* 93, 677–81, 2007.
34. Rangel-Castro, J. I., Staffas, A., and Danell, E. The ergocalciferol content of dried pigmented, and albino *Cantharellus cibarius* fruit bodies, *Mycol. Res.* 106:70–73, 2002
35. Food and Nutrition Board/Institute of Medicine. *Dietary Reference Intakes for Calcium, Phosphorus, Magnesium, Vitamin D, and Fluoride*, Washington, DC, National Academy Press, 1997, pp. 250–87.
36. National Institutes of Health, Osteoporosis and Related Bone Diseases–National Resource Center, 2006. Osteoporosis Overview. http://www.osteo.org/osteoporosis. Accessed 08/13/2008.
37. National Institutes of Health, Consensus Development Panel on Osteoporosis Prevention, Diagnosis, and Therapy. Osteoporosis prevention, diagnosis, and therapy, *J. Am. Med. Assoc.* 285, 320–23, 2001.
38. Bischioff-Ferrari, H. A., Willet, W. C., Wong, J. B., Giovannucci, E., Dietrich, T., and Dawson-Hughes, B., Fracture prevention with vitamin D supplementation: A meta analysis of randomized controlled trials, *JAMA.* 293, 2257–64, 2005.

39. Holick, M. F., High prevalence of vitamin D inadequacy and implications for health, *Mayo. Clin. Proc.* 81, 353–73, 2006.
40. Holick, M. F., Vitamin D deficiency, *N. Engl. J. Med.* 357, 266–81, 2007.
41. Brustad, M., Alsaker, E., Engelsen, O., Aksnes, L., and Lund, E., Vitamin D status of middle-aged women at 65–71°N in relation to dietary intake and exposure to ultraviolet radiation, *Pub. Hlth. Nutr.* 7, 327–35, 2004.
42. Zadshir, A., Tareen, N., Pan, D., Norris, K., and Martins, D., The prevalence to hypovitaminosis D among US adults: Data from the NHANES III, *Ethn. Dis.* 15, S5–97–S5–101, 2005.
43. Nuti, R., Martini, G., Valenti, R., Gambera, D., Gennari, L., Salvadori, S., and Avanzati, A., Vitamin D status and bone turnover in women with acute hip fracture, *Clin. Orthop.* 422, 208–13, 2004.
44. Bischoff-Ferrari, H. A., Dietrich, T., Orav, E. J. and Dawson-Hughes, B., Positive association between 25-hydroxy vitamin D levels and bone mineral density: A population-based study of younger and older adults, *Am. J. Med.* 116, 634–9, 2004.
45. Holick, M. F., Vitamin D status: Measurement, interpretation, and clinical application, *Ann. Epidemiol.* 2008. In press.
46. Zerwekh, J. E., Blood biomarkers of vitamin D status, *Am. J. Clin. Nutr.* 87, 1087S–91S, 2008.
47. Bikle, D. D., Gee, E., Halloran, B., and Haddad, J. G., Free 1,25-dihydroxyvitamin D levels in serum from normal subjects, pregnant subjects, and subjects with liver disease, *J. Clin. Invest.* 74, 1966–71, 1984.
48. Bischoff-Ferrari, H. A. and Dawson-Hughes, B., Where do we stand on vitamin D? *Bone* 41, S13–S19, 2007.
49. Talwar, S. A., Aloia, J. F., Pollack, S., and Yeh, J. K., Dose response to vitamin D supplementation among postmenopausal African American women, *Am. J. Clin. Nutr.* 86, 1657–62, 2007.
50. Hathcock, J. W., Shao, A., Vieth, R., and Heaney, R., Risk assessment for vitamin D, *Am. J. Clin. Nutr.* 85, 6–18, 2007.
51. Holick, M. F., Vitamin D: Importance in the prevention of cancers, type 1 diabetes, heart disease, and osteoporosis, *Am. J. Clin. Nutr.* 79, 362–71, 2004
52. McCarty, C. A., Sunlight exposure assessment: Can we accurately assess vitamin D exposure from sunlight questionnaires? *Am. J. Clin. Nutr.* 87, 1097S–110S, 2008.
53. van der Maei, A. E. F., Blizzard, L, Ponsonby, A. L., and Dwyer, T., Validity and reliability of adult recall of past sun exposure in a case-control study of multiple sclerosis, *Cancer Epidemiol. Biomarkers Prev.* 15, 1538–44, 2006.
54. Brot, C., Vestergaard, P., Kolthoff, N., Gram, J., Hermann, AP., and Sorensen, O. H., Vitamin D status and its adequacy in healthy Danish perimenopausal women: Relationships to dietary intake, sun exposure and serum parathyroid hormone, *Br. J. Nutr.* 86, S97–S103, 2001.
55. Autier, P. and Gandini, S., Vitamin D supplementation and total mortality, *Arch. Intern. Med.* 167, 1730–7, 2007.
56. Scragg, R., Sowers, M., and Bell, C., Serum 25-hydroxyvitamin D, ethnicity, and blood pressure in the National Health and Nutrition Examination Survey, *Am. J. Hypertens.* 20, 713–9, 2007.
57. Wang, T. J., Pencina, M. J., Booth, S. L., Jacques, P. F., Ingelsson, E., Lanier, K., et al., Vitamin D deficiency and risk of cardiovascular disease, *Circulation* 117, 503–11, 2008.
58. Giovannucci, E., Liu, Y., Hollis, B. W., and Rimm, E. B., 25-Hydroxyvitamin D and risk of myocardial infarction in men. *Arch. Int. Med.* 168, 1174–80, 2008
59. Lappe, J., Travers-Gustafson, D., Davies, K., Recker R., and Heaney, R., Vitamin D and calcium supplementation reduces cancer risk: Results of a randomized trial, *Am. J. Clin. Nutr.* 85, 1586–91, 2007.

60. Cross, H.S., Pavelka, M., Slavik, J., and Peterlik, M., Growth control of human colon cancer cells by vitamin D and calcium *in vitro, J. Natl. Cancer Inst.* 84,1355–7, 1992.
61. Zinser, G. M., Suckow, M., and Welsh, J., Vitamin D receptor (VDR) ablation alters carcinogen-induced tumorigenesis in mammary gland, epidermis and lymphoid tissues, *J. Steroid. Biochem. Mol. Biol.* 97, 153–164, 2005.
62. Indra, A. K., Castaneda, E., Antal, M. C., Jiang, M., Messaddeq, N., Meng, X., et al., Malignant transformation of DMBA/TPA-induced papillomas and nevi in the skin of mice selectivity lacking retinoid-X-receptor alpha in epidermal keratinocytes, *J. Invest. Dermatol.* 127, 1250–60, 2007.
63. Holick, C. N., Stamford, J. L., Kwon, E. M., Ostrander, E. A., Nejentsev, S., and Peters, U., Comprehensive association analysis of the vitamin D pathway genes, VDR, CYP27B1 and CYP24A1 in prostate cancer, *Cancer Epidemiol. Biomarkers Prev.* 16, 1990–9, 2007.
64. Li, H., Stampfer, M. J., Hollis, J. B. W., Mucci, L. A., Gaziano, J. M., Hunter, D., et al., A prospective study of plasma vitamin D metabolites, vitamin D receptor polymorphisms, and prostate cancer, *PLoS. Med.* 4, e103, 0562–71, 2007.
65. Otani, T., Iwasaki, M., Sasazuki, S., Inoue, M., and Tsugane, S., Japan Public Health Center Prospective Study Group. Plasma vitamin D and risk of colorectal cancer: The Japan Public Health Center Based Prospective Study, *Br. J. Cancer.* 97, 446–51, 2007.
66. Freedman, D. M., Looker, A. C., Chang, S., and Graubard, B., Prospective study of serum vitamin D and cancer mortality in the United States, *J. Natl. Cancer Inst.* 99, 1594–1602, 2007.
67. Gorham, E. D., Garland, C. F., Garland, F. C., Grant, W. B., Mohr, S. B., Lipkin, M., et al., Optimal vitamin D status for colorectal cancer prevention, *Am. J. Prev. Med.* 32, 210–6, 2007.
68. Garland, C. F., Grant, W. B., Mohr, S. B., Goham, E. D., and Garland, F. C., What is the dose–response relationship between vitamin D and cancer risk? *Nutr. Rev.* 65, S91–5, 2007.
69. Garland, C. F., Gorham, E. D., Mohr, S. B., Grant, W. B., Giovannucci, E., Lipkin, M., et al., Vitamin D and prevention of breast cancer: Pooled analysis, *J. Steroid. Biochem. Mol. Biol.* 103, 708–11, 2007.
70. Kemmler, W., Engelke, K., vonStengel, S., Weineck, J., Lanber, D., and Kalender, W. A., Long term four year exercise has a positive effect on menopausal risk factors: the Erlangen Fitness Osteoporosis Prevention Study, *J. Strength Cond. Res.* 21: 232–9, 2007.
71. Hagberg, J. M., Zmuda, J. M., McCole, S. D., Rodgers, K. S., Ferrell, R. E., Wilund, K. R., and Moore, G. E., Moderate physical activity is associated with higher bone mineral density in postmenopausal women, *J. Am. Geriatr. Soc.* 49, 1411–7, 2001.
72. Roddam, A. W., Neale, R., Appleby, P., Allen, N. E., Tipper, S., and Key, T. J., Association between plasma 25-hydroxyvitamin D levels and fracture risk. The EPIC-Oxford Study, *Am. J. Epidemiol.* 166, 1327–36, 2007.
73. Chatard, J. C., Boutet, C., Tourny, C., Garcia, S., Berthouze, S., and Guezennec, C. Y., Nutritional status and physical fitness of elderly sportsmen, *Eur. J. Appl. Physiol.* 77, 157–63, 1998.
74. Papanek, P. E, The female athlete triad: An emerging role for physical therapy, *J. Orthop. Sports. Phys. Ther.* 33, 594–614, 2003.
75. Hosomi, A., Arita, M., Sato, Y., Kiyose, C., Ueda, T., Igarashi, O., et al., Affinity for alpha-tocopherol transfer protein as a determinant of the biological activities of vitamin E analogs, *FEBS Lett.* 409, 105–108, 1997.
76. Traber, M. G., Vitamin E, in *Modern Nutrition in Health and Disease*, 9th ed. Shils, M. E., Olson J. A., Shike, M., and Ross A. C., Eds., Williams & Wilkins, Baltimore, 1999, pp. 347–62.

77. Food and Nutrition Board, Institute of Medicine, Vitamin E, in *Dietary Reference Intakes for Vitamin C, Vitamin E, Selenium and Carotenoids,* National Academy Press, Washington, D. C., 2000, pp. 186–283.
78. Sattler, S. E., Gilliland, L., Magellanes-Lundback, M., Pollard, M., and DellaPenna, D., Vitamin E is essential for seed longevity and for preventing lipid peroxidation during germination, *Plant Cell* 16: 1419–32, 2004.
79. Traber, M. G. and Atkinson, J., Vitamin E, antioxidant and nothing more, *Free Radic. Biol. Med.* 43, 4–15, 2007.
80. Freedman J. E. and Keaney Jr., J. F., Vitamin E inhibition of platelet aggregation is independent of its antioxidant activity, *J. Nutr.* 131, 374S–7S, 2001.
81. Singh, U., Devaraj, S., and Jialal, I., Vitamin E, oxidative stress, and inflammation, *Ann. Rev. Nutr.* 25, 151–74, 2005.
82. Evans, H. M. and Bishop, K. S., On the existence of a hitherto unrecognized dietary factor essential for reproduction, *Science* 56, 650–51, 1922.
83. Hill, K. E., Montine, T. J., Motley, A. K., Li, X., May, J. M., and Burk, R. F., Combined deficiency of vitamins E and C causes paralysis and death in guinea pigs, *Am. J. Clin. Nutr.* 77, 1484–88, 2003.
84. U.S Department of Agriculture, Agricultural Research Service, 2007. What We Eat in America, NHANES, 2003–2004, Nutrient Intakes from Food: Mean Amounts Consumed per Individual, One Day, www.ars.usda.gov/ba/bhnrc/fsrg. Accessed 08/13/2008.
85. Horwitt, M. K., Harvey, C. C., Duncan, G. D., and Wilson, W. C., Effects of limited tocopherol intake in man with relationships to erythrocyte hemolysis and lipid oxidations, *Am. J. Clin. Nutr.* 4, 408–19, 1956.
86. ATBC (Alpha-Tocopherol, Beta-carotene) Cancer Prevention Study Group, The effect of vitamin E and beta-carotene on the incidence of lung cancer and other cancers in male smokers, *N. Eng. J. Med.* 330, 1029–35, 1994.
87. Bjelakovic, G., Nikolova, D., Gluud, L. L., Simonetti, R. G., and Gluud C., Mortality in randomized trials of antioxidant supplements for primary and secondary prevention, *J. Am. Med. Assoc.* 297, 842–57, 2007.
88. Vivekananthan, D. P., Penn, M. S., Sapp, S. K., Hsu, A., and Topol, E. J., Use of antioxidant vitamins for the prevention of cardiovascular disease: Meta-analysis of randomized trials, *Lancet* 361, 2017–23, 2003.
89. Slatore, C. G., Littman, A. J., Au, D. H., Satia, J. A., and White, E., Long-term use of supplemental multivitamins, vitamin C, vitamin E, and folate does not reduce the risk of lung cancer, *Am. J. Resp. Crit. Care Med.* 177, 524–30, 2008.
90. Traber, M. G., How much vitamin E? Just enough! *Am. J. Clin. Nutr.* 84, 959–60, 2006.
91. Traber, M. G., Frei, B., and Beckman J. S., Vitamin E revisited: Do new data validate benefits for chronic disease prevention? *Curr. Opin. Lipidol.* 19, 30–8, 2008.
92. Wright, M. E., Lawson, K. A., Weinstein, S. J., Pietinen, P., Taylor, P. R., Virtamo, J., and Albanes, D., Higher baseline serum concentrations of vitamin E are associated with lower total and cause-specific mortality in the Alpha-Tocopherol, Beta-carotene Cancer Prevention Study, *Am. J. Clin. Nutr.* 84, 1200–7, 2006.
93. Wagner, K. H., Kamal-Eldin, A., and Elmadfa, I. Gamma-tocopherol–an underestimated vitamin? *Ann. Nutr. Metab.* 48, 169–88, 2004.
94. Schneider, C., Chemistry and biology of vitamin E, *Mol. Nutr. Food Res.* 49, 7–30, 2005.
95. Handelman, G. J., Machlin, L. J., Fitch, K., Weiter, J. J., Dratz, E. A., and Frank, O., Oral α-tocopherol supplements decrease plasma γ-tocopherol levels in humans, *J. Nutr.* 115, 807–13, 1985.

96. Cooney, R. V., Franke, A. A., Harwood, P. J., Hatch–Pigott, V., Custer, L. J., and Mordan, L. J., Gamma-tocopherol detoxification of nitrogen dioxide: Superiority to α-tocopherol, *Proc. Natl. Acad. Sci. USA*, 90, 1771–5, 1993.
97. Chin, S.-F., Hamid, A. N. A., Latiff, A. A., Zakaria, Z., Mazlan, M., Yusof, Y. A. M., et al., Reduction of DNA damage in older healthy adults by Tri E Tocotrienol supplementation, *Nutrition* 24, 1–10, 2008.
98. Ji, L. L., Antioxidants and oxidative stress in exercise, *Proc. Soc. Exp. Biol. Med.* 222, 283–92, 1999.
99. Rjetjens, S. J., Beelen, M., Koopman, R., van Loon, L. J. C., Bast, A., and Haenen, G. R. M. M., A single session of resistance exercise induces oxidative damage in untrained men, *Med. Sci. Sports Exerc.* 39, 2145–51, 2007.
100. Chang, C.-K., Tseng, H.-F., Hsuuw, Y.-D., Chan, W.-H., and Shieh, L.-C., Higher LDL oxidation at rest and after rugby game in weekend warriors, *Ann. Nutr. Metab.* 46, 103–7, 2002.
101. Mastaloudis, A., Leonard, S., and Traber, M. G., Oxidative stress in athletes during extreme endurance exercise, *Free Radic. Biol. Med.* 31, 911–22, 2001.
102. Mastaloudis, A. and Traber, M. G., Vitamin E, in *Sports Nutrition*, 2nd ed., Driskell, J. A. and Wolinsky, I., Eds., CRC Press, Boca Raton, 2006, pp. 183–200.
103. Mastaloudis, A., Yu, T.-W., O'Donnel, R. P., Frei, B., Dashwood, R. H., and Traber, M. G., Endurance exercise results in DNA damage as detected by the comet assay, *Free Rad. Biol. Med.* 36, 966–75, 2004.
104. Thune, I. and Furberg, A.-S., Physical activity and cancer risk: dose–response and cancer, all sites and site-specific, *Med. Sci. Sports Exerc.* 33, S530–50, 2001.
105. Mastaloudis, A., Morrow, J., Hopkins, D., Devaraj, S., and Traber, M. G., Antioxidant supplementation prevents exercise-induced lipid peroxidation, but not inflammation, in ultramarathon runners, *Free Rad. Biol. Med.* 36, 1329–41, 2004.
106. Mastaloudis, A., Traber, M. G., Carstensen, K., and Widrick, J. J., Antioxidants did not prevent muscle damage in response to an ultramarathon run, *Med. Sci. Sports Exerc.* 38, 72–80, 2006.
107. Knez, W. L., Jenkins, D. G., and Coombes, J. S., Oxidative stress in half and full Ironman triathletes, *Med. Sci. Sports Exerc.* 39, 283–8, 2007.
108. Aguilo, A., Tauler, P., Sureda, A. Cases, N., Tur, J. A., and Pons, A., Antioxidant diet supplementation enhances aerobic performance in amateur sportsmen, *J. Sports Sci.* 25, 1203–10, 2007.
109. Tauler, P., Aguilo, A., Gimeno, I., Fuentespine, E., Tur, J. A., and Pons, A., Response of blood cell antioxidant enzyme defences to antioxidant diet supplementation and to intense exercise, *Europ. J. Nutr.* 45, 187–95, 2006.
110. Dumont, J. F., Peterson, J., Haytowitz, D., and Booth, S. L., Phylloquinone and dehydrophylloquinone contents of mixed dishes, processed meats, soups, and cheeses, *J. Food. Comp. Analysis.* 16, 595–603, 2003.
111. Okano, T., Shimomura, Y., Yamane, M., Suhara, Y., Kamao, M., Shigiura, M., and Nakagawa, K., Conversion of phylloquinone (vitamin K1) into menaquinone-4 (vitamin K_2): Two possible routes for menaquinone-4 accumulation in cerebra of mice, *J. Biol. Chem.* 283, 11270–9, 2008.
112. Davidson, R. T., Foley, A. L., Enggelke, J. A., and Suttie, J. W., Conversion of dietary phylloquinone to tissue menaquinone-4 in rats is not dependent on gut bacteria, *J. Nutr.* 128, 220–3, 1998.
113. Badr, M., Yoshihara, H., Kauffman, F., and Thurman, R., Menadione causes selective toxicity to periportal regions of the liver lobules, *Toxicol. Lett.* 35, 241–6, 1987.
114. Chang, M., Shi, M., and Forman, H. J., Exogenous glutathione protects endothelial cells from menadione toxicity, *Am. J. Physiol. Lung Cell Mol. Physiol.* 262, L637–43, 1992.

115. Marchionatti, A. M., Perez, A. V., Diaz de Barboza, G. E., Pereira, B. M., and Tolosa de Talamoni, N. G., Mitochondrial dysfunction is responsible for the intestinal calcium absorption inhibition induced by menadione, *Biochim. Biophys. Acta.* 1780, 101–7, 2008.
116. Schurgers, L. J. and Vermeer, C., Determination of phylloquinone and menaquinones in food, *Haemostasis* 30, 298–307, 2000.
117. Food and Nutrition Board, Institute of Medicine; Vitamin K. *Dietary reference intakes for vitamin A, vitamin K, Arsenic, Molybdenum, Nickel, Silicon, Vanadium, and Zinc.* Washington D. C: National Academy Press, 2001, 162–96.
118. Ronden, J. E., Thijssen, H. H. W., and Vermeer, C., Tissue distribution of K-vitamers under different nutritional regimens in the rat, *Biochim. Biophys. Acta.* 1379, 16–22, 1998.
119. Joyce, D. E. and Grinnell, B. W., Recombinant human activated protein C attenuates the inflammatory response in endothelium and monocytes by modulating nuclear-factor-kappaB, *Crit. Care Med.* 30, S288–93, 2002.
120. Feistritzer, C., Sturn, D. H., Kaneider, N. C., Djanani, A., and Wiedermann, C. J., Endothelial protein C receptor-dependent inhibition of human eosinophil chemotaxis by protein C, *J. Allergy Clin. Immunol.* 112, 375–81, 2003.
121. Cranenburg, E. C. M., Schurgers, L. J., and Vermeer, C., Vitamin K: The coagulation vitamin that became omnipotent, *Thromb. Haemost.* 98, 120–5, 2007.
122. U.S Department of Agriculture, Agricultural Research Service, 2007. What We Eat in America, NHANES, 2003–2004, Nutrient Intakes from Food: Mean Amounts Consumed per Individual, One Day, www.ars.usda.gov/ba/bhnrc/fsrg. Accessed 08/13/2008.
123. Booth, S. L., Tucker, K. L., McKeown, N. M., Davidson, K. W., Dallal, G. E., and Sadowski, J. A., Relationships between dietary intakes and fasting plasma concentrations of fat-soluble vitamins in humans, *J. Nutr.* 127, 587–92, 1997.
124. Thane, C. W., Wang, L. Y., and Coward, W. A., Plasma phylloquinone (vitamin K1) concentration and its relationship to intake in British adults aged 19–64 years, *Br. J. Nutr.* 96, 1116–24, 2006.
125. McKeown, N. M., Jacques, P. F., Gundberg, C. M., Peterson, J. W., Tucker, K. L., Kiel, D. P., et al., Dietary and nondietary determinants of vitamin K biochemical measures in men and women, *J. Nutr.* 132, 1329–34, 2002.
126. Guthrie, H. A. and Picciano, M. F; *Human Nutrition*, Molsby–Year Book, Inc., Missouri, 1995, chap. 11.
127. Shearer, M. J., The roles of vitamins D and K in bone health and osteoporosis prevention, *Proc. Nutr. Soc.* 56, 915–37, 1997.
128. Binkley, N. C., Krueger, D. C., Engelka, J. A., Foley, A. L., and Suttie, J. W., Vitamin K supplementation reduces serum concentrations of under-γ-carboxylated osteocalcin in healthy young and elderly adults, *Am. J. Clin. Nutr.* 72, 1523–8, 2000.
129. Booth, S. L., Lichtenstein, A. H., O'Brien-Morse, M., McKeown, N. M., Wood, R. J., Saltzman, E., and Gundberg, C. M., Effects of a hydrogenated form of vitamin K on bone formation and resorption, *Am. J. Clin. Nutr.* 74, 783–90, 2001.
130. Feskanich, D., Weber, P., Willett, W. C., Rockett, H., Booth, S. L., and Colditz, G. A., Vitamin K intake and hip fractures in women: A prospective study, *Am. J. Clin. Nutr.* 69, 74–9, 1999.
131. Booth, S. L., Broe, K. E., Gagnon, D. R., Tucker, K. L., Hannan, M. T., McLean, R. R., et al., Vitamin K intake and bone mineral density in women and men, *Am. J. Clin. Nutr.* 77, 512–6, 2003.
132. Zittermann, A., Effects of vitamin K on calcium and bone metabolism, *Curr. Opin. Clin. Nutr. Metab. Care.* 4, 483–7, 2001.

133. Cockayne, S., Adamson, J., Lanham-New, S., Shearer, M. J., Gilbody, S., and Torgerson, D. J., Vitamin K and the prevention of fractures: Systematic review and meta-analysis of randomized controlled trials, *Arch. Intern. Med.* 166, 1256–61, 2006.
134. Binkley, N. C., Krueger, D. C., Kawahara, T. N., Engelka, J. A., Chappell, R. J., and Suttie, J. W., A high phylloquinone intake is required to achieve maximal osteocalcin gamma-carboxylation, *Am. J. Clin. Nutr.* 76, 1055–60, 2002.
135. Braam, L. A., Knapen, M. H., Geusens, P., Brouns, F., Hamulyak, K., Gerichhausen, M. J., and Vermeer, C., Vitamin K_1 supplementation retards bone loss in postmenopausal women between 50 and 60 years of age, *Calcif. Tissue Int.* 73, 21–6, 2003.
136. Schurgers, L. J., Teunissen, K. J. F., Hamulyak, K., Knapen, M. H. J., Vik, H., and Vermeer, C., Vitamin K-containing dietary supplements: Comparison of synthetic vitamin K-1 and natto-derived menaquinone-7, *Blood* 109, 3279–83, 2007.
137. Erkkilä, A. T. and Booth S. L., Vitamin K intake and atherosclerosis, *Curr. Opin. Lipidol.* 19, 39–42, 2008.
138. Shea, M. K., Booth, S. L., Massaro, J. M., Jacques, P. E., D'Agostine, R. B., Dawson-Hughes, B., et al., Vitamin K and vitamin D status: Association with inflammatory markers in the Framingham Offspring Study, *Am. J. Epidemiol.* 167, 313–20, 2008.
139. Braam, L. A., Hoeks, A. P., Brouns, F., Hamulyak, K., Gerichhausen, M. J., and Vermeer, C., Beneficial effects of vitamin D and K on the elastic properties of the vessel wall in postmenopausal women: A follow-up study, *Thromb. Haemost.* 91, 373–80, 2004.
140. Schurgers, L. J., Spronk, H. M. H., Soute, B. A. M., Schiffers, P. M., DeMey, J. G. R., and Vermeer, C., Regression of warfarin-induced medial elastocalcinosis by high intake of vitamn K in rats, *Blood* 109, 2823–31, 2007.
141. Cario-Toumaniantz, C., Boularan, C., Schurgers, L. J., Heymann, M. F., Le Cunff, M., Leger, J., et al., Identification of differentially expressed genes in human varicose veins: Involvement of matrix Gla protein in extracellular matrix remodeling, *J. Vasc. Res.* 44, 444–59, 2007.
142. Craciun, A. M., Wolf, J., Knapen, M. H., Brouns, F., and Vermeer, C., Improved bone metabolism in female elite athletes after vitamin K supplementation, *Int. J. Sport Med.* 19, 479–84, 1998.
143. Buettner, G. R., The pecking order of free radicals and antioxidants: Lipid peroxidation, alpha-tocopherol, and ascorbate, *Arch. Biochem. Biophys.* 300, 535–43, 1993.
144. Hamilton, I. M., Gilmore, W. S., Benzie, I. F. F., Mulholland, C. W., and Strain, J. J., Interactions between vitamins C and E in human subjects, *Br. J. Nutr*, 84, 261–7, 2000.
145. Bruno, R. S., Ramakrishnan, R., Montine, T. J., Bray, T. M., and Traber, M. G., α-Tocopherol disappearance is faster in cigarette smokers and is inversely related to their ascorbic acid status, *Am J, Clin. Nutr.* 81, 95–103, 2005.
146. Bruno, R. S., Leonard, S. W., Atkinson, J., Montint, T. J., Ramakrishnan, R., Bray, T. M. and Traber, M. G., Faster plasma vitamin E disappearance in smokers is normalized by vitamin C supplementation, *Free Rad. Biol. Med.* 40, 689–97, 2006.
147. Arnrich, L. and Arthur, V. A., Interactions of fat-soluble vitamins in hypervitaminoses, *Ann. NY Acad. Sci.* 355, 109–18, 1980.
148. Kusin, J. A., Redde, V., and Sivakumar, B., Vitamin E supplements and the absorption of a massive dose of vitamin A, *Am. J. Clin. Nutr.* 27, 774–6, 1974.
149. Jimenez-Lara, A. M. and Aranda, A., Interaction of vitamin D and retinoid receptors on regulation of gene expression, *Hormone Res.* 54, 301–5, 2000.
150. Traber, M. G., Frei, B., and Beckman, J. S., Vitamin E revisited: Do new data validate benefits for chronic disease prevention? *Curr. Opin. Lipidol.* 19, 30–8, 2008
151. Booth, S. L., Golly, I., Sacheck, J. M., Roubenoff, R., Dallal, G. E., Hamada, K., and Blumberg, J. B., Effect of vitamin E supplementation on vitamin K status in adults with normal coagulation status, *Am. J. Clin. Nutr.* 80, 143–8, 2004.

152. Campbell, W. and Geik, R., Nutritional considerations for the older athlete, *Nutrition.* 20, 603–8, 2004.
153. American College of Sports Medicine, American Dietetic Association, and Dietitians of Canada, Joint position statement: Nutrition and athletic performance, *Med. Sci. Sports Exerc.* 32, 2130–45, 2000.
154. Blum, M., Dolnikowski, G., Seyoum, E., Harris, S. S., Booth, S. L., Peterson, J., et al., Vitamin D_3 in fat tissue, *Endocrine* 33, 90–4, 2008.

6 Vitamin C

Herb E. Schellhorn and Yi Li

CONTENTS

I. INTRODUCTION

The role of dietary antioxidants, and particularly vitamin C, in general health have been the subject of considerable debate. The rapid turnover of vitamin C, its interaction with other physiological antioxidants and its rapid depletion during imposed oxidative stress (such as would likely occur during exercise), make study of this important vitamin complex. While the effects of acute vitamin C deficiency are well known and characterized (scurvy) and can be readily "treated" with relatively small amounts of supplements, the levels of vitamin C that may be optimal for long-term health are difficult to determine. There is considerable evidence, though not completely unequivocal, that high levels of vitamin C may have some beneficial effect in preventing biological damage and can thus be a potentially important element of strategies to promote good health. Vitamin C has several known biological roles, all of which are of relevance to exercise and good health. In addition, vitamin C has some surprising physiological functions that have recently been described and these too may be relevant for exercise and aging.

What type of scientific information is most valuable in estimating nutritional requirements? Given that the focus of this volume is on the middle-aged segment of the population, a large proportion of which will likely survive into old age, it is important to have long-term well-controlled studies to assess biological effects. However, short-term studies focusing on important biological markers that are good prognosticators of long-term health should also be considered in formulating dietary requirements.[1]

Vitamin C is a subject of considerable interest because of its many physiological roles and its potential relevance to chronic diseases, including cancer and heart disease. As a key soluble antioxidant, it is important in neutralizing excess free radicals generated during normal metabolism and during exercise. Despite many years of intense research, we are still discovering new facets of biological function for vitamin C and, as such, our current assessment of research must be considered limited and incomplete.

Several relevant reviews on vitamin C and exercise are available, including a consideration of interactions with vitamin E,[2] the value of nutritional supplements, including vitamin C in preventing muscle damage,[3] and detailed reviews of antioxidants and exercise.[4,5]

II. CHEMICAL STRUCTURE AND PURIFICATION/SYNTHESIS

A. Chemical Structure

The most common and naturally occurring form of vitamin C is L-ascorbic acid (Figure 6.1). It exists as white crystal with a molecular weight of 176.1 g/mol. L-ascorbic acid is freely soluble in water. Once dissolved in water, its two enolic hydroxyl groups can be sequentially deprotonated, giving rise to two pKa values, pKa1= 4.17 and pKa2= 11.57 (Figure 6.1). Vitamin C can also exist as dehydroascorbic acid (DHA), which is the oxidized form of ascorbic acid. While structurally similar to ascorbic acid, DHA exhibits some unique physiological properties and is

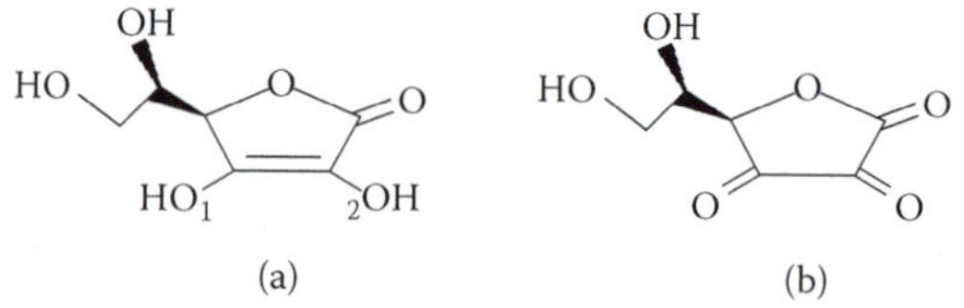

(a) (b)

FIGURE 6.1 Molecular structure of L-ascorbic acid (A) and dehydroascorbic acid (B). L-ascorbic acid has a molecular weight of 176.1 g/mol. It carries two acidic hydrogen atoms with pKD values of 4.17 and 11.57, respectively. Dehydroascorbic acid is the oxidized form of ascorbic acid. It ia another naturally occurring structure of vitamin C.

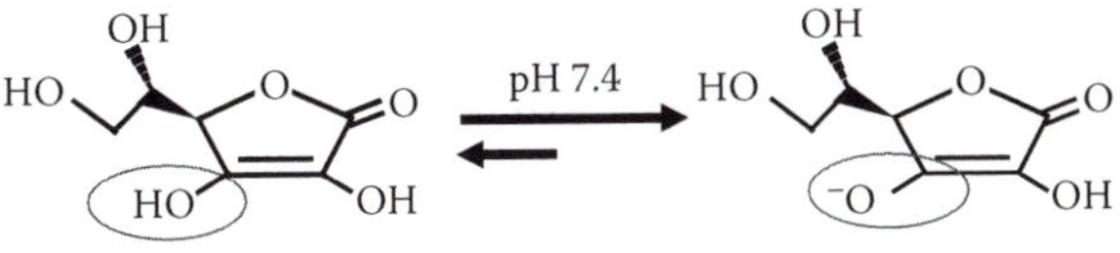

FIGURE 6.2 Formation of ascorbate from ascorbic acid in solution at physiological pH. In solution, L-ascorbic acid is readily deprotonated at physiological pH (7.4) to form ascorbate.

transported by a different mechanism, which will be discussed in detail in Section V, Figure 6.4. At physiological pH (pH 7.4), L-ascorbic acid is readily deprotonated at the first and more acidic hydroxyl group (pKa1= 4.17) to form ascorbate, a salt of ascorbic acid (Figure 6.2).

When encountering single-electron carrying compounds in solution, including free radicals and reactive oxygen species, ascorbate can donate one electron to these compounds and itself become ascorbyl radical. Unlike other single-electron radicals, ascorbyl radical is extremely inert. This is attributable to its unique molecular structure, in which the unpaired electron is delocalized in the pi molecular orbital of the ascorbyl ring and thus stabilized by a resonance structure (Figure 6.3). Therefore, this simple redox reaction replaces reactive radicals with a relative unreactive compound, and as a consequence, offers antioxidant protection to the biological system.

B. Synthesis

In animals, vitamin C is synthesized from L-gulonolactone by the enzyme gulonolactone oxidase. Plants use a different pathway utilizing enzyme L-galactolactone dehydrogenase to synthesize vitamin C.[6] L-ascorbic acid is synthesized from L-glucose in a series of biological reactions. In most mammals, it is produced in the liver using glucose extracted from the hepatic glycogen storage. The rate-limiting reaction of vitamin C biosynthesis is the oxidation of gulonolactone by gulonolactone oxidase (GULO).

Unlike most mammals, humans do not have functional GULO, and, as a result, cannot produce vitamin C. This nutritional defect is caused by inactivating mutations of the gene encoding GULO. Because of this defect, humans are dependent on dietary vitamin C intake for metabolic needs.

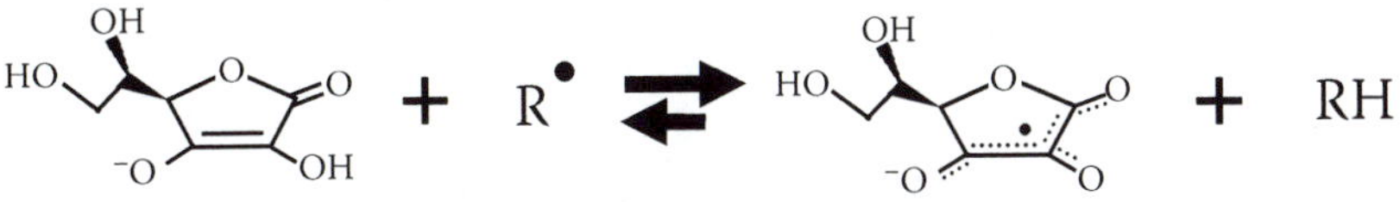

FIGURE 6.3 Neutralization of single-electron carrying radicals (R) by ascorbate, which donates a single electron to free radicals in solution, resulting in a reduced form of these radicals (RH). Ascorbate itself becomes a singular electron-carrying ascorbyl radical, which, unlike other radicals, is unreactive, as the electron is stabilized by resonance.

III. BASIS FOR BIOCHEMICAL DEFICIENCY IN HUMANS AND OTHER PRIMATES

In most mammals, vitamin C is normally synthesized from glucose. In mammals that lack the terminal biosynthetic step, the precursor is decarboxylated to form xylulose that can be used in other synthetic pathways. Primates and guinea pigs independently lost the ability to synthesize vitamin C 40 million years ago.[7] The loss in both cases is due to a mutation in the gene for the enzyme that catalyzes the terminal step in the above pathway—GULO. The gene has since become a so-called pseudogene (a highly mutated gene that no longer codes for a functional protein). Reasons for the evolutionary loss of this function have been the subject of considerable speculation[8]—the loss must have been benign, or even selected for, since this mutation is found in all primates. In an evolutionary sense, the loss likely had little effect on the reproductive success of primate populations because the amounts of vitamin C required for growth are very low (much lower than required for antioxidant function) and could be easily obtained in the diet. It has been estimated that most nonhuman primates easily obtain 1–2 grams per day in their diet.[9] In contrast, humans generally consume far less because they consume fewer foods that are rich in vitamin C (such as fruits) and also because cooking food inactivates vitamin C. As a result, even in North America, many individuals do not obtain even the relatively low levels (~60 mg per day) thought to be adequate for human nutrition[10] (it should be noted that the current standard, the Dietary Reference Intake (DRI), is now 90 mg per day for males and 75 mg per day for females,[11] although even this level could be considered inadequate for satisfying dietary antioxidant needs). Primates, particularly humans in the Western world, occupy a very different world from the one in which the inactivating mutation first arose. Rather than bacterial and virus-mediated mortality, the principal causes of death in Western society today are primarily heart disease[7] and cancer,[10] both of which are influenced by diet and, relevant to this review, are suspected to be aggravated by inadequate consumption of dietary oxidants such as vitamin C.[12] The RDA levels, based on the need to alleviate the symptoms of scurvy,[13] are likely far below those required for antioxidant function.[10] This difference in levels has two potentially important consequences for middle age—(1) insufficient levels may aggravate oxidative damage that occurs as a result of increased respiration that accompanies increased exertion, and (2) high levels above those normally obtained in the diet may, at least theoretically, offer protection against high levels of reactive oxygen species (ROS).

IV. PHYSIOLOGICAL FUNCTIONS OF VITAMIN C

Vitamin C plays important roles in a broad spectrum of physiological processes. The lack of sufficient vitamin C intake in humans results in a well-defined set of symptoms, including fatigue, poor wound healing, depression and tooth loss, which are collectively referred to as scurvy. If left untreated, the individual would die within months.

A. Collagen Biosynthesis

Collagen is the major component of the extracellular matrix. A longitudinal protein, collagen fiber aggregates to form a tough, rope-like structure that provides structural support for various tissues. It confers strength and elasticity to the skin. Aging-related degradation of collagen is a common cause for wrinkles and poor wound healing in aging populations. In addition, collagen is the major component of cartilage and bone, and is responsible for the fracture-resistant property of these structures. Therefore, insufficient collagen synthesis may contribute to increased bone fracture and poor post-fracture recovery in aging humans.

Vitamin C is a cofactor for collagen biosynthesis.[14] It functions as an electron donor for proline hydroxylase, lysine hydroxylase and procollagen-proline 2-oxoglutarate 3-dioxygenase, which are responsible for posttranslational modification and maturation of collagen. Inadequate intracellular vitamin C levels result in formation of defective collagen, leading to collagen deficiency in the body. This deficiency manifests itself in characteristic scurvy symptoms such as bleeding gums, skin deterioration, and tooth loss. In its early stages, these symptoms can be alleviated by consumption of vitamin C-containing foods, such as lemons and oranges, a regimen commonly used during 18th-century sea voyages.

B. L-Carnitine Biosynthesis

Carnitine is essential for fat metabolism. It carries long chain fatty acids from the cytosol into the mitochondrial matrix, where these fatty acids can be broken down to provide metabolic energy.[15]

L-carnitine is produced from amino acids L-lysine and L-methionine. Vitamin C functions as a cofactor in carnitine biosynthesis in a similar manner as in collagen maturation. It is the electron donor of two carnitine synthetic enzymes, *N*-trimethyl-L-lysine hydroxylase and γ-butyrobetaine hydroxylase.[15] Vitamin C deficiency results in decreased levels of carnitine in the body, and, in turn, impaired fatty acid metabolism, which is manifested as fatigue and lethargy.[16] These symptoms are also commonly documented in cases of scurvy. Supplementation of vitamin C by dietary means has been shown to restore carnitine synthesis in animals.[16]

C. Iron Absorption

Iron is the vital component of the hemoglobin of the red blood cell, which transports oxygen in the body for energy metabolism. Iron deficiency is the cause of iron deficiency anemia, characterized by diminished capacity of the red blood cell to carry oxygen into body tissues. Similar to hemoglobin, myoglobin, which is responsible for oxygen storage in muscle cells, also relies on iron to trap the oxygen molecule. Therefore, iron deficiency also leads to poor energy metabolism in muscle cells, resulting in fatigue and inability to exercise for prolonged periods.[17]

Although iron deficiency anemia is multifactorial, poor iron absorption is the most common cause for this ailment. Vitamin C has been shown to facilitate iron absorption from the diet in a dose-dependent manner.[17] An electron-donating agent, ascorbic acid reduces ferric iron (Fe^{3+}) to the more soluble ferrous form (Fe^{2+}), which is then absorbed in the small intestine.[18] In addition to acting on iron directly, vitamin C also potentiates the activity of ferric reductase, which catalyzes the conversion of ferric iron to the more absorbable ferrous iron.[19] Therefore, diets rich in vitamin C and iron may counteract the effect of iron deficiency anemia.

D. Conversion of Dopamine to Norepinephrine

Norepinephrine deficiency can cause depression and hypochondria, which are commonly observed in scurvy patients.[20] Ascorbic acid is a cofactor for dopamine hydroxylase and peptidylglycine amidating monooxygenase, which are enzymes involved in norepinephrine biosynthesis.[20] Therefore, adequate levels of vitamin C may be important for preventing these psychiatric disorders.

E. Role as a Key Biological Antioxidant

Antioxidants are reducing compounds that protect the biological system from oxidative damage caused by ROS and nitrogen species (RNS). ROS and RNS ar produced as the byproducts of normal mitochondrial respiratory processes involving oxygen as the terminal electron acceptor. Incomplete utilization of oxygen gives rise to free radicals, which are compounds carrying unpaired electrons; they are toxic to various components of the biological system. Commonly, biological ROS and RNS include superoxide, hydrogen peroxide, and hydroxyl radical. In addition, some ROS are produced as a defense mechanism against invading pathogens. For example, superoxide is produced by NADPH-oxidase to destroy engulfed microorganisms in phagocytes.

ROS and RNS are detrimental to the biological system, as they can induce irreversible oxidative damage to various cellular structures and macromolecules, including DNA, lipids, and proteins. Accumulating with age, ROS is believed to be one of the major causes for aging and age-related degenerative diseases, including cancer, heart disease, and neurodegeneration.

Oxidative damage caused by ROS results in redox imbalance inside the cell, which, in turn, triggers redox-sensitive signaling pathways leading to tumorigenesis. Indeed, many key oncogenic pathways have been shown to be responsive to the reduction–oxidation state of the cell, and their alteration may lead to abnormalities in various cellular processes including uncontrollable proliferation,[21] growth of new blood vessels or angiogenesis,[22] and inhibition of programmed cell death or apoptosis,[23] all of which contribute to the formation of tumors. Moreover, ROS and RNS also induce genomic instability, as DNA, the major component of chromosomes, is extremely susceptible to oxidative damage by these compounds. Reaction between DNA molecule and ROS, such as hydroxyl radical, results in oxidative modification of the genetic material, leading to mutagenesis and carcinogenesis.[24,25]

Oxidative stress induced by ROS and RNS is also a cause for the initiation and progression of heart disease. For example, superoxide produced by vascular cells[26] oxidizes low-density lipoprotein (LDL), resulting in highly reactive oxidized LDL (oxLDL), which triggers a sequence of atherosclerotic events. First, oxLDL enters macrophages in the blood and transforms them into cholesterol lipid-laden foam cells.[27,28] These cholesterol-laden macrophages adhere to the blood vessel wall and start to accumulate in blood vessels.[29,30] These cells elicit multiple inflammatory responses in the circulatory system[31,32] and induce programmed cell death of endothelial cells composing the vessel wall.[33,34] These events mark the onset of atherosclerosis and cardiovascular dysfunction.

ROS also alters the nitric oxide (NO) biosynthetic pathway. Endothelial NO is essential for modulating cardiovascular homeostasis and protecting the vascular system. It simulates relaxation of the vascular smooth muscle, allowing vasodilatation and unhindered blood flow.[35] NO also prevents inflammation[36,37] and programmed cell death in endothelial cells,[33,38] where mechanisms counteract the effects of atherosclerosis, thus preventing the onset of cardiovascular disease.

However, NO synthesis is susceptible to ROS attack. For example, superoxide alters NO synthetic pathway by oxidative modification of an essential element. This has two effects: (1) reduction of endothelial NO, and, consequently, diminished protection offered by NO, and (2) further production of ROS and RNS by the hijacked NO pathway.[39] Indeed, impaired endothelium-dependent vessel relaxation is commonly observed in individuals with endothelial dysfunction.[40]

Oxidative modification of macromolecules by ROS and RNS has been proposed as a mechanistic basis for aging-related neurodegeneration. The brain consumes disproportionately large quantities of oxygen and is composed of oxidation-prone fatty acids. Therefore, it is extremely sensitive to oxidative damage.[41] ROS in the brain triggers an inflammatory response and elicits damage to protein and lipid components, which contributes to the onset of neurodegenerative disease such as Alzheimer's. As these age-related degenerative diseases, including cancer, heart disease, and neurodegeneration, are attributable to accumulation of ROS and RNS over time, reduction of ROS and RNS levels in the body is essential for delaying and preventing the onset of these diseases, especially in aging populations.

Vitamin C is an ideal biological antioxidant. When encountering ROS and RNS, vitamin C donates a single electron to these molecules, hence reducing them to their unreactive state. Vitamin C itself becomes a single electron carrying ascorbyl free radical. However, unlike other free radicals such as superoxide or hydroxyl radical, ascorbyl free radical is relatively inert, as the reactive electron is delocalized and stabilized by the unique molecular structure (Figure 6.3). Ascorbic acid can be readily replenished from ascorbyl radical by thioredoxin reductase using NADPH as electron donor, and enters subsequent cycles of ROS quenching. Vitamin C is soluble in biological fluid such as the blood, and, as such, can destroy blood-borne ROS and RNS before they reach tissues and cause damage. In addition, vitamin C is nontoxic and can be used therapeutically to maintain the antioxidant–oxidant balance in the body. Indeed, a large number of studies have shown that ascorbic acid protects the biological system against oxidative damage induced by various ROS and RNS.

Vitamin C prevents oxidative damage to DNA,[42–45] lipids,[46,47] and protein.[46,48,49] Consumption of vitamin C-rich diets is inversely related to the levels of oxidative DNA damage.[50–53] Not only does vitamin C offer structural protection to biological molecules, it also modulates redox-sensitive signal transduction pathways, leading to increased cell cycle arrest and programmed cell death in response to DNA damage[54,55] and attenuation of cell proliferation.[56–58] These mechanisms together give rise to the antitumorigenic effect of ascorbic acid.

At physiological concentrations, ascorbic acid protects LDL from oxidative modification by (1) quenching ROS and RNS in the blood and (2) enhancing the resistance of LDL to oxidation,[59] and, in effect, attenuates the levels of harmful oxLDL in circulation.[60–62] In addition, ascorbic acid mitigates the effects of oxLDL on the biological system. For instance, it protects smooth muscle cells and macrophages from oxLDL-induced cell death[63,64] and attenuates oxLDL-related atherogenic inflammation.[65,66] Inside the cells, vitamin C protects normal NO synthesis.[67,68] Adequate concentrations of vitamin C are also essential to maintain the structural integrity of the aorta.[69,70] As vitamin C potentiates the antioxidant capacity of the biological systems and offers protection for various cellular components, it has been hypothesized to attenuate the process of aging and progression of age-related degenerative diseases.[71,72]

V. VITAMIN C TRANSPORT

Humans acquire vitamin C from our diets or dietary supplements as we cannot produce it in our bodies. Absorption of vitamin C occurs in the small intestine and is mediated by specific sodium-vitamin C co-transporters (SVCT1). Once transported into the intestinal epithelial cells, ascorbic acid diffuses into the surrounding capillary bed and then enters the circulatory system[73–75] (Figure 6.4).

In the kidney, ascorbic acid in the blood is filtered in bulk from the blood into the renal tubule by a general filtration mechanism. When passing down the renal tubule, it is reabsorbed back into the blood through renal epithelial cells by the same class of vitamin C transporters (SVCT1). The difference in the amounts of vitamin C leaving the blood by general filtration and those returning to the blood by reabsorption constitutes renal excretion (Figure 6.4).

Vitamin C is carried by the blood to body tissues and is imported from the blood into cells by two classes of transporters, depending on cell type. For example, vitamin C is transported into muscle cells in its oxidized form, dehydroascorbic acid, by glucose transporter (GLUT), but is imported into the brain by SVCT2 transporter in the form of ascorbic acid or ascorbate.[76]

VI. MEASUREMENT OF VITAMIN C

Vitamin C can be readily assayed in biological fluids in several ways including spectrophotometric analysis,[77] electrochemical detection (ECD)[78] and, following derivatization, by fluorescence.[79] A fluorescence assay has been recently adapted to microtiter plates, facilitating high throughput analysis that should be useful for comparative analysis.[80] Key considerations in an assay of vitamin C are the inherent instability of the vitamin, the presence of interfering compounds, and the need for high sensitivity to assess low concentrations. As ECD and fluorescence detection are extremely sensitive and specific, these are the preferred methods for assay. The factors affecting measurement of vitamin C, including stability and interfering compounds, have been thoroughly considered in the development of assay protocols using ECD.[78]

	Transporter	Mechanism	Distribution	Regulation
A	GLUT1 GLUT3 GLUT4	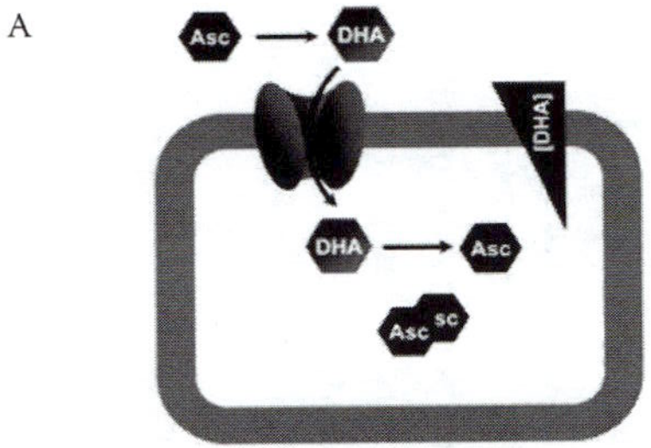	Osteoblast, astrocyte, muscles cells, and retinal cells	Glucose: Competitive inhibition Insulin: Stimulates transport
B	SVCT1 SVCT2	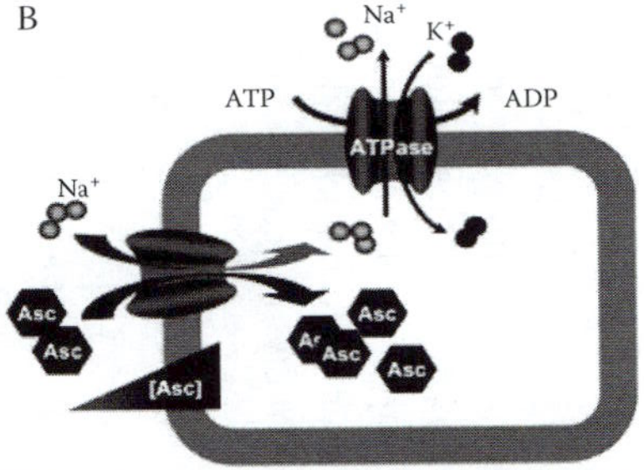	Intestinal, renal, and liver epithelial cells Brain, retinal, and placental cells	Ascorbate: Substrate feedback inhibition of SVCT1 expression Ascorbate: Substrate feedback inhibition of SVCT2 expression

FIGURE 6.4 Major mechanisms for vitamin C transport, their regulation and distribution of transporters in mammals. Vitamin C is transported by both glucose transporter (GLUT) in an energy-independent, three-step mechanism (A) and by secondary active sodium vitamin C co-transporters (SVCT) in an ATP-dependent manner (B). Transport via GLUT requires extracellular oxidation of ascorbate to dehydroascorbate (DHA), which is imported by GLUT and reduced back to ascorbate in the cell. The concentration gradient of DHA is maintained (A). Ascorbate can be coupled to sodium ions and transported directly by SVCT. The excess intracellular sodium ion is actively exported in exchange for extracellular potassium ions through a sodium-potassium ATPase. (Li, Y and Schellhorn, H. E. 2007. *J. Nutr.* 137. pp. 2171–2184.[72] With permission.)

VII. ROLE IN EXERCISE

A. Vitamin C and General Effects on Exercise

The role of vitamin C as an antioxidant is particularly relevant to exercise physiology, because high levels of ROS produced during exercise can be neutralized by high levels of this vitamin. ROS, as a normal product of respiration, are produced as a consequence of the neutrophil-mediated respiratory burst that accompanies the release of cytokines from tissue damaged during exercise.[81] This results in the release of creatine kinase, a muscle-specific enzyme, which can be readily assayed as a quantitative marker for muscle damage.[82] The potential for dietary antioxidants to prevent this damage would offer the possibility of reducing the negative effects of eccentric exercise.* Vitamin C alone, or in combination with vitamin E, has been examined in a meta-analysis to assess potential beneficial effects of alleviating exercise-induced muscle soreness.[3] While results do not exclude a beneficial role for vitamin C, other micronutrients are probably as important in preventing damage.

B. Vitamin C and Exercise in Middle Age

There are many potential ways in which vitamin C may be relevant for exercise in middle-aged individuals. Because it is required for epinephrine and norepinephrine synthesis, lack of vitamin C may cause feelings of fatigue or lack of energy that may affect athletic performance. As an antioxidant, vitamin C may be important in ameliorating the effects of oxidative stress caused during extreme exercise. Because exercise induces muscle damage at the cellular level, inflammation can occur as a consequence, and neutrophil activation in response to inflammation may generate reactive oxygen species, which can be reduced or eliminated by vitamin C. Vitamin C supplementation prior to exercise can reduce indicators of oxidative stress including protein carbonylation and oxidation of glutathione in young males,[83] and it is likely that similar results would be observed with middle-aged athletes.

Loss of bone mineral density (BMD), which can occur toward the end of middle age and extend into old age, can be affected by both age and nutrition. Levels of dietary vitamin C in elderly women (> 60 years) are inversely correlated with BMD[84] but show little correlation in men.

VIII. BODY RESERVES

Much of our knowledge regarding vitamin C cycling in humans comes from controlled diet studies. In healthy human males, normal body stores of vitamin C are approx. 20mg/kg body weight.[85] Metabolism and excretion result in a turnover of 60 mg/day vitamin C with a half-life in the body of about 10 days.[85] High levels of dietary vitamin C (~2g per day) result in high excretion rates of up to 80% of the

* Eccentric exercise can be defined as muscle contraction while the muscle fibers are extending (e.g., stretching or weight resistance training that involves muscle extension).

ingested vitamin.[85] The effects of vitamin C deprivation on the time required to display overt symptoms of scurvy are extremely variable.

IX. DIETARY AND SUPPLEMENTAL SOURCES

The amounts of vitamin C that are required for collagen biosynthesis are minimal; greater than 10 mg per day will prevent scurvy. The best sources of vitamin C are citrus fruits, peppers, paprika, and rosehips (Table 6.1). Animal sources of vitamin C, especially cooked meat, are invariably low in vitamin C because vitamin C is oxidized by tissue stores of iron and is decomposed by heat. High-dose oral supplementation (3g every 4 h) can lead to sustained higher levels of serum vitamin C of 130 μM, which is probably an upper limit due to inefficient absorption.[86] Current recommended dietary levels of vitamin C are 75 mg and 90 mg per day for males and females respectively. Levels for pregnant and lactating women are higher and age dependent. Current levels for all populations can be obtained from the Institute of Medicine (www.iom.org).

X. POSSIBLE TOXICITY

Toxicity levels of vitamin C that exceed the DRI are few. High levels of intake (2g/day) may cause kidney stones in some individuals but most are not affected.[87] Relevant for toxicity considerations, the levels of serum vitamin C that can be attained are inherently limited by the inefficient intestinal absorption of this nutrient and by the fact that it is readily excreted by the kidneys because of its high solubility. Gastrointestinal disorders may also be a consequence of high chronic use but the literature on this is equivocal.

Despite the slight risk for these conditions, there is considerable evidence that moderate pharmacological levels (those that are slightly above normal dietary intake) are not harmful to healthy individuals. Vitamin C, administered in conjunction with several other antioxidants, has been shown to be effective at preventing macular degeneration of the eye in the comprehensive Age-Related Eye Disease Study (AREDS).[88] The AREDS formulation, containing 500 mg Vitamin C given twice per day, has been thoroughly tested on thousands of middle-aged individuals over many years without significant adverse effects.

Because vitamin C promotes iron uptake, dietary supplementation may potentially cause toxicity through accumulation of high levels of iron (which can be a potent pro-oxidant). In normal healthy individuals this not likely to be a concern,[89] but may be a consideration for individuals who have hemachromatosis (a homozygous genetic condition that can have a frequency as high as one per 200 individuals.[90] It is important to note that some of the negative effects associated with this high vitamin C consumption may be subject to a great degree of variability among individuals that is poorly understood.

TABLE 6.1

Dietary Sources of Vitamin C

Source (Size)	Vitamin C, mg
Fruit	
Strawberries (255g, 1 cup, sliced)	95
Kiwi fruit (76g, 1 medium)	75
Orange (131g, 1 medium)	70
Cantaloupe (138g, 1/4 medium)	60
Mango (207g, 1 cup, sliced)	45
Watermelon (286g, 1 cup)	23
Peaches, frozen, sliced, sweetened (250g, 1 cup)	234
Juice	
Orange concentrate (213g, 1 Cup)	294
Orange (248g, 1 Cup)	124
Grapefruit concentrate (207g, 1 Cup)	248
Fortified Juice (with added vitamin C)	
Grape concentrate (216g,1 cup)	179
Cranberry cocktail (253g, 1 cup)	107
Vegetables	
Pepper, red or green	
Raw (149g, 1 cup)	120
Cooked (136g, 1 cup)	100
Broccoli, cooked (156g, 1 cup)	120
Brussels sprouts, cooked (156, 1 cup)	97
Cabbage	
Red, raw (70g, 1 cup)	40
White, raw (70g, 1 cup)	22
Cauliflower (54, 1 cup)	24
Potato, baked (156g, 1 medium)	20

Modified from: Levine, M., Rumsey, S.C., Daruwala, R., Park, J.B., and Wang, Y.H. 1999. *JAMA* 281, 1415–1423.

XI. INTERACTIONS WITH OTHER NUTRIENTS AND DRUGS

As an antioxidant, vitamin C works in conjunction with other small antioxidant molecules such as vitamin E, uric acid, and glutathione to prevent oxidative damage. Few controlled studies have specifically examined vitamin C in isolation. Relative to young individuals, middle-aged persons have reduced elasticity of veins and arteries that may be affected by reduced collagen synthesis. Vitamin C has a relatively low redox potential and can thus reduce other physiological antioxidants, including the oxidized forms of vitamin E,[91] uric acid,[92] sulfhydryl groups, and glutathione.[93] By abstracting electrons from these other antioxidants or directly from ROS, the relatively stable ascorbyl radical is formed, which can either react with another ascorbyl radical to form dehydroascorbate and ascorbate or it can simply be excreted. Reflecting its key role as a direct and indirect soluble antioxidant, reduced vitamin C is depleted in plasma exposed to peroxides.

XII. FUTURE RESEARCH NEEDS

Few studies have examined the effect of vitamin C in control populations of middle-aged individuals. An enormous literature examines the effects of vitamin C on the performance of elite athletes, particularly at the college level, presumably because of the ready availability of subjects for study. More information is needed on the effects of vitamin C supplements on athletic performance in middle-aged individuals. Such studies would include more precise age-cohort group studies to determine the effects of sufficiency or deficiency over extended time periods of supplementation. Currently, very few studies have examined cohort groups of middle-aged individuals in relation to matched young individuals. Such studies might give an indication of how parameters associated with aging are influenced by dietary vitamin C.

A further complication in studying vitamin C and exercise is that very few appropriate laboratory animals can be used as models because most animals can make their own vitamin C. Thus, the rat and mouse, which are commonly used in the study of the effects of other vitamins on exercise, cannot be employed for vitamin C studies. The guinea pig has been used, but there is not much information available. Animals are particularly useful for modeling vitamin C effects because their relatively short life span facilitates examination of the effects of chronic sufficiency or deficiency on performance. In addition, controlled animal studies permit the isolation of vitamin C effects from other confounding variables (such as other dietary antioxidants).

XIII. CONCLUSIONS

In view of the increased RDA and the importance of other micronutrients in vitamin C-containing foods, middle-aged individuals engaged in regular vigorous exercise should consume a dietary regimen that includes sufficient fresh fruits and vegetables to ensure adequate intake of vitamin C and other important antioxidants. The use of dietary supplements may provide an additional benefit in improving physiological indices, but additional research on the effects of sustained supplementation is required before substantive recommendations can be made. The potential for deleterious consequences of dietary supplementation with moderately high levels of vitamin C (1–2g/day) is negligible or nonexistent, making the use of supplements a decision based on informed personal choice.

REFERENCES

1. Ames, B.N., Mccann, J.C., Stampfer, M.J., and Willett, W.C., Evidence-based decision making on micronutrients and chronic disease: long-term randomized controlled trials are not enough. *Am. J. Clin. Nutr.* 86, 522–523, 2007.
2. Evans, W.J., Vitamin E, vitamin C, and exercise. *Am. J. Clin. Nutr.* 72, 647S–652S, 2000.
3. Bloomer, R.J., The role of nutritional supplements in the prevention and treatment of resistance exercise-induced skeletal muscle injury. *Sports Med.* 37, 519–532, 2007.
4. Urso, M.L. and Clarkson, P.M., Oxidative stress, exercise, and antioxidant supplementation. *Toxicology* 189, 41–54, 2003.
5. Clarkson, P.M. and Thompson, H.S., Antioxidants: What role do they play in physical activity and health? *Am. J. Clin. Nutr.* 72, 637S–646S, 2000.
6. Smirnoff, N., L-ascorbic acid biosynthesis. *Vitam. Horm.* 61, 241–266, 2001.
7. Hu, F.B. and Willett, W.C., Optimal diets for prevention of coronary heart disease. *JAMA* 288, 2569–2578, 2002.
8. Nandi, A., Mukhopadhyay, C.K., Ghosh, M.K., Chattopadhyay, D.J., and Chatterjee, I.B., Evolutionary significance of vitamin C biosynthesis in terrestrial vertebrates. *Free Radical Biol. Med.* 22, 1047–1054, 1997.
9. Milton, K., Nutritional characteristics of wild primate foods: Do the diets of our closest living relatives have lessons for us? *Nutrition* 15, 488–498, 1999.
10. Ames, B.N., Gold, L.S., and Willett, W.C., The causes and prevention of cancer. *Proc. Natl. Acad. Sci. USA* 92, 5258–5265, 1995.
11. Institute of Medicine, Vitamin C. Dietary reference intakes for vitamin C, vitamin E, selenium, and carotenoids. National Academy Press, Washington, D.C., 2000, 95.
12. Sato, P. and Udenfriend, S., Scurvy-prone animals, including man, monkey, and guinea pig, do not express the gene for gulonolactone oxidase. *Arch. Biochem. Biophys.* 187, 158–162, 1978.
13. Carr, A.C. and Frei, B., Toward a new recommended dietary allowance for vitamin C based on antioxidant and health effects in humans. *Am. J. Clin. Nutr.* 69, 1086–1107, 1999.
14. Murad, S., Grove, D., Lindberg, K.A., Reynolds, G., Sivarajah, A., and Pinnell, S.R., Regulation of collagen synthesis by ascorbic acid. *Proc. Natl. Acad. Sci. USA* 78, 2879–2882, 1981.
15. Rebouche, C.J., Ascorbic-acid and carnitine biosynthesis. *Am. J. Clin. Nutr.* 54, S1147–S1152, 1991.
16. Ha, T.Y., Otsuka, M., and Arakawa, N., The regulatory effect of ascorbate on the carnitine synthesis in primary cultured guinea pig hepatocytes. *J. Nutr. Sci. Vitamin.* 37, 371–378, 1991.
17. Hallberg, L., Brune, M., and Rossander, L., Effect of ascorbic-acid on iron absorption from different types of meals—Studies with ascorbic-acid-rich foods and synthetic ascorbic-acid given in different amounts with different meals. *Human Nutr.* 40A, 97–113, 1986.
18. Levine, M., Rumsey, S.C., Daruwala, R., Park, J.B., and Wang, Y.H., Criteria and recommendations for vitamin C intake. *JAMA* 281, 1415–1423, 1999.
19. Herbert, V., Shaw, S., and Jayatilleke, E., Vitamin C-driven free radical generation from iron. *J. Nutr.* 126, S1213–S1220, 1996.
20. Diliberto, E.J., Daniels, A.J., and Viveros, O.H., Multicompartmental secretion of ascorbate and its dual role in dopamine beta-hydroxylation. *Am. J. Clin. Nutr.* 54, S1163–S1172, 1991.

21. Catarzi, S., Degl'Innocenti, D., Iantomasi, T., Favilli, F., and Vincenzini, M.T., The role of H_2O_2 in the platelet-derived growth factor-induced transcription of the gamma-glutamylcysteine synthetase heavy subunit. *Cell. Mol. Life Sci.* 59, 1388–1394, 2002.
22. Hughes, G., Murphy, M.P., and Ledgerwood, E.C., Mitochondrial reactive oxygen species regulate the temporal activation of nuclear factor kappa B to modulate tumour necrosis factor-induced apoptosis: evidence from mitochondria-targeted antioxidants. *Biochem. J.* 389, 83–89, 2005.
23. Souici, A.C., Mirkovitch, J., Hausel, P., Keefer, L.K., and Felley-Bosco, E., Transition mutation in codon 248 of the p53 tumor suppressor gene induced by reactive oxygen species and a nitric oxide-releasing compound. *Carcinogenesis* 21, 281–287, 2000.
24. Marnett, L.J., Oxyradicals and DNA damage. *Carcinogenesis* 21, 361–370, 2000.
25. Cooke, M.S., Evans, M.D., Dizdaroglu, M., and Lunec, J., Oxidative DNA damage: Mechanisms, mutation, and disease. *FASEB J.* 17, 1195–1214, 2003.
26. Griendling, K.K., Sorescu, D., and Ushio-Fukai, M., NAD(P)H oxidase: Role in cardiovascular biology and disease. *Circ. Res.* 86, 494–501, 2000.
27. de Villiers, W.J.S. and Smart, E.J., Macrophage scavenger receptors and foam cell formation. *J. Leukoc. Biol.* 66, 740–746, 1999.
28. Li, A.C. and Glass, C.K., The macrophage foam cell as a target for therapeutic intervention. *Nat. Med.* 8, 1235–1242, 2002.
29. Parthasarathy, S., Quinn, M.T., Schwenke, D.C., Carew, T.E., and Steinberg, D., Oxidative modification of beta-very low-density lipoprotein: Potential role in monocyte recruitment and foam cell formation. *Arteriosclerosis* 9, 398–404, 1989.
30. Quinn, M.T., Parthasarathy, S., Fong, L.G., and Steinberg, D., Oxidatively modified low density lipoproteins: A potential role in recruitment and retention of monocyte/macrophages during atherogenesis. *Proc. Natl. Acad. Sci. USA* 84, 2995–2998, 1987.
31. Ross, R., Atherosclerosis is an inflammatory disease. *Am. Heart J.* 138, S419–S420, 1999.
32. Stoll, G. and Bendszus, M., Inflammation and atherosclerosis: Novel insights into plaque formation and destabilization. *Stroke* 37, 1923–1932, 2006.
33. Dimmeler, S., Haendeler, J., Galle, J., and Zeiher, A.M., Oxidized low-density lipoprotein induces apoptosis of human endothelial cells by activation of CPP32-like proteases: A mechanistic clue to the "response to injury" hypothesis. *Circulation* 95, 1760–1763, 1997.
34. Harada-Shiba, M., Kinoshita, M., Kamido, H., and Shimokado, K., Oxidized low density lipoprotein induces apoptosis in cultured human umbilical vein endothelial cells by common and unique mechanisms. *J. Biol. Chem.* 273, 9681–9687, 1998.
35. Ignarro, L.J., Buga, G.M., Wood, K.S., Byrns, R.E., and Chaudhuri, G., Endothelium-derived relaxing factor produced and released from artery and vein is nitric-oxide. *Proc. Natl. Acad. Sci. USA* 84, 9265–9269, 1987.
36. Decaterina, R., Libby, P., Peng, H.B., Thannickal, V.J., Rajavashisth, T.B., Gimbrone, M.A., et al., Nitric oxide decreases cytokine-induced endothelial activation: Nitric oxide selectively reduces endothelial expression of adhesion molecules and proinflammatory cytokines. *J. Clin. Invest.* 96, 60–68, 1995.
37. Cornelis, R.S., van Vliet, M., Vos, C.B., Cleton-Jansen, A.M., van de Vijver, M.J., Peterse, J.L., et al., Evidence for a gene on 17p13.3, distal to TP53, as a target for allele loss in breast tumors without p53 mutations. *Cancer. Res.* 54, 4200–4206, 1994.

38. Khan, B.V., Harrison, D.G., Olbrych, M.T., Alexander, R.W., and Medford, R.M., Nitric oxide regulates vascular cell adhesion molecule 1 gene expression and redox-sensitive transcriptional events in human vascular endothelial cells. *Proc. Natl. Acad. Sci. USA* 93, 9114–9119, 1996.
39. Vasquez-Vivar, J., Kalyanaraman, B., Martasek, P., Hogg, N., Masters, B.S.S., Karoui, H., et al., Superoxide generation by endothelial nitric oxide synthase: The influence of cofactors. *Proc. Natl. Acad. Sci. USA* 95, 9220–9225, 1998.
40. Lapu-Bula, R. and Ofili, E., From hypertension to heart failure: Role of nitric oxide-mediated endothelial dysfunction and emerging insights from myocardial contrast echocardiography. *Am. J. Cardiol.* 99, 7D–14D, 2007.
41. Floyd, R.A., Antioxidants, oxidative stress, and degenerative neurological disorders. *Proc. Soc. Exp. Biol. Med.* 222, 236–245, 1999.
42. Lutsenko, E.A., Carcamo, J.M., and Golde, D.W., Vitamin C prevents DNA mutation induced by oxidative stress. *J. Biol. Chem.* 277, 16895–16899, 2002.
43. Noroozi, M., Angerson, W.J., and Lean, M.E., Effects of flavonoids and vitamin C on oxidative DNA damage to human lymphocytes. *Am. J. Clin. Nutr.* 67, 1210–1218, 1998.
44. Pflaum, M., Kielbassa, C., Garmyn, M., and Epe, B., Oxidative DNA damage induced by visible light in mammalian cells: Extent, inhibition by antioxidants and genotoxic effects. *Mutat Res* 408, 137–146, 1998.
45. Sweetman, S.F., Strain, J.J., and McKelvey-Martin, V.J., Effect of antioxidant vitamin supplementation on DNA damage and repair in human lymphoblastoid cells. *Nutr. Cancer* 27, 122–130, 1997.
46. Barja, G., Lopez-Torres, M., Perez-Campo, R., Rojas, C., Cadenas, S., Prat, J., and Pamplona, R., Dietary vitamin C decreases endogenous protein oxidative damage, malondialdehyde, and lipid peroxidation and maintains fatty acid unsaturation in the guinea pig liver. *Free Radical Biol. Med.* 17, 105–115, 1994.
47. Kimura, H., Yamada, Y., Morita, Y., Ikeda, H., and Matsuo, T., Dietary ascorbic acid depresses plasma and low density lipoprotein lipid peroxidation in genetically scorbutic rats. *J. Nutr.* 122, 1904–1909, 1992.
48. Cadenas, S., Rojas, C., and Barja, G., Endotoxin increases oxidative injury to proteins in guinea pig liver: Protection by dietary vitamin C. *Pharmacol. Toxicol.* 82, 11–18, 1998.
49. Hoey, B.M. and Butler, J., The repair of oxidized amino-acids by antioxidants. *Biochem Biophys Acta* 791, 212–218, 1984.
50. Deng, X.S., Tuo, J.S., Poulsen, H.E., and Loft, S., Prevention of oxidative DNA damage in rats by Brussels sprouts. *Free Radical Res.* 28, 323–333, 1998.
51. Fraga, C.G., Motchnik, P.A., Shigenaga, M.K., Helbock, H.J., Jacob, R.A., and Ames, B.N., Ascorbic acid protects against endogenous oxidative DNA damage in human sperm. *Proc. Natl. Acad. Sci. USA* 88, 11003–11006, 1991.
52. Rehman, A., Bourne, L.C., Halliwell, B., and Rice–Evans, C.A., Tomato consumption modulates oxidative DNA damage in humans. *Biochem. Biophys. Res. Commun.* 262, 828–831, 1999.
53. Thompson, H.J., Heimendinger, J., Haegele, A., Sedlacek, S.M., Gillette, C., O'Neill, C., et al., Effect of increased vegetable and fruit consumption on markers of oxidative cellular damage. *Carcinogenesis* 20, 2261–2266, 1999.
54. Reddy, V.G., Khanna, N., and Singh, N., Vitamin C augments chemotherapeutic response of cervical carcinoma HeLa cells by stabilizing P53. *Biochem. Biophys. Res. Commun.* 282, 409–415, 2001.

55. Catani, M.V., Costanzo, A., Savini, I., Levrero, M., De Laurenzi, V., Wang, J.Y.J., et al., Ascorbate up-regulates MLH1 (Mut L homologue-1) and p73: Implications for the cellular response to DNA damage. *Biochem. J.* 364, 441–447, 2002.
56. Bowie, A.G. and O'Neill, L.A., Vitamin C inhibits NF-kappa B activation by TNF via the activation of p38 mitogen-activated protein kinase. *J. Immunol.* 165, 7180–7188, 2000.
57. Carcamo, J.M., Pedraza, A., Borquez-Ojeda, O., and Golde, D.W., Vitamin C suppresses TNF alpha-induced NF kappa B activation by inhibiting I kappa B alpha phosphorylation. *Biochemistry* 41, 12995–13002, 2002.
58. Han, S.S., Kim, K., Hahm, E.R., Lee, S.J., Surh, Y.J., et al, L-ascorbic acid represses constitutive activation of NF-kappaB and COX-2 expression in human acute myeloid leukemia, HL-60. *J. Cell. Biochem.* 93, 257–270, 2004.
59. Retsky, K.L., Freeman, M.W., and Frei, B., Ascorbic acid oxidation product(s) protect human low density lipoprotein against atherogenic modification. Anti- rather than prooxidant activity of vitamin C in the presence of transition metal ions. *J. Biol. Chem.* 268, 1304–1309, 1993.
60. Retsky, K.L. and Frei, B., Vitamin C prevents metal ion-dependent initiation and propagation of lipid peroxidation in human low-density lipoprotein. *Biochem Biophys Acta* 1257, 279–287, 1995.
61. Martin, A. and Frei, B., Both intracellular and extracellular vitamin C inhibit atherogenic modification of LDL by human vascular endothelial cells. *Arterioscler Thrombosis Vasc Biol* 17, 1583–1590, 1997.
62. Alul, R.H., Wood, M., Longo, J., Marcotte, A.L., Campione, A.L., Moore, M.K., and Lynch, S.M., Vitamin C protects low-density lipoprotein from homocysteine-mediated oxidation. *Free Radical Biol. Med.* 34, 881–891, 2003.
63. Siow, R.C.M., Sato, H., Leake, D.S., Pearson, J.D., Bannai, S., and Mann, G.E., Vitamin C protects human arterial smooth muscle cells against atherogenic lipoproteins: Effects of antioxidant vitamins C and E on oxidized LDL-induced adaptive increases in cystine transport and glutathione. *Arterioscler. Thrombosis Vasc. Biol.* 18, 1662–1670, 1998.
64. Asmis, R. and Wintergerst, E.S., Dehydroascorbic acid prevents apoptosis induced by oxidized low-density lipoprotein in human monocyte-derived macrophages. *Eur. J. Biochem.* 255, 147–155, 1998.
65. Griffiths, H., Rayment, S., Shaw, J., Lunec, J., and Woollard, K., Dietary supplementation with vitamin C but not vitamin E reduces constitutive expression of ICAM-1 in peripheral blood monocytes of normal subjects with low plasma vitamin C levels. *Free Radical Biol. Med.* 35, S35–S35, 2003.
66. Mo, S.J., Son, E.W., Rhee, D.K., and Pyo, S., Modulation of TNF-alpha-induced ICAM-1 expression, NO and H2O2 production by alginate, allicin and ascorbic acid in human endothelial cells. *Arch. Pharmacol. Res.* 26, 244–251, 2003.
67. Marui, N., Offermann, M.K., Swerlick, R., Kunsch, C., Rosen, C.A., Ahmad, M., et al., Vascular cell-adhesion molecule-1 (Vcam-1) gene transcription and expression are regulated through an antioxidant sensitive mechanism in human vascular endothelial cells. *J. Clin. Invest.* 92, 1866–1874, 1993.
68. Baker, R.A., Milstien, S., and Katusic, Z.S., Effect of vitamin C on the availability of tetrahydrobiopterin in human endothelial cells. *J. Cardiovasc. Pharm.* 37, 333–338, 2001.
69. Maeda, N., Hagihara, H., Nakata, Y., Hiller, S., Wilder, J., and Reddick, R., Aortic wall damage in mice unable to synthesize ascorbic acid. *Proc. Natl. Acad. Sci. USA* 97, 841–846, 2000.

70. Nakata, Y. and Maeda, N., Vulnerable atherosclerotic plaque morphology in apolipoprotein E-deficient mice unable to make ascorbic acid. *Circulation* 105, 1485–1490, 2002.
71. Li, Y. and Schellhorn, H.E., Can ageing-related degenerative diseases be ameliorated through administration of vitamin C at pharmacological levels? *Med. Hypotheses* 68, 1315–1317, 2007.
72. Li, Y. and Schellhorn, H.E., New developments and novel therapeutic perspectives for vitamin C. *J. Nutr.* 137, 2171–2184, 2007.
73. Takanaga, H., Mackenzie, B., and Hediger, M.A., Sodium-dependent ascorbic acid transporter family SLC23. *Pflugers Arch* 447, 677–682, 2004.
74. Hornig, D., Weber, F., and Wiss, O., Site of intestinal absorption of ascorbic acid in guinea pigs and rats. *Biochem. Biophys. Res. Commun.* 52, 168–172, 1973.
75. Malo, C. and Wilson, J.X., Glucose modulates vitamin C transport in adult human small intestinal brush border membrane vesicles. *J. Nutr.* 130, 63–69, 2000.
76. Korcok, J., Dixon, S.J., Lo, T.C.Y., and Wilson, J.X., Differential effects of glucose on dehydroascorbic acid transport and intracellular ascorbate accumulation in astrocytes and skeletal myocytes. *Brain Res* 993, 201–207, 2003.
77. Kallio, H., Yang, B.R., and Peippo, P., Effects of different origins and harvesting time on vitamin C, tocopherols, and tocotrienols in sea buckthorn (Hippophae rhamnoides) berries. *J. Agric. Food Chem.* 50, 6136–6142, 2002.
78. Lykkesfeldt, J., Loft, S., and Poulsen, H.E., Determination of ascorbic-acid and dehydroascorbic acid in plasma by high-performance liquid chromatography with coulometric detection: Are they reliable biomarkers of oxidative stress? *Anal. Biochem.* 229, 329–335, 1995.
79. Nakagawa, H., Asano, A., and Sato, R., Ascorbate-synthesizing system in rat liver microsomes. II. A peptide-bound flavin as the prosthetic group of L-gulono-gamma-lactone oxidase. *J. Biol. Chem.* 77, 221–232, 1975.
80. Vislisel, J.M., Schafer, F.Q., and Buettner, G.R., A simple and sensitive assay for ascorbate using a plate reader. *Anal. Biochem* 365, 31–39, 2007.
81. Steinberg, J.G., Ba, A., Bregeon, F., Delliaux, S., and Jammes, Y., Cytokine and oxidative responses to maximal cycling exercise in sedentary subjects. *Med. Sci. Sport Exer.* 39, 964–968, 2007.
82. Dawson, B., Henry, G.J., Goodman, C., Gillam, I., Beilby, J.R., Ching, S., et al., Effect of Vitamin C and E supplementation on biochemical and ultrastructural indices of muscle damage after a 21 km run. *Int. J. Sports. Med.* 23, 10–15, 2002.
83. Goldfarb, A.H., Patrick, S.W., Bryer, S., and You, T., Vitamin C supplementation affects oxidative-stress blood markers in response to a 30-minute run at 75% VO2max. *Int. J. Sport Nutr. Exerc. Metab* 15, 279–290, 2005.
84. Kaptoge, S., Welch, A., McTaggart, A., Mulligan, A., Dalzell, N., Day, N.E., et al., Effects of dietary nutrients and food groups on bone loss from the proximal femur in men and women in the 7th and 8th decades of age. *Osteoporos. Int.* 14, 418–428, 2003.
85. Kallner, A., Hartmann, D., and Hornig, D., Steady-state turnover and body pool of ascorbic acid in man. *Am. J. Clin. Nutr.* 32, 530–539, 1979.
86. Padayatty, S.J., Sun, H., Wang, Y.H., Riordan, H.D., Hewitt, S.M., Katz, A., et al., Vitamin C pharmacokinetics: Implications for oral and intravenous use. *Ann. Internal Med.* 140, 533–537, 2004.
87. Massey, L.K., Liebman, M., and Kynast-Gales, S.A., Ascorbate increases human oxaluria and kidney stone risk. *J. Nutr.* 135, 1673–1677, 2005.

88. Kassoff, A., Kassoff, J., Buehler, J., Eglow, M., Kaufman, F., et al., A randomized, placebo-controlled, clinical trial of high-dose supplementation with vitamins C and E, beta carotene, and zinc for age-related macular degeneration and vision loss: AREDS Report No. 8. *Arch. Opthamol.* 119, 1417–1436, 2001.
89. Gerster, H., High-dose vitamin C: A risk for persons with high iron stores? *Int. J. Vitam. Nutr. Res.* 69, 67–82, 1999.
90. Beutler, E., Hemochromatosis: Genetics and pathophysiology. *Annu. Rev. Med.* 57, 331–347, 2006.
91. Sharma, M.K. and Buettner, G.R., Interaction of vitamin C and vitamin E during free radical stress in plasma: An ESR study. *Free Radical Biol. Med.* 14, 649–653, 1993.
92. Frei, B., Stocker, R., and Ames, B.N., Small antioxidant defenses in human extracellular fluids. In Scandalios, J. G., Ed., *Molecular Biology of Free Radical Scavenging Systems, Cold Spring Harbor Press,* NY, 1992.
93. Sipe, H.J., Jr., Jordan, S.J., Hanna, P.M., and Mason, R.P., The metabolism of 17 beta-estradiol by lactoperoxidase: A possible source of oxidative stress in breast cancer. *Carcinogenesis* 15, 2637–2643, 1994

7 B-Vitamins

George U. Liepa, Sandra D. Pernecky, Steven J. Pernecky, and Stephen J. McGregor

CONTENTS

I. INTRODUCTION

B vitamins are organic molecules that must be supplied in foods because they cannot be produced in the body. They are best known for their co-enzymatic roles in energy and protein metabolism as well as immune functions. The B vitamins are all water soluble and include vitamins B_1 (thiamin), B_2 (riboflavin), B_3 (nicotinic acid), B_5 (pantothenic acid), B_6 (pyridoxine, pyridoxal, pyridoxamine), B_7 (biotin), B_9 (folic acid, folacin, pteroyl glutamic acid), and B_{12} (cyanocobalamin). Each vitamin will be referred to by its most common name throughout this chapter.

Recommended intakes of the B vitamins will be identified as Recommended Dietary Intakes (RDA) or Adequate Intakes (AI) as defined by the United States Department of Agriculture (USDA).[1] The RDA represents the average daily intake of a nutrient that meets the requirements of approximately 98% of all healthy people and is listed related to age and gender. The estimated average requirement is calculated from scientific evidence. When there is not enough scientific evidence about a nutrient to determine a specific estimated average requirement for an RDA, an AI is estimated. Whereas the AI is based on current scientific research, further research is needed to determine a more exact amount of the specific nutrient. The AI is also designed to meet the needs of all healthy children and adults.[1] The Dietary Reference Intake (DRI) values are provided in Table 7.1; they are reference values that incorporate the RDA and AI as quantitative estimates of nutrient intakes to be used for planning and assessing diets for healthy people.[1] The upper limits for most of the vitamins in Table 7.1 are not determinable, although the few upper limits that are given are as little as about twice (niacin and folic acid) and about 20 times (pyridoxine) the DRI.[2]

This chapter will present background material about each of the B vitamins including information about normal absorption, metabolism, functions, deficiencies, toxicities, and recommended intakes. The impact of exercise on vitamin status and effects of vitamin supplementation on performance will be discussed for each of the B vitamins.

TABLE 7.1

Dietary Reference Intakes: Recommended Intakes for Individuals

	Males		Females		Upper Limits Males/Females
Vitamin	**31–50yrs**	**51–70yrs**	**31–50yrs**	**51–70yrs**	**19–70yrs**
Thiamin (Vit B_1), mg/d	1.2	1.2	1.1	1.1	ND
Riboflavin (Vit. B_2), mg/day	1.3	1.3	1.1	1.1	ND
Niacin (Vit B_3), mg/d	16	16	14	14	35[d]
Panthothenic acid (Vit B_5), mg/d	5[a]	5[a]	5[a]	5[a]	ND
Pyridoxine (Vit B_6), mg/d	1.3	1.7	1.3	1.5	100
Biotin (Vit B_7), μg/d	30[a]	30[a]	30[a]	30[a]	ND
Folic acid (Vit B_9), μg/d	400	400	400[b]	400	1,000[d]
Cobalamin (Vit. B_{12}), μg/d	2.4	2.4	2.4	2.4[c]	ND

[a] AI values (the values without this footnote are RDA values).

[b] Consumption of 400 μg of folic acid from supplements is recommended for all women capable of becoming pregnant.

[c] It is recommended that those older than 50 years consume foods fortified with B_{12} or a supplement containing B_{12} because up to 30% of this group malabsorbs food-bound B_{12}.

[d] 'The UL for niacin and folic acid apply to synthetic forms obtained from supplements, fortified foods, or a combination of the two

II. THIAMIN (VITAMIN B_1)

Thiamin plays a critical role in energy metabolism. It is highly soluble in water and stable to both heat and oxidation at < pH 5.0. The structural formula of thiamin is shown in Figure 7.1.

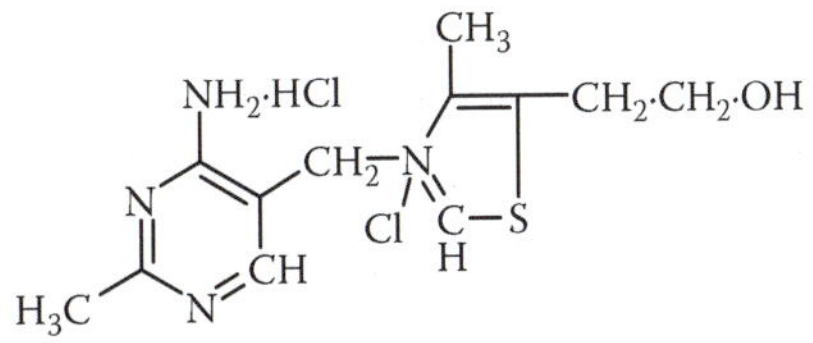

FIGURE 7.1 Thiamin.

Because of its structure, thiamin can form ester linkages with various acid groups, allowing for the formation of its active forms (Thiamin pyrophosphate [TPP], Thiamin monophosphate [TMP], and Thiamin triphosphate [TTP]). The three enzymes that are known to participate in the formation of these phosphate esters are (1) thiamin pyrophosphokinase, which catalyzes the formation of TPP from thiamin and ATP (2) TPP-ATP phosphoryl transferase, which catalyzes the formation of TTP from TPP and adenosine triphosphate (ATP) and (3) thiamin pyrophosphatase, which hydrolyzes TPP to form TMP. The percentages of the three active forms of thiamin found in the body are: TPP (80%), TTP (10%), and TMP and thiamin (10%). Higher concentrations are found in the skeletal muscle (50%), heart, liver, kidneys, and brain.[3]

The absorption of thiamin takes place in the upper part of the small intestine (i.e., duodenum). Oral thiamin is well absorbed and rapidly converted to its phosphorylated forms. It has been shown that when the upper section of the small intestine is removed due to ulcers or injury, thiamin absorption is significantly affected by alkaline pH, found in the lower intestinal tract. After absorption, thiamin is carried by the hepatic portal system to the liver. In normal adults, 20% to 30% of thiamin in the plasma is protein bound in the form of TPP. The biological half-life of ^{14}C-thiamin in the body is 9 to 18 days.[4] Since thiamin is not stored in large amounts in any tissue, a continuous supply from the diet is necessary.

Thiamin deficiency in animals and humans affects the cardiovascular, muscular, nervous and gastrointestinal systems, with end results including cardiac failure, muscular weakness, peripheral and central neuropathy, and gastrointestinal malfunction. This broad-based impact is primarily due to the fact that thiamin is required for glucose metabolism with the help of the coenzyme NAD (nicotinamide adenine dinucleotide). Thiamin pyrophosphate plays a vital role in the energy metabolism of the cells by participating in the conversion of pyruvate to acetyl coenzyme and CO_2 by the enzyme pyruvate dehydrogenase and also by promoting the conversion of a 5-carbon compound in the tricarboxylic acid (TCA) cycle to a 4-carbon compound. It is clear that the main metabolic function of thiamin is in oxidative decarboxylation. Clinically, thiamin deficiency has been shown to cause beriberi, heart disease and, in alcoholics, Wernicke-Korsakoff Syndrome. Polyneuropathy is a common problem with this deficiency because failure of energy metabolism predominantly affects neurons and their functions in selected areas of the central nervous system.

Thiamin deficiency is more common in the elderly. It is also noted to occur in alcoholics. It has been postulated that thiamin deficiency induced by excess alcohol intake or liver disease may affect levels of apoenzyme transketolase or its cofactor binding and thus prevent the formation of TPP. However, it has been observed that in well-nourished alcoholics, sufficient amounts of thiamin are maintained in the organs and there is no abnormality in the maintenance of appropriate concentrations of phosphorylated species of thiamin. Acute thiamin deficiency was recently reported in foreign workers who complained of weakness and lower limb edema. One worker died of refractory metabolic acidosis and shock. Thiamin deficiency is also more common in subjects taking diuretics, as thiamin is readily excreted in the urine.[3]

Various biochemical tests are available to detect thiamin deficiency. These include urinary thiamin excretion, thiamin concentrations in cerebral spinal fluid (CSF), erythrocyte transketolase activity (ETKA) and thiamin pyrophosphate effect (TPPE) on ETKA. Presently there is no known data that indicates that thiamin has toxic effects when large amounts are consumed in the diet or via long-term supplementation.

Thiamin is present in a variety of animal and vegetable food products. However, the best sources are ready-to-eat breakfast cereals; enriched, fortified, or whole grain bread and bread products; lean pork; ham products; and some fortified meat substitutes. A number of compounds are known to be thiamin antagonists or anti-thiamin factors. These include alcohols, polyphenols, flavonoids, and thiaminase (a heat-labile enzyme found in certain foods).[3] Alcohol has been shown to inhibit intestinal ATPase, which is involved in thiamine absorption.[3] The RDA for thiamine in the United States is 1.2 mg/d for males 31 to 70 years old, and 1.1 mg/d for females 31 to 70 years old.[1]

A. Thiamin and Exercise

Considering the important role thiamin derivatives play in the metabolism of carbohydrates and amino acids it is hypothetically plausible that thiamin could be a performance-limiting nutrient for the physically active individual. In particular, the conversion of pyruvate to acetyl-CoA during the complete oxidation of glucose is a vital process for the maintenance of high rates of ATP provision during periods of intense aerobic activity. However, no available data supports the concept that low endogenous thiamin levels impair performance, or that supplemental thiamin provision improves performance in otherwise healthy individuals.

In a classic study by Keys et al., exogenous administration of thiamin at four different levels (0.23, 0.33, 0.53 and 0.63 mg/1000 kcal) over a period of 12 weeks in healthy young men resulted in no differences in performance or physiological parameters during treadmill exercise.[5] Later, Webster et al. examined the effects of supplementation with two thiamin derivatives, allithiamin and tetrahydrofurfuryl disulfide (TTFD).[6,7] In the first study, six highly trained cyclists were given allithiamin and pantethine or placebo, and no differences were observed in physiological or performance measures when subjects performed a laboratory 50 km bout at 60% VO_{2max} followed by a 2000-m maximal trial. In another study, supplementation with TTFD for 4 days in healthy young males did not affect maximal oxygen uptake in a graded exercise test or physiological or performance measures during a 2000-m performance trial lasting approximately 200 seconds.[6] Both of the aforementioned studies by Webster et al. were performed in a randomized, double blind, crossover design and should therefore account for any confounders such as training status or dietary habits. Further, a performance trial of 200 seconds in duration should be sufficiently long to elicit both maximal glycolytic and aerobic metabolism.[8–10] Therefore, the studies of Webster et al. address both experimental and metabolic requirements necessary to determine an effect of thiamin supplementation in healthy or trained individuals.

Despite the aforementioned studies indicating that thiamin supplementation does not benefit performance in healthy nonthiamin-deficient young adults, the effects of thiamine deficiency are less clear. In particular, Van der Beek et al. used a metabolic diet and restricted the intake of thiamin to 55% of the Dutch RDA, while riboflavin and vitamin B_6 were restricted to the same extent in two other groups. The remaining vitamins were supplemented to twice the RDA in all three groups.[11] Although no significant difference could be attributed entirely to thiamin, collectively, the vitamin restricted groups exhibited a significantly reduced VO_{2max}, onset of blood lactate accumulation (OBLA), VO_2 at OBLA, peak power and mean power. Therefore, the authors argued that restriction of B vitamins leading to short-term deficiency results in impaired mitochondrial function and performance decrements. In contrast, in a double-blind crossover design study of thiamin restriction leading to subclinical thiamin deficiency (urinary excretion 27 microgram thiamin/g creatinine) for 5 weeks, again in healthy young males, no performance decrement was observed.[12]

An important question that remains to be addressed is: Does physical activity increase the requirement for thiamin in active older individuals? There is evidence in young athletes that caloric restriction in sports such as gymnastics and wrestling may impart inadequate thiamin intake.[13] To our knowledge, there is no data with regard to the thiamin status of older athletes, therefore, it is plausible that thiamin deficiency may be present, and if so, performance in aerobic activities may be impaired. Clearly, further research is indicated in this area.

III. RIBOFLAVIN (VITAMIN B_2)

Riboflavin plays a critical role in protein metabolism and is a key component of the oxidative phosphorylation enzyme system that is intimately involved in the production of cellular energy. Its chemical structure is shown in Figure 7.2.

Riboflavin is primarily absorbed in the proximal small intestine and uptake is facilitated by bile salts. Transport in the blood is accomplished via attachment to protein complexes (i.e., albumin). Very little riboflavin is stored in the body, therefore, urinary excretion of metabolites (7 and 8 hydroxymethylflavins; i.e., 7 alpha hydroxyriboflavin) reflect dietary intake.

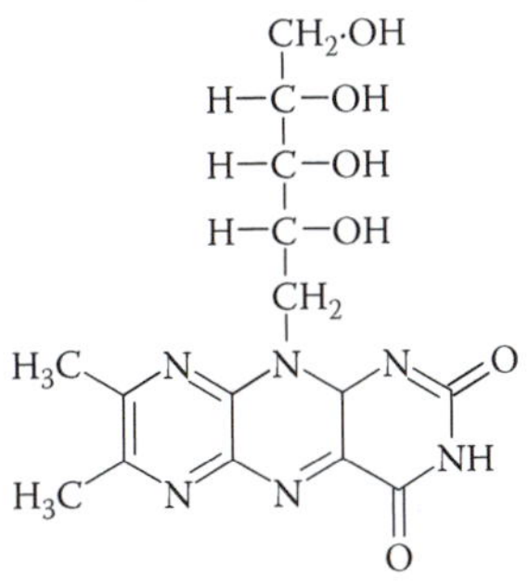

The coenzyme forms of riboflavin are flavin mononucleotide (FMN) and flavin adenine dinucleotide (FAD). Riboflavin is converted to its coenzyme forms within the cellular cytoplasm of most tissues, but particularly in the small intestine, liver, heart, and

FIGURE 7.2 Riboflavin.

kidney. In this process, FMN forms of riboflavin are complexed with specific active enzymes to form several functional flavoproteins, but most of it is further converted to FAD. Thus, the biosynthesis of flavo-coenzymes is tightly regulated and dependent on riboflavin status. Thyroxine and triiodothyroxine stimulate FMN and FAD synthesis in mammalian systems. Riboflavin has been shown to participate in oxidation-reduction reactions in numerous metabolic pathways and in energy production via the respiratory chain. A variety of chemical reactions are catalyzed by flavoproteins.[4]

When a riboflavin deficiency occurs, its symptoms include sore throat, cheilosis, angular stomatitis, glossitis, seborrheic dermatitis, and normocytic normochromic anemia. Riboflavin deficiencies have rarely been reported, and toxicities are almost never reported. On the other hand, electroencephalographic abnormalities have been mentioned as a very rare side effect of excessive riboflavin intake.[4]

Riboflavin is present in a variety of foods. Some of the best sources are milk, enriched breads and cereals, and organ meats. The RDA for riboflavin in adult males is 1.3 mg/d whereas in adult females it is 1.1 mg/d.[1]

A. Riboflavin and Exercise

Because riboflavin is responsible for providing key components of the electron acceptors FAD and FMN, which play a role in energy provision by the mitochondrial electron transport chain, it is expected that riboflavin would be an important nutrient for active and athletic individuals. From an ergogenic standpoint though, there is little evidence indicating a benefit to riboflavin supplementation. However, there is a great deal of evidence that exercise places a stress on riboflavin status in active individuals. For example, when Soares et al. put untrained, healthy young men on a metabolic diet with sufficient riboflavin content and exercised them for 18 days, riboflavin status declined during the exercise phase relative to the nonexercise metabolic diet.[14] Further, there was a reduced excretion of riboflavin metabolites in the urine. The authors suggested these data indicated an increased requirement for riboflavin during the exercise phase of the study. Despite the proposed increased riboflavin requirement and decreased status, economy of running and gross mechanical efficiency of cycling were not affected. Interestingly though, the delta mechanical efficiency (DME; change in oxygen cost relative to change in power) of cycling was inversely related to urinary excretion of riboflavin, while DME was directly related to hemoglobin levels.[14] The significance of these relationships was not determined.

In a series of metabolic studies performed by Belko et al., it was determined that initiation of an exercise program or dieting increases the requirement for riboflavin to maintain healthy status.[15–17] In particular, in the case of aerobic exercise 25–50 min/d, 6 d/week, almost 50% more riboflavin was required to maintain healthy status compared with the nonexercise condition.[15] Further, when diet and exercise were combined, the riboflavin requirements were greater than with either dieting or exercise alone.[16–18] In older active women (e.g. 50–67 yr) exercise induced the same elevated requirement for riboflavin that was observed in younger individuals.[19] In this study, Winters used a similar design to that of Belko,[15] except that in the former case, subjects completed a two-level crossover design at 0.6 micrograms/kcal and

0.9 micrograms/kcal. During the exercise phases, they cycled on an ergometer for 20 to 25 min/d, 6 d/week. This exercise protocol was sufficient to increase VO_{2max}, but was not affected by riboflavin treatment. Riboflavin excretion decreased, while endogenous status was impaired. Therefore, it is likely that older active individuals require more riboflavin than current guidelines, and these requirements are exacerbated if the interaction of diet is introduced with exercise.

IV. NIACIN (VITAMIN B_3)

Niacin, the term that is commonly used for nicotinic acid, is the metabolic precursor to nicotinamide. It is best known for its role as a component of two active coenzymes: nicotinamide adenine dinucleotide (NAD) and nicotinamide adenine dinucleotide phosphate (NADP), which play key roles in energy metabolism. The structure of niacin is shown in Figure 7.3. This vitamin can also be made in the body from tryptophan, a relatively common amino acid.

Niacin absorption occurs readily in the intestine. Approximately 25% of niacin is carried through the blood bound to protein. Niacin is easily absorbed by adipocytes, however, it is poorly stored in the body and excess amounts are generally excreted in the urine as niacin and nicotinamide metabolites.

Niacin functions primarily as a constituent of key nucleotide-containing enzymes that play critical roles in oxidation-reduction reactions as well as ATP synthesis and ADP-ribose transfer reactions. NAD is converted into NADP in the mammalian liver. NADP can also be converted to NAD. NAD plays a critical role in catabolic reactions, where it transfers the potential free energy stored in micronutrients such as carbohydrates, lipids, and proteins to NADH, which is then used to form ATP, the primary energy currency of the cell. NADP-dependent enzymes are preferentially involved in anabolic reactions such as the synthesis of fatty acids and cholesterol.

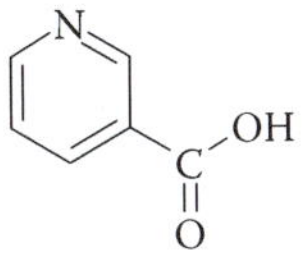

N
OH
C
O

FIGURE 7.3 Niacin.

Another key role played by NAD is in DNA repair. By serving as an ingredient in the formation of a DNA polymerase (poly [ADP Ribose] polymerase; PARP) it plays a critical role in DNA maintenance. It has been suggested that proper repair of DNA damage would require functional PARP and abundant NAD. The current hypothesis is that if a small amount of DNA damage occurs, PARP activity can repair it, whereas if more DNA damage occurs, a functional PARP would trigger apoptosis (cell death), probably via NAD depletion.[19a]

Increased niacin intake has been proposed to be of benefit for a wide variety of disorders including diabetes, atherosclerosis, arthritis, and cataracts. High doses of niacin have been used to prevent the development of atherosclerosis and to reduce recurrent complications such as heart attacks and peripheral vascular disease. Niacin is commonly used to lower elevated LDL cholesterol and triglyceride levels in the blood and is more effective in increasing HDL levels than other cholesterol-lowering medications. One study also found that the combination of niacin and the cholesterol-lowering drug Simvastatin (Merck and Company, Whitehouse Station, NJ) may slow the progression of heart disease, reducing risk of a heart attack, and even death.[20] Although niacin has been shown to boost HDL cholesterol and decrease triglyceride and LDL cholesterol concentrations, there has been some concern that it may raise blood glucose concentrations. In a recent study involving 125 diabetics and 343 controls, it was shown that high doses of niacin (roughly 3000 mg/d) increased blood glucose concentrations in both groups, but hemoglobin A1C concentration (considered a better measure of blood glucose over time) actually decreased in the diabetics over a 60-week follow-up period.[21]

Some preliminary studies have also suggested that nicotinamide may improve symptoms of arthritis, including increased joint mobility and a reduced need for anti-inflammatory medications. Researchers speculate that dietary niacin may aid in cartilage repair (damage to joint cartilage causes arthritis) and suggest that it may be used safely along with nonsteroidal anti-inflammatory medications to reduce inflammation.[22] It has also been suggested that long-term use (at least 3 years) may slow the progression of arthritis. Niacin, along with other nutrients, is also important for the maintenance of normal vision and the prevention of cataracts.[23] Severe niacin/tryptophan deficiency has historically been associated with the development of pellagra. This disease has four primary symptoms that are often referred to as the four "D"s (diarrhea, dermatitis, dementia, and death).

The Food and Nutrition Board of the Institute of Medicine has set the tolerable upper intake level (UL) of niacin at 35 mg/d because of high intakes' being associated with flushing of the face, arms, and chest. This limit is not meant to apply to patients under a physician's care who are being treated for hypercholesterolemia.[1]

Sources for niacin include mixed dishes with a high composition of meat, fish, or poultry, enriched and whole grain breads, and fortified ready-to-eat cereals. The 1998 RDAs for niacin for men and women are 19 and 15 mg of NE (niacin equivalents)/d respectively.[1] American women and men consume an average of 700 mg and 1100 mg of tryptophan respectively per day, which represents 47 and 58 niacin equivalents for women and men respectively.

A. Niacin and Exercise

Considering the key role niacin, nicotinamide, and nicotinic acid (NA) play in ATP generation (NAD^+ is involved in the generation of approximately 28 of the 36 ATPs derived from the complete oxidation of 1 mole of glucose) the relative paucity of data regarding the interaction of niacin and exercise is surprising.[24] One primary factor in this problem is likely the lack of a reliable marker of niacin metabolism. Regardless, some investigators have studied the interaction between niacin and exercise, primarily by looking at the effects of niacin supplementation. For example, Heath et al. administered 4 g/d of nicotinic acid to trained runners who then performed submaximal runs at approximately 60% VO_{2max} at the start, midpoint, and end of a 3-week treatment.[25] Nicotinic acid administration resulted in a significantly higher respiratory exchange ratio (RER), indicating reduced fat utilization and increased carbohydrate utilization, compared with the baseline run. In addition, circulating free fatty acids and glycerol were significantly reduced after supplementation with

NA. Interestingly, additional alterations in fat metabolism included significantly reduced serum concentrations of total cholesterol and increased concentrations of HDL cholesterol as a result of NA administration. There were no differences in performance in the trials, but performance differences would be unlikely at a controlled submaximal intensity (60% VO_{2max}) in trained runners. Thus, it appears as though NA supplementation results in decreased lipolysis and fatty acid utilization and increased carbohydrate utilization at submaximal exercise intensities.

Later, Murray et al. confirmed the effects of NA supplementation on lipid utilization, and extended findings by incorporating a performance trial.[26] Subjects cycled for 2 hr at 68% VO_2 peak and subsequently completed a 3.5-mile laboratory performance trial. Two of four conditions studied in this work were the addition of the use of water + NA or carbohydrate/electrolyte + NA beverages by participants. The two other conditions were the addition of water only and carbohydrate/electrolyte only. As in the study by Heath,[25] administration of either of the NA-containing beverages impaired lipolysis to the extent that subject's circulating free fatty acid levels were not significantly different from the rest. Administration of the water + NA beverage resulted in a similar performance time to that of subjects consuming water only, and it was significantly slower than performance times of subjects who used carbohydrate/electrolyte + NA or carbohydrate/electrolyte only. Thus, it is clear that NA administration inhibits lipolysis during exercise, which is generally considered an unfavorable metabolic condition.[27] In summary, niacin administration does not seem to improve performance and may actually be ergolytic if lipolysis and fat utilization are important components of the exercise to be undertaken.

Due to the aforementioned lack of a reliable biomarker for niacin metabolism, there is no data concerning the niacin status of active individuals, either young or older.

V. BIOTIN (VITAMIN B_4)

Biotin (see Figure 7.4), which acts as an energy metabolism co-enzyme, is necessary for maintaining a variety of normal functions in the body. Biotin is primarily absorbed from the small intestine; however, it has also been shown to be absorbed via the colon after it is synthesized by enteric flora. Biotin plays an important role in cells as a carbon dioxide carrier and has been shown to deliver a carbon molecule that is used in the formation of the tricarboxylic acid cycle (TCA) intermediate oxaloacetate from pyruvate, which is a vital process for keeping the TCA cycle functioning. Biotin also plays critical roles in gluconeogenesis, fatty acid synthesis, and fatty acid and amino acids breakdown. Hymes and Wolf proposed that biotin, by binding to histones, may also play a role in DNA replication and transcription.[28]

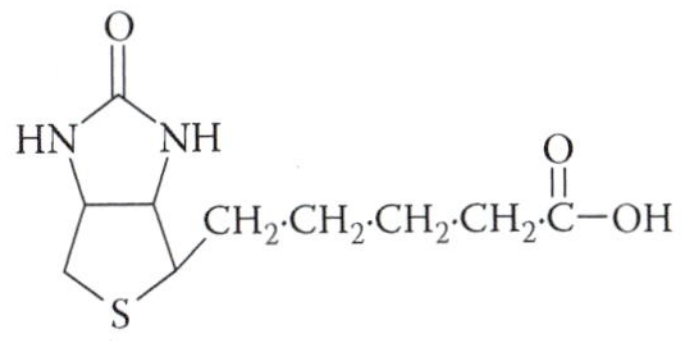

Biotin is needed for normal growth and the maintenance of healthy hair, skin, nerves, bone marrow, and sex glands. Biotin deficiency symptoms include hair loss and the development of a scaly rash around the mouth, eyes, nose, and genital area. Depression

FIGURE 7.4 Biotin.

and lethargy, as well as numbness and tingling in the extremities, have also been observed. In addition, biotin deficiency has been associated with noninsulin-dependent diabetes mellitus. When these subjects are provided with biotin there is a significant decrease in fasting blood glucose concentrations. It has been proposed that biotin may increase glucose conversion to fatty acids and also may increase insulin secretion.[29]

The Food and Nutrition Board of the Institute of Medicine did not establish a tolerable upper level of intake for biotin since it is not known to be toxic.[1] One case report of a negative reaction (development of eosinophilic pleuropericardial effusion) was noted for an elderly woman who consumed large quantities of biotin (10 mg/d) and pantothenic acid (300 mg/d) for 2 months.[30]

Recommendations for daily intake have not been established, but the AI for Americans has been determined to be 30 μg/d.[1] Biotin is not normally included in food composition tables and its level within many foods is unknown. It is present in small amounts in fruits and most meats. A good food source of biotin is liver. Certain drugs interact with biotin and thereby alter the amounts needed in the diet. Specific families of drugs include some anticonvulsants, which have an impact on both absorption and excretion, and antibiotics, which destroy bacteria in the gastrointestinal tract that normally produce biotin.

A. Biotin and Exercise

Biotin's relationship to exercise has been studied only in conjunction with pantothenic acid. Both B vitamins were provided as part of a vitamin/mineral supplement to athletes who were involved in either basketball, gymnastics, rowing, or swimming over a 7- to 8-month period. While these athletes were going through their training, they were provided with either a placebo or the vitamin/mineral supplement. No evidence of improved athletic performance was shown for the supplement group.[31]

VI. PANTOTHENIC ACID (VITAMIN B_5)

Pantothenic acid, an important cofactor of coenzyme A (CoA), is essential for the completion of biologic acetylation reactions as illustrated by the formation of sulfonamide in the liver and choline in the brain. The structure of pantothenic acid is shown in Figure 7.5.

Pantothenic acid is ingested in its CoA form and is then hydrolyzed in the intestine to pantothenic acid, which is then absorbed into the bloodstream. Pantothenate containing CoA is essential for the maintenance of the respiratory TCA cycle, fatty acid synthesis, and the degradation of a variety of other compounds. All of the enzymes required for CoA synthesis are present in cell cytoplasm. Mitochondria are the final

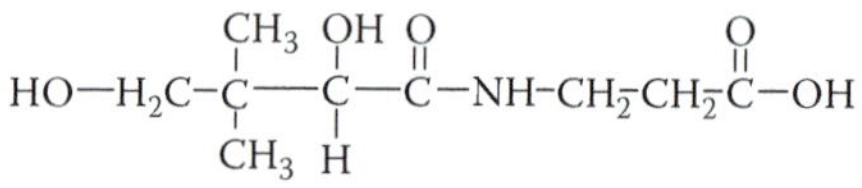

$$HO{-}H_2C{-}C(CH_3)_2{-}CH(OH){-}C(=O){-}NH{-}CH_2{-}CH_2{-}C(=O){-}OH$$

FIGURE 7.5 Pantothenic acid.

site of CoA synthesis, since 95% of CoA is found in mitochondria and CoA does not cross the mitochondria membranes. Multiple hydrolytic steps liberate pantothenic acid from CoA and allow for it to eventually be excreted in the urine. Pantothenic acid has also been shown to be required for the synthesis of key amino acids (methionine, leucine and arginine).[3]

Pantothenic acid deficiencies are rare in humans because this vitamin is found in so many sources of our diet. Severe malnutrition leads to pantothenic acid deficiency, whose symptoms include painful burning sensations in the feet and numbness in the toes. When pantothenic acid antagonists are provided along with a pantothenic acid-deficient diet, headaches, fatigue, and insomnia have been noted.

The Food and Nutrition Board of the Institute of Medicine did not establish a tolerable upper level intake (UL) for pantothenic acid since it is well tolerated in large amounts and has no known toxic effects in humans.[1] Very high intakes of calcium D-pantothenate have been shown to result in diarrhea.[32]

Because inadequate data is available to set an RDA for pantothenic acid the Food and Nutrition Board of the Institute of Medicine has set an Adequate Intake (AI) of 5 mg/d for male and female adolescents as well as adults.[1] Sources of this vitamin include liver, egg yolk, yogurt, avocados, milk, sweet potatoes, broccoli, and cooked chicken.

A. Pantothenic Acid and Exercise

Very little research has been done in which pantothenic acid's impact on exercise has been evaluated. In a study done by Nice et al., the effects of pantothenic acid on run time were analyzed using male distance runners.[33] A group of conditioned men consumed either pantothenic acid supplements or a placebo for 2 weeks. When the men were asked to run to exhaustion, run times were similar for the two groups and no differences were noted in either pulse rates or blood biochemical parameters. In a separate study, highly trained male runners took supplements of pantothenic acid (2 gm) or a placebo for 2 weeks.[34] During exercise, both blood lactate concentrations and oxygen consumption decreased. In a study by Webster, cyclists who received thiamin/pantothenic acid supplements did not show enhanced performance or altered exercise metabolism.

VII. PYRIDOXINE (VITAMIN B_6)

Vitamin B_6, which plays a critical role in protein metabolism, occurs in three forms in the body (pyridoxine, pyridoxal, and pyridoxamine). All three forms are relatively stable in an acidic medium but are not heat stable under alkaline conditions. The active coenzyme forms are pyridoxal 5' phosphate (PLP) and pyridoxamine-5-phosphate (PMP) (see Figure 7.6).

All forms of vitamin B_6 are absorbed in the upper part of the small intestine. They are phosphorylated within the mucosal cells to form PLP and PMP. PLP can be oxidized further to form other metabolites that are excreted in the urine. Vitamin B_6 is stored in muscle tissues.

PLP plays an important role in amino acid metabolism. It has the ability to transfer amino groups from compounds by removing an amino acid from one

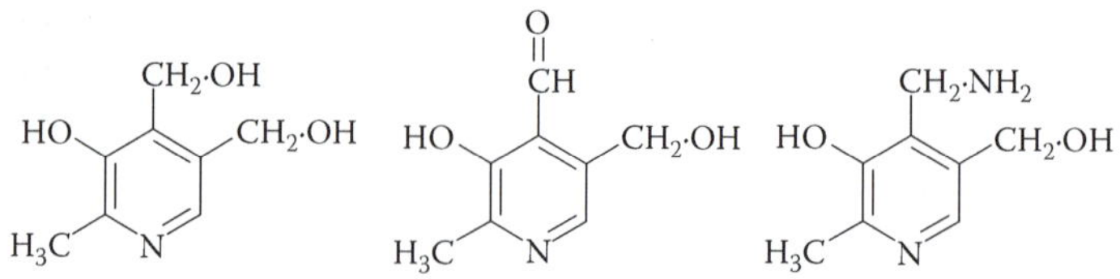

FIGURE 7.6 Pyridoxine, pyridoxal, and pyridoxamine.

component and adding to another. This allows the body to synthesize nonessential amino acids when amino groups become available. Pyridoxal 5 phosphate's ability to add and remove amino groups makes it invaluable for protein and urea metabolism. Vitamin B_6 is transferred in the blood, in both plasma and red blood cells. PLP and PMP can both be bound to albumin, with PLP binding more tightly, or to hemoglobin in the red blood cell. The liver is the primary organ that is responsible for the metabolism of vitamin B_6 metabolites. As a result, the liver supplies the active form PLP to the blood as well as to other tissues. The three non-phosphorylated forms of vitamin B_6 are converted to their respective phosphorylated forms by pyridoxine kinase, with zinc and ATP as cofactors. Pyridoxamine 5' phosphate and pyridoxine 5' phosphate can then be converted to PLP by flavin mononucleotide (FMN) oxidase.

It has been shown in both animal and human studies that a low intake of vitamin B_6 causes impaired immune function due to decreased interleukin-2 production and lymphocyte proliferation. It has also been demonstrated that PLP inhibits the binding of steroid receptors to DNA and may therefore impact on endocrine-mediated diseases. It has been suggested that reactions between physiologic concentrations of PLP and receptors for estrogen, androgen, progesterone, and glucocorticoids are dependent on adequate levels of vitamin B_6 in an individual.[34a]

A number of vitamin B_6 antagonists have been identified including certain food additives, oral contraceptives, and alcohol.[35] When alcohol is broken down in the body, acetaldehyde is produced and knocks PLP loose from its enzyme, which is broken down and then excreted. Thus, alcohol abuse causes a loss of vitamin B_6 from the body. Some drugs have been shown to be vitamin B_6 antagonists, including cycloserine, ethionarnide, furfural, hydralazine, isoniazid, isonicotinic acid, L-Dopa, penicillamin, pyrazinamide, theophylline, and thiosemicarbizones.[36] Another drug that acts as a vitamin B_6 antagonist is isonicotinic acid hydrazide (INH), a potent inhibitor of the growth of the tuberculosis bacterium. INH binds and inactivates the vitamin, inducing a vitamin B_6 deficiency. In a number of disease states, it has been shown that apparent alterations of vitamin B_6 metabolism can cause concomitant alterations in tryptophan metabolism. These alterations have been observed in patients with asthma, diabetes, breast and bladder cancer, renal disease, coronary heart disease, and sickle cell anemia.

High-protein diets have been shown to alter vitamin B_6 requirements because vitamin B_6 coenzymes play important roles in amino acid metabolism. The RDA for vitamin B_6 is 1.3 mg/d for females and adult males up to the age of 50 and 1.7 mg/d for those who are 51 and older.[1] When vitamin B_6 is deficient in the diet, symptoms include weakness, irritability, and insomnia. Advanced symptoms include growth failure, impaired motor function, and convulsions.

Vitamin B_6 toxicity can arise if one routinely takes large doses of B_6 over a lengthy period of time, and so a UL of 100 mg/d has been established. Toxicity may involve irreversible sensory neuropathy and nerve damage. Intakes of 200 mg/d or less show no evidence of damage, but levels of 500 to 1,000 mg/d have been associated with sensory damage.[37]

Excellent food sources include fortified ready-to-eat cereals, white potatoes (with skin) and other starchy vegetables, meats, fish, poultry, highly fortified soy-based meat substitutes, beef liver, and other organ meats.

A. Pyridoxine and Exercise

There have been numerous reports of vitamin B_6 deficiency in active adults. Rokitzki et al. looked at 57 strength and power athletes and assessed vitamin B_6 status by a combination of food records and biochemical tests of vitamin B_6 metabolites.[38] From these criteria, it was determined that approximately 5% of the athletes exhibited vitamin B_6 deficiency, although more than 60% had vitamin B_6 intakes below the German government's recommendations. In this case though, the investigators argued that the biomarkers of vitamin B_6 were not sufficiently reliable, and by another method (urinary-PA excretion) 18% of study participants had reduced vitamin B_6 status. In another study, 18 of 42 healthy, college-age participants were considered vitamin B_6 deficient prior to a placebo-controlled supplementation study.[39] Administration of a multivitamin supplement alleviated poor vitamin status, but did not affect lactate kinetics during a laboratory trial. Similarly, Telford et al. reported more than half of 86 athletes they studied exhibited impaired vitamin B_6 status, and that vitamin deficit was rectified by supplementation with a multivitamin over the course of an 8-month intensive training program.[40] In older sedentary females, Manore et al. observed a vitamin B_6 deficiency that was alleviated when subjects were placed on a metabolic diet.[41] Thus, it appears that vitamin B_6 deficiency may be present in some active or athletic individuals, and that supplementation can bring B_6 status back into normal range.

The acute effects of exercise on vitamin B_6 appear to be a generally observed increase in plasma PLP levels during the first few minutes of exercise, but a return to pre-exercise levels shortly after the cessation of exercise.[42] For example, when trained or untrained subjects performed cycling exercise for 20 min at 80% VO_{2max}, PLP levels were significantly higher immediately following exercise than at the start, and levels returned to baseline 1 hour after exercise.[41] Manore has proposed that increased plasma PLP during exercise could lead to increased excretion and loss of vitamin B_6 through the formation of 4-PA and loss in the urine. Although transient losses of vitamin B_6 can occur as a result of acute exercise, there is no data indicating supplementation with vitamin B_6 improves performance.[41]

VIII. FOLIC ACID (VITAMIN B_9)

Folic acid, or folate, consists of a pteridine base that is attached to one molecule each of P-aminobenzoic acid (PABA) and glutamic acid. Folacin is the generic term that is used for folic acid and related substances that act like folic acid. The structure is shown in Figure 7.7.

Folic acid has been shown to be involved in the transfer of 1-carbon units, as well as the metabolism of both nucleic acids and amino acids. Because of this, symptoms of deficiencies include anemia as well as an increase in serum homocysteine concentrations.

Folate derivatives in the diet are cleaved by specific intestinal enzymes to prepare monoglutamyl folate (MGF) for absorption. Most MGF is reduced to tetrahydrofolate (THF) in the intestinal cells by the enzyme folate reductase. This enzyme uses NADPH as a donor of reducing equivalents. Tetrahydrofolate polyglutamates are the functional coenzymes used in tissues. The folate coenzymes participate in reactions by carrying 1-carbon compounds from one molecule to another. Thus, glycine can be converted to a 3-carbon amino acid, serine with the help of folate coenzymes. This action helps convert vitamin B_{12} to one of its active coenzyme forms and helps synthesize the DNA required for all rapidly growing cells. Enzymes on the intestinal cell surface, while hydrolyzing polyglutamate to monoglutamate, attach a methyl group. Special transport systems then help to deliver monoglutamate to the liver and other body cells. Folate is stored only in polyglutamate forms. When the need arises, it is converted back to monoglutamate and released. Excess folate is disposed of by the liver into bile fluid and stored in the gall bladder until it is released into the small intestine. An important role served by methyl THF is the methylation of homocysteine to methionine. Methylcobalamin serves as a cofactor along with vitamin B_{12}; if these vitamins are missing, folate becomes trapped inside cells in its methyl form, unavailable to support DNA synthesis and cell growth.

Since folate is repeatedly reabsorbed, any injury to gastrointestinal tract cells causes an interference with absorption and folate is lost from the body. The cells lining the gastrointestinal tract are the most rapidly renewed cells in the body, so not only will the folate be lost, but also other nutrients will not be absorbed.

Folate deficiency impairs both cell division and protein synthesis. Deficiencies of this vitamin are found most often in elderly people whose primary symptom is megaloblastic anemia. Another symptom is an increase in homocysteine concentrations. Deficiencies can also occur in patients who have cancer, skin-destroying diseases,

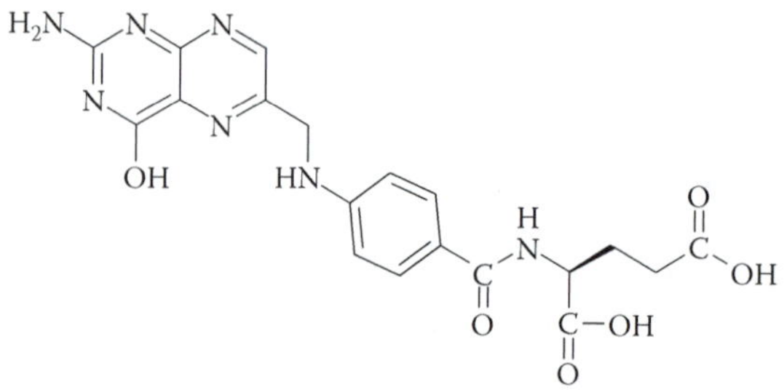

FIGURE 7.7 Folacin.

and severe burns. Of all the vitamins, folate is most vulnerable to interactions with drugs, since some drugs have chemical structures similar to the vitamin.

High intake of folate from foods has not been shown to have negative side effects. The Food and Nutrition Board of the Institute of Medicine recommends that adults limit their intake of Vitamin B_{12} to 1 mg/d in the treatment of megaloblastic anemia and that caution be taken to ensure that the B_{12} deficiency does not mask a folate deficiency.[1] This is critical since misdiagnosis can result in irreversible neurological damage.

The RDA for folate in Dietary Folate Equivalents (DFE) is 400 μg/d in both male and female adults.[1] Since animals cannot synthesize PABA or attach glutamic acid to pteroic acid, folate must be obtained from the diet. Common sources of folate are fortified ready-to-eat cereal, enriched noodles, pasta, rice, bread, spinach, lentils, and legumes.[1]

No adverse effects have been associated with excessive intake of folate from food sources.

A. Folic Acid and Exercise

There is little data regarding the effects of exercise on folic acid status in active individuals or athletes. There has been interest in the vitamin in endurance sports, and Singh et al. determined ultra-marathoners participating in a 100-mile run exhibited sufficient folic acid intake based on questionnaires.[43] Similarly, few studies have looked at the effects folic acid supplementation has on exercise performance. There have been numerous studies that have investigated folic acid as a component of multivitamin or multicomponent nutritional interventions, but the effects specifically attributable to folic acid in these types of studies are difficult to infer.[44–47] One study did examine the folic acid status of female marathon runners (n = 85), of whom 33% had deficient serum folic acid levels, but only 2% exhibited overt anemia. After 1 week of supplementation with 5 mg/d of folic acid, folic acid levels had returned to normal. In tests of endurance performance (e.g., VO_{2max}, treadmill time to exhaustion, and running velocity at the lactate turnpoint), no improvements were observed after the supplementation period. In a more complicated analysis of a relatively large cohort (1139 F/ 931 M) of middle-aged (35–60 yr) French adults, it was determined that increasing folic acid intake and physical activity were two important factors that played a role in controlling total homocysteine levels of males, but neither of these factors altered homocysteine in females.[48] Furthermore, recent evidence from Herrmann et al. indicates that, although exercise is thought to chronically reduce homocysteine levels acutely, exercise increases homocycteine levels, and this is associated with low folic acid levels in some recreational athletes.[49] This was confirmed by König et al., who observed acute elevation in homocysteine levels in trained males following a sprint triathlon.[50] Training for 30 days leading up to the competition did not affect homocysteine levels, although when analyzed based on training volume, athletes who trained the most (14.9 hr/week) had significantly lower homocysteine levels than those who trained the least (9.1 hr/week). Statistical analysis showed that acute elevations in homocysteine following the triathlon were inversely related to baseline training volume and plasma folate.[50] Similarly, Rousseau et al. determined homocysteine levels were inversely proportional to folic acid intake, but in contrast to conventional wisdom, they were not related to the mode of training (e.g., aerobic vs. intermittent or anaerobic).[51] Although there is no evidence of folic acid deficiency in active older individuals, the important link between folic acid, homocysteine, and heart disease may warrant further attention in this area.

IX. CYANOCOBALAMIN (VITAMIN B_{12})

Vitamin B12 (cobalamin; see Figure 7.8) is synthesized exclusively by microorganisms.

Although vitamin B_{12} is absent from plants it is synthesized by bacteria and is stored by the liver in animals as methyl cobalamin, adenosyl cobalamin, and hydroxyl cobalamin. Intrinsic factor (a highly specific glycoprotein in gastric secretions) is necessary for absorption of vitamin B_{12}. After absorption, the vitamin is bound by a plasma protein (transcobalamin II) that transports it to various tissues. It is also stored in the liver in this form. The active coenzyme forms of vitamin B_{12} are methyl cobalamin and deoxy-adenosyl cobalamin. In the blood, free cobalamin is released into the cytosol of cells as hydroxycobalamin. It is then either converted in the cytosol to methyl cobalamin or it enters mitochondria where it is converted to 5-deoxy-adenosyl cobalamin. The methyl group that is bound to cobalamin is eventually transferred to homocysteine to form methionine and the remaining cobalamin then removes the methyl group from N^5-methyl tetrahydrofolate to form tetrahydrofolate (THF). Thus, in this metabolic process, methionine is stored and tetrahydrofolate (THF) is available to participate in purine and pyrimidine nucleotide synthesis.[4]

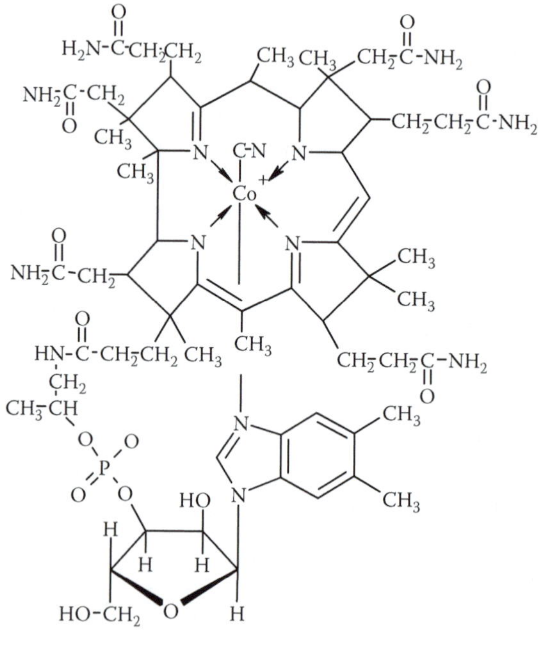

FIGURE 7.8 Cobalamin.

A deficiency of vitamin B_{12} leads to the development of megaloblastic anemia, which can be caused by pernicious anemia, a condition in which an autoimmune inflammation occurs in the stomach that leads to a breakdown in the cells lining the stomach. Because the final result is a decrease in acid production, Vitamin B_{12} cannot be released from food. Treatment of pernicious anemia requires B_{12} injections or high-dose supplementation. Approximately 2% of all adults over 60 years of age have pernicious anemia.[52] True vegetarians are at risk of B_{12} deficiency because this vitamin is found only in foods of animal origin. A deficiency of this vitamin causes impairment in the methionine synthase reaction. Anemia is the result of impaired DNA synthesis, thus preventing cell division and formation of the nucleus of new erythrocytes with consequent accumulation in the bone marrow of megaloblastic red blood cells.

A number of drugs have been shown to decrease absorption of vitamin B_{12}, including gastric-acid inhibitors (Tagamet [GlaxoSmithKline], Pepcid [Merck], and Zantac [Warner Lambert]) and proton pump inhibitors (omeprazole and lansoprazole).[53] Other drugs that inhibit absorption of vitamin B_{12} include: cholestyramine (cholesterol binding agent), neomycin (antibiotic) and colchicine (gout treatment). A drug that is used in the treatment of adult onset diabetes (Metformin [Mylan Laboratories]) requires use with calcium-containing foods to allow for B_{12} absorption.[54]

The RDA for Vitamin B_{12} is 2.4 μg/d for adolescent and adult males and females.[1] Food sources are found naturally only in animal products, but some plant foods are fortified with vitamin B_{12}. Food sources include: fortified ready-to-eat cereals, shellfish, some fortified meat alternative products, organ meat, beef, fin fish (i.e., salmon, trout, tuna, etc.), and milk.

No toxic effects have been associated with intake of vitamin B_{12}.

A. Cyanocobalamin and Exercise

As with folic acid, there is an apparent relationship between vitamin B_{12}, exercise, and homocysteine levels. The study by Herrmann et al. showed not only that endurance exercise acutely elevates homocysteine levels, but that a large proportion (25%) of recreational athletes examined exhibited hyperhomocysteinemia associated with low vitamin B_{12} levels.[49] In other studies by the same group, data indicate there may be a complicated interaction between exercise, vitamin B_{12}, and homocysteine levels that requires further investigation.[55,56] Again, owing to the important relationship between homocysteine levels and heart disease, this may be an area of concern to older athletes.

Although vitamin B_{12} may have important links to homocysteine levels in individuals who exercise, there is no evidence that supplementation with this vitamin improves performance.[57,58] Therefore, it is unclear whether vitamin B_{12} supplementation is warranted in older athletes.

X. B VITAMIN INTAKE

It is critical that B vitamins be included in the diet in adequate amounts as specified by the RDA or AI. Many B vitamins work in concert with each other, for example if B_{12} deficiency is suspected, folate status should also be checked. People who are especially at risk of B vitamin deficiency are those who have a history of alcoholism or those who have had a nutrient-deficient diet such as the elderly, poor, or those who are malnourished due to disease or malabsorption. If deficiencies are found, these should be corrected with supplemental B vitamins either individually or as a multiple vitamin.

When an oral diet is inadequate, B vitamins can be provided as a supplement in a multivitamin form that taken orally. Most commercially available enteral (tube-feeding) formulas have adequate amounts of B vitamins at a minimal level of formula intake. Higher levels of formula based on increased caloric needs should not pose a toxicity problem for B vitamins. Patients who receive parenteral nutrition as their sole or major source of nutrition support should be receiving an intravenous multivitamin product with adequate amounts of B vitamins.[59,60] Individual B vitamins are also available in various forms to accommodate the absorptive capacity of the patient with wounds. If a nutrient deficiency is suspected or confirmed, supplementation will be necessary to bring the level to within normal limits.

XI. FUTURE RESEARCH AND CONCLUSIONS

It is difficult to make a general statement that applies to all B vitamins in relationship to their use by exercising adults. Although few studies show increased performance with supplementation, some studies have shown that exercise induces certain B vitamin deficiencies. Also, B vitamin requirements seem to increase with age in exercising adults. Since B vitamins have been shown to help lower homocysteine—one of the primary biomarkers for coronary heart disease—and since they are major players in energy metabolism, it is recommended that special attention be paid to ensure adequate intake in athletes and exercising adults in general. Surveys show that large numbers of athletes take vitamin supplements. It is suggested that at a minimum, sound nutritional habits be emphasized among exercising adults to ensure that B vitamins are consumed in adequate amounts. It is unfortunate that at the present time most of the data related to B vitamins and exercise pertain to short-term exercise. More studies are needed to see how long-term B vitamin intake affects athletic performance.

REFERENCES

1. Dietary Reference Intakes (DRI) and Recommended Dietary Allowances (RDA), http://www.nal.usda.gov/fnic/etext/000105.html. Accessed 01/20/08.
2. Grandjean, A.C., Vitamin/Mineral Supplements. *Strength Cond. J.* 25, 76–78, 2003.
3. DeBiasse, M.A., What is optimal nutritional support? *New Horiz.* 2, 122–130, 1994.
4. Shils, M. E., Olson, J.A., Shike, M., and Ross, C., in *Modern Nutrition in Health and Disease*, 9th ed., Lippincott, Williams, and Wilkins, Baltimore, 1999, chap. 21.
5. Keys, A., Henschel, A.F., Michelsen, O., and Brozek, J.M., The performance of normal young men on controlled thiamin intakes, *J. Nutr.* 26, 399, 1943.
6. Webster, M.J., Scheett, T.P., Doyle, M.R., and Branz, M., The effect of a thiamin derivative on exercise performance, *Eur. J. Appl. Physiol. Occup. Physiol.* 75, 520–524, 1997.

7. Webster, M.J., Physiological and performance responses to supplementation with thiamin and pantothenic acid derivatives, *Eur. J. Appl. Physiol. Occup. Physiol.* 77, 486–91, 1998.
8. Gastin, P.B., Energy system interaction and relative contribution during maximal exercise, *Sports Med.* 31, 725–41, 2001.
9. Spencer, M.R. and Gastin, P.B., Energy system contribution during 200– to 1500–m running in highly trained athletes, *Med. Sci. Sports Exerc.* 33, 157–162, 2001.
10. Whipp, B.J., Rossiter, H.B., and Ward, S.A., Exertional oxygen uptake kinetics: A stamen of stamina? *Biochem. Soc. Trans.* 30, 237–247, 2002.
11. van der Beek, E.J., van Dokkum, W., Wedel, M., Schrijver, J., and van den Berg, H., Thiamin, riboflavin and vitamin B6: Impact of restricted intake on physical performance in man, *J. Am. Coll. Nutr.* 13, 629–640, 1994.
12. Wood, B., Gijsbers, A., Goode, A., Davis, S., Mulholland, J., and Breen, K., A study of partial thiamin restriction in human volunteers, *Am. J. Clin. Nutr.* 33, 848–861, 1980.
13. Short, S.H. and Short, W.R., Four-year study of university athletes' dietary intake, *J. Am. Diet. Assoc.* 82, 632–645, 1983.
14. Soares, M.J., Satyanarayana, K., Bamji, M.S., Jacob, C.M., Ramana, Y.V., and Rao S.S., The effect of exercise on the riboflavin status of adult men, *Br. J. Nutr.* 69, 541–551, 1993.
15. Belko, A.Z., Obarzanek, E., Kalkwarf, H.J., Rotter, M.A., Bogusz, S., and Miller, D., Effects of exercise on riboflavin requirements of young women, *Amer. J. Clin. Nutr.* 37, 509–517, 1983.
16. Belko, A.Z., Obarzanek, E., Kalkwarf, H.J., Rotter, M.A., Bogusz, S., and Miller, D., Effects of aerobic exercise and weight loss on riboflavin requirements of moderately obese, marginally deficient young women, *Amer. J. Clin. Nutr.* 40, 553–561, 1984.
17. Belko, A.Z., Van Loan, M., Barbieri, T.F., and Mayclin. P., Diet, exercise, weight loss, and energy expenditure in moderately overweight women, *Int. J. Obesity* 11, 93–104, 1987.
18. Belko, A.Z., Meredith, M.P., Kalwarf, H.J., Obarzanek, E., Weinberg, S., and Roach, R., Effects of exercise on riboflavin requirements: biological validation in weight reducing women, *Amer. J. Clin. Nutr.* 41, 270–277, 1985.
19. Winters, L.R., Yoon, J.S., Kalkwarf, H.J., Davies, J.C., Berkowitz, M.G., Haas, J., and Roe, D.A., Riboflavin requirements and exercise adaptation in older women. *Biochem. Soc. Trans.* 56, 526–532, 1992.
19a. Kirkland, J. B., Niacin, in *Handbook of Vitamins*, 4th ed., Zempleni, J. (Ed.) CRC Press (Taylor & Francis), 2007, Ch. 6.
20. Brown, B.G., Zhao, X.Q., Chait, A., Fisher, L.D., Cheung, M.C., Morse, J.S., et al., Simvastatin and niacin, antioxidant vitamins, or the combination for the prevention of coronary disease, *NEJM* 345, 1583–1592, 2001.
21. Garg, A., Lipid-lowering therapy and macrovascular disease in diabetes mellitus. *Diabetes* 41 (Suppl 2), 111–115, 1992.
22. Jonas, W.B., Rapoza, C.P., and Blair, W.F., The effect of niacinamide on osteoarthritis: A pilot study, *Inflammation Res.* 45, 330–334, 1996.
23. Jacques, P.F., Chylack, L.T., Jr., Hankinson, S.E., Khu, P.M., Rogers, G., Friend, J., et al., Long-term nutrient intake and early age related nuclear lens opacities, *Arch. Ophthalmol.* 119, 1009–1019, 2001.
24. McArdle, W.D., Katch, F.I., and Katch, V.L., *Exercise Physiology: Energy, nutrition, and human performance*, 5th ed., Lippincott, Williams, and Wilkins, Baltimore, MD, 2001.

25. Heath, E.M., Wilcox, A.R., and Quinn, C.M., Effects of nicotinic acid on respiratory exchange ratio and substrate levels during exercise, *Med. Sci. Sports Exerc.* 25, 1018–1023, 1993.
26. Murray, R., Bartoli, W. P., Eddy, D.E., and Horn M.K., Physiological and performance responses to nicotinic-acid ingestion during exercise, *Med. Sci. Sports Exerc.* 27, 1057–1062, 1995.
27. Horowitz, J., in *Exercise Metabolism*, Hargreaves, M., and Spriet, L., Eds.: Champaign, IL, 2005, p 125.
28. Hymes, J., and Wolf, B., Human biotinadase isn't just for recycling biotin, *J. Nutr.* 129 (suppl), 485s, 1999.
29. Romero-Navarro, G., Cabrera-Valladares, G., German, M.S., Matschinsky, F.M., Velazquez, A., Wang, J., and Fernandez-Mejia, C., Biotin regulation of pancreatic glucokinase and insulin in primary cultural rat islets and in biotin-deficient rats, *Endocrinology* 140, 4594–4600, 1999.
30. Debourdeau, P.M., Djezzar, S., Estival, J.L., Zammit, C.M., Richard, R.C., and Castot, A.C., Life-threatening eosinophilic pleuropericardial effusion related to vitamins B5, *Ann. Pharmacother.* 35, 424–6, 2001.
31. Thomas, E.A., Pantothenic acid and biotin, in *Sports Nutrition,* Wolinsky, I., and Driskell, J.A., Eds., CRC Press, Boca Raton, 1997, chap. 7.
32. Flodin, N., *Pharmacology of micronutrients*, Alan R. Liss, New York, 1988.
33. Nice, C., Reeves, A.G., Brink-Johnson, T., and Noll, W., The effects of pantothenic acid on human exercise capacity, *J. Sports Med.* 24, 26, 1984.
34. Litoff, D., Scherzett, H., and Harrison, J., Effects of pantothenic acid supplementation on human exercise, *Med. Sci. Sports Exerc.* 17, 287, 1985.
34a. Natori, Y., and Oka, T., Vitamin B6 modulation of gene expression, *Nutr. Res.* 17, (7), 1199–1207, 1997.
35. Rucker, R.B., Murray, J., and Riggins, R.S., Nutritional copper deficiency and penicillamine administration: Some effects on bone collagen and arterial elastin crosslinking, *Adv. Exp. Med. Biol.* 86B, 619–648, 1977.
36. Osiecki, H., *The Physician's Handbook of Clinical Nutrition*, 5th ed., Bioconcepts Publishing, Kelvin Grove, Queensland, Australia, 1998.
37. Bender, D.A., Non-nutritional uses of vitamin B6, *Brit. J. Nutr.* 8, 7–20, 1999.
38. Rokitzki, L., Sagredos, A.N., Reuss, F., Cufi, D., and Keul, J.A., Assessment of vitamin B6 status of strength and speedpower athletes, *J. Am. Coll. Nutr.* 13, 87–94, 1994.
39. Fogelholm, M., Ruokonen, I., Laakso, J.T., Vuorimaa, T., and Himberg, J.J., Lack of association between indices of vitamin B1, B2, and B6 status and exercise-induced blood lactate in young adults, *Int. J. Sports Nutr.* 3, 165–176, 1993.
40. Telford, R.D., Catchpole, E.A., Deakin, V., McLeay, A.C., and Plank, A.W., The effect of 7 to 8 months of vitamin/mineral supplementation on the vitamin and mineral status of athletes, *Int. J. Sport Nutr.* 2, 123–134, 1992.
41. Manore, M.N., Leklem, J.E., and Walter, M.C., Vitamin B-6 metabolism as affected by exercise in trained and untrained women fed diets differing in carbohydrate and vitamin B-6 content, *Am. J. Clin. Nutr.* 46, 995–1004, 1987.
42. Manore, M.M., Vitamin B6 and exercise *Int. J. Sport Nutr.* 4, 89–103, 1994.
43. Singh, A., Evans, P., Gallagher, K.L., and Deuster, P.A., Dietary intakes and biochemical profiles of nutritional status of ultramarathoners, *Med. Sci. Sports Exerc.* 25, 328–334, 1993.
44. Carrero, J. J., Fonolla, J., Marti, J.L., Jimenez, J., Boza, J.J., and Lopez-Huertase, E., Intake of fish oil, oleic acid, folic acid, and vitamins B-6 and E for 1 year decreases plasma C-reactive protein and reduces coronary heart disease risk factors in male patients in a cardiac rehabilitation program, *J. Nutr. Health Aging* 137, 384–390, 2007.

45. Hu, F.B., Stampfer, M.J., Soloman, C., Liu, S., Colditz, G.A., and Speizer, F.E., Physical activity and risk for cardiovascular events in diabetic women, *Ann. Intern. Med.* 134, 96–105, 2001.
46. Kopp-Woodroffe, S. A., Manore, M. M., Dueck, C. A., Skinner, J.S., and Matt, K.S., Energy and nutrient status of amenorrheic athletes participating in a diet and exercise training intervention program, *Int. J. Sport Nutr.* 9, 70–88, 1999.
47. Volek, J.S., Gómez, A. L., Love, D.M., Weyers, A. M., Hesslink, R., Jr., Wise, J.A., and Kraemer ,W.J., Effects of an 8-week weight-loss program on cardiovascular disease risk factors and regional body composition, *Eur. J. Clin. Nutr.* 56, 585–592, 2002.
48. Mennen, L.I., de Courcy, G.P., Guilland, J.C., Ducros, V., Bertrais, S., Nicolas, J.P., et al., Homocysteine, cardiovascular disease risk factors, and habitual diet in the French Supplementation with Antioxidant Vitamins and Minerals Study, *Am. J. Clin. Nutr.* 76, 1279–1289, 2002.
49. Herrmann, M., Schorr, H., Obeid, R., Scharhag, J., Urhausen, A., Kindermann, W., and Herrmann, W., Homocysteine increases during endurance exercise, *Clin. Chem. Lab. Med.* 41, 1518–1524, 2003.
50. König, D., Bissé, E., Deibert, P., Müller, H.M., Wieland, H., and Berg, A., Influence of training volume and acute physical exercise on the homocysteine levels in endurance-trained men: Interactions with plasma folate and vitamin B12, *Ann. Nutr. Metab.* 47, 114–8, 2003.
51. Rousseau, A.S., Robin, S., Roussel, A.M., Ducros, V., and Margaritis, I., Plasma homocysteine is related to folate intake but not training status, *Nutr. Metab. Cardiovasc. Dis.* 15, 125–133, 2005.
52. Thiamine deficiency and its prevention and control in major emergencies, World Health Organization, Geneva, 1999. http://www.helid.desastres.net/?e=d-000who--000--1-0--010---4-----0--0-10l--11en-5000---50-about-0---01131-001-110utfZz-8-0-0&a=d&cl=CL1.9&d=Js2900e. Accessed Aug. 22, 2008.
53. Kasper, H., Vitamin absorption in the elderly, *Int. J. Vit. Nutr. Res.* 69, 169–172, 1999.
54. Herbert, V., Vitamin B 12, in *Present Knowledge in Nutrition*, 7th ed., ILSI Press, Washington D.C., 1996, pp 191–205.
55. Herrmann, M., Obeid, R., Scharhag, J., Kindermann, W., and Herrmann, W., Altered vitamin B12 status in recreational endurance athletes, *Int. J. Sport. Nutr. Exer. Metab.* 15, 433–441, 2005.
56. Herrmann, M., Wilkinson, J., Schorr, H., Obeid, R., Georg, T., Urhausen, A., et al., Comparison of the influence of volume-oriented training and high-intensity interval training on serum homocysteine and its cofactors in young, healthy swimmers, *Clin. Chem. Lab. Med.* 41, 1525–1531, 2003.
57. Lukaski, H.C., Vitamin and mineral status: Effects on physical performance, *Nutrition* 20, 632–644, 2004.
58. Tin May, T., Ma Win, M., Khin S.A., and Mya-Tu, M., The effect of vitamin B12 on physical performance capacity, *Br. J. Nutr.* 40, 269–273, 1978.
59. American Medical Association Department of Foods and Nutrition. Multivitamins for parenteral use: A statement by the Nutrition Advisory Group, *J. Parenter. Enteral. Nutri.* 3, 258, 1979.
60. Parenteral multivitamin products: drugs for human use; drug efficacy study implementation: *Fed. Reg.* 65: 21200–21201 (21 CFR 5.70), 2000.

Section IV

Minerals

8 Major Minerals—*Calcium, Magnesium, and Phosphorus*

Forrest H. Nielsen

CONTENTS

I. INTRODUCTION

Calcium, phosphorus, and magnesium are elements integral to the function of the musculoskeletal system. These three elements are interrelated in the formation and transduction of energy and the maintenance of healthy bone. Thus, intakes of these nutrients that are neither too low nor excessive are needed to allow people of all ages, including those aged ~30–60 years, to participate in regular exercise and enjoy recreational physical activities.

II. CALCIUM

A. General Properties

Calcium, the fifth most abundant element in the biosphere, is an alkaline earth metal with an atomic weight of 40.08. Calcium does not exist in nature as a metal, but the divalent calcium cation (Ca^{2+}) in minerals and solutions is common. Chloride and sulfate salts of Ca^{2+} are water-soluble; most other inorganic Ca^{2+} salts are only slightly soluble in water. The properties of Ca^{2+} (ionic radius of 0.99 angstroms; forms coordination bonds with up to 12 oxygen atoms) has made it the ion of choice to fit into the folds of peptide chains for the maintenance of tertiary structure. Its ionic size and ability to bind reversibly to cell proteins have made Ca^{2+} the most common signal transmitter across the cell membrane and an activator of a number of functional proteins.

B. Metabolic Functions

Calcium has three major metabolic functions. In addition to the fundamental function as a second messenger, coupling intracellular responses to extracellular signals, and as an activator of some functional proteins,[1,2]calcium is indispensable for skeletal function.[1]

In the role as signaling or messenger ion, Ca^{2+} mediates vascular contraction and vasodilation, muscle contraction, nerve transmission, and hormone action. In response to a chemical, electrical, or physical stimulus, extracellular Ca^{2+} enters the cell or increases intracellularly through release from internal stores such as endoplasmic or sarcoplasmic reticulum.[1,2] Increased intracellular Ca^{2+} stimulates a specific cellular response, such as activation of a kinase to phosphorylate a protein, that results in a physiological response.[2]

A number of enzymes, including several proteases and dehydrogenases, are activated or stabilized by bound calcium independent of changes in intracellular Ca^{2+}.[3]

Muscle contraction exemplifies the roles that Ca^{2+} plays in signaling and enzyme function. When a muscle fiber receives a nerve stimulus to contract, the initial signal transduction Ca^{2+} enters the cell from the extracellular space upon membrane depolarization.[1] This Ca^{2+} activates intracellular release of Ca^{2+} from the internal storage sites (sarcoplasmic reticulum for muscle) that binds and activates proteins of the contraction complex. Two significant proteins that bind $Ca^{2+}$are troponin c, which initates a series of steps that lead to muscle contraction, and calmodulin, which activates enzymes that break down glycogen for contraction energy.[3] Relaxation occurs when various ionic pumps reduce cytosol Ca^{2+} by moving it to storage sites and into the extracellular space.

About 99% of total body calcium is found in bones and teeth. Bone crystals have a composition similar to hydroxyapatite [$Ca_{19}(PO_4)_6OH)_2$], which contains about 39% calcium. The crystals, which have the ability to resist compression, are arrayed in a protein matrix, which has the ability to withstand tensile loads. Alterations in either the inorganic (hydroxyapatite) or organic (protein matrix) components can result in changes in bone strength.[4] The skeleton must undergo continuous remodeling throughout life (it is replaced every 10–12 years[5]) to adapt its internal microstructure to changes in the mechanical and physiological environment. Additionally, bone is renewed continuously to repair microdamage to minimize the risk of fracture.

C. Body Reserves

Calcium is the most abundant mineral element in the body. Calcium accounts for 1 to 2% of body weight, or 920–1000 g in an adult female and ~1220 g in an adult male.[2] Approximately 1% of total body calcium is found in extracellular fluids, intracellular structures, and cell membranes. Extracellular Ca^{2+} concentrations are about 10,000 times higher than intracellular Ca^{2+}concentrations (about 100 nM). Bones and teeth contain the other 99% of body calcium. The calcium in bone is a large reserve available for times of inadequate intakes to assure the maintenance of extracellular calcium concentrations. Changes in the bone calcium reserve while maintaining extracellular calcium occurs through bone turnover. Thus, a decrease in skeletal calcium reserves is equivalent to a decrease in bone mass, and an increase in reserves is equivalent to an increase in bone mass.[5]

D. Metabolism (Absorption and Excretion)

Calcium absorption occurs through two independent routes, transcellular and paracellular.[6] The transcellular route, localized in the proximal duodenum, is an active or saturable transfer that involves the calcium-binding protein calbindin. Biosynthesis of calbindin D_{9k} is totally vitamin D-dependent. Thus, transcellular absorption of calcium is dependent upon vitamin D. Paracellular transfer occurs throughout the small intestine, and is a nonsaturable diffusion process that is a linear function of the calcium concentration in the intestinal contents. When calcium intake is moderately high, the paracellular route accounts for at least two thirds of the total calcium absorbed.[6] About 20–25% of calcium ingested is absorbed with intakes between 600 and 1000 mg (15–25 mmol)/d.[6]

Regardless of the source of calcium, calcium absorption efficiency decreases with increasing intake, but total calcium absorbed continues to increase.[7] Calcium absorption is more efficient when consumed in divided doses throughout the day.[2] Contrary to the earlier suggestion that protein decreases calcium balance,[8] it has been shown that calcium retention is not reduced by high dietary protein from sources such as meat.[9] Calcium absorption declines with age.[7]

Mechanisms for calcium transport in the intestine also exist in the nephron.[3,6] Most of the calcium arriving in the kidney is reabsorbed by the passive, paracellular mechanism. Active calcium reabsorption is mediated by calbindin D_{28k} and occurs mainly in the distal convoluted tubule.[6] Both active and passive transport systems respond to extracellular Ca^{2+} concentration that is detected by Ca^{2+}-sensing receptors, and is stimulated by parathyroid hormone and 1,25-dihydroxy vitamin D.[3] The urinary calcium output of a 70-kg man is about 200–280 mg (5–7 mmol)/d or about 0.3% of the filtered load.[6,7]

Calcium in stool comes from food and endogenous (cellular debris and body fluids) calcium entering the intestinal tract and escaping absorption.[6] The quantity of endogenous calcium lost in stool daily is about the same as that lost in urine.[6]

E. Dietary and Supplemental Sources

Milk products, the most calcium-dense foods in Western diets, contain about 300 mg (7.5 mmol) calcium per serving (e.g., 8 oz milk or yogurt, or 1.5 oz cheddar cheese).[10] Unfortunately, milk is being replaced by sweetened soft drinks and juices that do not contain much calcium; Americans drank about 2.5 times more soft drinks than milk in 2001.[7] Grains are not particularly rich in calcium, but when consumed in large quantities can provide a substantial portion of dietary calcium.[7] After milk, the second most important food sources of calcium for Mexican-American and Puerto Rican adults are corn tortillas and bread, respectively.[11]

In addition to content, calcium sources should be evaluated based on bioavailability.[8] About 32% of calcium in milk and dairy products is absorbed.[8] Fractional absorption of calcium from low-oxalate vegetables such as broccoli (61%), bok choy (54%), and kale (49%) is higher than from milk.[8] Calcium bioavailability is typically reduced by oxalate and phytate in foods, but food products from soybeans, rich in both oxalate and phytate, have relatively high calcium bioavailability.

Although the best source of calcium is food, calcium supplements are often consumed to prevent or treat bone loss that can lead to osteoporosis and fractures. Common salts used in supplements include calcium carbonate, citrate, citrate malate, lactate, gluconate, fumarate, malate fumarate, glubionate, tricalcium phosphate, dicalcium phosphate, bone meal, oyster shell, coral and algal calcium, and dolomite.[7] Some supplements (e.g., bone meal, dolomite) may have heavy metal (e.g., lead) contaminants and thus should be avoided. Calcium salts, regardless of solubility, have fractional calcium absorption values similar to that of milk, with the exception of calcium citrate malate, which is slightly higher.[8]

F. Status Assessment

As indicated above, the skeleton is a source of calcium that assures critical cellular functions and maintains extracellular fluid concentrations. If serum calcium is more than 10% away from the population mean, disease (e.g., hypo- or hyperthyroidism) probably is the cause.[3,6] Thus, there is no good biochemical indicator of calcium status for the healthy middle-aged adult. Determination of the amount of bone mineral is the best current method for assessing calcium status, but this determination may be affected by other factors such as weight, gonadal hormone status, and other dietary factors (e.g., vitamin D, magnesium levels). Total-body bone mineral can be estimated by using dual x-ray absorption, microcomputed tomography, or peripheral quantitative computed tomography.[12] Numerous blood and urine tests indicate whether bone is being lost or formed after a dietary modification or a pharmacologic intervention. However, tests such as serum osteocalcin and bone-specific alkaline phosphatase for bone formation, and urinary type I collagen cross-linked N-telopeptides, type I C-telopeptide breakdown products, pyridinoline, deoxypyridinoline, and helical peptide for bone resorption, do not predict fracture risk or calcium status well.[13]

Many middle-aged Americans do not consume adequate intakes (AI) of calcium. Mean usual calcium intakes from food calculated for males and females, respectively, from NHANES 2001–2002 data,[14]were for ages 31–50 years, 1021 and 755 mg, and for ages 51–60 years, 874 and 701 mg. Calcium intake data (four standardized 24-h dietary recalls collected 3–6 wks apart) for 4680 men and women aged 40–59 years in Japan, China, United Kingdom, and the United States indicated mean daily calcium intakes of 605, 356, 1013, and 882 mg, respectively.[15]

G. Toxicity

Evidence that health can be harmed in healthy adults by excessive intakes of calcium is limited. Now that the treatment of peptic ulcers with antacids plus large quantities of milk is rarely prescribed, the occurrence of a syndrome termed milk-alkali disease is rare. Symptoms of this syndrome, which causes hypocalcemia, are lax muscle tone, constipation, large urine volumes, nausea, and ultimately, confusion, coma, and death.[2] A review in 1997 revealed only 26 reported cases of milk-alkali disease without renal disease associated with high calcium intakes since 1980.[10]

Nephrolithiasis (kidney stones) has been associated with excessive calcium intake.[10] However, numerous other factors have been associated with nephrolithiasis, including high intakes of oxalate, protein, vegetable fiber, and phosphorus and low intakes of magnesium.[10] As a result, it has been suggested that excess calcium intake may play only a contributing role in the development of nephrolithiasis.[10]

Studies of whether high calcium intakes negatively affect the metabolism of some minerals, particularly iron, magnesium and zinc, have been inconclusive. For example, although 400 mg (10 mmol) of calcium significantly decreased iron absorption in a single meal, calcium supplementation at 1200 mg (30 mmol)/d for 6 months did not decrease iron status in 11 iron-replete adults.[16]High calcium intakes apparently result in a reduced magnesium status in rats[17] but not in humans.[18]High calcium was found to decrease zinc balance in one human study,[19]but increased milk consumption and calcium phosphate supplementation did not decrease zinc absorption in another.[20]

H. Interactions with Other Nutrients and Drugs

As calcium and sodium share the same transport system in the kidney proximal tubule, sodium can have a negative effect on calcium metabolism. Every 1000 mg (43 mmol) of sodium excreted by the kidney results in an additional loss of 26.3 mg calcium (26.3 mmol).[2] This additional loss apparently is not offset by changes in calcium absorption because a high sodium intake results in bone loss.[2,21]Thus, a high sodium intake has a negative effect on the calcium economy.

Dietary protein also increases urinary calcium loss, apparently through an increased urinary acid load caused by the presence of phosphoric and sulfuric acids from the breakdown of phosphorus- and sulfur-containing amino acids.[21,22] However, dietary protein does not decrease calcium retention because of offsetting changes in endogenous secretion or absorption of calcium.[23]

An over-the-counter drug that can increase calcium loss is aluminum-containing antacid.[24] Therapeutic doses of aluminum-containing antacids can increase daily urinary excretion by 50 mg (1.25 mmol) or more.[21]

Some non-digestible oligosaccharides (e.g. inulin) enhance calcium absorption and bone mineralization.[25,26]Vitamin D has long been recognized as an effecter of both absorption and excretion of calcium (see Section II.D). Vitamin D induces the formation of calcium-binding calbindins that facilitate active transport in the intestine and kidney.

A large number of drugs have been developed for the prevention or treatment of osteoporosis. These drugs act by increasing the availability of calcium from the gastrointestinal tract, decreasing the rate of bone resorption, or increasing the rate of bone formation.[22] It is beyond the scope of this review to discuss each drug individually. Most drugs, however, are antiresorptive agents;they include estrogens, selective estrogen receptor modulators (SERMS), isoflavones (act like weak SERMS or weak estrogen agonists), bisphosphonates, and calcitonin.[22] Some experimental anabolic agents that have promise for stimulating bone formation are parathyroid hormone, growth hormone, and insulin-like growth factor-1.[22] Calcium ingested in supra nutritional amounts will increase the amount of calcium crossing the intestinal tract.[7]

I. EFFECTS OF DEFICIENCY OR EXCESS ON PHYSICAL PERFORMANCE

The maintenance of extracellular Ca^{2+} by the mobilization of skeletal calcium stores means that nutritional calcium deficiency almost never manifests itself as a shortage of Ca^{2+} in critical cellular or physiological processes.[5] Thus, for the physically active healthy individual, the only concern about calcium intake is an amount that will maintain bone health. If bone renewal during remodeling or turnover is slower than bone loss, osteoporosis may occur. If bone repairing is slower than microdamage accumulation, stress fractures may occur. In a large case-controlled study of hip fracture risk in women in Europe, fracture risk declined until calcium intake rose to an estimated 500 mg (12.5 mmol)/d.[27] Most studies with adults showing a positive influence of high dietary calcium in decreasing bone loss or fracture risk also had supplemental vitamin D as an experimental co-variable. Calcium supplementation alone of individuals consuming more than 500 mg (12.5 mmol) Ca/d has not been shown to decrease fracture risk.[27–30]

As indicated in the Section II.G, an excessive intake of calcium that would affect physical performance is unlikely for a healthy middle-aged individual.

J. Dietary Recommendations

Calcium intake recommendations vary widely worldwide, with the United States among the highest.[10] In the United States, a Recommended Dietary Allowance (RDA) was not established for calcium because of concerns that included uncertainties in the precision and significance of balance studies, and lack of concordance between mean calcium intakes and experimentally derived values predicted as necessary for a desirable amount of calcium retention.[10] As a result, only AI were established for middle-aged adults; these were 1000 mg (25 mmol)/d for ages 31–50 years, and 1200 mg (30 mmol)/d for ages 51–60 years.[10] The calcium dietary reference intake in the United Kingdom for adults aged 30–60 years is a much lower 700 mg (17.5 mmol)/d[31]. In India, the recommended dietary allowance for calcium is 400 mg (10 mmol)/d for adults.[32] Recently, an analysis of primary calcium balance data from tightly controlled metabolic feeding studies indicated an RDA of 1035 mg (25.8 mmol)/d for men and 741 mg (18.5 mmol)/d for women.[33] Several countries and organizations, including the United States and the European Community have established 2500 mg (62.4 mmol)/d as the upper limit (UL) for calcium.[34]

K. Future Research Needs

Perhaps the most pressing need is for a marker of calcium status more determinate than the estimation of calcium reserve in the skeleton. In addition, the effect of lifestyle choices on calcium requirements needs further definition. For example, about 65% of the U.S. population is either overweight or obese.[35] Weight loss, which is recommended to prevent comorbid conditions, may cause bone loss.[35] Recommendations for calcium intakes during weight loss need clarification because they apparently will vary with initial body weight, age, gender, physical activity, and conditions of dieting.[35] An example of age's affecting calcium loss during weight loss is that premenopausal overweight women did not lose bone during moderate weight loss with adequate (1 g/d) or higher calcium intakes (1.8 g/d),[36] but postmenopausal overweight women lost bone during moderate weight loss while consuming 1 g calcium/d.[37] Consuming 1.7 g calcium/d only mitigated the bone loss in postmenopausal women.

L. Summary

Calcium is a critical ion for vascular contraction and vasodilation, muscle contraction, nerve transmission, hormone action, and bone growth and maintenance in the physically active middle-aged adult. However, the skeleton maintains extracellular calcium so that a nutritional calcium deficiency almost never manifests itself as a shortage of Ca^{2+} for critical cellular physiological processes. Thus, the major calcium concern for the physically active healthy middle-aged individual is an intake that will prevent bone loss and fractures. Calcium intakes near the AI (1.0 g for ages 31–50 years and 1.2 g for ages 50–60 years) will assure bone health if there are no other health problems, lifestyle conditions, or nutrient deficiencies affecting bone turnover. Consuming greater amounts of calcium is unlikely to have any further benefit for physically active middle-aged adults.

III. MAGNESIUM

A. General Properties

Magnesium, the eighth most abundant element on earth,[38] is an alkaline earth metal with an atomic weight of 24.31. Magnesium does not exist in nature as a metal, but the divalent magnesium cation (Mg^{2+}) is common in minerals and solutions. It is the second most abundant cation in seawater.[38] One compound, magnesium sulfate (Epsom salts) is obtained from the wastewater (bittern) of solar salt production. Cooling diluted bittern to between –5° and –10° C precipitates up to 70% of the magnesium sulfate that is removed by filtration. Small amounts of Mg^{2+} contribute to the tartness and taste of natural waters. Mg^{2+}, although chemically similar to Ca^{2+}, does not bond as well as calcium to proteins, but still is involved in over 300 enzyme reactions through binding enzyme substrates or directly with enzymes.[38] Magnesium is second to potassium as the most abundant intracellular cation. The ratio of extracellular to intracellular $Mg^{2+}$is 0.33, which contrasts markedly with the ratio of 10,000 for Ca^{2+}. Thus, unlike calcium, magnesium is not a common signal transmitter from the outside to the inside of cells. However, magnesium through affecting cell membrane receptors and protein phosphorylation is a critical cation for cell signaling.

B. Metabolic Functions

Magnesium is needed for enzymatic reactions vital to every metabolic pathway.[10,38–40] These reactions include those involving DNA, RNA, protein, and adenylate cyclase synthesis, cellular energy production and storage, glycolysis, and preservation of cellular electrolyte composition. Magnesium has two functions in enzymatic reactions. It binds directly to some enzymes to alter their structure or to serve in a catalytic role (e.g., exonuclease, topoisomerase, RNA polymerase, DNA polymerase). Magnesium also binds to enzyme substrates to form complexes with which enzymes react. The predominant role of magnesium is involvement in ATP utilization. An example of this role is the reaction of kinases with MgATP to phosphorylate proteins. Magnesium exists primarily as MgATP in all cells. Magnesium at the cell membrane level regulates intracellular calcium and potassium, and thus is a controlling factor in nerve transmission, skeletal and smooth muscle contraction, cardiac excitability, vasomotor tone, blood pressure, and bone turnover.

C. Body Reserves

Magnesium is the fourth most abundant cation in the body.[38] The adult human body contains about 25 g (1028 mmol) of magnesium, which is about equally divided between bone and soft tissue.[39] Less than 1% of the total body magnesium is in blood. Approximately one-third of skeletal magnesium is exchangeable, and acts as a pool for maintaining normal concentrations of extracellular magnesium. The other two-thirds of skeletal magnesium is an integral part of bone mineral crystals. This magnesium is not readily labile and thus is not available for metabolic needs during periods of magnesium deficiency. Normal serum magnesium concentrations, which are tightly regulated, range from 1.8 to 2.3 mg/dL (0.74–0.95 mmol/L).

D. Metabolism (Absorption and Excretion)

Magnesium is absorbed throughout the intestinal tract, but the greatest amount is absorbed in the distal jejunum and ileum.[38] Between 40% and 60% of ingested magnesium is absorbed by using both passive paracellular and active transport mechanisms.[39] Net magnesium absorption increases with increasing intake, but fractional magnesium absorption falls. About 90% of intestinal magnesium absorption is through the paracellular route when the dietary intake is adequate. A greater fractional absorption through the active transport system occurs when dietary intake is low. Thus, absorption mechanisms contribute to magnesium homeostasis.

The kidney, however, is the primary organ regulating magnesium homeostasis. About 10% of the total body magnesium is normally filtered through the glomeruli of an healthy adult, with only 5% of the filtered magnesium's being excreted.[38]About 90–95% of magnesium is reabsorbed through a paracellular mechanism in the proximal convoluted tubules and the loops of Henle, the other 5–10% is reabsorbed by an active transcellular pathway in the distal convoluted tubules.[38] Renal magnesium excretion decreases to as low as 12–24 mg (0.5-0.1.0 mmol)/d when dietary intakes are deficient. When body stores are normal, excess absorbed magnesium is almost entirely excreted.

E. Dietary and Supplemental Sources

Green leafy vegetables, whole grains, and nuts are the richest sources of magnesium.[39] Milk (about 100 mg [4.11 mmol] Mg/L) and milk products provide moderate amounts of magnesium. A variety of magnesium salts are used as supplements, including oxide, hydroxide, citrate, chloride, gluconate, lactate, and aspartate. The fractional absorption of magnesium from these supplements depends on the solubility in the intestinal fluid. For example, highly soluble magnesium citrate is much better absorbed than poorly soluble magnesium oxide.[41]

F. Status Assessment

Low serum magnesium is the most common method for diagnosing severe magnesium deficiency. However, plasma or serum magnesium is a poor indicator of subclinical magnesium deficiency because exchangeable skeletal magnesium and urinary responses to changes in magnesium intake maintain extracellular magnesium at a rather constant level even while tissue magnesium is decreasing. Thus, normal serum and plasma magnesium concentrations have been found in individuals with low magnesium in erythrocytes and tissues.[38]

Efforts to find an indicator of subclinical magnesium status (also called chronic latent magnesium deficiency[38,42]) have not yielded a cost-effective one that has been well validated. Among the tests evaluated as an indicator of magnesium status are serum ionized magnesium, urinary magnesium excretion, sublingual cellular magnesium, erythrocyte magnesium, and the magnesium load test.

At present, the magnesium load test is the test of choice to diagnose a total body deficit of magnesium. This test determines the percentage of magnesium retained over a given period of time after the parenteral administration of a magnesium load.[38,42]Retention of a greater percentage than that (22–25%) by individuals with adequate magnesium status indicates some body magnesium depletion.[38] This test is invasive, time-consuming, and expensive; requires hospitalization or close supervision for about 24 hours after magnesium infusion; and requires careful urine collection for laboratory analysis.

The ionized fraction (61%) in serum is the physiologically active form of magnesium that serves as a metabolic cofactor for many enzymatic reactions. Measurement of this fraction has been suggested as appropriate for assessing magnesium status. However, this test has the same problem as the determination of total serum magnesium in measuring subclinical magnesium deficiency. For example, the magnesium load test and serum total and ionized magnesium concentration were determined in 44 critically ill persons.[43] Of the 19 subjects who were determined to be magnesium deficient by the magnesium load test, only two had serum total or ionized magnesium concentrations below the reference interval. One review found that the determination of ionized magnesium concentration had limited value in assessing magnesium status in disorders associated with chronic latent magnesium deficiency.[44]

A 24-hour magnesium excretion in urine that is more than 10–15% of the amount ingested suggests adequate magnesium status.[38] When deficient amounts of magnesium are ingested or absorbed, there is a rapid and progressive reduction in the urinary excretion of magnesium (see Section III.D). Thus, a low urinary excretion of magnesium can occur while serum magnesium is normal and before total body reduction results in changes that become biochemically and clinically significant. Thus, urinary magnesium excretion is best used to corroborate other tests indicating a subclinical magnesium deficiency.

In experimental magnesium deficiency, a decrease in erythrocyte, or erythrocyte membrane, magnesium has been used to indicate a decrease in magnesium status.[45,46]However, standard reference intervals have not been established that allow the use of this test for status assessment.

The measurement of magnesium in sublingual epithelial cells may be a method that can assess a subclinical magnesium deficiency.[47] At present, this expensive test determines cellular magnesium by using energy-dispersive X-ray analysis, thus it has been used mainly in research studies. Comparing this test with the magnesium load test would help validate the use of sub-lingual cellular magnesium as an indicator of magnesium status.

The U.S. National Health and Nutrition Examination Survey (NHANES) 2001–2002 data set indicated that the majority of adults in the survey consumed less than the Estimated Average Requirement (EAR) for magnesium.[14] For example, 64% of women aged 51–70 years did not attain the magnesium EAR. Daily intakes of 10% adult males and females were 206 and 148 mg (8.47 and 2.39 mmol) magnesium, respectively.[14] Thus, a significant number of middle-aged adults routinely have magnesium intakes that may result in a deficient status. However, it should be noted that a recent survey of the dietary behavior of German adults engaging in different levels of physical activity found that the median magnesium density was higher in the diets of active persons.[48]

G. Toxicity

Severe magnesium toxicity results in high serum magnesium (hypermagnesmia). Signs of hypermagnesmia include lethargy, confusion, nausea, diarrhea, appetite loss, muscle weakness, breathing difficulty, low blood pressure, and irregular heart rhythm.[38,39] Hypermagnesmia is most commonly associated with the combination of impaired renal function and high intakes of nonfood sources of magnesium such as magnesium-containing laxatives and antacids. Thus, hypermagnesmia is not an issue for the healthy middle-aged physically active adult.[38,39]

The major effect of excessive magnesium intake without hypermagnesmia is diarrhea.[10,39] Nausea and abdominal cramping may also occur.

H. Interactions with Other Nutrients and Drugs

Protein intake affects magnesium balance and retention. Low dietary protein (30 mg/d) resulted in negative magnesium balance in adult females when dietary magnesium was less than 180 mg (7.4 mmol)/d; a higher protein intake prevented the negative balance.[49] Magnesium absorption by adolescent boys was lower when dietary protein was low (43 mg/d) than when high (93 mg/d).[50] In addition, low dietary protein with a magnesium intake of 240 mg (9.87 mmol)/d resulted in negative magnesium retention, which did not occur when dietary protein was high.[50] High protein intakes that increase renal acid load also may decrease magnesium retention through increased renal loss.[51]

A high zinc intake decreases magnesium absorption and balance. Zinc supplementation at 142 mg (2.17 mmol)/d decreased magnesium absorption and balance in adult males.[52] A more moderate zinc intake (53 mg [0.81 mmol]/d) decreased magnesium balance in postmenopausal women.[53]

High dietary phosphorus was found to decrease magnesium absorption.[38] The decreased absorption may have been the result of the formation of insoluble magnesium phosphate. Magnesium absorption also may be decreased through the binding with phosphate groups of phytate in high-fiber foods.[54] The interaction between magnesium and phosphorus may be more than an effect on absorption. Magnesium supplementation ameliorates the kidney calcification[55] and bone loss[56] induced by high dietary phosphorus in experimental animals. In postmenopausal women, a deficient magnesium intake (~107 mg [4.40 mmol]/d) increased urinary excretion of phosphorus, but apparent phosphorus absorption increased, so no change in phosphorus balance occurred.[57]

Another factor that may negatively affect magnesium requirement is vitamin B_6 deficiency. Young women depleted of vitamin B_6 exhibited negative magnesium balance because of increased urinary excretion.[58]

There is a relationship between magnesium and calcium, but this apparently is not at the intestinal level. High calcium intakes (up to 2400 mg/d) were found to have no effect on magnesium absorption or retention,[59,60] and high magnesium intakes (up to 826 mg/d) were found to have no effect on calcium absorption.[61] However, moderate magnesium deprivation increased calcium balance or retention in postmenopausal women, with a decreased urinary calcium excretion contributing most to the increased balance.[57,62] The increased retention suggests that moderate magnesium deficiency increases intracellular calcium.

Although not a nutrient, short-chain fructo-oligosaccharides (e.g., inulin) increases the intestinal absorption of magnesium by about 25%.[25,63] Vitamin D may also have a limited effect on magnesium absorption. Pharmacologic doses have been found to increase magnesium absorption in animals.[64] However, the increased absorption may be counteracted by an increase in urinary magnesium excretion induced by vitamin D.

There are some drugs, particularly those used for controlling hypertension, that affect magnesium metabolism. Diuretics such as furosemide and ethacrynic acid have been shown to cause marked renal wasting of magnesium.[38] On the other hand, angiotension converting enzyme (ACE) inhibitors may increase cellular and serum magnesium.[65] Increased intracellular magnesium may result in heart arrhythmia.[66]

I. Effects of Deficiency or Excess on Physical Performance

Subclinical or chronic latent magnesium deficiency most likely affects physical performance. A subclinical magnesium deficiency impaired exercise performance in untrained postmenopausal women in a controlled metabolic unit study.[45] Heart rate and oxygen consumption increased significantly during submaximal exercise when the women were fed 150 mg (6.17 mmol) compared with 320 mg (13.16 mmol) magnesium/d. Young men consuming about 250 mg (10.28 mmol) magnesium/d (most likely a deficient intake) and participating in a strength-training program showed a greater increase in peak knee-extension torque when fed a 250-mg (10.28) magnesium supplement/d than when fed a placebo.[67] Moderately trained adults consuming about 250 mg (10.28 mmol) magnesium/d and taking a supplemental 250 mg (10.28 mmol) magnesium/d (instead of a placebo) had improved cardiorespiratory function during a 30-minute submaximal exercise test.[68] An animal study gave similar results. Marginally magnesium-deficient rats exhibited reduced exercise capacity or endurance on a treadmill.[69] Subclinical magnesium deficiency also may result in muscle spasms or cramps. For example, magnesium supplementation resolved muscle cramps, normalized neuromuscular excitability and decreased lactate dehydrogenase and creatine kinase activities in a physically active individual determined to be magnesium-deficient.[70] In another case, magnesium supplementation resolved muscle cramps in a tennis player with hypomagnesmia.[71] There is a lack of reports showing that magnesium supplementation improves performance of individuals with established adequate magnesium status. Thus, differences in magnesium status may be the reason for conflicting reports about the effect of magnesium supplementation on exercise performance.

Magnesium deficiency may amplify some undesirable effects of exercise. Reactive oxygen species production or oxidative stress occurs during exercise.[72] Magnesium deficiency has been shown to increase reactive oxygen species or oxidative stress in experimental animals.[73] The increase apparently induces ultrastructural damage in skeletal muscle (i.e., swollen mitochondria and disorganized sarcoplasmic reticulum).[73] In addition, dietary magnesium deficiency has been shown to induce a pro-oxidant/pro-inflammatory response to rodents characterized by enhanced free radical (lipid radicals and nitric oxide) production, accumulation of oxidation products and pro-oxidant metals, depletion of endogenous antioxidants (e.g., glutathione), and elevated inflammatory mediators (e.g., substance P).[74,75] These findings suggest that a relationship may exist between oxidative stress induced by exercise and subclinical magnesium deficiency such that one may amplify the adverse effects of the other.

Controlled metabolic unit studies with postmenopausal women have shown that a subclinical magnesium deficiency may induce arrythmias and changes in potassium metabolism that may affect heart function.[46,62,76] Additionally, a chronic low intake of magnesium may contribute to hypertension, bone loss leading to osteoporosis, and insulin resistance and impaired insulin secretion leading to diabetes mellitus. Impaired heart function and fracture risk induced by a chronic latent magnesium deficiency are noteworthy concerns for middle-aged physically active adults.[38]

Severe magnesium deficiency, which is not likely to occur in the physically active middle-aged adult, usually is the result of dysfunctional states resulting in its malabsorption or excessive excretion; it results in numerous signs and symptoms.[38] Loss of appetite, nausea, vomiting, fatigue, and weakness are early signs of magnesium deficiency. As deficiency becomes more severe, numbness, tingling, muscle contractions and cramps, seizures, personality changes, and coronary spasms (angina pectoris) occur. As indicated earlier, an excessive intake of magnesium that would affect physical performance is unlikely for a healthy middle-aged individual.

J. Dietary Recommendations

The lack of usable data has made it difficult to establish a sound recommendation for magnesium. In 1997, the U.S. Food and Nutrition Board set the magnesium RDA for men and women between ages 30 and 60 years at 420 and 320 mg (17.28 and 13.16 mmol)/d,[10] respectively. These RDAs are consistent with the recommendation of 6 mg (0.25 mmol)/kg body weight/d suggested by Seelig[77] and Durlach.[78] The U.S. RDAs were based almost exclusively on findings from one poorly controlled balance study performed in 1984.[79] In that study, subjects consumed self-selected diets in their home environment and were responsible for the collection of their urine, feces, and duplicate diet and beverage samples used in the balance determinations. The samples were collected only 1 week each season for 1 year. There was much overlap in the magnesium intakes that resulted in negative and positive magnesium balance. For example, four of 10 women aged 35–53 years were in positive balance or equilibrium with intakes ranging from 182 to 258 mg (7.49 to 10.61 mmol)/d; the other six women were in negative balance with intakes ranging from 164 to 301 mg (6.75 to 12.38 mmol)/d. Three of seven men aged 35–53 years were in equilibrium with intakes ranging from 286 to 418 mg (11.76 to 17.19 mmol)/d; the four men were in negative balance with intakes ranging from 157 to 344 mg (6.46 to 14.15 mmol)/d.

Because of the tenuous nature of the data used, the magnesium RDAs for the United States and Canada have been appropriately questioned. For example, an expert consultation for the Food and Agriculture Organization/World Health Organization (FAO/WHO) concluded that evidence was lacking for nutritional magnesium deficiency occurring with the consumption of diets supplying a range of magnesium intakes sometimes considerably less than the RDA for the United States and Canada or the United Kingdom equivalent to the RDA called Recommended Nutrient Intake (RNI).[80] Thus, the expert consultation subjectively set RNIs for magnesium at 220 and 260 mg (9.05 and 10.69 mmol)/d for women and men, respectively, including those between ages 30 and 60 years.

Some recent reports suggest that the RNIs set by the FAO/WHO consultation may be valid. Based on balance data and findings of heart rhythm changes and impaired physiologic function in postmenopausal women fed slightly less than 200 mg (8.23 mmol)/magnesium/d under controlled metabolic unit conditions,[45,76] consistent intakes less than the RNIs set by the FAO/WHO probably would result in chronic latent magnesium deficiency. Balance data from 27 different tightly controlled metabolic unit studies revealed that neutral magnesium balance, without considering surface losses, occurred at an intake of 165 mg (6.79 mmol)/d with a 95% prediction interval of 113 and 213 mg (4.65 and 8.76 mmol)/d.[81] These recent findings suggest that middle-aged physically active adults should strive for dietary magnesium intakes of over 220 mg (9.05 mmol)/d.

The U.S. Food and Nutrition Board determined that magnesium ingested as a naturally occurring substance in foods would not exert any adverse effects.[10] Because the primary initial manifestation of excessive magnesium intake from nonfood sources is diarrhea, the Board used diarrhea as sensitive hazard to set the UL for magnesium. For middle-aged adults, the UL was set at 350 mg (14.6 mmol) of *supplementary* magnesium.

K. Future Research Needs

The most pressing research need is for biochemical indicators that provide an accurate and specific assessment of magnesium status. These status assessment indicators then can be used to determine the extent of subclinical or chronic latent magnesium deficiency in apparently healthy populations, including middle-aged physically active adults. There also is a need to assess the relationships between dietary magnesium intakes, indicators of magnesium status, and possible adverse health outcomes such impaired physical performance, bone loss and arrhythmias. Findings from the assessment of the relationships would help determine intervention strategies to improve magnesium status and determine their impact on specific health outcomes.

L. Summary

Magnesium is needed for enzymatic reactions vital to every metabolic pathway including cellular energy production and storage, glycolysis, and preservation of cellular electrolyte composition. Magnesium also is a controlling factor in nerve transmission, skeletal and smooth muscle contraction, cardiac excitability, blood pressure, and bone turnover. Based on dietary surveys, subclinical or chronic latent magnesium deficiency may occur in significant numbers in middle-aged adults. Subclinical magnesium deficiency has been found to impair energy utilization and exercise performance in adults. Additionally, subclinical magnesium deficiency may amplify some undesirable effects of exercise including oxidative stress; it may impair heart function and result in bone loss. Unfortunately, there is no practical biochemical indicator that provides an accurate and specific assessment of subclinical magnesium status. However, balance studies indicate that intakes of more than 220 mg (9.05 mmol) magnesium/d are needed to prevent adverse effects of chronic latent magnesium deficiency. An intake near the RDA set by the U.S. Food and Nutrition Board (420 and 320 mg [17.28 and 13.16 mmol]/d for men and women, respectively) should assure adequate magnesium status for almost all physically active middle-aged adults. Consuming greater amounts of magnesium is unlikely to have any further benefit, thus there is no reason to exceed the U.S. UL of 350 mg (14.40 mmol) supplementary magnesium/d.

IV. PHOSPHORUS

A. General Properties

Phosphorus (atomic number 15 and atomic weight of 30.97) is too reactive to exist in nature in its elemental form. About 0.12% of the earth's crust is phosphorus, which often is found combined with oxygen as inorganic or organic phosphates. Inorganic phosphates have the same basic orthophosphate tetrahedron structure, which is 1 phosphorus atom surrounded by 4 oxygen atoms with either a monovalent or a divalent anionic charge. The predominant species of inorganic phosphate in all biological fluids and tissues is the divalent anion, HPO_4^{2-}. At normal blood pH, the ratio of HPO_4^{2-} ions to $H_2PO_4^{1-}$is 4 to 1. Phosphate ions in blood serve as a buffer of blood pH and as a regulator of whole body acid–base balance through facilitating the renal excretion hydrogen ions by shifting from HPO_4^{2-} to $H_2PO_4^{1-}$. Phosphate ions contribute about 50% to daily urinary hydrogen ion excretion, or titratable acidity.[82]

B. Metabolic Functions

Phosphorus is involved in virtually every aspect of metabolism.[82,83] It is an integral part of structural molecules including phospholipids and phosphoproteins. Membranes that surround all cells and separate intracellular organelles from cytoplasm are primarily a bilayer of phospholipids. Glucose, the ultimate energy source for most cellular activities, must be phosphorylated before entering into the glycolytic pathway. Energy storage and use is in the form of phosphorus-containing compounds ATP and creatine phosphate. Cyclic AMP and cyclic GMP are intracellular second messengers regulating many biochemical processes including the actions of many hormones. DNA and RNA contain phosphate groups linking deoxyribose and ribose along the backbone of these molecules, respectively. Phosphorus is a critical component of virtually all enzyme reactions, often in the form of a co-enzyme such MgATP and nicotinamide adenine dinucleotide, and the addition or removal of phosphate moieties changes the catalytic activity of many enzymes. In extracellular fluids, about 30% of phosphorus exists as inorganic ions that help maintain osmotic pressure and acid–base balance. The highly anionic organic phosphate, 2,3-diphosphoglycerate binds to hemoglobin to facilitate the release of oxygen to tissues. In bones and teeth, phosphorus is a component of crystalline hydroxyapatite $[Ca_{10}(PO_4)_6OH)_2]$. Over 50% of bone mineral mass is the phosphate ion.

C. Body Reserves

The adult human body contains about 850 g (27.45 mol) of elemental phosphorus (about 1.1% of total body weight) with about 85% in the skeleton, 14% in the soft tissues, and 1% in extracellular fluids, intracellular structures, and cell membranes.[82] Phosphate is the most abundant anion in the cell. The hydroxyapatite in bone crystals has a constant calcium:phosphate ratio of about 2:1. Bone acts as a reservoir for exchangeable phosphate ions. The flux between plasma and bone phosphate ion is very high, about 5 g (1614 mmol)/d.[82] Bone mineral phosphate ion efflux and influx occurs through ionic exchange and active bone resorption. Bone usually has a slow turnover rate so dynamic ion exchange is the primary bone mechanism for maintaining phosphate ion concentrations in plasma and extracellular fluids. The kidney (see below) is the other major regulator of phosphate balance in the body. The kidney and bone keep serum phosphate concentration, which has circadian rhythm, between 2.5 to 4.5 mg/dL (0.87 to 1.45 mmol/L).[82]

D. Metabolism (Absorption and Excretion)

Most phosphorus absorption occurs as the inorganic phosphate ion because intestinal phosphatases hydrolyze most organic phosphorus in foods to this form.[10] Phosphorus is highly bioavailable (55–70%) from most food sources.[10] Foods containing phosphorus as phytate, the storage form of phosphorus in plant seeds (e.g., beans, peas, nuts, cereals), is an exception. The hydrolysis of phytate depends on exogenous phytase provided by yeasts, colonic bacteria, and foods. For example, leavening with yeast that produces phytase increases phosphorus bioavailability from breads.[82] Because a number of factors influence the presence of phytase, phosphorus bioavailability from food phytate is quite variable.[10] Milk casein contains a phosphopeptide that also is resistant to enzymatic hydrolysis.[83] Absorption of phosphate ions occurs throughout the small intestine, primarily by facilitated diffusion. Active transport of phosphate becomes important only when phosphorus intake is low or the demand for phosphorus is greatly increased.[82]

The kidney is the primary organ regulating phosphorus homeostasis. Humoral phosphaturic factors (phosphatonins), parathyroid hormone, and 1,25-hydroxy vitamin D influence the reabsorption of filtered phosphate ions.[82] The kidneys reabsorb about 80% of filtered phosphate ions, with 60% reabsorbed in the proximal convoluted tubule, 15–20% in the proximal straight tubule, and less than 10% in the distal segments of the nephron.[82]

An uncompensated change in absorption, excretion, or exchange with bone mineral will result in either hypophosphatemia or hyperphosphatemia.[82] Hypophosphatemia also can induced by exercise or changes in arterial blood acid–base balance, which redistribute phosphate from extracellular fluids to intracellular sites.[82]

E. Dietary and Supplemental Sources

Phosphorus is found in nearly all foods, where it occurs as a mixture of inorganic phosphate and various organic phosphorus compounds. Foods high in protein are generally high in phosphorus. About 15 mg (0.48 mmol) of phosphorus is consumed with every gram of protein. Thus, meat and dairy products are major contributors to the daily intake of phosphorus.

The phosphorus content of the U.S. food supply has increased in recent years because phosphate salts are added to processed foods for non-nutrient functions (moisture retention, smoothness, and binding), and cola soft drinks are acidulated with phosphoric acid.[82] As a result, the median phosphorus intakes by females and males in the United States exceed the RDA (700 mg [22.6 mmol]/d for middle-aged adults) by 300 and 800 mg (9.69 and 25.83 mmol)/d.[10]

Phosphorus in supplement form for most people usually occurs as an anion component of another nutrient (e.g., calcium phosphate) in supplements. However, there are reports that supplemental phosphorus may have some ergogenic properties.[84] As a result, supplemental phosphorus in the forms of high-energy bars and shakes, creatine monophosphate, and sodium phosphate may be consumed to enhance athletic performance and build muscle mass. If these supplements are consumed, the daily intake of phosphorus can easily exceed the UL for phosphorus (4000 mg [129.2 mmol]/d). For example, consumption of some high-energy bars and shakes, or creatine monophosphate supplements at the manufacturer's recommended daily dose alone, can provide up to 3000 mg (96.9 mmol) phosphorus/d.[82]

F. Status Assessment

Serum phosphorus concentration is generally used as an indicator of phosphorus status. Normal concentrations for adults are 2.5–4.5 mg/dL (0.87–1.45 mmol/L). However, the concentration of phosphorus in serum can be falsely elevated or depressed, which results in concentrations that appear normal when body stores are low, or concentrations that appear low when body stores are adequate. For example, consuming laxatives containing high amounts of sodium phosphate and phosphate loading for ergogenic purposes elevate serum phosphate concentrations.[84] Exercise, which results in the redistribution of phosphate from extracellular fluids to intracellular sites, decreases serum phosphate concentrations.[82] Other factors that decrease serum phosphorus concentrations include respiratory alkalosis, various disease states, and changes in hormonal status.[83] For example, individuals with insulin-dependent diabetes mellitus have fluctuating serum phosphorus concentrations because insulin decreases serum phosphorus concentrations. Thus, assessing phosphorus status by using serum phosphorus concentrations requires awareness of possible factors, especially the large number that cause hypophosphatemia without phosphorus deficiency,[83] affecting values obtained.

G. Toxicity

Excessive phosphorus intake from any source is expressed as hyperphospathemia.[10] Essentially all phosphorus toxicity effects are caused by elevated inorganic phosphate in the extracellular fluid.[10]

A potential problem caused by excessive phosphorus intake is nonskeletal tissue calcification (ectopic or metastatic calcification), particularly of the kidney. This calcification occurs when calcium and phosphorus concentrations of the extracellular fluid exceed limits of calcium phosphate solubility. Metastatic calcification of the kidney is not known to occur through dietary means alone in persons with adequate renal function, but occurs often in patients with end-stage renal disease and is associated with increased all-cause and cardiovascular mortality and vascular calcification.[85]

Hyperphosphatemia also can induce changes in the hormonal regulation of calcium metabolism and utilization. Hyperphosphatemia induced by phosphate loading results in decreased extracellular fluid-ionized calcium, and increased circulating parathyroid hormone and 1,25-dihydroxy vitamin D concentrations.[86–88] These changes in calcium-regulating hormones can cause impairment of adaptive mechanisms for adequate calcium absorption and the removal of calcium and phosphorus from bone. If these changes continue for an extended period, bone loss may occur. Clinical evidence indicating parathyroid hormone-induced bone loss in individuals with healthy kidneys consuming high amounts of phosphorus is lacking. However, support is supplied by findings from epidemiological and animal studies. In a cross-sectional study with perimenopausal women, a significant positive relationship between bone mineral density and dietary calcium:phosphorus ratio was found.[89] Experimental animals fed diets with a low dietary calcium:phosphorus ratio when calcium intake was adequate or deficient exhibited secondary hyperparathyroidism and bone resorption.[90] In humans, however, phosphorus supplements have been found to decrease bone turnover markers.[91] Thus, the long-term consequences of a low calcium:phosphorus ratio or a high phosphorus intake are unclear. Although calcium intakes are often low, the U.S. Food and Nutrition Board concluded that current phosphorus intakes experienced by the U.S. population are unlikely to adversely affect bone health.[10]

H. Interactions with Other Nutrients and Drugs

In the United States, phosphorus intake is consistently higher than calcium intake in the absence of calcium supplementation; as indicated in the toxicity section, the significance of this fact is controversial. The intestinal absorption of phosphate ions may be enhanced by 1,25-dihydroxy vitamin D when phosphorus intakes are low, but the evidence supporting this interaction comes only from limited animal studies.[92] The magnesium interaction section above describes the interaction between phosphorus and magnesium, which results in high dietary phosphorus decreasing magnesium absorption, and magnesium supplementation ameliorating kidney calcification and bone loss induced by high dietary phosphorus in experimental animals.

Drugs that can cause hypophosphatemia include corticosteroids, diuretics, and phosphate-binding antacids.[83] A deficient phosphorus intake while ingesting diuretics or a phosphate-binding drug could have pathological consequences. For example, dietary phosphorus deprivation while consuming the phosphate-binding aluminum hydroxide gel can result in severe and potentially fatal phosphorus deficiency.[83]

I. Effects of Deficiency Or Excess on Physical Performance

When inorganic phosphorus concentrations in extracellular fluid are low, cellular dysfunction occurs. The consequences of hypophosphatemia include anorexia, anemia, muscle weakness, bone pain, osteomalacia, increased susceptibility to infection, paresthesias, ataxia, confusion, and even death.[93] The muscle weakness, which particularly involves proximal muscle when prolonged or severe, can result in muscle fiber degeneration. A deficient phosphorus intake also becomes potentially limiting for bone growth. However, the typical abundance of phosphorus in the diet minimizes the risk of hypophosphatemia and its consequences in healthy adults. Near total starvation is required to produce phosphorus deficiency by only dietary deprivation that manifests as hypophosphatemia.[10]

As indicated in the toxicology section, excessive phosphorus intakes induce an increase in circulating parathyroid hormone that may impair the adaptive mechanism needed for adequate calcium absorption and optimal bone accretion. However, based on the determination by the U.S. Food and Nutrition Board,[10] bone health is unlikely to be adversely affected by usual phosphorus intakes of middle-aged healthy, physically active adults in the United States.

One form of high phosphorus intake called phosphate loading has received much attention as an ergogenic aid. Phosphate loading is the consumption of 4 to 10 g/d of sodium or calcium phosphate supplements for 3 to 4 days prior to engaging in athletic events. Phosphate loading increases serum phosphate about 10% and the increase apparently can enhance the synthesis of ATP and creatine phosphate, which are depleted rapidly with high-intensity exercise, and the synthesis of 2,3-diphosphoglycerate to facilitate oxygen release to tissues.[84] An extensive review[84] found reports showing that phosphate loading also elevated intracellular phosphate concentrations that promoted glycolysis, attenuated anaerobic threshold, enhanced cardiovascular efficiency or performance, increased peripheral extraction of oxygen and maximal oxygen uptake, and improved endurance exercise performance or efficiency. The review noted that not all studies found ergogenic benefits with phosphate loading, and suggested that the reason for this may have been differences in the type and amount of phosphate ingested, the experimental design and procedures used, and the type of exercise evaluated. It also was stated that single-dose acute (e.g., 1.5 g sodium phosphate 2.5 hours before athletic competition) and chronic calcium phosphate supplementation (e.g., 3.7 g sodium phosphate for 6 or more days) provided little ergogenic benefits, and phosphate loading was of some benefit mainly to athletes performing high-intensity or endurance exercise.

J. Dietary Recommendations

The U.S. Food and Nutrition Board[10] established DRIs for phosphorus based on the amount needed to maintain serum inorganic phosphate at the bottom end of the normal range (2.5 to 2.8 mg/dL or 0.8 to 0.9 mmol/L). The RDA set for men and women aged 30–60 years was 700 mg/d. The UL was set at 4.0 g (130 mmol)/d based on the finding that the upper boundary of adult normal serum phosphate concentration (4.5 mg/dL or 1.45 mmol/L) is reached at a daily phosphorus intake of 3.5 g (113 mmol).

K. Future Research Needs

For the middle-aged physically active adult, how bone mineral mass is affected by different dietary phosphorus intakes needs further clarification. This clarification should include the determination of high phosphorus intakes on mineral elements needed for bone maintenance, including magnesium, iron, copper, and zinc. In addition, the effects of phosphate loading in moderately or untrained adults under varying exercise conditions should be determined.

L. Summary

Phosphorus is involved in virtually every aspect of metabolism. It is a component of the bone mineral hydroxyapatite; cell membranes in the form of phospholipids; molecules involved in energy storage and production; cellular messenger mechanisms; and virtually all enzyme reactions. Bone, which acts as reservoir for exchangeable phosphate ions, and the kidney, through regulating urinary excretion, loosely maintain serum phosphate concentrations between 2.5–4.5 mg/dL (0.87–1.4 mmol/L). Serum phosphorus concentration is generally used as an indicator of phosphorus status, but with caution because other factors can cause falsely high or low values. These factors include exercise, respiratory alkalosis, various disease states, and hormonal status. Low serum phosphorus (hypophosphatemia) may cause muscle weakness, and a low dietary phosphorus intake may potentially limit bone growth. However, the typical abundance of phosphorus in the diet (median intakes 300–800 mg [9.69–25.83 mmol]/d greater than RDA of 700 mg [22.6 mmol]/d) minimizes the risk of hypophosphatemia. Near total starvation is required to produce phosphorus deficiency by dietary deprivation alone. High serum phosphorus (hyperphosphatemia) can cause nonskeletal tissue calcification, but is not known to occur through dietary means in persons with adequate renal function. A high dietary phosphorus:calcium ratio induces changes in hormonal regulation of calcium metabolism and utilization that may cause bone loss. However, clinical evidence for bone loss in individual with healthy kidneys is lacking. Thus, current phosphorus intakes by healthy physically active adults are unlikely to have adverse effects. Phosphate loading (4–10 g/d of sodium phosphate for 3–6 days prior athletic events) may have some ergogenic benefit for endurance or intensely exercising athletes, but is unlikely to benefit adults participating in moderate physical activity. Thus, phosphorus nutrition is not a concern for the physically active middle-aged adult with normal renal function, and the consumption of bars or supplements in an attempt to increase energy in the form of creatine phosphate or ATP is unlikely to enhance exercise performance.

V. Conclusions

Calcium, magnesium and phosphorus are essential elements critically important for the function of the musculoskeletal system, including the formation and transduction of energy and the maintenance of healthy bone. The major calcium concern for physically active healthy middle-aged adults is to consume enough calcium to prevent bone loss and fractures; an intake at the AI level (1.0–1.2 g [25–30 mmol]/d) should accomplish this. Phosphorus intakes in the United States indicate that neither phosphorus deficiency nor excess is a nutritional concern for healthy middle-aged adults. Based on dietary surveys, subclinical or chronic latent magnesium deficiency, which impairs energy utilization and exercise performance, may occur in significant numbers of middle-aged adults. Subclinical magnesium deficiency may also impair heart function, result in bone loss, and amplify oxidative stress induced by exercise. Balance studies indicate that intakes of more than 220 mg (9.05 mmol) magnesium/d are needed to prevent adverse effects of chronic latent magnesium deficiency. Consuming amounts greater than the RDA for magnesium (420 mg and 320 mg [17.28 and 13.16 mmol]/d for men and women, respectively) is unlikely to provide any exercise performance benefits for healthy physically active middle-aged adults.

REFERENCES

1. Awumey, E. M. and Bukoski R. D., Cellular functions and fluxes of calcium. In *Calcium in Human Health*, Weaver, C. M. and Heaney, R. P., Eds., Humana Press, Totowa, 2006, chap. 3.
2. Weaver, C. M., Calcium. In *Present Knowledge in Nutrition,* Vol. 1, 9th ed., Bowman, B. A. and Russell, R. M., Eds., ILSI Press, Washington, DC, 2006, chap. 29.
3. Weaver, C. M. and Heaney R. P., Calcium. In *Modern Nutrition in Health and Disease, 10th ed.,* Shils, M. P., Shike M., Ross, A. C., Caballero, B., and Cousins, R. J., Eds., Lippincott Williams & Wilkins, Baltimore, 2006, chap. 9.
4. Rubin, C. and Rubin, J., Biomechanics and mechanobiology of bone. In *Primer on the Metabolic Bone Diseases and Disorders of Mineral Metabolism, 6th ed.*, Favus, M. J., Ed., American Society for Bone and Mineral Research, Washington, DC, 2006, chap. 6.
5. Heaney, R. P., Bone as the calcium nutrient reserve. In *Calcium in Human Health*, Weaver, C. M. and Heaney, R. P., Eds., Humana Press, Totowa, 2006, chap. 2.

6. Bronner, F., Calcium in exercise and sport. In *Macroelements, Water, and Electrolytes in Sports Nutrition*, Driskell, J. and Wolinsky, I., Eds., CRC Press, Boca Raton, 1999, chap. 2.
7. Weaver, C. M. and Heaney, R. P., Food sources, supplements, and bioavailability. In *Calcium in Human Health*, Weaver, C. M. and Heaney, R. P., Eds., Humana Press, Totowa, 2006, chap. 9.
8. Weaver, C. M., Proulx, W. R., and Heaney, R., Choices for achieving adequate dietary calcium with a vegetarian diet, *Am. J. Clin. Nutr.* 70, 543S–548S, 1999.
9. Kerstetter, J. E., Wall, D. E., O'Brien, K. O., Caseria, D. M., and Insogna, K. L., Meat and soy protein affect calcium homeostasis in healthy women. *J. Nutr.* 136, 1890–5, 2006.
10. Food and Nutrition Board. Institute of Medicine, *Dietary Reference Intakes for Calcium, Phosphorus, Magnesium, Vitamin D, and Fluoride*, National Academy Press, Washington, DC, 1997.
11. Looker, A. C., Harris, T. B., Madans, J. H., and Sempos, C. T., Dietary calcium and hip fracture risk: The NHANES I Epidemiologic Follow-Up Study, *Osteoporosis Int.* 3, 177–84, 1993.
12. MacNeil, J. A. and Boyd, S. K., Accuracy of high-resolution peripheral quantitative computed tomography for measurement of bone quality, *Med. Eng. Phys.* 29, 1096–105, 2007.
13. Bauer, D. C., Biochemical markers of bone turnover: The study of osteoporotic fracture. In *Bone Markers: Biochemical and Clinical Perspectives*, Eastell, R., Ed., Martin Dunitz, London, 2001, chap. 21.
14. Moshfegh, A., Goldman, J., and Cleveland, L., What We Eat in America, NHANES 2001–2002: Usual Nutrient Intakes from Food Compared to Dietary Reference Intakes, U. S. Department of Agriculture, Agricultural Research Service.
15. Zhou, B. F., Stamler, J., Dennis, B., Moag-Stahlberg, A., Okuda, N., et al., Nutrient intakes of middle-aged men and women in China, Japan, United Kingdom, and United States in the late 1990s: The INTERMAP study. *J. Hum. Hypertens.* 17, 623–30, 2003.
16. Minihane, A. M., and Fairweather-Tait, S. J., Effect of calcium supplementation on daily nonheme-iron absorption and long-term iron status, *Am. J. Clin. Nutr.* 68, 96–102, 1998.
17. Evans, G. H., Weaver, C. M., Harrington, D. D., and Babbs, C. F., Jr., Association of magnesium deficiency with blood pressure lowering effects of calcium. *J. Hypertension* 8, 327–37, 1990.
18. Andon, M. B., Ilich, J. Z., Tzagoumis, M. A., and Matkovic, V. Magnesium balance in adolescent females consuming a low- or high-calcium diet, *Am. J. Clin. Nutr.* 63, 950–3, 1996.
19. Wood, R. J. and Zheng, J. J., High dietary calcium intake reduces zinc absorption and balance in humans, *Am. J. Clin. Nutr.* 65, 1803–1809, 1997.
20. Wood, R. J. and Zheng, J. J., Milk consumption and zinc retention in postmenopausal women, *J. Nutr.* 120, 398–403, 1990.
21. Heaney, R. P., Nutrition and risk for osteoporosis. In *Osteoporosis,* 3rd ed., Marcus, R., Feldman, D., Nelson, D. A., and Rosen, C. J., Eds., Elsevier, Amsterdam, 2008, chap. 31.
22. Anderson, J. J. B. and Ontjes, D. A., Nutritional and pharmacological aspects of osteoporosis. In *Handbook of Clinical Nutrition and Aging*, Bales, C. W., and Ritchie, C. S., Eds., Humana Press, Totowa, 2004, chap. 29.
23. Kerstetter, J. E., O'Brien, K. O., Caseria, D. M., Wall, D. E., and Insogna, K. L., The impact of dietary protein on calcium absorption and kinetic measures of bone turnover in women, *J. Clin. Endocrinol. Metab.* 90, 26–31, 2005.
24. Spencer, H., Kramer, L., Norris, C., and Osis, D., Effect of small doses of aluminum-containing antacids on calcium and phosphorus metabolism, *Am. J. Clin. Nutr.* 36, 32–40, 1982.

25. Coudray, C., Bellanger, J., Castiglia-Delavaud, C., Rémésy, C., Vermorel, M., and Rayssignuier, Y., Effect of soluble or partly soluble dietary fibre supplementation on absorption and balance of calcium, magnesium, iron and zinc in healthy young men, *Eur. J. Clin. Nutr.* 51, 375–80, 1997.
26. Abrams, S. A., Griffin, I. J., Hawthorne, K. M., Liang, L., Gunn, S. K., Darlington, G., and Ellis, K. J., A combination of prebiotic short- and long-chain inulin-type fructans enhances calcium absorption and bone mineralization in young adolescents, *Am. J. Clin. Nutr.* 82, 471–6, 2005.
27. Dawson-Hughes, B., Calcium and vitamin D for bone health in adults. In *Nutrition and Bone Health*, Holick, M. F. and Dawson-Hughes, B, Eds., Humana Press, Totowa, 2004, chap. 12.
28. Shea, B., Wells, G., Cranney, A., Zytaruk, N., Robinson, V., Ortiz, Z., et al., Meta-analysis of therapies for postmenopausal osteoporosis: VII. Meta-analysis of calcium supplementation for the prevention of postmenopausal osteoporosis, *Endocrin. Rev.* 23, 552–9, 2002.
29. Jackson, R. D., LaCroix, A. Z., Gass, M., Wallace, R. B., Robbins, J. et al., Calcium plus vitamin D supplementation and the risk of fractures, *New Engl. J. Med.* 354, 669–683, 2006.
30. Cumming, R. G. and Nevitt, M. C., Calcium for prevention of osteoporotic fractures in postmenopausal women, *J. Bone Miner. Res.* 12, 1321–9, 1997.
31. Francis, R. M., What do we currently know about nutrition and bone health in relation to United Kingdom public health policy with particular reference to calcium and vitamin D? *Br. J. Nutr.* 7, 1–5, 2007.
32. Harinarayan, C. V., Ramalakshmi, T., Prasad, U. V., Sudhakar, D., Srinivasarao, P. V., Sarma, K. V., and Kumar E. G., High prevalence of low dietary calcium, high phytate consumption, and vitamin D deficiency in healthy south Indians, *Am. J. Clin. Nutr.* 85, 1062–7, 2007.
33. Hunt, C. D. and Johnson, L. K., Calcium requirement: new estimations for men and women by cross-sectional statistical analyses of calcium balance data from metabolic studies, *Am. J. Clin. Nutr.* 86, 1054–1063, 2007.
34. Looker, A. C., Dietary calcium: Recommendations and intakes around the world. In *Calcium in Human Health*, Weaver, C. M. and Heaney, R. P., Eds., Humana Press, Totowa, 2006, chap. 8.
35. Shapses, S. A. and Riedt, C. S., Bone, body weight, and weight reduction: What are the concerns? *J. Nutr.* 136, 1453–1456, 2006.
36. Riedt, C. S., Schlussel, Y., von Thun, N., Ambia-Sobhan, H., Stahl, T., Field, M. P., et al., Premenopausal overweight women do not lose bone during moderate weight loss with adequate or higher calcium intake, *Am. J. Clin. Nutr.* 85, 972–980, 2007.
37. Riedt, C. S., Cifuentes, M., Stahl, T., Chowdhury, H. A., Schlussel, Y., and Shapses, S. A., Overweight postmenopausal women lose bone with moderate weight reduction and 1 g/d calcium intake, *J. Bone Miner. Res.* 20, 455–463, 2005.
38. Rude, R. K. and Shils, M. E., Magnesium. In *Modern Nutrition in Health and Disease, 10th ed.,* Shils, M. E., Shike, M., Ross, A. C., Caballero, B., and Cousins, R. J., Eds., Lippincott Williams & Wilkins, Philadelphia, 2006, chap. 11.
39. Volpe, S. L., Magnesium. In *Present Knowledge in Nutrition,* Vol. 1, 9th ed., Bowman, B. A., Russell, R. M., Eds., ILSI Press, Washington, DC, 2006, chap. 31.
40. Brilla, L. R. and Lombardi, V. P., Magnesium in Exercise and Sport. In *Macroelements, Water, and Electrolytes in Sports Nutrition,* Driskell, J. A. and Wolinsky, I., Eds., CRC Press, Boca Raton, 1999, chap. 4.
41. Walker, A. F., Marakis, G., Christie, S., and Byng, M., Mg citrate found more bioavailable than other Mg preparations in a randomized, double-blind study, *Magnes. Res.* 16, 183–91, 2003.

42. Elin, R. J., Laboratory evaluation of chronic latent magnesium deficiency. In *Advances in Magnesium Research: Magnesium and Health*, Rayssiguier, Y., Mazur, A., and Durlach, J., Eds., John Libbey & Company, Eastleigh, U. K., 2001, chap. 35.
43. Hébert P., Mehta, N., Wang, J., Hindmarsh, T., Jones, G., and Cardinal, P., Functional magnesium deficiency in critically ill patients identified using a magnesium-loading test, *Crit. Care Med.* 25, 749–755, 1997.
44. Sanders, G. T., Huijgen, H. J., and Sanders, R., Magnesium in disease: A review with special emphasis on the serum ionized magnesium, *Clin. Chem. Lab. Med.* 37, 1011–1033, 1999.
45. Lukaski, H. C. and Nielsen, F. H., Dietary magnesium depletion affects metabolic responses during submaximal exercise in postmenopausal women, *J. Nutr.* 132, 930–935, 2002.
46. Nielsen, F. H., Milne, D. B., Klevay, L. M., Gallagher, S., and Johnson, L., Dietary magnesium deficiency induces heart rhythm changes, impairs glucose tolerance, and decreases serum cholesterol in post menopausal women, *J. Am. Coll. Nutr.* 26, 121–132, 2007.
47. Silver, B. B., Development of cellular magnesium nano-analysis in treatment of clinical magnesium deficiency, *J. Am. Coll. Nutr.* 23, 732S–7S, 2004.
48. Beitz, R., Mensink, G. B. M., Henschel, Y., Fischer, B., and Erbersdobler, H. F., Dietary behavior of German adults differing in levels of sport activity, *Pub. Health Nutr.* 7, 45–52, 2004.
49. Hunt, M. S. and Schofield, F. A., Magnesium balance and protein intake level in adult human female, *Am. J. Clin. Nutr.* 22, 367–73, 1969.
50. Schwartz, R., Walker, G., Linz, M. D., and MacKellar I., Metabolic responses of adolescent boys to two levels of dietary magnesium and protein: I. Magnesium and nitrogen retention, *Am. J. Clin. Nutr.* 26, 510–8, 1973.
51. Rylander, R., Remer, T., Berkemeyer, S., and Vormann, J., Acid–base status affects renal magnesium losses in healthy, elderly persons, *J. Nutr.,* 136, 2374–7, 2006.
52. Spencer, H., Norris, C., Williams, D., Inhibitory effects of zinc on magnesium absorption in man, *J. Am. Coll. Nutr.* 13, 479–84, 1994.
53. Nielsen, F. H. and Milne, D. B., A moderately high intake compared to a low intake of zinc depresses magnesium balance and alters indices of bone turnover in postmenopausal women, *Eur. J. Clin. Nutr.,* 58, 703–10, 2004.
54. Coudray, C. and Rayssiguier, Y., Impact of vegetable products on intake. Intestinal absorption and status of magnesium. In *Advances in Magnesium Research: Nutrition and Health*, Rayssiguier, Y., Mazur, A. and Durlach, J., Eds., John Libbey & Company, Eastleigh, U. K., 2001, chap. 16.
55. Kasaoka, S., Kitano, T., Hanai, M., Futatsuka, M., and Esashi, T., Effect of dietary magnesium level on nephrocalcinosis and growth in rats, *J. Nutr. Sci. Vitaminol.* 44, 503–14, 1998.
56. Katsumata, S. I., Matsuzaki, H., Uehara, M., and Suzuki, K., Effect of dietary magnesium supplementation on bone loss in rats fed a high phosphorus diet, *Magnes. Res.* 18, 91–6, 2005.
57. Nielsen, F. H., Milne, D. B., Gallagher, S., Johnson, L., and Hoverson, B., Moderate magnesium deprivation results in calcium retention and altered potassium and phosphorus excretion by postmenopausal women, *Magnes. Res.* 20, 19–31, 2007.
58. Turnlund, J. R., Betschart, A. A., Liebman, M., Kretsch, M. J., and Sauberlich, H. E., Vitamin B6 depletion followed by repletion with animal- or plant-source diets and calcium and magnesium metabolism in young women, *Am. J. Clin. Nutr.* 56, 905–10, 1992.

59. Leichsenring, J. M., Norris, L. M., and Lamison, S. A., Magnesium metabolism in college women: Observations on the effect of calcium and phosphorus intake levels, *J. Nutr.* 45, 477–85, 1951.
60. Greger, J. L., Smith, S. A., and Snedeker, S. M., Effect of dietary calcium and phosphorus levels on the utilization of calcium, phosphorus, magnesium, manganese, and selenium by adult males, *Nutr. Res.* 1, 315–325, 1981.
61. Spencer, H., Fuller, H., Norris, C., and Williams, D., Effect of magnesium on the intestinal absorption of calcium in man, *J. Am. Coll. Nutr.* 13, 485–92, 1994.
62. Nielsen, F. H., The alteration of magnesium, calcium and phosphorus metabolism by dietary magnesium deprivation in postmenopausal women is not affected by dietary boron deprivation, *Magnes. Res.* 17, 197–210, 2004.
63. Coudray, C., Bellanger, J., Vermorel, M., Sinaud, S., Wils, D., Feillet-Coudray, et al., Two polyol, low digestible carbohydrates improve the apparent absorption of magnesium but not of calcium in healthy young men, *J. Nutr.* 133, 90–3, 2003.
64. Hardwick, L. L., Jones, M. R., Brautbar, N., and Lee, D. B., Magnesium absorption: Mechanisms and the influence of vitamin D, calcium and phosphate, *J. Nutr.* 121, 13–23, 1991.
65. Rubio-Luengo, M. A., Maldonado-Martin, A., Gil-Extremera, B., Gonzáles-Gómez, L. and de Dios Luna del Castillo, J., Variations in magnesium and zinc in hypertensive patients receiving different treatments, *Am. J. Hypertens.* 8m 689–95, 1995.
66. Averbukh, Z., Berman, S., Efrati, S., Manevits, E., Rosenberg, R., Malcev, E., et al., Blockade of rennin-angiotensin system reduces QT dispersion and improves intracellular Ca/Mg status in hemodialysis patients, *Nephron. Clin. Pract.* 104, c176–84, 2006.
67. Brilla, L. R. and Haley, T. F., Effect of magnesium supplementation on strength training in humans, *J. Am. Coll. Nutr.* 11, 326–9, 1992.
68. Ripari, P., Pieralisi, G., Giamberardino, M. A., Resina, A., and Vecchiet, L., Effects of magnesium pidolate on cardiorespiratory submaximal effort parameters, *Magnes. Res.* 2, 70–4, 1992.
69. McDonald, R. and Keen, C. L., Iron, zinc and magnesium nutrition and athletic performance, *Sports Med.* 5, 171–84, 1988.
70. Dragani, L., D'Aurelio, A., and Vecchiet, L., Clinical, haematological, and neurophysical evidence of muscle damage from magnesium deficiency in athletes: A case report. In Golf, S., Dralle, D., Vecchiet, L., Eds. John Libbey & Company, London, 1993, chap. 33.
71. Liu, L., Borowski, G., and Rose, L. I., Hypomagnesmia in a tennis player, *Phys. Sportsmed.* 11, 79–80, 1983.
72. Laires, M. J. and Monteiro, C., Magnesium status: influence on the regulation of exercise–induced oxidative stress and immune function in athletes. In *Advances in Magnesium Research: Nutrition and Health*, Rayssiguier, Y., Mazur, A., Durlach, J., Eds., John Libbey & Company, Eastleigh, U. K., 2001, chap. 74.
73. Rock, E., Astier, C., Lab, C., Vignon, X., Gueux, E., Motta, C., and Rayssiguier, Y., Dietary magnesium deficiency in rats enhances free radical production in skeletal muscle, *J. Nutr.* 125, 1205–10, 1995.
74. Weglicki, W. B., Mak, I. T., Dickens, B. F., Stafford, R. E., Komarov, A. M., Gibson, B., et al., Neuropeptides, free radical stress antioxidants in models of Mg-deficient cardiomyopathy. In *Magnesium: Current Status and New Developments–Theoretical, Biological and Medical Aspects*, Theophanides, T. and Anastassopoulou, J., Eds. Kluwer Academic Publishers, Dordrecht, Netherlands,1997, pp. 169–78.
75. Kramer, J. H., Mak, I. T., Phillips, T. M., and Weglicki, W. B., Dietary magnesium intake influences circulating pro-inflammatory neuropeptide levels and loss of myocardial tolerance to postischemic stress, *Exp. Biol. Med.* 228, 665–73, 2003.
76. Klevay, L. M. and Milne, D. B., Low dietary magnesium increases supraventricular ectopy, *Am. J. Clin. Nutr.* 75, 550–4, 2002.

77. Seelig, M. S., Magnesium requirements in human nutrition, *Magnesium–Bull.* 3, 26–47, 1981.
78. Durlach, J., Recommended dietary amounts of magnesium: Mg RDA, *Magnes. Res.* 2, 195–203, 1989.
79. Lakshmanan, F. L., Rao, R. B., Kim, W. W., and Kelsay, J. L., Magnesium intakes, balances, and blood levels of adults consuming self-selected diets, *Am. J. Clin. Nutr.* 40, 1380–9, 1984.
80. Food and Agriculture Organization/World Health Organization, Magnesium. In *Human Vitamin and Mineral Requirements: Report of a Joint FAO/WHO Expert Consultation, Bangkok, Thailand.* FAO/WHO, Geneva, pp. 223–33, 2002.
81. Hunt, C. D. and Johnson, L. K., Magnesium requirements: New estimations for men and women by cross–sectional statistical analyses of metabolic magnesium balance data, *Am. J. Clin. Nutr.* 84, 843–52, 2006.
82. Anderson, J. J. B., Klemmer, P. J., Watts, M. L., Garner, S. C., and Calvo, M. S., Phosphorus. In *Present Knowledge in Nutrition,* 9th ed., Vol. 1, Bowman, B. A. and Russell, R. M., Eds., ILSI Press, Washington, DC, 2006, chap. 30.
83. Knochel, J. P., Phosphorus. In *Modern Nutrition in Health and Disease,* 10th ed., Shils, M. E., Shike, M., Ross, A. C., Caballero, B. and Cousins, R. J., Eds., Lippincott Williams & Wilkins, Baltimore, 2006, chap. 10.
84. Kreider, R. B., Phosphorus in exercise and sport. In *Macroelements, Water, and Electrolytes in Sports Nutrition*, Driskell, J. and Wolinsky, I., Eds., CRC Press, Boca Raton, 1999, chap. 3.
85. Kooienga, L., Phosphorus balance with daily dialysis. *Semin. Dial.* 20, 342–5, 2007.
86. Calvo, M. S. and Heath, H. III, Acute effects of oral phosphate-salt ingestion on young adults, *Am. J. Clin. Nutr.* 47, 1025–9, 1988.
87. Calvo, M. S., Kumar, R., and Heath, H. III, Elevated secretion and action of serum parathyroid hormone in young adults consuming high phosphorus, low calcium diets assembled from common foods, *J. Clin. Endocrinol. Metab.* 66, 823–9, 1988.
88. Anderson, J. J. B., Nutritional biochemistry of calcium and phosphorus, *J. Nutr. Biochem.* 2, 300–9, 1991.
89. Brot, C., Jørgensen, N., Madsen, O. R., Jensen, L. B., and Sørensen, O. H., Relationships between bone mineral density, serum vitamin D metabolites and calcium:phosphorus intake in healthy perimenopausal women, *J. Intern. Med.* 245, 509–16, 1999.
90. Anderson, J. J. B., Calcium, phosphorus and human bone development, *J. Nutr.* 126, 1153S–8S, 1996.
91. Heaney, R. P., Sodium, potassium, phosphorus, and magnesium. In *Nutrition and Bone Health*, Holick, M. F., Dawson-Hughes, B., Eds., Humana Press, Totowa, 2004, chap. 20.
92. Peterlik, M. and Wasserman, R. H., Effect of vitamin D on transepithelial phosphate transport in chicken intestine, *Am. J. Physiol.* 244, E379–88, 1978.
93. Lotz, M. Zisman, E., and Bartter, F. C., Evidence for a phosphorus-depletion syndrome in man, *N. Engl. J. Med.* 278, 409–15, 1968.

9 Iron

Emily M. Haymes

CONTENTS

I. INTRODUCTION

Because of the multiple roles it plays in metabolism, iron is one of the most important trace minerals found in the body. It is also the trace mineral found in the greatest amount in humans. Most of the iron is found inside erythrocytes as part of the hemoglobin molecule. Oxygen binds to the iron in hemoglobin for transport through the blood from the lungs to the rest of the cells in the body. Iron is also found inside the mitochondria of cells, where it plays a critical role in the production of energy via the electron transport system. Because of its critical roles in aerobic metabolism, iron deficiency and anemia can reduce an individual's endurance. Iron deficiency anemia is the most common nutritional deficiency found throughout the world, including North America.

II. IRON METBOLISM

A. Iron in the Human Body

The total amount of iron in the body is estimated to range from 40 mg/kg for women to 50 mg/kg for men.[1] Approximately two thirds of this iron is found in hemoglobin as heme iron. There are four heme groups in each hemoglobin molecule and 250,000 hemoglobin molecules per erythrocyte. In other words, there are one million hemoglobin atoms in each erythrocyte and each heme iron can bind to a single oxygen molecule. Hemoglobin concentration is slightly lower in women (132–135 g/l of blood) than in men (144–154 g/l of blood). The total heme iron content of the blood is somewhat lower in women than men. As a result, women have a lower maximal oxygen carrying capacity than men.

Heme iron is part of the myoglobin molecule found in skeletal muscles. Myoglobin's role is to assist in transferring oxygen molecules through muscle to the mitochondria. The cytochromes in the mitochondria also contain heme iron proteins as well as iron-sulfur proteins. These proteins are involved in the transfer of electrons in the electron transport system that results in the formation of adenosine triphosphate (ATP) in aerobic metabolism. There are also other iron-containing enzymes that are found in the cytoplasm and mitochondria of cells. It is estimated that 10% of the body's iron is found in myoglobin and 5% is in iron-containing enzymes.[2]

The remaining iron is found in the iron stores in the red bone marrow, liver, and spleen. Iron is stored as ferritin and hemosiderin in reticuloendothelial cells in the red bone marrow and spleen and in both reticuloendothelial cells and hepatocytes in the liver. It is estimated that men have 1000 mg of iron stored while women have 300 mg of stored iron.

B. Iron Homeostasis

1. Absorption

Iron is absorbed in the first part (duodenum) of the small intestine. Food iron is composed of heme iron and nonheme iron. Meats, fish, and poultry contain both heme and nonheme iron, while dairy products and plants contain only nonheme iron. The iron in nonheme iron is in the ferric state (+3) and must be converted to the ferrous state (+2) before absorption can occur. The divalent metal transporter-1 (DMT1) transports nonheme iron across the duodenal mucosal cell membrane. Iron is then exported into the capillaries via ferroportin. Hepcidin, a recently discovered peptide, regulates the release of iron into the blood by interacting with ferroportin.[3] Binding of hepcidin results in the degradation of ferroportin and prevents iron release into the blood.

Heme iron is absorbed at a higher rate by the mucosal cells than nonheme iron. Recent research has reported the existence of a heme iron transporter that is believed to transport heme iron into the intestinal mucosal cells.[4] Once inside the cell, the iron is released from heme and becomes part of the nonheme iron, which can be exported by ferroportin to the blood.

2. Transport

Iron is transported in the plasma bound to the protein transferrin. Iron must be oxidized to the ferric state by ceruloplasmin, a copper-containing oxidase present in plasma, before it can bind to the surface of the protein. A low percentage of iron bound to transferrin, known as the transferrin saturation, is used as an indicator of iron deficiency clinically.

Transferrin-iron can bind to transferrin receptors (TfR) on cell membranes and enter the cell by endocytosis. Cells that require large amounts of iron will have a greater number of TfR on their cell surface than those with little need for iron. Because TfR concentration in the plasma is correlated to the number of TfR on cells, elevated TfR is also used as an indicator of iron deficiency.

3. Excretion

Four pathways are used to excrete iron from the body: gastrointestinal tract, urinary tract, desquamation of epidermal cells and sweat, and in women, loss of blood through the menses. The gastrointestinal tract is the primary site of iron excretion due to the high rate of enterocyte turnover every 2 days and blood loss. Estimated iron loss in the feces is 0.51 mg/d.[5]

Small amounts of iron, averaging 0.1 mg/d, are excreted through the urinary tract. The amount of iron lost when epidermal cells of the skin are desquamated has been measured at 0.24 mg/d using the uptake of a radioactive isotope of iron (Fe^{55}) by the skin cells.[5] Collection of whole body skin cell desquamation and sweat in men resulted in iron losses of 0.33 mg/d, slightly higher than measured with the iron isotope technique.[6] In women, blood loss through the menses is a major source of iron loss until menopause occurs. It has been estimated that the iron loss in the menses averages 0.6 mg/d.[7]

The total amount of iron excreted daily by men is estimated to be about 0.9 mg/d. In women prior to menopause total iron loss is estimated to be 1.4 mg/d.[1] Postmenopausal women have total iron losses similar to those of men.

III. ASSESSMENT OF IRON STATUS

Three stages are used in the assessment of iron status: iron depletion, iron deficiency without anemia, and iron deficiency anemia. Iron depletion indicates that the body's iron stores have been depleted. The most widely used biomarker of iron depletion is the serum ferritin concentration less than 12 μg/l.[8,9] Under normal physiological conditions there is a direct relationship between the bone marrow iron stores and concentration of ferritin in the blood. However, there are exceptions, such as when a person has an infection or an inflammatory disease. In this case, serum ferritin concentrations will be elevated, even though iron stores are depleted.

As the iron content of the body continues to decrease, other biomarkers of iron status begin to change in addition to the low ferritin level. The serum transferrin saturation, or percentage of iron bound to transferrin, falls below the normal range.

Serum transferrin saturations less than 16% are used as an indicator of iron deficiency. Two other biomarkers may also be used as indicators: elevated free erythrocyte protoporphyrin concentration (FEP) and elevated serum transferrin receptor concentration (sTfR). When bone marrow iron is depleted, less hemoglobin will be formed and more heme protoporphyrin groups will be released. An FEP greater than 70 μg/dL erythrocytes also is used as a clinical indicator of iron deficiency. Depleted iron stores also reduce the amount of iron available to the tissues and the number of transferrin receptors on cells increases. Elevated sTfR greater than 8.5 mg/L is used as another indicator of iron deficiency.[1] An alternative method for determining tissue iron deficiency that uses the log (sTfR/serum ferritin) has been shown to provide a quantitative measure of body iron stores.[10]

Iron deficiency anemia is diagnosed by low hemoglobin concentrations, <120 g/l for women and <130 g/l for men.[1] Not all cases of anemia are due to iron deficiency. Chronic inflammatory diseases are accompanied by reduced iron transport to the red bone marrow, however, serum ferritin concentration will be elevated. Below-normal hemoglobin concentrations accompanied by serum ferritin concentrations less than 30 μg/l are used clinically to diagnose iron deficiency anemia.[11]

IV. IRON STATUS OF THE PHYSICALLY ACTIVE

A. Iron Status

The prevalence of low serum ferritin in the U.S. population has been reported to be less than 5% in men between the ages of 31 and 70 years old and women ages 51–70 years.[1] In women 31 to 50 years, 16% were found to have low serum ferritin levels.[1] Numerous studies have found low serum ferritin concentrations in 20% or more of young women athletes.[12–17] Very few of these athletes were found to be anemic. These competitive athletes were engaged in endurance sports including distance running and cross-country skiing. Several of these studies also included male athletes and found 8% to 11% had low serum ferritin concentrations.[12,16,17]

One recent study of male and female recreational athletes, ages 18–41 years, examined iron status.[18] Most of the male athletes had normal iron status, however, 4% were iron deficient and 2% were diagnosed with iron deficiency anemia. Among the female athletes, 30% were identified as iron deficient and an additional 11% had iron deficiency anemia. Many of the athletes in this study were cyclists. An earlier study of male and female joggers and runners, ages 16–78 years, reported 40% of the females and 13% of the males had hemoglobin concentrations below 130 g/l.[19] Among males ages 17–53 yr who participated in a variety of sports, lower ferritin concentrations were found in athletes with higher training frequencies.[20] Mean serum ferritin was 31 μg/l in the males who trained 10–14 times per week.

Middle-aged adults who undergo resistance training have experienced decreases in iron status. Murray-Kolb and colleagues found women ages 51–69 had significantly lower serum ferritin concentrations and higher sTfR/serum ferritin ratios following 12 weeks of resistance training.[21] Men in the same study experienced significant increases in serum transferrin receptor and the sTfR/serum ferritin ratio following training. Although the total iron intake of the men and postmenopausal women exceeded the RDA, the bioavailable iron intake was significantly lower for the women, suggesting this might have been a contributing factor.

Another study of middle-aged overweight males who completed 12 weeks of resistance training found no significant difference in serum ferritin but a significant increase in transferrin saturation following training.[22] Studies with younger males undergoing resistance training have reported significant decreases in serum ferritin after 6 to 8 weeks of training.[23,24] A third study of younger males and females found serum ferritin was decreased after resistance training only in males with normal ferritin levels but not in males or females with low ferritin levels.[25]

There also is some evidence of iron stores' being depleted in females involved in aerobic fitness-type programs. Blum et al.[26] found significant decreases in serum ferritin concentrations of females ages 22–51 following 13 weeks of an aerobic exercise program. Pratt and colleagues studied females ages 56–67 who participated in aerobic training or control groups.[27] No significant changes were observed in serum ferritin or transferrin saturation following training in either group, but hemoglobin concentration increased significantly.

Female runners ages 27–34, who ran 70 km/wk in preparation for a marathon, had mean ferritin concentration of 30 μg/l during training.[28] Serum ferritin concentration was significantly increased for 3 days after the marathon. Serum iron concentration has been observed to decrease significantly for 24 hours following a triathlon accompanied by a significant increase in C-reactive protein.[29] Fallon and colleagues studied a group of male and female ultramarathon runners age 41–76, who completed a 1600-km ultramarathon over 16 days.[30] Serum ferritin was significantly increased and serum iron and transferrin saturation were significantly decreased by the fourth day through the end of the race. White blood cell counts were also increased significantly during the run, suggesting an acute phase response during exercise. Recent research has found that the cytokine interleukin-6 can increase hepcidin release that is followed by decreases in serum iron.[31] Elevated urinary excretion of hepcidin has recently been observed 24 hours following a marathon in female distance runners age 26-45.[32]

B. Iron Excretion

1. Gastrointestinal Bleeding

Excretion of iron through several avenues has been found to increase during exercise and may explain why some individuals experience a depletion of iron stores during training. Several studies of distance runners found evidence of gastrointestinal bleeding during marathon runs.[33–35] The amount of hemoglobin lost during the runs ranged from 1.51–2.25 mg/g of stool.[34–35] Lampe and colleagues (1991) found women increased fecal hemoglobin from 0.94 to 1.6 mg/g stool after a marathon.[33] Estimated iron loss during the run was an additional 0.8 mg/g stool. During training, these women runners lost significantly more hemoglobin/d in the stool than sedentary women.

The reason for increased gastrointestinal bleeding during exercise is not well understood. One possibility is that shunting of blood from the splanchnic circulation to the skeletal muscles during higher-intensity exercise leads to rebound hyperemia and bleeding into the gastrointestinal tract. There is evidence of increased transit time through the gastrointestinal tract during the marathon, which could be responsible for some of the increase in hemoglobin loss in the feces.[33] Two other possible reasons for blood loss in the gastrointestinal tract include use of analgesic drugs and failure of mechanisms to protect the mucosa from gastric acid.[34,36]

2. Sweat Iron

Iron excretion in the sweat during exercise has been quantified by several investigators. During exercise, it decreases over time with the highest concentration found in first sweat collection.[37–39] Brune and colleagues (1986) found a similar decrease in the iron content of whole body sweat during rest in a hot environment.[40] They suggested that much of the iron lost in the early sweat was due to contamination from the external environment and cellular debris in the sweat pores.

Whole-body sweat collection is impractical during prolonged exercise. Paulev and colleagues took serial sweat samples over 30 min during running and found the sweat iron concentration decreased from 0.20 mg/l to 0.13 mg/l.[37] Waller and Haymes found the arm sweat iron concentration was significantly lower at 60 min than after 30 min and DeRuisseau et al. (2002) found lower sweat iron concentrations from the arm during the second hour of exercise than the first.[38–39]

The concentration of iron in sweat decreases during exercise in the heat, probably due to the greater volume of sweat produced, however the total amount of iron lost in the sweat is not different between neutral and hot environments.[38] Wheeler et al. (1973) measured daily whole-body dermal iron loss in men with and without 2 h exercise.[41] Mean dermal iron loss was 0.38 mg/d with normal physical activity and 0.32 mg/d with the addition of 2 h exercise. Sweat iron concentration also was lower with exercise (0.13 mg/L) than with habitual physical activity (0.20 mg/L).

3. Urinary Iron Loss

Urinary iron loss is normally quite low even in athletes. Magnusson and colleagues (1984) found iron excreted in the urine to be slightly higher (0.18 mg/d) in elite distance runners than the average daily iron loss.[42] There are reports of loss of hemoglobin and red blood cells in the urine following distance running.[43–44] Known as exercise-induced hematuria, the presence of hemoglobin in the urine may be due to hemolysis of the red blood cells during exercise. Free hemoglobin in the plasma is usually bound by haptoglobin and removed in the liver, but excessive hemolysis may result in elevated plasma hemoglobin and hemoglobin excretion in the urine. Increased hemolysis can occur in the feet during running. Elevated plasma hemoglobin concentrations have been observed following running and cycling, with greater increases found in the runners.[45]

4. Menstrual Blood Loss

Blood loss through the menses averages approximately 30 ml per menstrual cycle or about 0.6 mg iron/d. However, approximately 25% of women with menstrual cycles lose 52 ml/cyle or more (>0.9 mg iron/d).[46] The additional blood lost through the menses places these women at greater risk of depleted iron stores and iron deficiency anemia. Postmenopausal women ages 51–70 have higher serum ferritin concentra-

TABLE 9.1

Prevalence of Low Ferritin, Iron Deficiency, and Iron Deficiency Anemia

Population	Age (Yr)	Sex (%)	Low Ferritin (%)	Iron Deficiency (%)	Iron Deficiency Anemia (%)
Recreational Athletes[18]	18–41	F	29		11
		M	4		2
Athletes[29]	17–53	M	6		10
Marathon Runners[15]	19–43	F	35		
Runners[12]	29±5	F	25		5
	36±8	M	8		6
Runners[13]	21±5	F	30	9	0
Nordic Skiers[17]	21±5	F	20	20	0
	23±4	M	11	0	0
U.S. Adults[1,47]	20–49	F	16*	11	5
	20–49	M	<5*	<1	<1
	50–69	F	<5	5	2
	50–69	M	<5	2	1

* Low Ferritin for age range 31–50 yr

Low Ferritin: Ferritin <12 μg/L; Iron Deficiency: Ferritin <12μg/L, Transferrin Saturation <16% or FEP >100 μg/dL RBC; Iron Deficiency Anemia: Hemoglobin <120 g/L for Females, <130 g/L of Males

tions and are at much lower risk of developing iron deficiency and iron deficiency anemia than are women between ages 31 and 50 (see Table 9.1).[1,47]

Serum ferritin concentrations of highly trained female distance runners who were amenorrheic and eumenorrheic were compared by Deuster et al.[48] (1986). Although no significant differences in serum ferritin were found between the two groups, amenorrheic runners were more likely to be iron depleted (46%) than the eumenorrheic runners (31%). Dietary iron intake was significantly correlated to serum ferritin concentration only among the amenorrheic runners, who also had significantly lower dietary fat intakes. Because low energy intake is associated with changes in lutenizing hormone release from the anterior pituitary and a shorter luteal phase,[49] lower fat intake in the amenorrheic runners may have been due to reduced energy intake.

C. Dietary Iron Intake

Among collegiate and adolescent female athletes iron depletion is most likely due to low dietary iron intake. The RDA for iron is 18 mg/d for women ages 19–50 yrs and 15 mg/d for girls ages 14–18 yr.[1] Most studies of young women athletes report mean daily iron intakes that are less than 18 mg/d, The RDA for males ages >19 yr is 8 mg/d and ages 14–18 yr is 11 mg/d.[1] Studies of food iron intake among male athletes report mean iron intakes that exceed the RDA.

Few studies have reported mean iron intakes that exceed the RDA for iron among female athletes. Elite female cross-country skiers had a mean dietary iron intake of 19.2 mg/d.[50] Highly trained female distance runners were found to have mean iron intakes of 41.9 mg/, but this included both dietary and supplemental iron.[15] Slightly less than 50% of the runners were taking iron supplements. Mean dietary iron intake of runners not taking supplemental iron was less than the RDA. Approximately 35% of the highly trained marathon runners in this study had depleted iron stores. Another study of female marathon runners found mean dietary iron intake of 14 mg/d.[28]

Some individuals who appear to have adequate iron intakes may be consuming foods that contain primarily nonheme iron. The absorption of nonheme iron is much lower (2–8%) than is the absorption of heme iron found only in meat, fish, and poultry. Heme iron absorption in the small intestine is approximately 23%. Two studies of female athletes found that those with low ferritin concentrations consumed diets low in heme iron and bioavailable iron.[13,51] Another study found female runners who had low serum ferritin consumed fewer servings of meat per week than those with normal ferritin concentrations.[14] These studies suggest consuming foods low in heme iron may contribute to the depletion of iron stores.

V. IRON SUPPLEMENTATION

A. Improving Iron Status

Numerous studies have shown that use of supplemental iron improves iron status in active individuals. Iron supplementation is standard treatment for iron deficiency anemia. Studies of active males and females with iron deficiency anemia have found significant increases in hemoglobin concentrations following iron supplementation.[52–53] Some subjects in these two studies were more than 40 years old.

Many studies of iron depleted athletes who received iron supplements found significantly increased serum ferritin concentrations.[54–61] However, only three of these studies found significant increases in hemoglobin concentration.[54,58–59] In all of these studies the female athletes had hemoglobin concentrations that were borderline anemia. Lyle and colleagues (1992) compared groups of college females receiving iron supplements, increased meat intake, or a placebo during aerobic training.[62] Significant increases in hemoglobin and serum ferritin were observed only in the group with increased meat intake. Decreases in hemoglobin and serum ferritin were found in college age females in the placebo group after the 12 week aerobic training program.[62]

Several recent studies also observed significant reductions in sTfR of iron deficient females during aerobic training following iron supplementation.[56,61] Zhu and Haas also found significant increases in serum ferritin and transferrin saturation in the subjects who received 135 mg Fe/d for 6 weeks.[61] Brutsaert and colleagues (2003) examined the effects of iron supplements in a group of iron depleted females aged 18–45 yr.[63] Both serum ferritin and transferrin saturation increased in the supplement group after 6 weeks of supplementation.

B. Performance Enhancement Effects

Celsing and colleagues demonstrated the importance of hemoglobin concentration to aerobic performance by repeatedly removing pints of blood from a group of male athletes in order to decrease hemoglobin below the normal range.[64] Both VO_{2max} and endurance were significantly decreased once the athletes were anemic. Replacement of each athlete's stored red blood cells immediately restored both VO_{2max} and endurance. Iron supplementation in anemic individuals has been found to reduce heart rate during submaximal exercise, but oxygen uptake was not significantly different. After iron treatment there was also a decrease in blood lactate following exercise.[52] Ohira et al. found lower heart rates at the same exercise intensity one week after iron treatment in males with iron deficiency anemia.[53]

Improvements in aerobic performance of iron depleted athletes who are not anemic following iron supplementation have only been observed in a few studies. Lamanca and Haymes found a significant increase in VO_{2max}/kg of body weight and a significant decrease in blood lactate during prolonged exercise after eight weeks of iron supplements.[58] Schoene and colleagues did not find a significant increase in VO_{2max} after supplementation, but post-exercise blood lactate decreased significantly.[59] Yoshida and colleagues found a significant improvement in 3000 m running velocity and the onset of blood lactate accumulation occurred at a higher velocity after iron supplementation.[60] Other studies did not find any significant changes in exercise performance following iron supplementation in iron depleted athletes.

In subjects undergoing aerobic training, the group receiving iron supplements improved their time to complete 10 km and 15 km in a cycling trial.[56] Significant decreases in sTfR and increases in serum ferritin and transferrin saturation were also found in the iron supplemented group. Brutsaert and colleagues found iron supplementation increased knee extensor endurance in women who were iron depleted.[63] Iron supplementation for 6 weeks also increased work efficiency in the iron depleted women.[2] Although not all studies of iron supplementation found improvements in physical performance, those with borderline anemia or tissue iron deficiency (elevated sTfR) were most likely to observe improved performance after iron supplementation.

C. Risk of Iron Overload

In the most recent revision of the recommended dietary allowances for iron the tolerable upper intake for iron was set at 45 mg/d for adults.[1] The most common adverse effects are gastrointestinal problems (e.g., constipation, diarrhea) associated with the use of large doses of iron supplements. Higher levels of iron can also inhibit the absorption of dietary zinc, especially when taking iron supplements.

Because iron is a transition metal it can contribute electrons to produce reactive oxygen species if the iron atoms are not bound to proteins. This is more likely to occur when transferrin saturation and iron stores are elevated. The risk of secondary iron overload is increased when red blood cell transfusions are given over a prolonged time in some forms of anemia.[11]

Hemochromatosis occurs when an excessive amount of iron is stored in the body. Hemochromatosis is classified as primary (hereditary) or secondary. Hereditary hemochromatosis is divided into the following types: HFE hemochromatosis (Type 1); juvenile hemochromatosis (Type 2); transferrin receptor deficiency (Type 3); ferroportin deficiency (Type 4).[11] Inborn and acquired disorders are responsible for the secondary hemochromatosis. Diagnosis of hemochromatosis is based on elevated serum ferritin concentration and transferrin saturation.[11]

VI. DIETARY IRON

A. Food Sources

Meat, fish, and poultry contain both heme and nonheme iron. Breads, cereals, and grain products are good sources of nonheme iron because iron is added to flour in the enrichment process. Some cereals are even fortified, as additional iron has been added in processing. Other sources of nonheme iron include legumes and vegetables.

In the U.S. diet most dietary iron comes from meat, fish, and poultry (35%) and from cereals and grains (33%). Vegetables and fruits contribute 16% of the food iron with lesser amounts provided by legumes and eggs (7%), fats, sweets, and drinks (5%) and milk and dairy products (4%).[65]

B. Iron Bioavailability

Heme iron bioavailability is approximately three times greater than for nonheme iron. The average absorption of heme iron is 23%. Amount of stored iron is the primary factor that affects the heme iron absorption. Individuals with depleted iron stores will have the highest absorption rate of heme iron. Not all of the iron found in meat, fish, and poultry is heme iron. In chicken, beef, and lamb, 50–60% of the iron will be heme iron, while liver, pork, and fish will have 30–40% heme iron.[66]

Bioavailability of nonheme iron is only 2–8% of the food iron. Absorption will be highest when the iron stores are depleted. Meat, fish, and poultry are enhancing factors that increase absorption of nonheme iron when they are present in the same meal. Ascorbic acid (vitamin C) is also an enhancing factor if it is consumed in the same meal with the nonheme iron and will increase its rate of absorption.

There are inhibitors of iron that reduce food iron bioavailability. Phytic acid, present in whole grains, nuts, and legumes reduces the amount of nonheme iron absorbed.[67] Polyphenols like tannic acid and gallic acid, which are found in red wine, tea, and coffee, also decrease the bioavailability of nonheme iron.[68] Calcium will inhibit both heme and nonheme iron absorption when taken in large amounts.[67–68] This would most likely occur when taking calcium supplements with a meal.

VII. CONCLUSIONS

There is evidence of low ferritin concentrations in some middle-aged athletes, particularly females. Premenopausal females are at a greater risk of developing depleted iron stores because of the iron lost through the menses. Use of iron supplements will increase the amount of iron stored in active individuals and are needed when iron deficiency anemia occurs. Iron supplements will improve aerobic performance in anemic individuals and may improve performance when hemoglobin levels are borderline anemia.

REFERENCES

1. Food and Nutrition Board, Institute of Medicine, *Dietary Reference Intakes for Vitamin A, Vitamin K, Arsenic, Boron, Chromium, Copper, Iodine, Iron, Manganese, Molybdenum, Nickel, Silicon, Vanadium and Zinc*, National Academy Press, Washington, DC, 2001.
2. Haas, J. D., The effects of iron deficiency on physical performance, in *Military Requirements for Military Personnel: Levels Needed for Cognitive and Physical Performance During Garrison Training*, Committee on Mineral Requirements for Cognitive and Physical Performance of Military Personnel, Food and Nutrition Board, National Academy Press, Washington, DC, 2006, 451–61.
3. Ganz, T., Hepcidin—a regulator of intestinal iron absorption and iron recycling by macrophages, *Best Practices & Res. Clinical Haem.* 18, 171–82, 2005.
4. Donovan, A., Roy, C. N., and Andrews, N. C., The ins and outs of iron homeostasis, *Physiology* 21, 115–23, 2006.
5. Green, R., Charlton, R., Seftel, H., Bothwell, T., Mayet, F., Adams, B., and Finch, C., Body iron excretion in man, *Am. J. Med.*, 45, 336–53, 1968.
6. Jacob, R. A., Sandstead, H. H., Munoz, J. M., Klevay, L. M., and Milne, D. B. Whole body surface loss of trace metals in normal males, *Am. J. Clin. Nutr.,* 34, 1379–82, 1981.
7. Hallberg, L. and Rossander-Hulten, L., Iron requirements in menstruating women, *Am. J. Clin. Nutr.* 54, 1047–58, 1991.
8. Expert Scientific Writing Group, Summary of a report on assessment of the iron nutritional status of the United States population, *Am. J. Clin. Nutr.* 42, 1318–30, 1985.
9. Cook, J. D., Skikne, B. S., Lynch, S. R., and Reusser, M. F. Estimates of iron sufficiency in the U. S. population, *Blood* 88, 726–31, 1986.
10. Cook, J. D., Flowers, C. H., and Skikne, B. S., The quantitative assessment of body iron, *Blood* 101, 3359–64, 2003.
11. Beutler, E., Hoffbrand, A. V., and Cook, J. D. Iron deficiency and overload. *Hematology Am. Soc. Hematol. Educ. Program*, 2003, 40–61.
12. Balaban, E. P., Cox, J. V., Snell, P., Vaughn, R. H., and Frenkel, E. P. The frequency of anemia and iron deficiency in the runner. *Med. Sci. Sports Exer.* 21, 643–8, 1989.
13. Haymes, E. M. and Spillman, D. M. Iron status of women distance runners. *Int. J. Sports Med.* 10, 430–3, 1989.
14. Pate, R. R., Miller, B. J., Davis, J. M., Slentz, C. A., and Klingshirn, L. A. Iron status of female runners, *Int. J. Sport Nutr.* 3, 222–31, 1993.
15. Deuster, P. A., Kyle, S. B., Moser, P. B., Vigersky, R. A., Singh, A., and Schoonmaker, E. B., Nutritional survey of highly trained women runners, *Am. J. Clin. Nutr.*, 45, 954–62, 1986.
16. Clement, D. B., Lloyd-Smith, D. R., MacIntyre, J. G., Matheson, G. O., Brock, R., and DuPont, M. Iron status of highly trained women runners, *J. Sports Sci.,* 5, 261–71, 1987.
17. Haymes, E. M., Puhl, J. L., and Temples, T. E. Training for cross-country skiing and iron status. *Med. Sci. Sports Exer.* 18, 162–7, 1986.
18. Sinclair, L. M. and Hinton, P. S., Prevalence of iron deficiency with and without anemia in recreationally active men and women, *J. Am. Diet. Assoc.* 105, 975–8, 2005.
19. Hunding, A., Jordal, R., and Paulev, P.-E., Runner's anemia and iron deficiency, *Acta Med. Scand.* 209, 315–8, 1981.

20. Dallongeville, J., Ledoux, M., and Brisson, G., Iron deficiency among active men, *J. Am. Coll. Nutr.* 8, 195–202, 1989
21. Murray-Kolb, L. E., Beard, J. L., Joseph, L. J., Davey, S. L.,Evans, W. J., and Campbell, W. W., Resistance training affects iron status in older men and women, *Int. J. Sport Nutr. Exer. Metab.* 11, 287–98, 2001.
22. Campbell, W. W., Beard, J. L., Joseph, L. J., Davey, S. L., and Evans, W. J., Chromium picolinate supplementation and resistive training by older men: Effects on iron status and hematologic indexes, *Am. J. Clin. Nutr.* 66, 944–9, 1997.
23. Lukaski, H. C., Bolonchuk, W. W., Siders, W. A., and Milne, D. B., Chromium supplementation and resistance training: Effects on body composition, strength, and trace element status of men, *Am. J. Clin. Nutr.* 63, 954–65, 1996.
24. Schobersberger, W., Tschann, M., Hasibeder, W., Steidl, M.,Herold, M., Nachnauer, H., and Koller, A. Consequences of 6 weeks of strength training on red cell O_2 transport and iron status, *Eur. J. Appl. Physiol.* 60, 163–8, 1990.
25. DeRuisseau, K. C., Roberts, L. M., Kushnick, M. P., Evans, A. M., Austin, K., and Haymes, E. M., Iron status of young males and females performing weight-training exercise, *Med. Sci. Sports Exer.* 36, 241–8, 2004.
26. Blum, S. M., Sherman, A. R., and Boileau, R. A., The effects of fitness-type exercise on iron status in adult women, *Am. J. Clin. Nutr.* 43, 456–63, 1986.
27. Pratt, C. A., Woo, V., and Chrisley, B. The effects of exercise on iron status and aerobic capacity in moderately exercising adult women, *Nutr. Res.* 16, 23–32, 1996.
28. Lampe, J. W., Slavin, J. L., and Apple, F. S., Poor iron status of women runners training for a marathon, *Int. J. Sports Med.* 7, 111–4, 1986.
29. Taylor, C., Rogers, G., Goodman, C., Baynes, R. D., Bothwell, T. H., Bezwoda, W. R. et al., Hematologic, iron-related, and acute phase protein responses to sustained strenuous exercise, *J. Appl. Physiol.* 62, 464–9, 1987.
30. Fallon, K. E., Slvyer, G., Slvyer K., and Dare, A., Changes in haematological parameters and iron metabolism associated with a 1600 kilometre ultramarathon, *Br. J. Sports Med.* 33, 27–31, 1999.
31. Nemeth, E., Rivera, S., Gabayan, V., Keller, C.,Taudorf, S., Pedersen, B. K., and Ganz, T., IL-6 mediates hypoferremia of inflammation by inducing the synthesis of the iron regulatory hormone hepcidin, *J. Clin. Invest.*,113, 1271–6. 2004.
32. Roecker, L., Meier-Buttermilch, R., Brechtel, L., Nemeth, E., and Ganz, T., Iron-regulatory protein hepcidin is increased in female athletes after a marathon, *Eur. J. Appl. Physiol.* 95, 569–71, 2005.
33. Lampe, J. W., Slavin, J. L., and Apple, F. S., Iron status of active women and the effect of running a marathon on bowel function and gastrointestinal blood loss, *Int. J. Sports Med.* 12, 173–9, 1991.
34. Robertson, J. D., Maughan, R. J., and Davidson, R. J. L., Faecal blood loss in response to exercise, *Br. Med. J.* 295, 303–5, 1987.
35. Stewart, J. G., Ahlquist, D. A., McGill, D. B., Ilstrup, D. M., Schwartz, S., and Owen, R. A., Gastrointestinal blood loss and anemia in runners, *Ann. Int. Med.,* 100, 843–5, 1984.
36. Cooper, B. T., Douglas, S. A., Firth, L. A., Hannagan, J. A., and Chadwick, V. S., Erosive gastritis and gastrointestinal bleeding in a female runner: Prevention of the bleeding and healing of the of the gastritis with H2-receptor antagonists, *Gastroenterology*, 92, 2019–23, 1987.
37. Paulev, P. E., Jordal, R., and Pedersen, N. S., Dermal excretion of iron in intensely training athletes, *Clin. Chim. Acta* 127, 19–27, 1983.
38. Waller, M. F. and Haymes, E. M. The effects of heat and exercise on sweat iron loss, *Med. Sci. Sports Exer.* 28, 197–203, 1996.

39. DeRuisseau, K. C., Cheuvront, S. N., Haymes, E. M., and Sharp, R. G., Sweat iron and zinc losses during prolonged exercise, *Int. J. Sport Nutr. Exer. Metab.* 12, 428–37, 2002.
40. Brune, M. D., Magnusson, B., Persson, H., and Hallberg, L., Iron losses in sweat, *Am. J. Clin. Nutr.* 43, 438–43, 1986.
41. Wheeler, E. F., El-Neil, H., Willson, J. O. C., and Weiner, J. S., The effect of work level and dietary intake on water balance and the excretion of sodium, potassium and iron in a hot climate. *Br. J. Nutr.* 30, 127–37, 1973.
42. Magnusson, B., Hallberg, L., Rossander, L., and Swolin. B., Iron metabolism and "sports anemia. " I. A study of several iron parameters in elite runners with differences in iron status, *Acta Med. Scand.,* 216, 149–55, 1984.
43. Boileau, M., Fuchs, E., Barry, J. M., and Hodges, C. V., Stress hematuria: Athletic pseudonephritis in marathoners, *Urology*, 15, 471–4, 1980.
44. Siegal, A. J., Hennekens, C. H., Solomon, H. S., and Van Boekel, B. Exercise-related hematuria: Findings in a group of marathon runners, *JAMA*, 241, 391–2, 1979.
45. Telford, R. D., Sly, G. J., Hahn, A. G., Cunningham, R. B., Bryant, C., and Smith, J. A., Footstrike is the major cause of hemolysis during running, *J. Appl. Physiol.*, 94, 38–42, 2003.
46. Hallberg, L., Hogdahl, A. M., Nilsson, L., and Rybo, G., Menstrual blood loss and iron deficiency, *Acta Med. Scand.*, 180, 639–50, 1966.
47. Looker, A. C., Dallman, P. R., Carroll, M. D., Gunter, E. W., and Johnson, C. W., Prevalence of iron deficiency in the United States, *JAMA*, 277, 973–6, 1997.
48. Deuster, P. A., Kyle, S. B., Moser, P. B., Vigersky, R. A., Singh, A., and Schoonmaker, E. B., Nutritional intakes and status of highly trained amenorrheic and eumenorrheic women runners, *Fert. Steril.* 46, 636–43, 1986.
49. Loucks, A. B., Energy availability, not body fatness, regulates reproductive function in women, *Exer. Sport Sci. Rev.* 31, 144–8, 2003.
50. Ellsworth, N. B., Hewitt, H. F., and Haskell, W. L., Nutrient intake of elite male and female Nordic skiers, *Phys. Sportsmed.* 13, 78–92, 1985.
51. Snyder, A. C., Dvorak, L. L., and Roepke, J. B., Influence of dietary iron sources on measures of iron status among female runners, *Med. Sci. Sports Exer.*, 21, 7–10, 1989.
52. Gardner, G. W., Edgerton, V. R., Barnard, R. J., and Bernauer, E. M., Cardiorespiratory, hematological and physical performance responses of anemic subjects to iron treatment, *Am. J. Clin. Nutr*. 28, 983–8, 1975.
53. Ohira, Y., Edgerton, V. R., Gardner, G. W., Gunawardena, K. A., Senewiratne, B., and Ikawa, S., Work capacity after iron treatment as a function of hemoglobin and iron deficiency, *J. Nutr. Sci. Vitaminol.* 27, 87–96, 1981.
54. Clement, D. B., Taunton, J. E., McKenzie, D. C, Sawchuk, L. L., and Wiley, J. P., High- and low-dosage iron supplementation in iron deficient, endurance trained females, in *Sport, Health and Nutrition*, Katch, F. I., Ed., Human Kinetics, Champaign, IL, 1986, 75–81.
55. Fogelholm, M., Jaakkola, L., and Lammpisjarvi, T., Effects of iron supplementation in female athletes with low serum ferritin concentration, *Int. J. Sports Med.* 13, 158–62, 1992.
56. Hinton, P. S., Giordana, C., Brownlie, T., and Haas, J. D., Iron supplementation improves endurance after training in iron-depleted, nonanemic women, *J. Appl. Physiol.* 88, 1103–11, 2000.
57. Klingshirn, L. A., Pate, R. R., Bourque, S. P., Davis, J. M., and Sargent, R. G., Effect of iron supplementation on endurance capacity in iron-depleted female runners, *Med. Sci. Sports Exer*. 24, 819–24, 1992.
58. Lamanca, J. J. and Haymes, E. M., Effects of iron repletion on VO_{2max}, endurance and blood lactate, *Med. Sci. Sports Exer*. 25, 1386–92, 1993.

59. Schoene, R. B., Escourrous, P., Robertson, H. T., Nilson, K. L., Parsons, J. R., and Smith, N. J., Iron repletion decreases maximal exercise lactate concentration in female athletes with minimal iron-deficiency anemia, *J. Lab. Clin. Med.* 102, 306–12, 1983.
60. Yoshida, T., Udo, M., Chida, M., Ichioka, M., and Makiguchi, K., Dietary iron supplement during severe physical training in competitive female distance runners, *Sports Training, Med. Rehab.*,1, 279–85, 1990.
61. Zhu, Y. I. and Haas, J. D., Response of serum transferrin receptor to iron supplementation in iron-depleted, nonanemic women, *Am. J. Clin. Nutr.* 67, 271–5, 1998.
62. Lyle, R. M., Weaver, C. M., Sedlock, D. A., Rajaram, S., Martin, B., and Melby, C. L., Iron status in exercising women: The effect of oral iron therapy vs. increased consumption of muscle foods, *Am. J. Clin. Nutr.* 56, 1649–55, 1992.
63. Brutsaert, T. D., Hernandez-Cordero, S., Rivera, J., Viola, T., Hughes, G., and Haas, J. D., Iron supplementation improves progressive fatigue resistance during dynamic knee extensor exercise in iron-depleted, nonanemic women, *Am. J. Clin. Nutr.* 77, 441–8, 2003.
64. Celsing, F., Blomstrand, E., Werner, B., Pihlstedt, P., and Ekblom, B., Effects of iron deficiency on endurance and muscle enzyme activity in man, *Med. Sci. Sports Exer.* 18, 156–61, 1986.
65. National Research Council, Committee on Diet and Health, *Diet and Health: Implications for Reducing Chronic Disease Risk*, National Academy Press, Washington, DC, 1989, 70–74.
66. Monsen, E. R., Hallberg, L., Layrisse, M., Hegsted, D. M., Cook, J. D., Mertz, W., and Finch, C. A., Estimation of available dietary iron, *Am. J. Clin. Nutr.* 31, 134–41, 1978.
67. Hunt, J. R., Bioavailability of iron, zinc, and copper as influenced by host and dietary factors, in *Mineral Requirement for Military Personnel: Levels Needed for Cognitive and Physical Performance During Garrison Training*, Committee on Mineral Requirements for Cognitive and Physical Performance of Military Personnel, Food and Nutrition Board, National Academy Press, Washington, DC, 2006, 265–77.
68. Hallberg, L. and Hulthen, L., Prediction of iron absorption: An algorithm for calculating absorption and bioavailability of dietary iron, *Am. J. Clin. Nutr.* 71, 1147–60, 2000.

10 Trace Elements Excluding Iron—Chromium and Zinc

Henry C. Lukaski and Angus G. Scrimgeour

CONTENTS

I. INTRODUCTION

The mounting public awareness of the increased risk of chronic disease associated with physical inactivity and nutritionally imbalanced diets is leading many

Americans to adopt healthful behaviors. Recommendations by public health organizations in the form of the Dietary Guidelines for Americans are available.[1] Middle-aged (30–60 yr) adults are accepting the advice to boost participation in physical activity with the participation increasing, albeit modestly, from 55% to more than 61% in the past 5 years.[2] Although considerable information exists about the health benefits of regular exercise in middle-aged adults,[3] little information is available indicating the impact of micronutrients consumed in less than recommended amounts or large amounts on physiological function or performance during regular aerobic or resistance activities.

Chromium and zinc are two minerals that are limited in the diets of middle-aged adults. National nutritional surveys estimate that 20% to 36% of middle-aged men and women fail to consume the recommended intake of zinc.[4] Similarly, chromium intakes are considered to be low because contemporary food processing depletes chromium.[5]

Although the public press touts chromium for its supportive role in protein, carbohydrate, and lipid metabolism, the benefits of supplemental chromium in response to exercise training are controversial.[6] Accumulating evidence supports the importance of adequate amounts of dietary zinc in promoting physiological function during exercise.[7] An argument for supplementation of physically active people with chromium and zinc is based on findings of substantially increased urinary losses of these minerals after strenuous physical exercise.[8] This chapter critically evaluates the roles of chromium and zinc in support of optimal physiological function in response to physical activity in middle-aged adults; it examines the effects of supplementation with chromium or zinc on various measures of performance and body composition in response to training; concludes with a consensus opinion on the value of chromium or zinc supplementation on exercise-related outcomes in middle-aged adults, and highlights recommendations for further research.

II. CHROMIUM

Chromium (Cr) exists in nature in many oxidation states ranging from Cr^{-2} to Cr^{+6}; the predominant forms are Cr^{+3} (trivalent) and Cr^{+6} (hexavalent). Trivalent chromium is nutritionally active and found in food, whereas hexavalent chromium is a toxic form that is produced during industrial processes.[9] Chromium is a putatively essential mineral that can play a role in carbohydrate and lipid metabolism;[5] it potentiates insulin binding to insulin-sensitive cells and facilitates gene expression.[6,10]

A. Chromium Homeostasis

1. Dietary Chromium

Chromium is widely distributed in the food supply but most foods contain only very small amounts (1–2 μg per serving). Good sources of chromium include whole-grain products, some fruits (grapes and bananas) and vegetables (broccoli and potatoes), meat (beef), and some spices (garlic and basil).[11] In contrast, foods high in simple sugars, such as sucrose and fructose, are low in chromium content.[12] Estimation of dietary chromium intake is problematic because of the high variability in reported chromium content of foods due to agricultural and processing practices.[9]

The lack of reliable data on the chromium content of foods and the paucity of controlled feeding studies in human contribute to the lack of a Recommended Dietary Allowance for chromium.[13] However, an Adequate Intake, which indicates the amount that healthy people typically consume, for chromium has been established at 35 μg and 25 μg for men and women, respectively.[13]

2. Absorption

Absorption of chromium from the intestines is low, with estimates ranging from 0.4% to 2.5% of the amount ingested, with the remainder excreted in feces.[14–17] Food components, such as vitamin C in fruits and vegetables and niacin in meats, poultry, fish, and grain products enhance the absorption of chromium.[18] Absorbed chromium is stored in the liver, spleen, soft tissues, and bone.[19] However, diets high in simple sugars (more than 35% of energy intake) increase urinary excretion of chromium.[12]

Inorganic (chloride) and organic (nicotinate, picolinate, and a histidine complex) compounds of trivalent chromium are available. However, the predominant chemical form promoted to enhance biological function, including performance enhancement and weight reduction is chromium picolinate because of its increased bioavailability compared with other trivalent chromium compounds.[20,21]

3. Factors Mediating Body Chromium

In addition to diet, other factors may contribute to depletion of chromium content of the body. Physiological states such as pregnancy and lactation increase chromium losses.[22] Acute strenuous exercise, infection, and physical trauma markedly increase chromium losses, principally in the urine, and can lead to chromium deficiency, especially when chromium intakes are low.[22,23] Aging also may reduce chromium in the body, as shown by decreased concentrations of chromium in the blood, hair, and sweat of older compared with younger adults.[13]

4. Assessment of Chromium Nutritional Status

Accurate and sensitive biochemical indicators of human chromium nutriture are lacking. Plasma or serum chromium concentrations do not reflect tissue chromium levels.[20,21] Serum chromium responds to chromium supplementation,[23,24] but does not correlate with functional biomarkers of chromium action *in vivo* such as serum glucose or insulin in the fasting state or after glucose load.[25] Similarly, urinary chromium concentration and output are responsive to chromium supplementation but are inadequate indicators of chromium status because they fail to correlate with glucose, insulin, or lipid concentrations.[25] Thus, assessment of chromium nutritional status remains elusive.

B. Chromium as an Ergogenic Aid in Middle-Aged Adults

Findings of marked increases in fat-free mass and concomitant decreases in fat in livestock supplemented with chromium picolinate (≥200 μg chromium) provided an incentive to determine the ergogenic effects and body composition changes of young adults during physical training.[9] Although preliminary findings in young adults suggested that chromium picolinate supplementation combined with physical training resulted in a gain in fat-free mass and loss of fat, subsequent studies did not confirm these initial results.[26] Differences in physical training modes, doses of chromium picolinate, failure to assess dietary chromium intake, methods of assessment of outcomes, and initial fitness levels of the subjects may have contributed to the inconsistent results.[24]

Studies in middle-aged and older adults, in whom impairments of glucose and insulin metabolism might be more prevalent than in younger and healthier adults, also have examined the effects of chromium picolinate supplementation. The goals of these studies were to ascertain whether supplemental chromium with or without regular physical activity affects body composition, physical performance, and some aspects of metabolism.

1. Chromium Supplementation and Body Composition

Excess body weight is associated with increased circulating insulin concentrations that are directly related to body fat content. The proposed link between trivalent chromium and facilitation of insulin action motivated investigators to determine the effects of supplemental chromium on weight loss and maintenance with an emphasis on reduction of body fat and preservation of lean body mass in a variety of experimental plans. In the studies with older adults, the amount of supplemental chromium far exceeded the dose of 200 μg/d used in the studies with young adults.[24] The investigators apparently reasoned that weight loss increased chromium needs to ameliorate any deficits in insulin utilization associated with excess adipose tissue.

Studies to determine the effects of supplemental chromium on weight loss have yielded contradictory results. Forty-four obese middle-aged women were matched by body mass index then randomized to receive either 400 μg chromium as chromium picolinate daily or placebo for 12 wk.[27] All women participated in an exercise component of the weight loss program, including 30 min of resistance training and 30 min of moderate-intensity walking daily, 2 d/wk. Only 20 women supplemented with chromium and 17 women receiving placebo completed the study. Neither body composition, determined by using underwater weighing, nor sum of the circumferences of the waist and hips, were affected by chromium supplementation compared with placebo. Plasma chromium concentration and urinary chromium excretion increased significantly only in the women supplemented with chromium. Muscular strength increased significantly regardless of treatment.

Two additional studies failed to provide reasonable evidence of a beneficial effect of chromium during weight loss. One hundred fifty-four obese middle-aged adults participated in a randomized, double-blind, placebo-controlled trial to determine the effects of chromium picolinate supplements on the composition of weight lost.[28] Volunteers received 200 or 400 μg of chromium daily or placebo for 72 d. Supplemental chromium was provided in a proprietary drink containing protein and carbohydrate. Volunteers were asked to consume at least two servings daily, but there was no control of the volume of the drink, and hence chromium intake, consumed by a subject. No instruction regarding dietary practices or physical activity was provided to the participants. Body composition was determined by using underwater weighing before and after treatment. Compared with the placebo group, significant decreases in body weight, fat weight, and body fatness were found for the chromium supplementation groups with no differential effect of chromium dose on these variables. Treatment did not significantly affect lean body mass. These findings are problematic because of the use of a body composition improvement index that accounts for fat loss (positive effect) and reduction of lean body mass (negative effect) that occurred during the trial. The investigators concluded that chromium supplementation facilitated significantly more positive changes in body composition compared with the results from the placebo. No effect of chromium level (200 vs. 400 μg/d) was found on the body composition improvement index.

In a second study, 122 obese middle-aged adults were randomized to receive a capsule containing either 400 μg of chromium (chromium picolinate) daily or placebo and participate in an exercise program for 90 d.[29] Subjects self-reported daily caloric intake and energy expenditure to fitness instructors. Although body fat, assessed with dual x-ray absorptiometry, decreased in both groups, the loss of fat was significantly greater in adults supplemented with chromium. Both treatment groups had non-significant loss of lean body weight. The investigators further adjusted the body composition data by calculating additional changes in fat weight on the basis that 3500 kcal energy expenditure reflected a 1 lb loss of body fat. After controlling for self-reported differences in energy intake and output, the subjects supplemented with chromium, as compared with the placebo group, lost significantly more weight (7.8 vs. 1.8 kg) and fat weight (7.7 vs. 1.5 kg) without loss of lean body mass.

Interpretation of the data from these studies[28,29] is confounded by some key concerns. Use of the body composition improvement index from self-reported energy expenditure rather than actual assessments of body composition is suspicious. Also, the lack of control and estimation of chromium intake and assessment of energy intake and expenditure restrict the interpretation of the findings. Similarly, calculation of loss of fat based on 3500-kcal energy expenditure associated with physical activity fails to acknowledge homeostatic adaptation in energy metabolism and produces uncertain conclusions. Therefore, conclusions from these results should be viewed with caution.

A double-blind, placebo-controlled pilot study evaluated the effects of trivalent chromium-bound niacin on weight loss and its composition in obese women.[30] Twenty African-American women were randomized to two groups that received either a total of 600 μg of chromium daily or placebo in a repeated measures, crossover designed trial. One group began with 200 μg/d of chromium supplementation administered three times daily (total supplemental chromium 600 μg/d) for 2 months, then a 1 month washout, followed by 2 months of placebo. Concurrently, the other group received placebo first then the chromium supplement. In the group treated with placebo first, body fat weight, assessed with bioelectrical impedance, decreased significantly more and lean body weight decreased significantly less with the chromium-bound niacin compared with placebo. In contrast, the group supplemented first with chromium lost significantly more fat weight and less lean body weight during the placebo compared with chromium supplementation. These findings suggest that although chromium-bound niacin had beneficial effects on fat loss and preservation of lean body weight when provided initially, placebo also was effective for weight loss. Because the rate of initial weight loss was independent of chromium supplementation, one can conclude that the effects were the result of a sequence effect.

Chromium also has been used in conjunction with other dietary components to augment weight loss. Thirty-three obese women who completed a 2-wk very low-calorie diet were randomized to receive a supplement containing chromium picolinate (200 μg), fiber (20 g), carbohydrate (50 g), and caffeine (100 mg), or placebo for 16 months.[31] The amount and course of the weight regain was similar between the groups with no differences in change in body composition by treatment. These results indicate that chromium, as a component of a multifactor supplement, was not useful in maintaining weight loss in weight-reduced adults.

The effect of different chromium-containing organic compounds has been evaluated in conjunction with exercise training in obese middle-aged adults. Grant et al.[32] studied 43 obese women who participated in a cross-training exercise program including step aerobics, cycling, and resistance training for 9 wk. They were randomly assigned to one of four treatment groups: chromium picolinate without exercise, exercise training supplemented with chromium picolinate, exercise training with placebo, and exercise training with chromium nicotinate. Chromium supplements, each containing 200 μg, were consumed as two capsules daily for a total chromium intake of 400 μg/d. Body weight increased significantly only in the nonexercising women supplemented with chromium picolinate. Thus, chromium picolinate supplementation was not effective in reducing body weight, positively affecting body composition assessed by using underwater weighing, nor on fasting glucose or insulin concentrations. However, in response to an oral glucose tolerance test, the area under the insulin curve was significantly reduced only in the women treated with chromium nicotinate and exercise. These findings suggest that chromium as nicotinate, not picolinate, may be beneficial in risk factor modification in obese adults.

Attempts to demonstrate the benefit of chromium on weight maintenance have not been successful. Twenty-one obese patients who successfully completed an 8-wk very low-calorie diet were supplemented with 200 μg of chromium daily either as chromium picolinate or chromium-enhanced yeast daily, or placebo for an 18-wk weight maintenance period.[33] Although body weight and body fatness, estimated from skinfold thicknesses, were not influenced by treatment, lean body mass significantly increased in the group supplemented with chromium picolinate compared with the other treatments. This finding suggests that chromium picolinate, but not chromium-enhanced yeast, promotes muscle retention, and may enhance muscle accretion during weight maintenance after weight loss.

Differences in experimental designs, including the dose and chemical form of chromium and lack of assessment of energy intake, complicate any interpretation of these findings. A recent study, however, has overcome many of these limitations and provides a clearer view of the effects of chromium supplementation on body weight and composition.[34] Eighty-three middle-aged women were matched by body mass index and randomized in a double-blind study to receive one of three treatment groups: chromium picolinate (200 μg), picolinic acid in an amount equivalent to the dose in the matched chromium picolinate, and placebo. After assessment of individual energy needs, the women consumed only food and beverages provided for 12 wk. The study tested the hypothesis that supplemental chromium promotes weight loss and selective loss of fat and gain of lean body mass when energy intake was constant. Body weight was maintained within 2% of admission values. Body composition, determined at admission and 12 wk by using dual x-ray absorptiometry, did not change significantly. Another outcome measure was frequency of increases in food (energy) intake needed to maintain body weight. Daily caloric intervention (increases) were needed statistically more in the placebo (48%) than in the chromium picolinate (20%) and picolinic acid (15%) groups. Thus, under conditions of constant energy intake, supplemental chromium (200 μg) affected neither body weight nor composition.

2. Compositional and Functional Effects in Older Adults

Advancing age has been associated with significant decreases in muscle mass and impairments in ambulatory function as well as decreased insulin sensitivity. Because of its putative role in anabolism as a potentiator of insulin action,[35] chromium supplementation independently and in conjunction with weight training has been hypothesized to increase muscle mass in the elderly.

Nineteen middle-aged and older healthy men and women were randomly assigned in a double-blind study and received either 1000 μg chromium as chromium picolinate or placebo for 8 wk.[36] Serum chromium concentrations increased significantly with supplementation. Body composition and insulin sensitivity were unchanged in both groups. Thus, chromium picolinate neither changed body composition nor improved insulin sensitivity in healthy older men and women.

The interaction of supplemental chromium and resistance training on body composition and strength gain has been determined. Eighteen healthy middle-aged men were randomly assigned (double-blind) to groups that consumed either 924 μg chromium as chromium picolinate or placebo daily for 13 wk while participating in a supervised resistance training program.[37] For 5-d sequences during each 3-wk testing period, the men consumed controlled diets designed to maintain constant chromium intake (~60 and ~100 μg chromium daily in a 2-d rotating menu). Lean body mass, muscle mass, and rates of strength gain increased independently of chromium supplementation.

A similar study was conducted in middle-aged women.[38] Seventeen sedentary women were randomized to groups that received either 924 μg chromium as chromium picolinate or placebo daily for 13 wk and participated in a supervised resistance training program. Resistance training significantly increased muscle strength of the muscle groups trained; these responses were not affected by chromium picolinate supplementation. Fat-free mass and body fatness were not changed by resistance training in the weight-stable women regardless of chromium supplementation.

3. Conundrum of Chromium

Lack of evidence describing the importance of supplemental chromium in promoting changes in body weight and composition raises question about the biological role of chromium on energy balance. If trivalent chromium potentiates insulin action,[5,35] it should stimulate anabolism. Thus, chromium should up-regulate protein synthesis and promote gain of muscle and lean body mass when energy balance is neutral or positive. However, the mechanism by which supplemental chromium is hypothesized to promote weight loss while decreasing fat and concomitantly increasing muscle or fat-free mass[39] is unknown and contradicts the anabolic function of chromium as a facilitator of insulin action. Thus, acceptance of the findings of decreased body weight and selective fat loss with supplemental chromium should be viewed guardedly until appropriately designed human trials have been undertaken and the results critically reviewed.

III. ZINC

Zinc is a transition element that forms stable complexes with side chains of proteins and nucleotides with a specific affinity for thiol and hydroxy groups and ligands containing nitrogen.[40] The zinc ion acts as a good electron acceptor, but does not participate in direct oxidation–reduction reactions. These characteristics explain the diverse biological functions of zinc in the regulation of body metabolism, which is bolstered by the requirement for zinc in more than 200 enzymes in various species.[41]

Zinc has several recognized functions in zinc-metalloenzymes including catalytic, structural, and regulatory roles.[42] Catalytic function specifies that zinc participates directly in facilitating the action of the enzyme. If the zinc is removed by chelates or other agents, the enzyme becomes inactive. Carbonic anhydrase is an enzyme in which zinc plays a catalytic role.[43]

In a structural role, zinc atoms are required to stabilize the tertiary structures of the enzyme protein and to maintain the integrity of the complex enzyme molecules, but it does not impact enzyme activity. Zinc plays a structural role in the enzymes superoxide dismutase and protein kinase c.[41]

The importance of zinc in biological systems is reflected by the various functions and activities on which zinc exerts a regulatory role.[40] Zinc is needed for macronutrient metabolism, and is required for nucleic acid and protein metabolism and, hence, cell differentiation and replication. Similarly, zinc is vital for glucose utilization, the secretion of insulin, and lipid metabolism. Zinc is also required for the production, storage, and secretion of individual hormones including growth and thyroid hormones, gonadotrophins and sex hormones, prolactin, and corticosteroids. Zinc status regulates the effectiveness of the interaction of some hormones at receptor sites and end-organ responsiveness.

Integrated biological systems also require zinc for optimal function. Adequate zinc intake is necessary for proper taste perception, reproduction, immuno-competence, skin integrity, wound healing, skeletal development, brain development, behavior, vision, and gastrointestinal function in humans.[13] Zinc, therefore, is a nutrient that regulates many physiological and psychological functions and is required in adequate amounts to promote human health and well-being.

A. Zinc in the Human Body

Zinc is an intracellular cation that is present in all organs, tissues, fluids, and secretions of the body. It is associated with all organelles of the cell but only 60% to 80% of cellular zinc is localized in the cytosol; the remainder is bound to membranes, which may be important in defining the effects of zinc deficiency on cellular function. The concentration of zinc in extracellular fluids is very low, with plasma zinc concentration only 65 nmol/L. If the body plasma concentration is 45 mL/kg body weight, then a 70-kg man has about 3 L of plasma, which contains 3 mg of zinc, or about 0.1% of the body zinc content.

The zinc concentration in various organs and tissues of the body is variable.[44] Although the concentration of zinc in skeletal muscle is not large, the substantial mass of skeletal muscle makes it the principal reservoir of zinc in the body. Bone and skeletal muscle account for almost 90% of the body zinc content.

The zinc concentration of muscles varies with their metabolic functions. The highest zinc concentrations are found in skeletal muscles that are highly oxidative, with a large proportion of slow-twitch fibers.[45] Rat soleus muscle, composed of 63% slow-twitch fibers, contains about 300 μg zinc per gram dry weight. Conversely, the extensor digitorum longus, which is primarily a fast-twitch glycolytic muscle, has only 100 μg of zinc per gram dry weight.[46] Dietary restriction of zinc generally does not significantly reduce the zinc concentration in skeletal muscles, except for small decreases (~5%) in the soleus. The size and number of various types of muscle fibers, however, may be reduced and their relative distribution altered in a muscle, with a characteristic decrease of the slow-twitch oxidative and an increase in the fast-twitch glycolytic fibers.[45,46] Thus, skeletal muscle, at least on a tissue level, is relatively unresponsive to changes in dietary zinc.

Because the concentration of zinc in bone is quite large relative to other body tissues and organs, and the amount of bone is substantial, the skeleton is the major depot of zinc. Restricted zinc intake adversely affects zinc concentration of bone, particularly in young, growing animals and to a lesser extent in older animals.[47] Bone zinc concentration is more responsive to dietary zinc level than other tissues, and it may better reflect the gradual decline in overall zinc status of the body compared with plasma zinc concentration, even in older animals.[47]

B. Zinc Homeostasis

1. Absorption

The amount of zinc in the body represents a dynamic balance between the zinc intake and losses.[40] Zinc is absorbed throughout the gastrointestinal tract, with highest rate of absorption in the jejunum and duodenum and only negligible amounts absorbed in the stomach and the large intestine. After a meal, the quantities of zinc in the intestines is the sum of zinc from food and beverages, and the zinc-containing endogenous secretions from the pancreas, gall bladder, and stomach that aid in digestion and cellular zinc flux into the gut.[47] Post-prandially, the amount of zinc in the lumen of the small intestine exceeds the quantity of zinc ingested because of endogenous secretions.

During digestion, secreted enzymes release zinc from food and endogenously secreted proteins. The free zinc can form coordination complexes with various exogenous and endogenous ligands, such as amino acids, organic acids, and phosphates. The amino acids histidine and cysteine have a high affinity for zinc, and are very efficiently absorbed, more so than zinc sulfate.[48] Other compounds such as iron and phytate, found in the intestine after a meal, can compete with zinc for mucosal binding sites or form insoluble complexes that inhibit zinc absorption.[49]

After a meal, zinc absorption follows the concentration gradient from the intestinal lumen to mucosal cells. Kinetic measurements indicate that the mucosal cell affinity for zinc uptake has a wide range, with highest rate under conditions of low zinc intake, which suggests an up-regulation of zinc transport when consumption is less than meets physiological needs.[40] Zinc uptake in the small intestine has saturable or active transport and passive components. Albumin is the major protein in the blood to transport zinc from the intestines to the liver. Evidence of an effect of acute or chronic physical activity on zinc absorption and homeostasis is not available.

Functional evidence reveals that at least 24 specific transporters are responsible for either zinc influx or efflux in mammalian cells. These transporters are designated as two gene families: the ZnT proteins and the Zip family.[50] ZnT transporters reduce intracellular zinc availability by promoting zinc efflux from cells, whereas Zip transporters increase intracellular zinc availability by promoting extracellular uptake of zinc. Evidence shows that human ZnT and ZIP genes exhibit either up-regulation or down-regulation in response to zinc intake and probably contribute to homeostatic control.[51] Information about the actions of these transporters in muscle or other tissues in response to physical activity is lacking.

The total body content of zinc is controlled partially by the regulation of the efficiency of intestinal absorption of zinc. Numerous studies in animals and humans have reported an inverse relationship between zinc intake and absorption.[52–54] Thus, the regulation of zinc absorption by the mucosal cell provides a general control of total body zinc.

2. Excretion

Control of zinc excretion in feces represents another regulatory mechanism for maintenance of body zinc. Secretion of pancreatic zinc-containing enzymes, mucosal cell loss into the gut, and transepithelial flux of zinc from the serosal to mucosal direction into the gastrointestinal tract is the major route of zinc excretion.[54] In normal dietary circumstances, the feces are the major route of zinc excretion. In healthy humans with an average zinc intake of 10 to 14 mg/d, more than 90% of dietary zinc is excreted in the feces.[52,55] Some of the zinc in the feces is from endogenous secretions. Studies indicate that 2.5 to 5 mg of zinc is secreted into the duodenum after a meal.[49] Much of the zinc secreted into the lumen of the gut is absorbed and returned to the body. The amount of zinc secreted into the gut varies with the zinc content of the meal. Endogenous zinc excretion in feces is directly related to dietary zinc intake. In humans, endogenous fecal zinc losses may range from 1 mg/d with very low zinc intakes (~1 mg/d) to 3 to 5 mg/d with usual zinc intakes (7 to 15 mg/d).[13,56] In contrast to intestinal absorption, endogenous fecal zinc excretion represents a sensitive control to balance zinc retention to metabolic needs.

Other routes of zinc excretion are present in humans. Less than 1 mg of zinc is excreted daily in the urine and is refractory to change with a wide range of zinc intake (4 to 25 mg/d).[55] Urinary zinc originates from the ultra-filterable portion of plasma zinc and represents a fraction of previously absorbed dietary zinc. Conditions that increase muscle breakdown (e.g., starvation or trauma) can raise urinary zinc excretion rates. Other losses of zinc include semen (1 mg/ejaculate), menses (0.1–0.5 mg per menstrual period), and parturition (100 mg/fetus and 100 mg/placenta).[40] Surface losses, which include sloughing of the skin, sweat, and hair, contribute up to 1 mg of zinc loss daily. A marked change in zinc intake results in parallel changes in surface zinc loss.[56] Surface losses at rest range from 0.3–0.4 to 0.4–0.5 and 0.7–0.8 mg with intakes of 3–4, 8–9 and 33–34 mg/d, respectively.[57]

Exercise in warm and hot environments increases zinc losses in sweat. Initial reports showed a mean zinc loss of 13.7 mg/d that decreased to 2.4 mg/d with acclimatization.[58] Other data confirm a reduction in sweat zinc concentrations either with repeated bouts of moderate physical activity in the heat or repeated collections during prolonged exposure.[59–62] Using the mean zinc concentration after acclimation, zinc losses in sweat during physical activity are estimated to be 3 to 4 mg/d.

The elimination of absorbed zinc from the human body has been described with a two-component model with an initial or rapid phase that has a half-life of 12.5 d and a slower turnover phase of about 300 d.[40] The initial phase represents liver uptake of circulating zinc and its quick release into the circulation. The slower turnover rate reflects the different rates of turnover in various organs, excluding the liver. The most rapid rates of zinc uptake and turnover occur in the pancreas, liver, kidney, and spleen, with slower rates in erythrocytes and muscle. Zinc turnover is slowest in bone and the central nervous system.

Manipulation of dietary zinc impacts zinc turnover. In rats, dietary zinc restrictions promote loss of zinc from bone but not soft tissues and organs. The turnover of the slow zinc pool in adult humans is increased by ingestion of pharmacologic amounts (100 mg) of zinc. An exchangeable zinc pool in humans is decreased in size when zinc intake is severely reduced, which may indicate the amount of zinc available to tissues and provide a biomarker of zinc status. The exchangeable zinc pool includes plasma zinc and perhaps liver zinc.[63]

3. Transport

Distribution of absorbed zinc to the extra-hepatic tissues occurs primarily in the plasma, which contains approximately 3 mg of zinc or about 0.1% of total body zinc. Zinc is partitioned among α_2-macroglobulin (40%), albumin (57%), and amino acids (3%) in plasma.[40] Zinc is bound loosely to albumin and amino acids; these fractions are responsible for transport of zinc from the liver to tissues. The amino acid-bound zinc constitutes the ultra-filterable fraction that is filtered at the kidneys and excreted in the urine. Because the total amount of zinc present in tissue is far greater than the zinc in the plasma, relatively small changes in tissue zinc content, such as the liver, can have striking effects on the plasma zinc concentration.

4. Assessment of Zinc Status

Routine assessment of human zinc nutritional status is hampered by the lack of accepted blood biochemical indicators of tissue zinc content. The ease of collection and measurement of plasma zinc concentration is practical and appealing. Because zinc homeostatic control is effective, plasma zinc concentrations are maintained within a narrow range (12–18 μM or 8–12 μg/100 mL) despite a broad amount of intake.[13] Restriction of dietary zinc will significantly reduce plasma zinc concentration.[64] Factors such as illness and consumption of food alter plasma zinc concentration and limit the usefulness of plasma zinc as a status indicator.[40] Nevertheless, studies of physically active people have used plasma zinc to characterize zinc nutritional status. Promising biomarkers of zinc status include the expression of some genes associated with zinc metabolism, such as metallothionein, in formed cells in the circulation.[65] This interesting approach has been used only in a few controlled studies[66,67] and awaits broader applications.

B. Zinc as an Ergogenic Agent

Zinc supplements have been used by physically active adults to improve performance for competition and military actions.[68,69] Analyses of usual dietary intakes reveal that zinc intakes can be low in some groups of athletes and soldiers during training.[70]

Early evidence indicated an important role of zinc in skeletal muscle performance. *Ex vivo* studies of frog skeletal muscle found that zinc added to the media improved muscle strength by increasing tension without tetanus and prolonging the contraction and relaxation periods of the muscle twitch.[71] The effects of supplemental zinc on muscle function were examined in adult male rats fed a chow diet and supplemented with modest amounts of zinc (2 or 4 mg/d) dissolved in water for 30 d. Rats supplemented with 4 mg zinc, as compared with 2 mg, performed significantly more work before fatigue.[72] These findings should be viewed with caution because there is no evidence that the observed change in performance resulted from an improvement in zinc status or increased activity of zinc-dependent enzymes.

1. Zinc Status as an Indicator of Function

Findings from observational studies in humans link poor zinc status with impaired physiological function. Serum zinc concentrations of adolescent gymnasts were significantly decreased compared with nonathletic, age- and gender-matched controls; half of the athletes were characterized as subclinically zinc deficient.[73] Serum zinc was significantly and positively correlated with adductor muscle strength in the gymnasts. Male professional soccer players with low compared with normal serum zinc concentrations had significantly decreased peak power output and increased blood lactate concentrations during peak cycle ergometer tests.[74] These findings, although not definitive, provide evidence that zinc status, as indicated by serum zinc concentration, may be a predictor of physical performance.

2. Zinc Supplementation and Performance in Middle-Aged Adults

Reports from controlled studies of the effects of zinc intake or supplementation on physiological function during exercise are limited. In a double-blind crossover study, middle-aged and older women received either 135 mg of zinc daily or placebo for 14-d periods with a 14-d washout period between treatments.[75] Zinc supplementation significantly increased lower-body isokinetic strength and endurance with no effect on strength or endurance with placebo treatment. These findings suggest that zinc consumed at a pharmacological dose may enhance performance of muscles that are glycolytic in function by acting on lactate dehydrogenase, a zinc metallo-enzyme.[43]

The effect of different levels of dietary zinc on muscle function was examined in more controlled studies. Men fed a formula-based diet containing low compared with adequate zinc content (1 vs. 12 mg/d) had significantly decreased serum zinc and zinc retention (e.g., diet minus losses in urine and feces); the reduced zinc status was associated with significant decreases in knee and shoulder extensor and flexor muscle strength.[76] Also, men fed whole-food diets low in zinc (3–4 mg/d) that were consistent with zinc intakes of endurance athletes[77] demonstrated significantly increased ventilation rates and decreased oxygen uptake, carbon dioxide output, and respiratory exchange ratio during prolonged submaximal cycle ergometer exercise.[64] The low-zinc diet resulted in significantly decreased serum zinc concentration and decreased zinc retention. The activity of carbonic anhydrase, a zinc-dependent enzyme, in erythrocytes decreased significantly when the low-zinc diet was consumed. The attenuated oxygen uptake and carbon dioxide elimination, as well as the decreased respiratory exchange ratio, are consistent with previous findings in zinc-deprived men.[78] Thus, subclinical zinc deficiency, evidenced by decreased concentrations of blood biochemical measures of zinc nutritional status and body zinc retention, adversely affects muscle strength and endurance and cardiorespiratory function.

IV. RESEARCH NEEDS

Secular trends indicate that the number of middle-aged adults will increase and many of them will have body weights in excess of the range proscribed for health. As these people adopt physical activity patterns to promote health, chromium and zinc will occupy increasingly important roles.

There is a burgeoning need to ascertain whether supplemental chromium has any beneficial effects on adults with impaired glucose, or on insulin metabolism in people with unhealthy body weight. Future studies must utilize combined dietary interventions, physical activity programs, and supplementation treatments that are properly designed to determine main and interactive effects of chromium supplementation and exercise on parameters of glucose utilization, insulin sensitivity, and body composition with appropriate technologies. An unresolved issue in the need to identify phenotypes that respond to chromium supplementation.

Future research should determine the amount of zinc required to optimize physical and mental function in middle-aged adults. Focused surveys of the relationships between traditional (intake and blood markers) and novel molecular markers of zinc nutritional status in parallel with objective measures of physical fitness (aerobic capacity and muscle strength and endurance) should be implemented. There also is a need to examine the effect of increasing physical activity patterns on the zinc needs of middle-aged and older adults. This work should include determination of the effects of different dietary levels of zinc (e.g., adequate intake, recommended dietary allowance, and supplemental levels) on zinc metabolism in adults undergoing different types of physical activity for health promotion such as endurance training for cardiovascular function and weight regulation and resistance training to combat sarcopenia. These investigations are needed to clearly determine whether current dietary recommendations for zinc are appropriate for the growing segment of the population that is aging and seeks to respond to current diet and physical activity guidelines for health maintenance.

V. CONCLUSIONS

Consensus for beneficial effects of chromium supplementation is conjectural because of inconsistent findings attributable to problems in experimental design. Many studies utilize samples of convenience and, thus, suffer from inadequate statistical power to test hypotheses. This limitation is significant because of the large within-subject variability in responses to supplementation and other interventions. There is a general lack of assessment of energy and chromium intakes before and during supplementation that limits interpretation of data on changes in body weight and composition. Determination of compliance regarding supplement consumption and adherence to training programs also is lacking in many studies. These concerns fuel the controversy surrounding the value of chromium supplementation as a weight loss aid. However, recent data from a randomized controlled trial in which energy intake was maintained throughout the study, showed no effect of supplemental chromium on weight and body composition change. This finding is the first evidence in support of the ruling of the U.S. Federal Trade Commission[79] that there is no basis for claims that chromium as chromium picolinate promotes weight loss and fat loss in humans. There is consensus, however, that supplemental chromium has no ergogenic benefit on muscle strength gain during resistance training in adults.

Zinc has biological roles in protein, carbohydrate, and lipid metabolism and, hence, is needed for health and optimal performance. Experimental evidence describing the interaction of zinc intake and physical activity in middle-aged adults is limited and, thus, needed. Recent evidence indicates that restricted zinc intake reduces traditional zinc status indicators, impairs muscle strength and endurance, and impairs cardiorespiratory function of adults. Nascent biomarkers for assessment of human zinc status hold promise for studying interactions between zinc intake and physical activity.

REFERENCES

1. US Department of Health and Human Services and US Department of Agriculture, Dietary Guidelines for Americans, 2005, http://www.healthierus.gov/dietaryguidelines.
2. National Center for Health Statistics, Health, United States 2006, with Chartbook on Trends in the Health of Americans, DHHS Publ. No. 2006-1232, US Government Printing Office, Washington, DC, 2006, 285, http://www.cdc.gov/nchs/fastats/exercise.htm.
3. The Practical Guide to Identification, Evaluation, and Treatment of Overweight and Obesity in Adults, NIH Publ. No. 02-4084, Bethesda, MD, NIH, NIDDK, 2002, http://www.nhlbi.nih.gov/guidelines/obesity/prctgd_c.pdf.
4. Moshfegy, A., Goldman, J., and Cleveland, L., What We Eat in America, NHANES 2001–2002: Usual Nutrient Intakes from Food Compared with Dietary Reference Intakes, US Department of Agriculture, Agricultural Research Service, 2005.
5. Anderson, R.A., Chromium, glucose intolerance and diabetes, *J. Am. Coll. Nutr.* 17, 548–55, 1998.
6. Vincent, J. B., Recent developments in the biochemistry of chromium (III), *J. Biol. Trace Elem. Res.* 99, 1–16, 2004.
7. Lukaski, H.C. Zinc, in *Sports Nutrition: Vitamins and Trace Elements, 2nd ed.*, Driskell, J.A. and Wolinsky, I, Eds., Taylor & Francis, Boca Raton, FL, 2006, 217–234.

8. Anderson, R.A., Polansky, M.M., and Bryden, N.A., Strenuous running: Acute effects on chromium, copper, zinc and selected variables in urine and serum of male runners, *Biol. Trace Elem. Res.* 6, 327–36, 1984.
9. Lukaski, H.C., Chromium as a supplement, *Ann. Rev. Nutr.* 19, 279–302, 1999.
10. Stoecker, B.J., Chromium. In *Modern Nutrition in Health and Disease, 10th ed.*, Shils, M.E., Shike, M., Ross, A.C., Caballero, B., and Cousins, R.J., Eds., Lippincott Williams & Wilkins, Philadelphia, PA, 2006, pp. 232–237.
11. Anderson, R.A., Bryden, N.A., and Polansky, M.M., Dietary chromium intake: Freely chosen foods, institutional diets and individual foods, *Biol. Trace Elem. Res.* 32, 117–21, 1992.
12. Kozlovsky, A.S., Moser, P.B., Resier, S., and Anderson, R.A., Effects of diets high in simple sugars on urinary chromium losses, *Metabolism* 35, 515–18, 1986.
13. National Research Council, Dietary Reference Intakes for Vitamin A, Vitamin K, Arsenic, Boron, Chromium, Copper, Iodine, Iron, Manganese, Molybdenum, Nickel, Silicon, Vanadium, and Zinc. A Report of the Panel on Micronutrients, Subcommittee on Upper Reference Levels of Nutrients and of Interpretations and Uses of Dietary Reference Intakes, and the Standing Committee on the Scientific Evaluation of Dietary Reference Intakes, National Academy of Sciences, Washington, DC, 2001.
14. Anderson, R.A., Polansky, M.M., Bryden, N.A., Patterson, K.Y., Veillon, C., and Glinsman, W.H., Effects of chromium supplementation on urinary chromium excretion of human subjects and correlation of chromium excretion with selected clinical parameters, *J. Nutr.* 113, 276–81, 1983.
15. Anderson, R.A. and Kozlovsky, A.S., Chromium intake, absorption and excretion of subjects consuming self-selected diets, *Am. J. Clin. Nutr.* 41, 1177–83, 1985.
16. Mertz, W., Chromium occurrence and function in biological systems, *Physiol. Rev.* 49, 163–239, 1969.
17. Offenbacher, E.G., Spencer, H., Dowling, H.J., and Pi-Sunyer, F.X., Metabolic chromium balances in men, *Am. J. Clin. Nutr.* 44, 77–82, 1986.
18. Offenbacher, E., Promotion of chromium absorption by ascorbic acid, *Trace Elem. Elec.* 11, 178–81, 1994.
19. Lim, T.H., Sargent, T., and Kusubov, N., Kinetics of trace element chromium (III) in the human body, *Am. J. Physiol.* 244, R445–54, 1983.
20. Olin, K.L., Stearns, D.M., Armstrong, W.H., and Keen, C.L., Comparative retention/absorption of ^{51}chromium (^{51}Cr) from ^{51}Cr chloride, ^{51}Cr nicotinate and ^{51}Cr picolinate in a rat model, *Trace Elem. Med.* 11, 182–6, 1994.
21. Anderson, R.A., Bryden, N.A.,Polansky, M.M., and Gautschi, K., Dietary chromium effects on tissue chromium concentrations and chromium absorption in rats, *J. Trace Elem. Exp. Biol.* 9, 11–25, 1996.
22. Anderson, R.A., Stress effects on chromium nutrition of humans and animals. In Biotechnology of the Feed Industry, *Proc. 10th Alltech Ann. Symp.*, Nottingham, England, 1994, 267–74.
23. Lukaski, H.C., Bolonchuk, W.W., Siders, W.A., and Milne, D.B., Chromium supplementation and resistance training: Effects on body composition, strength and trace element status of men, *Am. J. Clin. Nutr.* 63, 954–65, 1996.
24. Lukaski, H.C., Effects of chromium(III) as a nutritional supplement. In *The Nutritional Biochemistry of Chromium*(III), Vincent, J.B., Ed., Elsevier, New York, NY, 2007, 71–84.
25. Offenbacher, E.G. and Pi-Sunyer, F.X., Beneficial effects of chromium-rich yeast on glucose tolerance and blood lipids in elderly subjects, *Diabetes* 29, 919–25, 1985.
26. Vincent, J.B., The potential value and toxicity of chromium picolinate as a nutritional supplement, weight loss agent and muscle development agent. *Sports Med.* 33, 213–30, 2003.

27. Volpe, S.L., Huang, H.W., Larpadisorn, K., and Lesser, I.I., Effect of chromium supplementation and exercise on body composition, resting metabolic rate and selected biochemical parameters in moderately obese women following an exercise program, *J. Am. Coll. Nutr.* 20, 293–306, 2001.
28. Kaats, G.R., Blum, K., Fisher, J.A., and Adelman, J.A., Effects of chromium supplementation on body composition: A randomized, double-masked, placebo-controlled study, *Curr. Ther. Res.* 57, 747–56, 1996.
29. Kaats, G.R., Blum, K., Pullin, D., Keith, S.C., and Wood, R., A randomized, double-masked, placebo-controlled study of the effects of chromium picolinate supplementation on body composition: a replication and extension of a previous study, *Curr. Ther. Res.* 59, 379–88, 1998.
30. Crawford, V., Scheckenbach, R., and Preuss, H.G., Effects of niacin–bound chromium supplementation on body composition in overweight African-American women, *Diabetes Obes. Metabol.* 1,331–7, 1999.
31. Pasman, W.J., Westerterp-Plantenga, M.S., and Saris, W.H.M., The effectiveness of long-term supplementation of carbohydrate, chromium, fibre, and caffeine on weight maintenance, *Int. J. Obes.* 21, 1143–51, 1997.
32. Grant, K.E., Chandler, R.M., Castle, A.L., and Ivy, J.L., Chromium and exercise training: effect on obese women, *Med. Sci. Sports Exerc.* 29, 992–8, 1997.
33. Bahadori, B., Wallner, S., Schneider, H., Wascher, T.C., and Toplak, H., Effects of chromium yeast and chromium picolinate on body composition in obese, non-diabetic patients during and after a very-low-calorie diet, *Acta Med. Austriaca* 24,185–7, 1997.
34. Lukaski, H.C., Siders, W.A., and Penland, J.G., Chromium picolinate supplementation in women: Effects on body weight, composition and iron status, *Nutrition* 23,187–95, 2007.
35. Lefavi, R. G., Anderson, R. A., Keith, R. E., Wilson, G. D., McMillan, J. L., and Stone, M. H., Efficacy of chromium supplementation in athletes: Emphasis on anabolism, *Int. J. Sport Nutr.* 2,111–22, 1992.
36. Amato, P., Morales, A.J., and Yen, S.S.C., Effects of chromium picolinate supplementation on insulin sensitivity, serum lipids, and body composition in healthy, non-obese older men and women, *J. Gerontol.* 55A, M260–3, 2000.
37. Campbell, W.W., Joseph, L.J.O., Davey, S.L., Cyr–Campbell, D., Anderson, R.A., and Evans, W.J., Effects of resistance training and chromium picolinate on body composition and skeletal muscle in older men, *J. Appl. Physiol.* 86, 29–39, 1999.
38. Campbell, W.W., Joseph, L.J.O., Anderson, R.A., Davey, S.L., Hinton, J., and Evans, W.J., Effects of resistance training and chromium picolinate on body composition and muscle size in older women, *Int. J. Sport Nutr. Exerc. Metabol.* 12,125–35, 1999.
39. Evans, G. W., The effect of chromium picolinate on insulin controlled parameters in humans, *Int. J. Biosci. Med. Res.* 11,163–80, 1989.
40. King, J.C. and Cousins R.J., Zinc, in *Modern Nutrition in Health and Disease, 10th ed.*, Shils, M.E., Shike, M., Ross, A.C., Caballero, B., and Cousins, R.J., Eds., Lippincott Williams & Wilkins, Philadelphia, PA, 2006, pp. 271–285.
41. Vallee, B.L. and Falchuk, K.H., The biochemical basis of zinc physiology, *Physiol. Rev.* 73, 79–118, 1993.
42. Vallee, B.L. and Auld, D.S., Active zinc binding sites of zinc metalloenzymes, *Matrix Suppl.* 1, 5–19, 1992.
43. International Commission on Radiological Protection, Report No. 23, Report of the Task Group on Reference Man. Pergamon Press, Oxford, 1975.
44. Maltin, C.A., Duncan, L., Wilson, A.B., and Hesketh, J.E., Effect of zinc deficiency on muscle fibre type frequencies in the post-weanling rat, *Br. J. Nutr.* 50, 597–604, 1983.

45. O'Leary, M.J., McClain, C.J., and Hegarty, P.V., Effect of zinc deficiency on the weight, cellularity and zinc concentration of different skeletal muscles in the post-weanling rat, *Br. J. Nutr.* 42, 487–95, 1979.
46. Hambidge, K.M., Casey, C.E., and Krebs, N.F., Zinc, in *Trace Elements in Human and Animal Nutrition*, Mertz, W. and Underwood, E.J., Eds., Academic Press, Orlando, 1986, 1–137.
47. Scholmerich, J., Freudemann, A., Kottgen, E., Wietholtz, H., Steiert, B., Lohle, E., et al., Bioavailability of zinc from zinc-histidine complexes: I. Comparison with zinc sulfate in healthy men, *Am. J. Clin. Nutr.* 45, 1480–6, 1987.
48. Dibley, M.J.C., Zinc, in *Present Knowledge in Nutrition*, Bowman, B.A. and Russell, R.M., Eds., ILSI Press, Washington, DC, 2001, 329–40.
49. Eide, D.J., Zinc transporters and cellular trafficking of zinc, *Biochim. Biophys. Acta* 1763, 711–22, 2006.
50. Cousins, R.J., Liuzzi, J.P., and Lichten, L.A. Mammalian zinc transport, trafficking and signals, *J. Biol. Chem.* 281, 24085–9, 2006.
51. Baer, M.T. and King, J.C., Tissue zinc levels and zinc excretion during experimental zinc depletion in young men, *Am. J. Clin. Nutr.* 39, 556–70, 1984.
52. Johnson, P.E., Zinc absorption and excretion in humans and animals. In *Copper and Zinc in Inflammation*, Milanino, R., Rainsford, K.D. and Velo, G.P., Eds., Kluwer Academic, Dordrecht, Netherlands, 1989, p. 103.
53. Mills, C.F., *Zinc in Human Biology*, Springer-Verlag, London, 1989, pp. 371–81.
54. King, J.C., Shames, D.M., and Woodhouse, L.R., Zinc homeostasis in humans, *J. Nutr.* 130, 1360S–1366S, 2000.
55. Hambidge, K.M. and Krebs, N.F., Interrelationships of key variables of human zinc homeostasis: Relevance to dietary zinc requirements, *Ann. Rev. Nutr.* 21, 429–52, 2001.
56. Prasad, A.S. and Schulbert, A.R., Zinc, iron and nitrogen content of sweat in normal and zinc-deficient men, *J. Lab. Clin. Med.* 62, 84–9, 1963.
57. Milne, D.B., Canfield, W.K., Mahalko, J.R., and Sandstead, H.H., Effect of dietary zinc on whole body surface loss of zinc: impact on estimation of zinc retention by balance method, *Am. J. Clin. Nutr.* 38, 181–6, 1983.
58. Consolazio, C.F., Nelson, R.A., Matoush, L.O., Hughes, R.C., and Urone, P., The Trace Mineral Losses in Sweat, US Army Medical Research and Nutrition Laboratory, Report #248, 1964.
59. Tipton, K., Green, N.R., Haymes, E.M., and Waller, M., Zinc losses in sweat of athletes exercising in hot and neutral environments, *Int. J. Sport Nutr.* 3, 261–71, 1993.
60. DeRuisseau, K.C., Chevront, S.N., Haymes, E.M., and Sharp, R.G., Sweat iron and zinc losses during prolonged exercise, *Int. J. Sport Nutr. Exerc. Metab.* 12, 428–37, 2002.
61. Chinevere, T.D., Kenefick, R.W., Cheuvront, S.N., Lukaski, H.C., and Sawka, M.N., Sweat mineral concentrations before and after heat acclimation, *Med. Sci. Sports Exer.* 40, 886–91, 2008.
62. Montain, S.J., Cheuvront, S.N., and Lukaski, H.C., Sewat mineral element responses during 7-h of exercise-heat stress, *Int. J. Sport Nutr. Exerc. Metab.* 17:574–82, 2007.
63. Hambidge, M., Human zinc homeostasis: Good but not perfect, *J. Nutr.* 133, 1438S–42S, 2003.
64. Lukaski, H.C., Low dietary zinc decreases erythrocyte carbonic anhydrase activities and impairs cardiorespiratory function in men during exercise, *Am. J. Clin. Nutr.* 81, 1045–51, 2005.
65. Cao, J. and Cousins, R.J., Metallothionein mRNA in monocytes and peripheral blood mononuclear cells and in cells from dried blood spots increases after zinc supplementation of men, *J. Nutr.* 130, 2180–7, 2000.

66. Cousins, R.J., Blanchard, R.K., Popp, M.P., Liu, L., Cao, J., Moore, J.B., and Green, C.L., A global view of the selectivity of zinc deprivation and excess on genes expressed in human THP-1 mononuclear cells, *Proc. Natl. Acad. Sci.* 100, 6952–6957, 2003.
67. Aydemir, T.B., Blanchard, R.K., and Cousins, R.J., Zinc supplementation of young men alters metallothionein, zinc transporter, and cytokine gene expression in leukocyte populations, *Proc. Natl. Acad. Sci.* 103, 1699–1704, 2006.
68. Deuster, P.A., Kyle, S.B., Moser, P.B., Vigersky, R.A., Singh, A., and Schoomaker, E.B., Nutritional survey of highly trained women runners, *Am. J. Clin. Nutr.* 44, 954–62, 1986.
69. Singh, A., Deuster, P.A., and Moser, P.B., Zinc and copper status in women by physical activity and menstrual status, J. *Sports Med. Phys. Fitness* 30, 29–36, 1990.
70. Lukaski, H.C. and Penland, J.G., Zinc, magnesium, copper, selenium, and calcium in assault rations: Roles in promotion of physical and mental performance, in Nutrient Composition of Rations for Short-Term, High-Intensity Combat Operations, Committee on Military Nutrition, Food and Nutrition Board, Institute of Medicine, National Academies Press, Washington, DC, 2006, pp. 256–70.
71. Isaacson, A. and Sandow, A., Effects of zinc on responses of skeletal muscle, *J. Gen. Physiol.* 46, 655–77, 1963.
72. Richardson, J.H. and Drake, P.D., The effects of zinc on fatigue of striated muscle, J. *Sports Med. Phys. Fitness* 19, 133–4, 1979.
73. Brun, J.F., Dieu-Cambrezy, C., Charpiat, A., Fons, C., Fedou, C., Micallef, J.P., et al., Serum zinc in highly trained adolescent gymnasts, *Biol. Trace Elem. Res.* 47, 272–8, 1995.
74. Khaled, S., Brun, J.F., Micallef, J.P., Bardet, L., Cassanas, G., Monnier, J.F. and Orsetti, A., Serum zinc and blood rheology in sportsmen (football players), *Clin. Hemorheol. Microcirc.* 17, 47–58, 1997.
75. Krotkiewski, M., Gudmundsson, M., Backstrom, P., and Mandroukas, K., Zinc and muscle strength and endurance, *Acta Physiol Scand.* 116, 309–11, 1982.
76. Van Loan, M.D., Sutherland, B., Lowe, N.M., Turnlund, J.R., and King, J.C., The effects of zinc depletion on peak force and total work of knee and shoulder extensor and flexor muscles, *Int. J. Sport Nutr.* 9, 125–35, 1999.
77. Micheletti, A., Rossi, R., and Rufini, S., Zinc status in athletes: Relation to diet and exercise, *Sports Med.* 31, 577–82, 2001.
78. Wada, L. and King, J.C., Effect of low zinc intakes on basal metabolic rate, thyroid hormones and protein utilization in adult men, *J. Nutr.* 116, 1045–53, 1986.
79. United States of America before Federal Trade Commission, Docket No. C–3758, 1997. http://www.ftc.gov/os/1997/07/nutrit~2.htm.

Section V

Fluids and Hydration

11 Fluids, Electrolytes, and Hydration

Douglas S. Kalman

CONTENTS

I. INTRODUCTION

Fluid balance is of importance to the middle-aged population—as it is to populations of all age groups. In the United States, the Institute of Medicine (IOM) in 2005 published official recommendations for water/hydration needs. This official recommendation is a new step within the paradigm of Recommended Dietary Allowances, as prior to 2004, the IOM stated that it was impossible to set a water recommendation.[1] Water is the largest constituent of the human body, accounting for around 60% of the weight of the human body. Water is essential for cellular homeostasis, playing important roles in both physiological and biochemical functions. Many factors impact daily hydration needs as well as our ability to hydrate.

The manner in which the body regulates and utilizes water in body hydration is of importance. For example, when we exercise, core body temperature increases. The increase in body temperature is coupled with heat dissipation. Heat dissipation will result in cutaneous vasodilation and change in heat transfer and exchange. If heat transfer via radiation and convection is not adequate in reducing the heat load, sweating will occur and heat will be lost by evaporation. If the water loss exceeds fluid intake, hypohydration leading to dehydration will occur.

Water is a macronutrient that most often is underappreciated. The IOM has established a level of water intake deemed to describe the Adequate Intake (AI). The AI is meant to "to prevent deleterious, primary acute, effects of dehydration, which include metabolic and functional abnormalities."[1] One should recognize that there is extreme difficulty in establishing a specific level of water intake that ensures adequate hydration and promotes optimal health under all potential conditions. Understanding the relationship between hydration states and optimal wellness, along with disease relationships, allows for the belief that there is a relationship between hydration and disease. Further, it is believed that hydration may play a role in the prevention of prolonged physical labor, urolithiasis, urinary tract infections, bladder cancer, constipation, pulmonary and bronchial disorders, heart disease, hypertension, venous thrombosis, and other conditions.[2,3]

This chapter provides information regarding the fluid needs of middle-aged adults as related to physical activity. Hydration needs and fluid balance will be discussed in some detail. Fluid guidelines for both the physically active adult and the non-active middle-aged adult are included. Fluid needs consist of the body's need for water as well as the electrolytes, particularly sodium, chloride, and potassium. A discussion of hydration needs over the life span is available elsewhere.[4]

II. WATER AS A FLUID COMPONENT

Water is an often-overlooked macronutrient. In light of the rising incidence and prevalence of overweight and obesity in developed nations, the majority of news reports and translation of nutrition-related research has focused on the energy-yielding macronutrients (carbohydrates, proteins, and fats) and not on hydration. The relationship between fluid intake and health is well known. A reduction in total body water stores by as little as 1% to 2% can adversely impact aerobic performance, orthostatic tolerance, and cognitive function. The body is composed of 50% to 70% water (the average of 60% is the norm in the literature) and water/fluid is stored or circulated. For example, blood contains about 93% water, muscle about 73% water, blood 93%, and fat mass about 10%. It is known that approximately 5–10% percent of total body water is turned over daily through obligatory losses (respiration, urine, and sweat). Respiratory water losses are typically recouped by the production of metabolic water formed by substrate oxidation. Fluid losses during and post-exercise also affect overall fluid balance. Thus, fluid balance is easiest thought of as achieving a balance between fluid output and intake. It has been reported that physically active adults who reside in warmer climates have daily water needs of six liters, with highly active populations needing even more to remain euhydrated.[5]

Water is the component of body fluids, present in the greatest amount. Fluids acts as solvent and a transport system within the body. Water plays a central role in thermoregulation and optimal health, and its acute status can affect many essential metabolic processes as well as physical performance and mental acuity.

Currently, the average fluid intakes of adults in the United States averages around 48 ounces per day, with 19% of the fluid intake coming from foods.[6] Therefore, Americans are typically underhydrated, based on the following IOM guidelines: the IOM recommends in general that men aged 19 to 70+ years consume 2.7 L/day and women aged 19 to 70+ ingest 2.7 L/d of all water sources daily (water, other liquids, and the water in foods).[1] IOM has established the following AI for sodium, chloride, and potassium:

adults 31–50 years, 1500 mg sodium, 2300 mg chloride, 4700 mg potassium; adults 51–70 years, 1300 mg sodium, 2000 mg chloride, 4700 mg potassium.[1]

III. WATER AND PHYSICAL ACTIVITY

Water is a multifunctional macronutrient. Regulation of body heat is one of the more important functions of water in the body. Water functions as a buffer; if there is high specific heat (the specific heat of water equals 1 when 1 kg of water is heated 1°C between 15 and 16°C). The body is about 60% fluid, therefore a 70-kg man will contain ~42 kg of water throughout his body.[7] For every 1°C rise in temperature in a 70-kg person, ~58 calories (actually kilocalories termed herein as calories) will be oxidized; thus, the heat buffering effect of water also results in increased metabolic rate.

Thermoregulation is of importance in exercise physiology (and thus physical activity) as evidenced by the evaporation of sweat. For each gram of sweat evaporated from the skin; the body expends 0.58 calories (or 2.43 kjoules).[7,8] Water not only has high specific heat, it also assists in the transfer of heat from areas of production to dissipation. Heat transport occurs with minimal change in actual blood temperature in an healthy individual.

All of the membranes of the body are readily transversed by water. Osmotic and hydrostatic gradients dictate the movement of water. Coupled with this, water also is affected by the activity of the adenosine triphosphatase (ATPase) sodium-potassium pump (Na-K pump). When a person who has not previously exercised very much exercises, fluid shifts occur and plasma volume expands. Fluid balance is tightly regulated by the body.

IV. REGULATION OF THIRST

The perception of thirst is subjective. The perception of being thirsty is also a subjective motivator to quench the thirst in animals, including humans.[9] Regulatory systems are in place to maintain body fluid levels, which ultimately are essential for long-term survival. Factors influencing fluid needs and the urge to drink include cultural and societal or habitual habits combined with internal psychogenic drive and regulatory controls to maintain fluid homeostasis. Regulatory control includes maintaining the fluid content of various bodily compartments, the osmotic gradient of the extracellular fluids, and the functioning of specific hormones to assist in the regulation.

Water is usually depleted from both the extracellular and intracellular compartments when the body loses water. These losses generally are not equal in volume. Sodium chloride (NaCl), which is the major solute of the extracellular fluid together with water, results in proportionately more extracellular fluid's being depleted than if water alone were lost. This can occur if there are fluid losses from the gastrointestinal tract (i.e., diarrhea). If the losses are of normal osmostic load (isotonic), then the depletion will be entirely from the extracellular fluid. However, if hypertonic fluid is added to the extracellular compartment, there will be an osmotic depletion of water from the intracellular compartment into the extracellular fluid, and this latter compartment will be expanded.

A range of compensatory responses can occur along with losses from the intra- or extracellular space. Understanding the effects of vasopressin secretion, stimulation of the renin-angiotensin-aldosterone system, sympathetic activation, and reduced renal solute and water excretion is important with regard to hydration in the athlete and others who are quite physically active. Hormonal responses to fluid losses, however, are not solutions to returning the athlete to a euhydrated state. The only means to return this individual to a euhydrated state is by hydrating him or her to the tune of 1.25 pt./lb. of body weight lost. Thirst can be thought of as the "vocal" component of the body's response to fluid shifts or losses.

The regulation of thirst includes osmoregulation. The osmotic pressure of the fluid (plasma osmolality) typically lies between 280–295 mosmol/kgH_20. Fluid losses as small as 1%–2% stimulates thirst. If the osmostic gradient is increased, the response will include thirst. Changes in NaCl or glucose induce this by their not crossing over cell membranes so easily. The osmotic differences between the intracellular and extracellular compartments are what dictate the flow of fluids (higher to lower concentration) occurring typically by osmosis (the diffusion of water). Osmosis is partially regulated by osmoreceptors (relative to vasopressin) in the brain and in the liver. The hypothalamus is the center of the brain from which thirst regulation is thought to emanate.

Thirst regulation is multifactorial. Within the central nervous system (CNS) osmotic, ionic, hormonal, and nervous signals are integrated and impact the perception of thirst. Overcoming hypohydration or dehydration following the ingestion of water or fluid involves additional physiological pathways and factors that are beyond the scope of this chapter. The fact that disease or metabolic disorder states can impact hydration status cannot be overlooked, even in the apparently healthy athlete.

V. HYDRATION IN HEALTH AND DISEASE

Body fluid losses occur from both the intracellular and extracellular compartments. The loss of NaCl causes greater losses from the extracellular space. In sweat, NaCl is lost at a rate of 7:1 compared with potassium.[9] Thus, fluid losses of 1%–2% of body weight or greater induce the need for fluid and electrolyte replacement. However, the importance of hydration state and health or disease prevention is often overlooked. In addition, aging may also be a risk factor for dehydration.

Most diseases have multifactorial origins. Lifestyle, genetics, environment, and other factors including the state of hydration are worthy of examination. Mild dehydration is a factor in the development of various conditions and diseases. Conditions associated with the negative impacts of hypohydration or dehydration include alterations in amniotic fluids, prolonged physical labor, cystic fibrosis, and renal toxicity secondary to dehydration, all of which alter how contrast agents are metabolized. The effects of chronic hypohydration or dehydration (systemic effects) include associations with (ranging from weak to mild) urinary tract infections, gallstones, constipation, hypertension, bladder and colon cancer, venous thromboembolism, cerebral infarcts, dental diseases, kidney stones, mitral valve prolapse, glaucoma, and diabetic ketiacidosis.[10] Evidence exists that rehydration and proper hydration assist with condition management, prevention, and the betterment of health. Recognizing the factors that can effect hydration is important. These factors include: high ambient temperature, relative humidity, high sweat losses (sweat rates), increased body temperature, exercise duration, training status of the individual, exercise intensity, high body fat percentage, underwater exercise, use of diuretic medications, and uncontrolled diabetes. The assessment of an athlete for hydration should include a review of all the aforementioned factors.

A goal with each individual, whether athlete or not, is euhydration. Hydration needs have been detailed by the IOM for both genders. However, the practicality of applying these recommendations every day is difficult for individuals. Easy "rule of thumb" hydration guidelines for general health are needed. Many dietitians tell their clients to shoot for a goal of drinking the equivalent in ounces to half their body weight. Hence, if you weigh 150 pounds, your goal hydration per day with normal activities is 50–75 ounces of nonalcoholic fluids.

VI. HYDRATION AS IT RELATES TO PHYSICAL AND ATHLETIC PERFORMANCE

The consistent conclusion across multiple studies, academic societies, and training associations is that dehydration can significantly impact performance and that this is magnified when the activity takes place in warm or hot conditions. Thus, fluid replacement guidelines have been established to minimize exertional dehydration. Dehydration is defined as a 2% loss of euhydrated body weight.[11] This negatively impacts athletic performance. Dehydration is associated with a reduction or an adverse effect upon muscle strength, endurance, coordination, mental acuity, and the thermoregulatory processes.

Water losses during exercise are affected by the aforementioned parameters, and since the interindividual variation in sweat rates is so wide, no universal recommendations are used. The closest universal rule is that for every pound of body weight lost between the initiation of exercise and the cessation, one replaces with 20 ounces per pound (1.25pt./lb.) of body weight lost (L. Armstrong, personal communication).

During prolonged exercise fluid and sodium losses occur. Human sweat contains 40–50 mmol sodium per liter.[11] For the most part, in the normal healthy person, large fluid losses are followed by large sodium losses. The typical sodium to potassium ratio of losses is 7:1. An athlete engaged in prolonged exercise can lose 5 liters of fluid per day with a range of 4,600 to 5,750 mg sodium and much smaller amounts of potassium. Heat-acclimated athletes benefit from enhanced sodium reabsorption, which results in better protection of plasma volume by reducing the sodium losses. The training state of the athlete is very important when contemplating fluid needs. Salt losses do not directly impact physical performance, however using salts in fluid replacement is proven to enhance the thirst response and aid in rehydration.

Hypohydration (1% bodyweight loss) also decreases the ability of athletes to perform. Athletes as a rule do not replace sweat/sodium losses enough during the event. The average marathon runner will lose up to 3% body weight and, if the run is in a temperate climate, the losses could be 5%. According to Maughan, elite marathoners tend to lose or sweat at a rate of 2L/h. This sweat rate exceeds the intestinal absorption capability of the gut.[12,13]

A plethora of studies clearly demonstrate a negative impact of hypohydration and dehydration on athletic performance (range from 1%–8% fluid losses). Studies using sports or situations designed to mimic a sport have noted a decrement in performance for soccer, basketball, running and racing, cycling, and others. In addition, better hydration is associated with lower esophageal temperature, heart rate, and ratings of perceived exertion–all factors that may impact performance.[14]

Exercise increases the metabolic rate and, since energy is converted into heat, water losses will occur. In cold climates (winter sports or outdoor sports in mild or cold climates) heat is lost via radiation and convection; as the temperature increases the losses are noticeable as sweat. The physiological response to exercise is to expand the blood volume and to increase the sensitivity for sweating to occur. Athletes and their coaches, trainers, and nutritionists must be cognizant of changes in osmolarity. Body temperature and the volume as well as the osmolarity can affect performance.

Other impacts of hypohydration or dehydration that should be a concern to athletes or their training staffs are the impact on cognition. The mental aspect of sports coupled with neuromuscular integration cannot be overstated. The neuropsychological impacts of hydration as well as the biological mechanisms and behavioral relationships are relatively new in research. Brain behavior and cognitive assessment are relatively new to the exercise physiology field as well, since many new cognitive assessment tools have become available. This is despite research since the 1940s on fluid and salt intake.[15,16] A review by Lieberman found that hypo- and dehydration were associated with increased fatigue, impaired discrimination, impaired tracking, impaired short-term memory, impaired recall and attention, decreased arithmetic ability, and a faster response time to peripheral visual stimuli.[16] The applications have been tested not only in academic exercise or psychology research, but in the military as well. Interestingly enough, dehydration induced by heat as compared with dehydration caused by exercise shows the same changes in cognitive performance, thus yielding that dehydration is the cause, not the exercise itself. Cognitive performance when one is dehydrated most often results in increased fatigue, tracking errors (vision–brain connection) along with a decrease in short-term memory. Ironically, when a person is hyperhydrated, short-term memory is increased while most of the other parameters mentioned remain neutral with no negative impacts.[17]

VII. MEASUREMENTS OF HYDRATION

No universal standard exists for measuring body hydration. At least 13 techniques are used for assessing hydration. Water is the body's currency, as it is the medium for circulatory function, biochemical reactions, temperature regulation, and other physiological processes. In addition, fluid turnover occurs as water is lost from fluid-electrolyte shifts, losses from the lungs, skin, and kidneys. Water is gained via the diet as well as fluid intake from energy-producing reactions.

Hydration assessment methods used in field and laboratory settings include:

- Stable isotope dilution
- Neutron activation analysis
- Bioelectrical impedance (BIA)

- Body mass change
- Plasma osmolality
- Plasma volume change
- Urine osmolality
- Urine specific gravity
- Urine conductivity
- Urine color
- 24-hour urine volume
- Salivary flow rate (osmolality, flow rate, protein content)
- Rating of thirst

One other tool that is used clinically is the Hydration Assessment (HA) Checklist.[20] This is a lengthy, in-depth assessment designed to screen for hydration problems. The HA checklist is most often used in clinical conditions and in the older population. Older adults, both in the community and in the nursing home, are grossly underhydrated, ingesting on average less than 33 ounces/d (~1000 cc/d), which is substantially lower than recommended. Of the ~half-gallon of fluid, few individuals consume plain water, an essential element supporting cellular and organ health, electrolyte balance, medication absorption and distribution as well as kidney, bladder, and integumentary functioning.

The following factors have been detailed in the literature as to why a single "gold standard" for measuring hydration is not possible:[21]

1. The physiological regulation of total body water volume (i.e., water turnover) and fluid concentrations is complex and dynamic. Renal, thirst, and sweat gland responses are involved to varying degrees, depending on the prevailing activities. Also, renal regulation of water balance (i.e., arginine vasopressin) is distinct from the regulation of tonicity.
2. The 24-hour fluid deficit varies greatly among sedentary individuals and athletes primarily due to the exercise and morphology. The deficit must be matched by food and fluid intake. The fluid portion of food is often overlooked.
3. Sodium and osmolyte consumption affects the daily water requirement. Regional customs impact the "normal" values used with biochemical assessment of hydration. For example, the mean 24-h urine osmolality in Germany is 860 mOsm/kg, in Poland it is 392 mOsm/kg, and in the United States it is in the range of 280 to 295 mOsm/kg.
4. The volume and timing of fluid intake alters measurement of hydration. Pure water or hypotonic solutions ingested rapidly can cause dilute urine prior to cellular equilibrium to occur.
5. One-time urine samples (spot) do not represent the true 24-hour void.
6. Experimental designs that differ in assessment techniques (blood versus urine).
7. Use of stable isotopes to assess hydration. However, it is not known if the isotopes are distributed throughout the body in a uniform fashion; thus, the assumption used in these techniques is faulty.

8. Exercise and physical labor (as well as pregnancy labor) increase blood volume while decreasing renal blood flow, thus altering the glomerular filtration rate affecting hydration.
9. Changes in osmolarity and osmolality can affect the readings for hydration on certain devices (i.e., Bioelectric Impedance Analysis).

In addition to the above, many questions exist regarding the use of plasma osmolality as a biomarker for hydration. These questions include the fact that plasma osmolality varies widely depending upon the physical condition being tested, environment of the test, the pre-exercise hydration state, and the intervention being evaluated.

Is there a way to meld laboratory techniques with those in the field so that trainers, coaches, and related personnel can better help athletes? The first item to discuss is the intervention and educational sessions that athletes should receive from appropriate professionals (i.e., exercise physiologist, registered dietitian, sports nutritionist, athletic trainer, etc.). Education is the key to preventing dehydration. Combining education with fluid stations on the field or in the general training area that are available to athletes at specific intervals (with or without *ad libitum* intake) may make euhydration an easier goal to maintain.

The field technique generally consists of using the combination of weighing the athlete before and after the training or competition and using the weight change as the guide for rehydration. This may just be the best standard when controlling for applicability, financial impact, and ease of education. The rehydration recommendation is 20 ounces per pound of body weight lost. Other techniques that can be used in combination with monitoring weight changes include using blood and urine testing if available. Testing for osmolality (both), sodium (both), and hematocrit levels (blood) are typical and inexpensive.

VIII. REHYDRATION WITH WATER VS. OTHER BEVERAGES

Normal hydration is achieved with a wide range of fluid intakes by humans across the life span. Maintaining fluid homeostasis during physical work and heat stress can be challenging. As stated earlier, body water composes 50% to 70% of body weight. Approximately 5%-10% of total body water is turned over daily via obligatory losses. The greater the fluid losses (from nonemergent situations, not medical or surgical), the longer the time it will take for rehydration (4% weight loss may take up to 24 h to rehydrate), thus need for prevention and use of foods or fluids that may aid when more expedient rehydration is of importance.[22]

Body water is maintained by matching daily water loss with intake. To a small degree, metabolic water production also contributes to body hydration (metabolic hydration yields ~250ml/d). IOM has established an adequate intake of water to be 3.7 L/d for men and 2.7 L/d for women.[1] The Continuing Survey of Food Intakes by Individuals (CSFII) concluded that adults living in the United States receive about 25% of their daily fluid intake from foods.[23]

Maintaining fluid and electrolyte balance means that active individuals need to replace the water and electrolytes lost in sweat. This requires active individuals, regardless of age, to strive to hydrate well before exercise, drink fluids throughout exercise, and rehydrate once exercise is over. As outlined by the American College of Sports Medicine (ACSM) and the National Athletic Trainers Association (NATA) generous amounts of fluids should be consumed 24 hours before exercise and 400–600 mL of fluids should be consumed 2 hours before exercise (this is ~6 to 10 oz).[23] Physically active individuals should attempt to drink ~150–350 mL (6–12 oz) of fluid every 15–20 minutes during exercise. If exercise is of longer duration than 1 hour or occurs in a hot environment, sport drinks containing carbohydrate and sodium could be used. When exercise is over, most active individuals have some level of dehydration. Drinking enough fluids to cover ~150% of the weight lost during exercise may be needed to replace fluids lost in sweat and urine. This fluid can be part of the postexercise meal, which should also contain sodium, either in foods or beverages, since diuresis (fluid losses) occurs when only plain water is ingested. Sodium helps the rehydration process by maintaining plasma osmolality and the desire to drink.

The fluid content of foods should not be underestimated or underappreciated by health professionals. High water content foods include: (given as percentage of water by weight) iceburg lettuce (96%), cooked squash (94%), pickles (92%), cantaloupe (90%), orange (87%), apple (86%), and pear (84%) as compared with beefsteaks (50%), Cheddar cheese (37%), white bread (36%), cookies (4%), and nuts (~2%). Therefore, including the goal of five to nine fruits and vegetables in the daily diet per the national recommendations also assists with hydration.[24]

Prior to exercise some athletes drink beverages that contain >100 mmol/L NaCl to temporarily induce hyperhydration and thus also aid in rehydration. The addition of glycerol to the typical sports beverage or oral rehydration solution at a dose of 1.0 to 1.5 g/kg/body weight (BW) also assists in inducing hyperhydration.[25]

Nonwater sources of hydration include caffeinated beverages. Caffeine is stated to be a mild diuretic, however, the vast evidence indicates that caffeinated beverages hydrate to the same degree over a 24-h period as does water. Fiala and associates[26] have found that caffeine is often rumored to be a mild diuretic, while noting that caffeine itself can enhance exercise performance (typical dose at 5 mg/kg). This study utilized 10 athletics who completed 2-a-day practices (2 hr/p = 4 hr/d) for 3 consecutive days at 23°C (73°F). This study utilized a randomized double-blind design offering of caffeine as a rehydration agent versus no caffeine (Coca-Cola® vs. the caffeine-free version). These researchers noted no evidence to show that caffeine intake impairs rehydration. No differential effects on urine or plasma osmolality, plasma volume, hematocrit, hemoglobin, or body weight were observed. The caffeine content of the cola was ~244 mg caffeine/d served in ~7cans/d of soda (~35 mg caffeine/12 oz.).[26] Grandjean and associates conducted a study with 18 men using a randomized crossover design with a free-living 24-hour capture design. The study tested four beverages (carbonated, caffeine caloric cola, non-caloric caffeinated cola, and coffee) and measured their respective effects on 24-h hydration status. These researchers collected urine for 24 h and analyzed for electrolytes, body weight, osmolality, hemoglobin, hematocrit, blood urea nitrogen, creatinine, and other biomarkers. The results clearly denoted no differences among the groups with regard to any variable. Thus, one can now consider caffeine-containing beverages to add to hydration.[27]

Recent data supports the inclusion of small amounts of protein with carbohydrates for hydration recovery. In 2001, in a double-blind study, 10 endurance-trained men ingested isocaloric carbohydrate (CHO, 152.7 g) and carbohydrate-protein (CHO-PRO, 112 g CHO with 40.7 g PRO) drinks following the consumption of a glycogen-lowering diet and exercise bout (run) and the ergogenic effects determined. Two dosages of one or the other of these drinks were ingested with a 60-min interval between dosages. The CHO-PRO trial resulted in the men's having significantly higher ($p<0.05$) serum insulin levels (60.84 vs. 30.1 mU/ml) 90 min into recovery than the CHO only trial. Furthermore, the time to run to exhaustion was longer during the CHO-PRO trial (540.7 ± 91.56 sec) than the CHO-only trial (446.1 ± 97.09 sec, $p<0.05$). In conclusion, the CHO-PRO drink following glycogen-depleting exercise may facilitate a greater rate of muscle glycogen resynthesis than a CHO-only beverage, may hasten the recovery process and improve exercise endurance during a second bout of exercise performed on the same day.[28] Subsequent studies have found that adding protein in the ratio of 1 part protein to every 4 parts carbohydrate has been found to induce exercise hydration on the magnitude of 15% better than the typical carbohydrate beverage and 40% more than water alone.[29,30]

A study by Seifert and associates[30] concluded that "contrary to popular misconception, adding protein to a carbohydrate-based sports drink … led to improved water retention by 15% over [a carbohydrate-only sports drink] and 40% over plain water." In this study, cyclists exercised until they lost 2% of their body weight (through sweating) and then drank either a carbohydrate-protein sports drink (Accelerade®), a carbohydrate-only sports drink (Gatorade®), or water. Over the next 3 hours, measurements were taken to determine how much of each beverage was retained in the body (vs. the amount lost through urination). The carbohydrate-protein sports drink was found to rehydrate the athletes 15% better than the carbohydrate-only sports drink and 40% better than water. All three drinks emptied from the stomach and were absorbed in the intestine at the same rate. In addition, there was no difference between the carbohydrate-protein drink and the carbohydrate-only drink in terms of effects on blood plasma volume. This suggests that the carbohydrate-protein drink resulted in increased water retention within and between cells. Therefore, a carbohydrate-protein sports drink may be a preferable choice over plain water and a carbohydrate-electrolyte sports drink, when rehydration and fluid retention are a concern.

An additional sports application study by Seifert and associates[31] found that "ingestion of a carbohydrate-protein beverage minimized muscle damage indices during skiing as compared to placebo and no fluid." Thirty-one recreational skiers were separated into three groups. All three groups skied 12 runs, which took about 3 hours. One group drank nothing. A second group drank 6 ounces of a placebo (flavored water) after every second run. A third group drank an equal amount of the carbohydrate-protein sports drink (Accelerade). After the 12th run, blood samples were taken from each skier and analyzed for two biomarkers of muscle stress (myoglobin and creatine kinase). The subjects that received the carbohydrate-protein sports drink showed no signs of muscle damage, while indicators of muscle damage increased by 49% in subjects receiving only water.[31] Thus, in this type of sport, using a carbohydrate-protein drink was found to be more beneficial than water for maintaining skeletal integrity and hydration.

Typically, hydration and rehydration for athletes is done with a 6% to 8% glucose-electrolyte solution. Newer research indicates that adding just a small amount of protein to this type of sports beverage not only enhances hydration and rehydration (or hydration maintenance), it also promotes muscle protein synthesis (which does not happen with CHO alone) and glycogen reaccumulation while reducing markers of muscle damage. Therefore, the use of these beverages is gaining popularity for the many benefits that appear to make them superior to the typical sports beverage during exercise and postexercise nutrition.

IX. FLUID REPLACEMENT RECOMMENDATIONS

Fluid replacement is essential for individuals who are vigorously active, as discussed earlier in this chapter. Fluid intake is increased by flavoring of the water or of the beverage. Research demonstrates that flavored beverages are ingested at a greater volume as compared to unflavored.[32] In general, the following fluid recommendations is used by sports nutritionists:[33,34]

- 16–20 oz. fluid: 1–2 hours pre-exercise.
- 10–16 oz. fluid: 15 minutes pre-exercise.
- 4–6 oz. fluid every 10–15 minutes during exercise.
- Generally increase fluid intake 24 hours prior to exercise event.

The fluid intake coming from food must also be considered, however, during the postexercise recovery period, hydration is best achieved by the ingestion of either the typical glucose-electrolyte solution or a carbohydrate-protein mixture. However, if the exercise has a duration of less than 60 to 75 min, then water (can be flavored) is recommended. There are no proven ergogenic effects or benefits from vitamin- or mineral-enriched waters except that they do provide absorbable nutrients at lower caloric costs than some foods.

Drinking beverages with sodium (20-50 $mEq{\cdot}L^{-1}$) or small amounts of salted snacks or foods containing sodium at meals will help stimulate thirst and retain the consumed fluids.[35] IOM recommends that fluid replacement beverages contain ~20–30 $meq{\cdot}L^{-1}$ sodium (chloride as the anion), ~2-5 $meq{\cdot}L^{-1}$ potassium, and 5-10% carbohydrate.[36] The need for these electrolytes ad carbohydrates depends on the specific exercise task (intensity and duration) and weather conditions.[37] These components can also be acquired from nonfluid sources such as energy bars and gels.

Athletes may consider noting the volume of their beverage intake so that they can become more familiar with how the body responds to rehydration. Doing this will allow the athlete to personalize his or her fluid intake noting just what types of beverages result in improved recovery as measured by hydration, return to normal body weight, subsequent exercise performance, and effects on mental abilities and cognition.

X. CONCLUSIONS

Fluid replacement is of importance to individuals of all ages. Physical performance increases the metabolic rate. Energy production leads to heat loss and fluid status is affected. Many individuals do not recognize the importance of the body's being hydrated. In cold climates, the thermoregulatory response includes enhanced heat production by a variety of means; all result in increased fluid losses. Exercising in temperate climates is actually a little easier on the body, as the accommodation response is to increase blood volume and sweating mechanism sensitivity. Athletes and their trainers and coaches must be cognizant about changes in body temperature and changes in blood volume—in other words, they need to have a good understanding of the physiological impacts of exercise and the climate. Elevated temperature is related to blood volume reduction and physical performance. Maintaining fluid balance reduces the effects of climate or blood volume on hydration status. For exercising lasting less than an hour, water or noncaloric fluid is recommended. It is not well known if "non-intensive" exercise requires that the rehydration solution include carbohydrate and electrolytes; most data notes no need for the calories and salts with short-term exercise bouts. If the exercise is longer in duration, maintaining hydration and rehydration is of great importance. The types of beverages that have been found to be beneficial in enhancing rehydration include carbohydrate-electrolyte solutions/beverages and carbohydrate-protein beverages. Caffeinated beverages with and without calories have also been found to aid in hydration and rehydration. In the immediate postexercise period, data are mounting that carbohydrate-protein beverages seem to be the superior postexercise rehydration and recovery beverage. Multiple applications of this carbohydrate-protein beverage will be a focus of future research. These beverages must be acceptable with regard to taste or they likely will not be ingested by athletes and others who are physically active. Therefore, overcoming taste issues for beverages that contain protein when used during exercise is an issue for researchers and food scientists to overcome. In conclusion, maintaining euhydration and understanding how to rehydrate after exercise is an important aspect of sports nutrition that is under-discussed and under-appreciated.

REFERENCES

1. Institute of Medicine and Food and Nutrition Board, *Dietary Reference Intakes for Water, Potassium, Sodium, Chloride and Sulfate*, National Academies Press, Washington, DC, 2005.
2. Health effects of mild dehydration, 2nd International Conference on Hydration throughout Life. Dortmund, Germany. October 8–9, 2001. *Eur. J. Clin. Nutr.* 57, Suppl. 2, 2003.
3. Manz, F., Hydration and disease. *J. Am. Coll. Nutr.* 26(5), 535s–41s, 2007.
4. Hydration and health promotion, ILSI North America Conference on Hydration and Health Promotion, November 29–30, 2006. *J. Am. Coll. Nutr.* 26, (5 Suppl.), 2007.
5. Welch, B. E., Bursick, E. R., and Iampietro, P. F., Relation of climate and temperature to food and water intake in man, *Metabolism* 7, 141–58, 1958.
6. Bullers, A. C., Bottled water: Better than tap? USFDA, Rockville, MD, 2002. www.fda.gov/fdac/features/2002/402_h2o. html. Accessed Sept. 12, 2008.

7. Senay, L. C., Water and electrolytes during physical activity, in *Nutrition in Exercise and Sport*, 3rd ed., CRC Press, Boca Raton, FL. 1998, pp 258–273.
8. Guyton, A. C., *Textbook of Medical Physiology*, 8th ed. W. B. Saunders, Philadelphia, 1991, p 799.
9. McKinley, M. J. and Johnson, A. K., The physiological regulation of thirst and fluid intake. *News in Physiol. Sci.* 19(1):1–6, 2004.
10. Manz, F., Hydration and disease. *J. Am. Coll. Nutr.* 26(5), 535s–41s, 2007.
11. Sharp, R. L., Role of sodium in fluid homeostasis with exercise, *J. Am. Coll. Nutr.* 25, 231s–9s, 2006.
12. Whiting, P. H. and Maughan, R. L., Dehydration and serum biochemical changes in marathon runners, *Eur. J. Appl. Physiol.* 52, 183–7, 1984.
13. Maughan, R. J., Fluid and electrolyte loss and replacement in exercise, *J. Sports Sci.* 9, 117–42, 1991.
14. Murray, B., Hydration and physical performance, *Am. Coll. Nutr.* 26(5), 542s–8s, 2006.
15. Grandjean, A. C. Dehydration and cognitive performance, *J. Am. Coll. Nutr.* 26(5), 549s–54s, 2006.
16. Lieberman, H. R. Hydration and cognition: A critical review and recommendations for future research, *J. Am. Coll. Nutr.* 26(5), 555s–61s, 2007.
17. Cian, C., Koulmann, N., Barraud, P., Raphel, C., Jimeniz, C., and Meli, B., Influence of variations on body hydration on cognitive function: Effect of hyperhydration, heat stress, and exercise-induced dehydration. *J. Psychophysiol.* 14, 29–36, 2000.
18. Posner, B. M., Jette, A. M., Smith, K. W., and Miller, D. R., Nutrition and health risks in the elderly: The nutritional screening initiative, *Am. J. Public Health* 83(7), 972–8, 1993.
19. Zembrzuski, C. D., A three-dimensional approach to hydration of elders: Administration, clinical staff, and in-service education. *Ger. Nurs.* 18(1), 20–6, 1997.
20. Zembrzuski, C. D., Hydration assessment checklist, *Ger. Nurs.* 18(1), 20–6, 1997.
21. Armstrong, L. E., Assessing hydration status: The elusive gold standard, *J. Am. Coll. Nutr.* 26(5), 575s–584s, 2006.
22. Kenefick, R. W. and Sawka, M., Hydration at the work site, *J. Am. Coll. Nutr.* 26(5), 597s–603s, 2006.
23. Heller, K. E., Sohn, W., Burt, B. A., and Eklund, S. A., Water consumption in the United States in 1995–1996 and implications for water fluoridation policy, *J. Publ. Health Dent.* 59, 3–11, 1999.
24. Departments of Health and Human Services and of Agriculture. Dietary Guidelines for Americans. http://www.health.gov/dietaryguidelines/dga2005/document/default.htm. Accessed May 13, 2008.
25. Shirreffs, S. M., Armstrong, L. E., and Cheuvront, S. N., Fluid and electrolyte needs for preparation and recovery from training and competition, *J. Sports Sci.* 22, 57–63, 2004.
26. Fiala, K. A., Casa, D. J., and Roti, M. W., Rehydration with a caffeinated beverage during the nonexercise periods of 3 consecutive days of 2-a-day practices, *Int. J. Sport Nutr. Exerc. Metab.* 14, 419–429, 2004.
27. Grandjean, A. C., Reimers, K. J., Bannick, K. E., and Haven, M. C., The effect of caffeinated, non-caffeinated, caloric and non-caloric beverages on hydration, *J. Am. Coll. Nutr.* 19(5), 591–600, 2000.
28. Niles, E. S., Lachowetz, T., Garfi, J., Sullivan, W., Smith, J. C., Leyh, B. P., and Headley, S. A. . Carbohydrate-protein drink improves time to exhaustion after recovery from endurance exercise. *J. Exerc. Physiol. online* 4(1), 45–52, 2001.
29. Ivy, J. L., Goforth, H. W., Jr., Damon, B. M., McCauley, T. R., Parsons, E. C., and Price, T. B., Early postexercise muscle glycogen recovery is enhanced with a carbohydrate-protein supplement, *J. Appl. Physiol.* 93(4),1337–44, 2002.

30. Seifert, J. G., Harmon, J., and DeClercq, P., Protein added to a sports drink improves fluid retention, *Intern. J. Sports Nut. Exerc. Metab.* 16, 420–9, 2006.
31. Seifert, J. G., Kipp, R. W., Amann, M. and Gazal, O., Muscle damage, fluid ingestion, and energy supplementation during recreational alpine skiing, *Intern. J. Sports Nutr. Exerc. Metab.* 15, 528–36, 2005.
32. Minehan, M. R., Riley, M. D., and Burke, L. M., Effect of flavor and awareness of kilojoule content of drinks on preference and fluid balance in team sports, *Int. J. Sports Nutr. Exerc. Metab.* 12, 81–92, 2002.
33. Pivarnik, J. M., Water and electrolytes during exercise, *Nutrition in Exercise and Sports*, CRC Press, Boca Raton, FL, 1989.
34. McArdle, W. D., Katch, F. I., and Katch, V. L., *Sports & Exercise Nutrition.* Lippincott Williams & Wilkens, Philadelphia, 1999, pp. 275–6.
35. Maughan, R. J., Leiper, J. B., and Shirreff, S. M., Restoration of fluid balance after exercise-induced dehydration: Effects of food and fluid intake, *Eur. J. Appl. Physiol.* 73, 317–25, 1996.
36. Committee on Military Nutrition Research, Food and Nutrition Board, Institute of Medicine, *Fluid Replacement and Heat Stress*, National Academy Press, Washington, DC, 1994.
37. Sawka, M. N., Burke, L. M., Eichner, E. R., Maughan, R. J., Montain, S. J., and Stachenfeld, N. S., American College of Sports Medicine Position Stand: Exercise and fluid replacement, *Med. Sci. Sports Exerc.* 39, 377–90, 2007.

Section VI

Other Commonly Consumed Substances

12 Caffeine and Tannins

Jay Kandiah and Valerie A. Amend

CONTENTS

I. CAFFEINE

A. Introduction

Although the use of caffeine and tannins from food and beverages has been in existence for many centuries, recently their recognition in the scientific arena has gained much popularity.[1,2] Several animal and human studies have demonstrated the effects of caffeine and or tannins in improving athletic performance and enhancing overall health status.[3–19] This chapter will focus primarily on research within the past 10 years and its implications on athletes. Even though scholarly evidence on the influence of caffeine/tannins in middle-aged recreational athletes is lacking, information extrapolated from research associated with other athletes will definitely add much-warranted value to the growing body of knowledge.

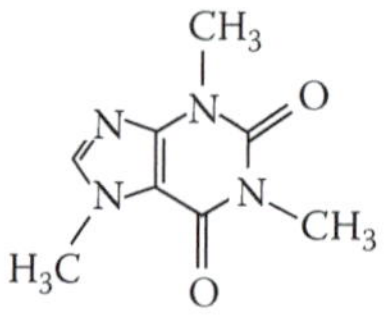

CH3 N N O N N CH3 H3C O

FIGURE 12.1 Structure of caffeine.

B. Structure

Caffeine (Figure 12.1) occurs naturally as a plant alkaloid.[1] It can be found in such species as *Caffea arabica, Thea sinenis*, and *Cola acuminate*; also known as coffee, tea, and cola, respectively.[1] Classification of caffeine as a methylxanthine puts it in the same family as theophyline and theobromine.[1]

C. General Properties

Caffeine, an odorless, bitter alkaloid, has no nutritional value, and is often classified as a drug.[1] Due to its lipophilic properties, caffeine has the ability to cross most cell membranes in the human body.[20] The drug's ability to cross the blood–brain barrier stimulates the central nervous system to release catecholamine, which causes a variety of physiological characteristics to be associated with this compound. [20]

D. Function and Metabolism

Caffeine is not stored in the body, but is excreted in the urine after ingestion.[21] Dunford and Doyle[22] stated that metabolism of caffeine occurs mainly in the liver using the cytochrome P450 enzyme system. It is degraded to dimethylxanthines, metabolites associated with increased metabolism. After consumption, the body quickly absorbs this drug. Keisler and Armsey[1] found that, in less than 20 minutes, 90% of the ingested substance is absorbed into the small intestine. According to Mangus et al.,[20] though half-life of caffeine may depend on an individual's metabolic ability, it usually takes between 2–15 hours. While a function of caffeine in the body is to inhibit adenosine's role as a vasodilator by binding to its receptors in the brain, it has been reported that this drug has reverse effect in the body.[1] Caffeine causes vasoconstriction and reduced blood flow, thereby increasing heart rate and blood pressure.[23] Since the effects of blood pressure may be more intense with hypertensive individuals, these factors should be taken into consideration before ingesting caffeine. Studies have also shown caffeine to increase mental acuity and epinephrine release.[23] Other factors, such as cigarette smoking and stress, may also exacerbate caffeine's effect on the cardiovascular system.[23] Although the hemodynamic effects of caffeine are similar between genders, the mechanism appears to be different. Research by Hartley et al.[24] found that, unlike females, in males, caffeine ingestion has resulted in increased vascular resistance. On the other hand, when women were given the same amount of caffeine as their male counterparts, they exhibited an increase in cardiac output due to higher stroke volume. Interestingly, these observations were not noted in men. Irrespective of gender, effects on the respiratory system, including bronchial dilation and pulmonary smooth muscle relaxation, have been observed among caffeine users.[1]

A viable area of interest among scientists has been caffeine's effect on the central nervous system (CNS) in enhancing athletic performance. Taylor et al.[25] reported that ingestion of caffeine prior to exercise is thought to provide a sudden burst of energy, and has been shown to increase metabolic rate. Mangus[20] indicated that stimulation of the CNS may prevent the brain from sensing fatigue caused by exercise. Strength in sports was attributed to increased calcium release into the muscle cells, thereby stimulating rapid and stronger contractions. In addition, stimulation of fatty acid has been possibly associated with fat oxidation and increased weight loss.[23] Unfortunately, to date the exact mechanism of caffeine's role in athletic performance has yet to be defined.

E. Dietary and Supplemental Sources

Caffeine, prevalent in chocolate, coffee, tea, colas, carbonated beverages, and chewing gum, occurs naturally or is synthetically produced.[26] Other items containing caffeine include over-the-counter stimulants, appetite suppressants, analgesics, cold and sinus medications, and some bottled waters.[1] New products reported by Dunford and Doyle [22] to be recently formulated to include caffeine include sports gels, sports candy such as Jolt Caffeine-Energy Gum and Buzz Bites, energy drinks, and some alcoholic beverages. In the United States, caffeine used to supplement foods must be stated on the ingredient list, while the exact amount in a food or beverage is often listed on the manufacturer's web site.[1] Approximately 75% of the caffeine consumed in the world is in the form of coffee. Research reveals an average American consumes 1–3 cups per day, and the amount of caffeine in coffee is based on the type and method of preparation.[26] Taylor et al.[25] found that 8 fluid ounces of coffee could provide between 65–150 milligrams of caffeine.

F. Nutrient Status Assessment and Dosage

Assessment for caffeine levels in the general population is administered by measuring urinary caffeine metabolites. Since metabolism of caffeine is affected by factors such as age, weight, and lean body mass, urinary excretion of caffeine is not a reliable assessment, especially for those involved in competitive sports.[20] Generally, ingesting 100 mg of caffeine will generate a 1.5 μg/ml urine concentration.[1] Table 12.1 shows sample products, caffeine content, and urinary metabolites within 2–3 hours of caffeine consumption. Due to genetic disposition, two athletes may produce different levels of urinary metabolites after ingesting the same amount of caffeine.[20] As such, the National Collegiate Athletic Association (NCAA) has an upper limit of 15μg/ml for those involved in athletic performances. In competitive sports, disqualification of athletes would arise after consumption of approximately 800 mg of caffeine prior to an event.[20] This would be equivalent to 6–8 cups of coffee or 7 Red Bulls. The ergogenic effects of caffeine start at levels as low as 250 mg. If athletes consumed less than the established standard of 15 μg/ml of urinary metabolites or 800 mg of caffeine, they might get some performance-enhancing effects without being disqualified.[20]

Caffeine use was banned entirely by the International Olympic Committee (IOC) until January 2, 2004.[23] Since then, the IOC has established an upper threshold limit

TABLE 12.1

Sample Products Containing Caffeine

Product	Dose of Caffeine	Urine concentration (Within 2–3 h)
1 cup coffee	80–135 mg	1.5 μg/ml
1 coke, 1 diet coke	45.6 mg	0.68 μg/ml
1 No doz caffeine pill	100 mg	1.5 μg/ml
1 Anacin	32 mg	0.48 μg/ml
1 Excedrin	65 mg	0.97 μg/ml

Adapted from:[27]

of 12 μg/ml, which could be achieved by ingesting 8 cups of coffee or 18 cans of coke, 8 NoDoz, 4 Vivarin, or 12 Excedrin pills. In addition, Mangus reported consumption of 3–6 mg/kg of body weight 1 hour prior to exercise has been demonstrated to elicit an ergogenic effect without violation of the IOC rules.[20]

In recreational athletes, ingestion of 180–450 mg of caffeine daily has exhibited properties such as improved mental and physical performance. Unfortunately, higher levels have resulted in undesirable side effects.[23]

G. Toxicity

In nonhabitual users, Rogers and Dinges[1] found ingestion of more than 180–450 mg of caffeine/d led to several side effects including: restlessness, anxiety, irritability, muscle tremors, sleeplessness, headaches, GI distress, arrhythmias, and seizures. However, habitual users may be less likely to experience the negative side effects associated with the drug.[29] Caffeine sensitivity is influenced by a variety of factors including body mass, previous history of consumption, age, smoking habits, illicit use of drugs, anxiety disorders, and stress.[20]

In athletes, caffeine may cause diuresis and lead to dehydration. Ingestion of less than 6 cups of coffee during long bouts of exercise caused delayed onset of diuresis.[23] Tachycardia, increased blood pressure, GI distress, and addiction toward caffeine have been associated with ingestion of this drug. Since exercise in itself increases heart rate, Kaminsky et al.[28] demonstrated that a combination of exercise and caffeine would exacerbate heart rate, thereby triggering a negative effect during athletic performance.

Withdrawal symptoms such as headache, fatigue, lethargy, and flu-like symptoms can be avoided if caffeine intake is weaned off gradually rather than stopped abruptly.[7] Table 12.2 provides tips to help alleviate caffeine withdrawal symptoms.

H. Interactions

Caffeine has a tendency to interact with a variety of drugs, resulting in a multitude of problems. Ephedra, a powerful stimulant, was banned in 2004 by the US Food

TABLE 12.2

Practical Tips to Lower Caffeine Content and Alleviate Withdrawal Symptoms

Read labels to know the amount of caffeine present in foods and beverages.
Reduce intake of caffeine gradually.
Replace caffeinated foods and beverages with decaffeinated versions.
Reduce brewing time of coffee and tea.
Check over-the-counter medications for caffeine content.

Adapted from:[29]

and Drug Administration.[12] Although the combined effect of these two drugs is to promote weight loss and increase performance, research has associated them with increased heart rate, blood pressure, cardiac infarction, and death.[29] Some antibiotics (e.g. ciproflaxin and norflaxin) may interfere with caffeine metabolism, resulting in delayed urinary caffeine excretion.[29] Theophyline, a bronchodilator, when taken together with caffeine may increase its concentration in the blood stream leading to nausea, vomiting, and heart palpitations.[29] Future research needs to focus on the interaction between caffeine and vitamins and minerals.

I. Effects on Physical Performance

Much research has been done to determine the effects of caffeine on physical performance. While studies have looked at glycogen sparing, CNS stimulation, catecholamine action, and free-fatty acid mobilization to explain the mechanism associated with the ergogenic effects of caffeine, there is insufficient consensus to postulate a theory to explain its benefits.[31] In the past, there have been very limited well-controlled randomized studies that have strongly associated caffeine consumption and athletic performance. Bruce et al.[33] looked at competitive rowing in a double blind placebo controlled study of 8 competitive rowers (mean age 22 ± 3 years). Caffeine supplementation (6–9mg) increased mean power and improved time in 2000-meter rowing events. Similarly, Stuart et al.[34] found significant improvements in speed and power in 9 competitive male rugby players (19–23 years) receiving 6 mg/kg caffeine. Of late, with the development of well-designed studies, there has been a strong relationship between caffeine ingestion and athletic performance.

Red Bull, an energy drink, is believed to enhance concentration, alertness, and improve reaction time.[6] To investigate the effectiveness of Red Bull, Forbes et al.[5] measured the effect of 2 mg/kg caffeine on muscle endurance and cycle performance of 15 young adults. Red Bull significantly improved upper body muscle endurance but had no significant effect on cycle performance. In addition, when compared with the placebo, Red Bull enhanced total bench press sets 34 ± 9 versus 32 ± 8 but failed to have any effect on cycle performance. Since Red Bull contains ingredients other than caffeine, researchers were unable to confirm the efficacy of caffeine. According to these results, Red Bull energy drink may be beneficial to those performing upper body exercises, but not necessarily for endurance activities. Further research needs to be performed to evaluate Red Bull's role in enhancing endurance activities.

In highly trained male cyclists, (27.5 ± 7 years) Cureton et al.[13] investigated the ergogenic effects of a sports drink containing caffeine. This double blind, placebo controlled, repeated measures experiment used 3 types of beverages, namely: (1) a placebo artificially flavored drink, (2) a 6% carbohydrate-electrolyte sports drink, and (3) a 7% carbohydrate-electrolyte sports drink with 195 mg/L of caffeine, 1.92 mg/L taurine, 46 mg/L carnitine, B vitamins, and sucralose. Results indicated, unlike the placebo, caffeine consumption significantly produced a greater amount of work, (218 ± 31 kJ vs. 190 ± 36 kJ), lower perceived rates of exertion, and less decreased maximal voluntary contraction strength. Similar observations were noted between caffeine ingestion and the 6% carbohydrate beverage. A meta-analysis of 414 participants, ages 27.1 ± 4.2 years, on enhancing exercise performance found that doses of 3–10 mg/kg had an impact on endurance.[14]

On the contrary, caffeine ingestion did not affect aerobic dance performance among recreationally active females (age 19–28).[11] There was no significant difference in VO_{2max}, VCO_{2max}, respiratory exchange ratio (RER), resting energy expenditure (REE), heart rate (HR), or perceived exertion in participants receiving the placebo, 3mg/kg, or 6-mg/kg-body weight of caffeine 1 hour prior to performance. Similarly, in college students, supplementation of 3.1 mg/kg caffeine and intense aerobic training had no effect on improvement in body composition.[9]

Interestingly, administration of 6 mg/kg of caffeine had no effect on initial sets of bench press or leg press.[10] However, after three sets, there was a significant increase in repetitions and higher peak heart rate. The authors attributed delay in fatigue to the involvement of either central or peripheral physiological mechanisms. Controversial findings were demonstrated by Lorino et al.[12] when 17 recreationally active adult males, (age 23.7 ± 2 years) received a placebo or 6-mg/kg caffeine, indicating that caffeine was ineffective on muscle power and athletic agility. Evidence from research findings is contradictory, which underlines a need for extensive research related to caffeinated products and their relationship to athletic performance.

J. Future Research Needs

With the growing body of knowledge related to several health benefits of caffeine, scientists should be encouraged to investigate the use of new caffeinated beverages and their influence on athletic performance. To ensure research linked to athletic performance, parameters that need to be taken into consideration in the development of scholarly endeavors would be variations in caffeine dose, use variety of age groups (e.g. middle age, older age), ethnically diverse populations, duration of research, side effects of caffeine, relationship of caffeine intake to health and athletic performance, and finally, the relationship between caffeine and other ergogenic aids.

II. TANNINS

I. Introduction

While caffeine has been the subject of much current research related to athletic performance, limited studies have investigated tannins use in physical activity. Contemporary research on this compound has focused mainly on health benefits of tea tannins such as in the prevention of cancer, inflammation, heart disease, hepatic necrosis, and dental cavities.[35] This section will speculate the role of tannins in athletic performance and goals for future research.

B. Structure

Tannins are intermediate- to high-molecular weight phenolic compounds.[36] Hydrolyzable tannins and proanthocyanidins (condensed tannins) are the two major groups of tannins found in plants.[36] Hyrolyzable tannins, found often in berries and nuts, contain a pylol (D-glucose) as the central core.[36] The hydroxyl groups are esterified, partially or completely, with phenolic groups such as gallic acid (Figure 12.2) to form gallotannins or ellagic acid to form ellagitanins.[37] Proanthocyanidins (commonly present in tea, coffee, red wine, and chocolate) are oligomers or polymers of catechins or epicatecins held together by C-C bonds, which are not cleaved by hydrolysis.[37] These are often referred to as condensed tannins, due to their more condensed chemical structure, and contain between 2 and 50 flavonoid units (Figure 12.3).[36] The major phenolic compounds found in green tea are the epicatechins including epigallocatechin-3-gallate (EGCG), epigallocatechin (ECG), and epicatechin (EC).[37] Another class of tannins, known as the derived tannins is formed during the manipulation and processing of tannins.[37] Derived tannins such as theaflavins in black tea have a benztropolone ring formed by the oxidation of the B ring ofEGC or EGCG.[37]

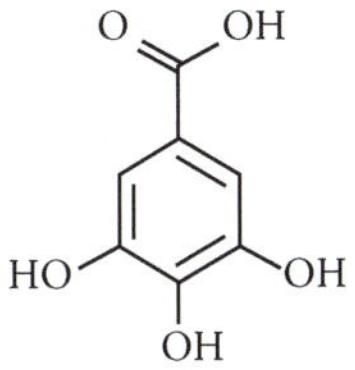

O OH
HO OH
OH

FIGURE 12.2 012x002.eps

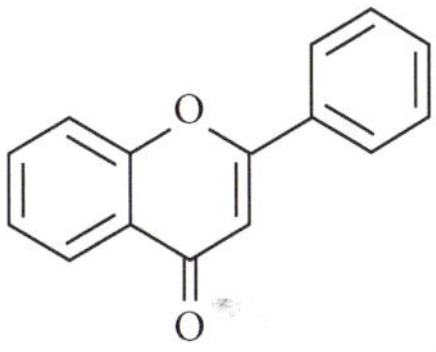

O
O

FIGURE 12.3 Flavone, base unit for condensed tannins.

C. General Properties

Tannins are soluble in water and are noted to interact with and form complexes with carbohydrates, proteins, polysaccharides, bacterial cell membranes, and enzymes.[36] They have high affinity for proline-rich proteins and salivary proline-rich proteins.[36] When bound to mouth proteins, they impart a distinctively astringent taste sensation.[38] Hydrolyzable tannins can be degraded by mild acids or bases to produce carbohydrates and phenolic acids, or by hot water and enzymes.[38] On the other hand, proanthocyanidins are non-hydrolyzable.[39]

D. Function and Metabolism

The metabolisms of the two main types of tannins differ greatly. While hydrolyzable tannins are absorbed after ingestion and bound to proteins, condensed tannins are unabsorbed from the gastrointestinal tract and are complexed to salivary proline-rich protein during transit from the alimentary canal. [39]

Tannins have been widely recognized for their antioxidant properties, especially their ability to scavenge reactive oxygen species.[15] Catechins also prevent low-density lipoprotein oxidation by recycling other antioxidants (e.g. vitamin E).[19] Though literature reveals inconsistencies in the efficacy of tea in the prevention of cardiovascular disease, there have been proposed mechanisms for its use. Tea polyphenols may have the ability to inhibit the oxidation of low-density lipoprotein (LDL) and decrease adenosine diphosphate (ADP)-induced platelet aggregation.[15] To date, no research has been conducted to examine the effectiveness of tea in preventing heart disease in athletes. However, the ability to inhibit LDL oxidation and reduce platelet aggregation may encourage physically active individuals to consider tea as an alternative to other ergogenic aids.[40]

E. Dietary and Supplemental Sources

The recommended intake for polyphenols is approximately 150–300 mg per day.[37] This can be found in 5 or more servings of fruits and vegetables, various supplemental forms of the compounds, or in teas.[37] Current interest in the health benefits of tea extract has led to its inclusion in nutritional supplements and topical ointments, while tea consumption remains a common source for tannins.[37] Originating in China, tea is made from the infusion of a plant, *Camellia sinensis*, native to Southeast Asia.[40] The tea plant, now cultivated in many countries around the world, is derived from the evergreen shrub of the Theaceae family.[40] Black tea, especially popular in Western countries, is the most commonly consumed tea in the world (78% of consumption). Green tea, responsible for 20% of total tea consumption, is a favorite in Asian, Middle Eastern, and North African countries. Oolong tea, much less common (2% of tea intake) is mainly consumed in Taiwan and southern China.[41] The composition of tea leaves reflects seasonal and climactic conditions, type of species, and horticultural practices.[42] The manufacturing and processing of the tea leaves is responsible for the differences in black, green, and oolong teas.[43] Green tea is produced by preventing fermentation. Freshly harvested tea leaves are pan fried or steamed to denature the enzymes, creating dry fresh tea leaves. During black tea manufacturing, fresh leaves are withered so that the moisture content is reduced 50%, resulting in a high concentration of polyphenols remaining in the leaves, which are then crushed and fermented. Oolong tea is processed similarly to black tea; however it is only partially fermented, resulting in a tea that consists of both green tea catechins and black tea theaflavins.[43]

F. Toxicity

Because most teas contain caffeine as well as tannins, those with sensitivity or allergies to either of these substances should avoid consumption as it may cause constipation and iron deficiency.[2] People with peptic ulcers may also need to avoid drinking this beverage as it can increase the production of stomach acid.[2]

G. Interactions

Interactions with tea have not been well studied. Since tannins often contain caffeine, simultaneous ingestion of certain drugs or herbal supplements along with products containing tannins may cause a variety of physiological effects. (Table 12.3)

H. Effects on Physical Performance

The effects of tannins on physical performance have not been the subject of extensive research. While the other benefits of tannins have been examined, further research is needed in the area of ergogenic potential of tannins and teas.

Tannins have been examined for their effect on balance performance,[44] platelet activation,[45] thermogenesis,[18] energy expenditure,[17] and metabolic parameters.[16] Tannins in tea have also recently been studied for a variety of other possible health benefits.[2] Short-term intervention strategies on human subjects with elevated blood pressure have revealed that black or green tea ingestion had no effect on lipid peroxidation.[46] These results indicate that the antioxidant properties of tea may aid in

TABLE 12.3

Drugs and Herbal Supplements plus Tannins and Physiological Effects

Drug or Herbal Supplement + Tannins	Physiological Effect
Ephedra	↑Blood pressure, stroke, heart attack, abnormal heart rhythms, insomnia, anxiety, headache, irritability, blurred vision
Benzodiazepines (e.g. ativan, valium)	↑Alertness
Disulfiram (e.g. antabuse)	↓Urinary excretion of caffeine
Oral contraceptives, HRT	↑Effectiveness of drug
Antibiotics (e.g. ciproflaxin, norflaxin. fluvoxamine)	↑Caffeine levels and length of time caffeine acts in the body
Dexamethasone (Decadron)	↑Urinary excretion of caffeine
Carbamazepine	↑Effectiveness of drug
Acetaminophen (aspirin)	↑Effectiveness of drug
Diuretics (furosemide)	↑Effectiveness of drug
Warfarin (coumadin)	↓ Effectiveness of drug
Guarnana (cola nut)	↑Effectiveness of drug
Yerba mate	↑Effectiveness of drug

Adapted from: [2]

the prevention of oxidative damage, possibly enhancing athletic performance. Other health benefits recently investigated include:[6]

- Asthma treatment
- Cancer prevention
- Dental cavities prevention
- Heart attack prevention
- Memory enhancement
- Mental performance alertness
- Methicillin-resistant staphylococcus aureus infection
- Osteoporosis prevention

I. Future Research Needs

Using well-controlled double blind randomized studies; researchers should investigate the effectiveness of tannins and their impact on athletic performance. Some areas of interest include tannins' influence on specific type of performance, inclusion of wide variety of population, and integration of gender. Potential avenues for research may include types of tannins, dose variations, time of day supplement or tannins were consumed, duration of supplementation, and inclusion or exclusion of exercise prior to tannin ingestion. Such research would contribute tremendously to the scientific community and the public at large.

III. CONCLUSIONS

Caffeine is found in a wide range of products and supplements and its potential as an ergogenic aid has been the subject of great curiosity in the sports community in the last several years. Caffeine's stimulant effects on the central nervous system and possible benefits to performance have facilitated much research in this area. Although many recent studies have shown a positive effect for athletes, others indicate no benefits to performance with caffeine supplementation, and there are side effects with excessive intake and drug interactions. Practical application to recreational athletes is still unclear, as there has been little to no research in this area. If recreational athletes are to experience benefits associated with athletic performance, exercise scientists and professionals interested in sports performance need to speculate, develop, and implement randomized controlled studies that would be applicable to the general public.

Tannins are phenolic compounds found naturally in many beverages, fruits, vegetables, and various other products. Although there are several ongoing studies, the potential health benefits of tannins, have yet to be well substantiated. It is hoped that, in the future, tannins' antioxidant capabilities may associate this important characteristic with athletic performance.

REFERENCES

1. Keisler, B. D. and Armsey, T. D., Caffeine as an ergogenic aid, *Cur. Sports Med. Rep.* 5, 215–119, 2006.
2. National Library of Medicine Website, Black Tea (*Camellia sinensis*). http://www.nlm.nih.gov/medlineplus/print/druginfo/natural/patient–black_tea.html. Accessed on 1/11/2008.
3. Roberts, A. T., de Jonge-Levitan, L., Parker, C. C., and Greenway, F. L., The effect of an herbal supplement containing black tea and caffeine on metabolic parameters in humans, *Alt. Med. Rev.* 10, 321–325.
4. Norager, C. B., Jensen, M. B., Weimann, A., and Madsen, M. R., Metabolic effects of caffeine ingestion and physical work in 75 year old citizens. A randomized, double blind, placebo-controlled, cross-over study, *Clin. Endocrinol.* 65, 223–228.
5. Forbes. S. C., Candow, D. G., Little, J. P., Magnus, C., and Chilibeck, P. D., Effect of Red Bull energy drink on repeated Wingate cycle performance and bench-press muscle endurance, *Int. J. Sport Nutr. and Exerc. Met.* 17, 433–444, 2007.
6. Alford, C., Cox, H., and Wescott, R., The effects of Red Bull energy drink on performance and mood, *Amino Acids.* 21, 139–150, 2000.
7. Jacobs, I., Pasternak, H., and Bell, D. G., Effects of ephedrine, caffeine, and their combination on muscular endurance, *Med. Sci. Sport. Exerc.* 35, 987–994, 2003.
8. Westerterp-Plantenga, M. S., Lejeune, M. P. G. M., Kovacs, E. M. R., Body weight loss and weight maintenance in relation to habitual caffeine intake and green tea supplementation, *Obesity Res.* 13, 1195–1204.
9. Malek, M. H., Housh, T. J., Coburn, J. W., Beck, T. W., Schmidt, R. J., and Housh, D. J., Johnson, G. O., Effects of eight weeks of caffeine supplementation and endurance training on aerobic fitness and body composition, *J. Strength Cond. Res.* 20, 751–755, 2006.
10. Green, M. J., Wickwire, P. J., McLester, J. R., Gendle, S., Hudson, G., Pritchett, R. C., Laurent, C. M., Effects of caffeine on repetitions to failure and ratings of perceived exertion during resistance training, *Int. J. of Sp. Phys. Perf.* 2, 250–259, 2007.
11. Ahrens, J. N., Lloyd, L. K., Crixell, S. H., and Walker, J. L., The effects of caffeine in women during aerobic-dance bench stepping, *Int. J. Sp. Nutr. and Exerc. Met.* 17, 27–34, 2007.
12. Lorino, A. J., Lloyd, L. K., Crixell, S. H., and Walker, J. L., The effects of caffeine on athletic agility, *J. Strength Cond. Res.* 20, 851–854, 2006.
13. Cureton, K. J., Warren, G. L, Millard-Stafford, M. L., Wingo, J. E., Trilk, J., Buyckx, M., Caffeinated sports drink: Ergogenic effects and possible mechanisms, *Int. J. Sport Nutr. Exerc. Met.* 17, 35–55, 2007.
14. Doherty, M. and Smith, Paul M., Effects of caffeine on exercise testing: A meta-analysis, *Int. J. Sport Nutr. Exerc. Met.* 14, 626–646, 2004.
15. Wiseman, S. A., Balentine, D. A., Kuo, M. C., and Schantz, S. P., Antioxidants in tea, *Crit. Rev. Food Sci. Nutr.* 37, 705–718, 1997.
16. Singh, I., Quinn, H., Mok, M., Southgate, R. J., Turner, A. H., Li, D., Sinclair, A. J., and Hawley, J. A., The effect of exercise and training on platelet activation: Do cocoa polyphenols play a role, *Platelets.* 17, 361–367, 2006.
17. Belza, A. and Jessen, A. B., Bioactive food stimulants of sympathetic activity: Effect on 24-h energy expenditure and fat oxidation, *Eur. J. Clin. Nutr.* 59, 733–741, 2005.
18. Dulloo, A. G., Seydoux, J., Girardier, L, Chantre, P., Vandermander, J., Green tea and thermogenesis: Interactions between catechin-polyphenols, caffeine, and sympathetic activity, *Int. J. Obesity.* 24, 252–258, 2000.
19. Zhu, Q. Y., Huang, Y., Tsang, D., Chen, Z. Y., Regeneration of α-tocopherol in human low density lipoprotein by green tea catechin, *J. Agric. Food Chem.,* 47, 2020–2025, 1999.

20. Mangus, B. C. and Throwbridge, C. A., Will caffeine work as an ergogenic aid? The latest research, *Ath. Ther. Tod.* 10, 57–62.
21. Caffeine in the Diet. UT Medical Center Website, http://www.utmedicalcenter.org/adam/health%20illustrated%20encyclopedia/1/002445.ht Accessed 1/9/2008.
22. Dunford, M. D. and Doyle, J. A., *Nutrition for Sport Exercise.* Thomson Wadsworth, U. S., 2008, pp. 323–326.
23. Supplement Watch Website, Caffeine. http://www.supplementwatch.com/suplib/supplementPrintFriendlyasp. Accessed 1/13/2008.
24. Hartley, T. R., Lovallo, W. R., Whitsett, T. L., Cardiovascular effects of caffeine in men and women, *Am. J. Cardiol. 93,* 1022–1026, 2004.
25. Taylor, L. W., Wilborn, C. D., Harvey, T., Wiseman, J., and Willoughby, D. S., Acute effect of ingesting Java Fit energy extreme functional coffee on resting energy expenditure and hemodynamic responses in male and female coffee drinkers, *J. Int. Soc. Sport Nutr.* 4:10, 2007.
26. National Library of Medicine Website, Medical Encyclopedia: Caffeine in the Diet. U. S. http://www.nlm.nih.gov.medlineplus/print/ency/article/002445.htm. Accessed 1/13/2008.
27. University of Michigan Health System Website, Caffeine and Athletic Performance. http://www.med.umich.edu/1libr/sma/sma_caffeine_sma.htm. Accessed 1/9/2008.
28. Kaminsky, L. A., Martin, C. A., Whaley, M. H., Caffeine consumption habits do not influence the exercise blood pressure response following caffeine ingestion, *J. Sports Med. Phys. Fitness.* 38, 53–58, 1998.
29. Caffeine: How Much is too Much? Mayo Clinic Website, http://www.MayoClinic.com. Accessed 1/9/2008.
30. UT Medical Center Website, Caffeine in the Diet. http://www.utmedicalcenter.org/adam/health%20illustrated%20encyclopedia/1/002445.ht Accessed 1/9/2008.
31. Williams, M., *Nutrition for Health, Fitness, & Sport,* New York: McGraw-Hill, 2007, pp. 485–491.
32. Graham, T., Caffeine, coffee, and ephedrine: Impact on exercise performance and metabolism, *Can. J. App. Phys.* 26, 103–119, 2001.
33. Bruce, C., Enhancement of 2000m-rowing performance after caffeine ingestion, *Med. Sci. Sports Exerc.* 32, 2000.
34. Stuart, G., Multiple effects of caffeine on simulated high intensity team-sport performance, *Med. Sci. Sports Exerc.* 37, 2005.
35. Manach, C., Scalbert, A., Morand, C., Remesey, C., and Jimenez, L., Polyphenols: Food sources and bioavailability, *Am. J. Clin. Nutr.* 79, 727–747, 2004.
36. Cornell Website, Tannins: Chemical Structure. http://www.ansci.cornell.edu/plants/toxicagents/tannin/chemical.html. Accessed 1/9/2008.
37. Supplement Watch Website, Flavonoids. http://www.supplementwatch.com/suplib/supplementPrintFriendly.asp. Accessed 1/9/2008.
38. Reidl, K. M., Carando, S., Alessio, H. M., McCarthy, M., and Hagerman, A. E., Antioxidant activity of tannins and tannin–protein complexes: Assessment *in vitro* and *in vivo.* American Chemical Society 88–200, 2002, chap 14.
39. Cornell Website, Tannins: Interaction with other Molecules. http://www.ansci.cornell.edu/plants/toxicagents/tannin/ineraction.html. Accessed 1/9/2008.
40. Higdon, J. V. and Frei, B., Tea catechins and polyphenols: Health effects, metabolism, and antioxidant functions, *Crit. Rev. Food Sci. Nutr.* 43, 89–143, 2003.
41. Katiyar, S. K., Mukthar, H., Tea in chemoprevention of cancer: Epidemiologic and experimental studies, *Int. J. Oncol.,* 8, 221–38, 1996.
42. Lin, J. K., Liang, Y. C., and Lin-Shiau, S. Y., Survey of catechins, gallic acid, and methylxantines in green, oolong, pu-erh and black teas, *J. Agric. Food Chem.* 46, 3635–3642, 1998.

43. Lin, Y.-S., Tsai, Y.-J., Tsay, J.-S., and Lin, J.-K., Factors affecting levels of tea polyphenols and caffeine in tea leaves, *J. Agric. Food Chem.,* 51, 1864–1873, 2003.
44. Zhou, B. and Lovegren, M., Effect of oolong tea on balance performance in naïve tea users–A pilot study, *J. Exerc. Phys. Online.* 10, 43–50, 2007
45. Singh, I., Quinn, H., Mok, M., Southgate, R. J., Turner, A. H., Li, D., Sinclair, A. J., and Hawley, J. A., The effect of exercise and training on platelet activation: Do cocoa polyphenols play a role, *Platelets.* 17, 361–367, 2006.
46. Hodgson, J. M., Croft, K. D., Mori, A., Burke, V., Beilin, L. J., and Puddey, I. B., Regular ingestion of tea does not inhibit *in vivo* lipid peroxidation in humans, *J. Nutr.* 132, 55–58, 2002.

13 Herbal Supplements

Jidong Sun and David W. Giraud

CONTENTS

I. INTRODUCTION

Herbal supplements have gained popularity and acceptance during the past decade. The Eisenberg Survey[1] of 1,539 adults showed that an increase in herbal supplement use from 2.5% in 1990 to 12.1% in 1997. The Slone Survey (http://www.bu.edu/slone/SloneSurvey/SloneSurvey.htm), a telephone survey investigating dietary supplement use among 8,470 adults, reported that the annual prevalence of herbal supplement use increased from 14.2% in 1998 to 18.8% in 2002. Although use among younger subjects (18–44 years old) was relatively low, the highest prevalence was in those aged 45 to 64 years, especially in women. Between 1998 and 2002, use of herbal supplement among women aged 45 to 64 years increased from 23.5% to 28.7%.[2]

Athletes or individuals who exercise regularly also take herbal supplements. Ziegler et al.[3] showed that 44% of male figure skaters and 48% of female figure skaters used some forms of herbal supplements. While male skaters were more likely to use ginseng, ginkgo, and other herbs, female skaters were more likely to use ginseng and echinacea. Herbold et al.[4] reported that 17% of female collegiate athletes used herbal supplements. Echinacea was the most frequently used herbal supplement (13.7%), followed by ginseng (6.2%) and Ciwujia (*Eleutherococcus*, 3.7%). Froiland et al.[5] reported 26% of college athletes used herbal supplements. Ginseng and echinacea were the most popular herbal supplements at 13% and 9.7%, respectively, followed by MaHuang/ephedra (6.3%) and ginkgo (3.9%). Morrison et al.[6] revealed that 19.4% of individuals who exercised at a commercial gym used herbal supplements. MaHuang/ephedra was consumed by 27.9% of participants at least once per week, followed by ginseng (16.2%) and other herbs (3.6%).

The main reasons given by male figure skaters for taking supplements were: to provide more energy (41%), to prevent illness or disease (34%), and to enhance performance (21%). Among female figure skaters, the main reasons given were: to prevent illness or disease (61%), to provide more energy (39%), and to make up for an inadequate diet (28%).[3] In his study, Froiland et al.[5] reported that over 40% of athletes took supplements for "their health" (43.5%), to improve strength and power (42.5%), to increase energy, or for weight or muscle gain (41.5%). Female athletes were more likely to take supplements for their health, while males were more likely to improve speed and agility, strength and power, or for weight/muscle gain. Consistent with the above findings, the primary motivations for using supplements among people who exercise at commercial gyms were to build muscle (49.1%), prevent future illness (38.4%), increase energy (36.1%), improve performance (24.4%), and gain strength (22.4%). Furthermore, more people over 45 years old consumed supplements to prevent future illness than people between the ages of 18 to 30 years.[6]

II. *PANAX GINSENG*

A. Introduction

Panax ginseng C.A. Meyer (Chinese or Korean ginseng) is a perennial herb from the *Araliaceous* family, indigenous to the mountainous forests of Eastern Asia (mainly China and Korea). The term "ginseng" usually refers to the dried root of *P. ginseng*. More than 10 *Panax* taxa (genus) are reported worldwide. Some of them are commercially available and are also labeled as ginseng, such as *P. quinquefolius* (American ginseng, mainly growing in rich woodlands in the eastern and central United States and Canada), *P. japonicus* (Japanese ginseng from India, southern China, and Japan), and *P. notoginseng* (common name "Sanchi" ginseng).[7,8] *Eleutherococcus* (or *Acanthopanax*) *senticosus*, also known as Siberian ginseng, is a thorny shrub belonging to the same family (*Araliaceae*) but is a different genus from the *Panax* species. The main active constituents of *E. senticosus* are eleutherosides, which are chemically distinct from ginsenosides.[7]

For thousands of years traditional Chinese medicine has relied upon *P. ginseng* to restore and enhance well-being. More recently, *P. ginseng* has gained popularity in the West, where it is used primarily to improve psychologic function, exercise performance, immune function, and conditions associated with diabetes.[9,10]

P. ginseng is available in many forms: whole root, root powder (white ginseng), steamed root powder (red ginseng), teas, tinctures, and standardized root extracts containing known and reproducible amounts of ginsenosides in every batch. When *P. ginseng* roots are washed after harvesting, peeled, and immediately dried (12% moisture or less), "white" ginseng is produced. Alternatively, roots may be steamed for 2 to 4 hours and then dried, producing cartilaginous, translucent, reddish roots called "red."[7,11] The chemical composition of commercial *P. ginseng* products is highly variable due to differences in the genetic nature of the plant source,[12] years of growth, season of harvest, and differences in the methods of drying and curing.[13,14]

Although there are several reviews[7,11,15] on the clinical trials of *P. ginseng*, the variation of commercial *P. ginseng* products creates a great difficulty in evaluating outcomes of well-controlled clinical research. Products used in those trials varied greatly in terms of plant species, part of plant utilized, type of preparation, purity, strength, and composition. Because of this variation, it is not surprising that the outcomes of those reviews tend to be mixed. A real progress in evidence-based research can be achieved only if the testing product is better defined and the product quality and consistency are improved.[16] This chapter includes human clinical data using only *P. ginseng*, not other *Panax* species or *E. senticosus*.

B. Ginsenosides

The main active constituents of the *Panax* genus are a group of over 30 different triterpenoid glycosides or saponins, also referred to as ginsenosides. Each ginsenoside has been named as ginsenoside Rx, where x is a, b_1, b_2, c, d, e, f, g_1, g_2, g_3, h_1, h_2, or o, according to its position on thin layer chromatograms.[7] Among the *Panax* genus, *P. ginseng* is rich in ginsenosides Rb_1, Rb2, Rc, Re, Rd, and Rg_1, while *P. quinquefolius* has little or no ginsenoside Rf and has a lower ratio of ginsenoside Rg_1 to Rb_1 than *P. ginseng.*[12,17,18] The roots of *P. japonicus* contain mainly different saponins, which are known as chikusetsu-saponins. Only two saponin glycosides are common to *P. japonicus, P. ginseng*, and *P. quinquefolius*, namely Rg_2 and Ro.[8]

Biological effects of *P. ginseng* might well be due to individual ginsenosides exerting pharmacological effects. Ginsenosides Rb_1, Rb_2, Rc, Rd, and Re have "anti-stress" effects. Rg_2 has inhibitory effects on platelet aggregation similar to those of aspirin, and Ro reportedly inhibits the conversion of fibrinogen to fibrin. Rb_1 increases RNA synthesis and Rg_1 stimulates DNA, protein, and lipid synthesis in rat bone marrow cells. Ginsenoside Rg_1 was reported to increase humoral and cell-mediated immune responses and increase the number of antigen-reactive T helper cells and T lymphocytes. Ginsenoside Rb_2 was reported to inhibit tumor angiogenesis and metastasis, whereas another study reported the same saponin to suppress the formation of sister-chromatid exchanges in human blood lymphocytes.[19]

The concentration of ginsenosides varies with the source. Cui et al.[20] assayed 50 commercial ginseng preparations sold in 11 countries. In 44 of those analyzed, the concentration of ginsenosides varied from 1.9% to 9.0%. Six products sold in Sweden, the United Kingdom, and the United States did not contain any specific ginsenosides. Harkey et al.[21] found that the total ginsenoside concentrations varied 15-fold (0.288–4.266% by wt) in powders and capsules and 36-fold (0.361–12.993 g/L) in liquid extracts from 16 commercial products labeled as containing *P. ginseng*. Recently, Krochmal et al.[16] analyzed nine *P. ginseng* products and reported that the amount of ginsenosides detected ranged from 44% to 261% of the label claim. G115 (Pharmaton, Lugano, Switzerland) is the most widely used standardized *P. ginseng* extract, which has been used in several clinical and pharmacological studies. It is a concentrated aqueous extract of *P. ginseng*, standardized to 4% ginsenosides. It is also marketed under the product name of Ginsana.[7,11]

C. Bioavailability and Metabolism of Ginsenosides

The absorption, distribution, excretion, and metabolism of ginsenosides, specifically of Rg_1 in the rat, have been investigated.[90] Oral doses of 100 mg/kg of the ginsenoside Rg_1 were administered to rats and 2% to 20% of the dose was found to be rapidly absorbed in the upper part of the gastrointestinal (GI) tract. Serum levels of Rg_1 peaked at 30 minutes after administration and reached maximum tissue levels (except for the brain) at 1.5 hours. Ginsenoside was excreted into rat urine and bile. Intravenous administration of Rg_1 did not lead to significant metabolism by the liver, but there was evidence of ginsenoside metabolism in the rat stomach and large intestine followed by rapid excretion through the urinary and biliary systems. The maximum concentrations in the liver and kidney were attained within 1.5 hours and were 3.5 ± 2.0 μg/g and 2.6 ± 1.5 μg/g, respectively. The levels identified in heart, lungs, and spleen were below 1.5 μg/g at all times after administration and at no time were they identified in the brain. Other studies revealed that metabolites of ginsenosides Rg_1, Rb_1, and Rb_2 in rat GI tract were mainly prosapogenins derived from hydrolysis of their sugar moieties.[19]

The absorption of ginsenoside Rb_1 and Rg_1 are relatively low, 0.1% and 1.9% of the dosage to rats, with the majority of the material in the small intestine.[22] When absorbed, ginsenosides are metabolized in the liver and assumed to be excreted into bile. Poor oral absorption of ginsenosides is believed to be associated with low solubility and membrane permeability, breakdown by stomach acid and digestive enzyme, or metabolism by bacteria in the small intestine. It has been reported that Rb_1 is broken down in gastric juice and transfer into compound K via ginsenoside Rd and F2 when incubated with human fecal microflora.[23] Ginsenosides are scarcely detectable in the brain, which suggests that they can hardly penetrate the blood–brain barrier, due to their high molecular weight (> 600) and hydrophilicity. On the other hand, the metabolites of ginsenosides, such as compound K, which have lower molecular weight and are less hydrophilic, have been found to be absorbed from the digestive tract.[22]

In humans, 1.2% of ingested ginsenosides (3 mg) was found in urine and less than 0.2% ingested amount (7 mg) was retained in the body. In a recent study, two health volunteers were given seven capsules of Ginsana (each containing 100 mg of G115 standardized to 4% gisenosides) and the hydrolyzed products, Rh_1 and Rf_1 were found in their plasma and urine. In addition, compound K, the main intestinal bacteria metabolite of ginsenosides, was also detected in plasma and urine. It was concluded that these metabolites might be responsible for the action of ginseng in humans.[24]

D. Effects on Physical Performance

Earlier research findings relative to the effects of *P. ginseng* on physical performance are equivocal. Vogler et al.[15] searched key databases from their respective inception to 1998 and retrieved five double-blind randomized placebo trials (Jada score > 3) investigating the effects of *P. ginseng* root extract on physical performance in young active volunteers during submaximal and maximal exercise. Three studies reported that administration of the standardized *P. ginseng* extract (200 mg or 300 mg/d for more than 8 wk) significantly decreased heart rate and increased in maximal oxygen uptake as compared with placebo. However, two studies found that the standardized *P. ginseng* extract (200 mg or 400 mg/d for 8 wk) failed to improve maximal work performance, oxygen uptake, respiratory exchange rate, and heart rate.

Bahrke and Morgan[7] analyzed human trials published between 1986 and 1999. Four trials found that *P. ginseng* improved endurance, recovery speed, reaction time, maximal oxygen uptake, heart rate, and strength, while seven trials failed to report significant change in maximal oxygen consumption or uptake, total workload, exhaustion time, and heart rate. It is speculated that the discrepancy in outcome from human trials might be associated with various methodological problems such as small sample size, varied treatment duration, combination of ginseng with other substances, lack of compelling "sourcing" data, and failure to demonstrate that human participants actually complied with the ginseng ingestion. Furthermore, other factors include the actual composition of ginseng preparations, delivery form (tablet, capsule, or liquid extract), and type plant (*P. ginseng*, *P. quinquefolius*, etc.) employed.

Recognizing the importance of dosage and duration of *P. ginseng* on the outcome of trials, Bucci[11] evaluated 34 controlled and uncontrolled human studies from 1973 to 1998 and found that the dosage and duration of *P. ginseng* accounted for most of the variation in the results. He noticed that properly controlled studies exhibiting statistically significant improvements in physical or psychomotor performance almost invariably used higher doses (usually standardized to ginsenoside content equivalent to ≥ 2 g dried root/d), longer durations of study (≥ 8 wk), and larger subject numbers with greater statistical power. Also evident was that those studies with lower doses, short durations, and small subject numbers were found to have no significant differences in performance, physiologic, or psychomotor measurements. He concluded that the *P. ginseng* supplement might enhance physical and mental performance if taken long enough and in sufficient doses. This appears valid for recreational athletes > 40 years of age, but less valid for younger athletes. Well-trained elite athletes may not notice any benefits beyond a placebo effect except possibly during times of increased physical stress. Ginseng does not appear to exert any acute effects on physical performance. Apparently the requirements needed to observe positive outcome are sufficient daily dose (≥ 2000 mg *P. ginseng* root powder or an equivalent amount of root extract with standardized ginsenoside content), sufficient duration for effects to develop (≥ 8 wk), and sufficient intensity of physical or mental activity (especially in untrained or older subjects).

Recently, Ziemba et al.[25] reported that *P. ginseng* improved psychomotor performance in strategic sports in a randomized double blind placebo-controlled study with young soccer players. It was showed that administration of 350 mg/d of ginseng for 6 weeks shortened reaction time at rest and during exercise, shifting the exercise load associated with the shortest reaction time toward higher exercise loads. In untrained adults, Kim et al.[26] found that 8 weeks' supplementation with *P. ginseng* extract (6 g/d) significantly increased exercise duration until exhaustion (by 1.5 min) and attenuated oxidant stress levels by measuring blood malondialdehyde, catalase, and superoxide dismutase levels. Authors concluded that ginseng has ergogenic properties in facilitating recovery from exhaustive exercise.

Furthermore, Rogers et al.[27] compared effects of creatine and creatine plus a botanical extract containing *P. ginseng* in 44 adults aged 55–84 years participating in a 12-week strength-training program. Participants consumed creatine only (3 g), creatine plus botanical extract (1.5 g with 10% ginsenosides), or placebo, and performed bench press, lateral pull down, biceps curl, leg press, knee extension, and knee flexion for 3 sets of 8–12 replicates on three days per week for 12 weeks. The one-repetition maximum for each exercise, body composition (full-body DEXA), blood lipids, and mood states were also evaluated before and after the intervention. Creatine plus *P. ginseng* produced significantly greater strength gains (bench press) and body fat reduction, compared with the creatine-only group. Creatine plus *P. ginseng* also improved blood lipids and self-reported vigor levels.

Many mechanisms of action have been proposed for *P. ginseng*. The traditional use is to restore *Qi*, or life energy. This herb is thought to be a tonic to increase vitality, health, and longevity, especially in older persons. Isolation of ginsenosides and administration to animals has revealed activities that stimulate the central nervous system as well as those that depress it. Other possible mechanisms for ginseng include increased production of corticotropin and cortisol in animals and humans, and anabolic actions (stimulation of deoxyribonucleic acid [DNA], ribonucleic acid [RNA], and protein synthesis in tissues) in animals. Ginseng has shown immunoenhancing effects in animals and humans and antioxidant activity *in vitro* and in animals. Ginsenosides are also credited with stimulation of nitric oxide production in immune system cells, vascular endothelial cells, arteries, and erectile tissue. Furthermore, ginsenosides can modulate acetylcholine release and re-uptake. Thus, it is believed that multiple mechanisms of ginsenosides attribute to its effects on physical performance.[11]

E. Effects on Cognitive and Mental Performance

While there is a good body of work regarding the cognitive enhancement effects of *P. ginseng*, the evidence of such effects following chronic administration is scarce in humans. Vogler et al.[15] searched key databases from their respective inception to 1998 and retrieved three double-blind randomized placebo trials (Jada score > 2) investigating the effects of *P. ginseng* root extract on psychomotor performance. Two studies reported significant improvements in mental arithmetic and abstraction tests with *P. ginseng*.

Using a 90-day double-blind placebo-controlled parallel-group dose-response study, Wesnes et al.[28] evaluated the effects of a *Ginkgo biloba/P. ginseng* combination on cognitive function in healthy volunteers with neurasthenic (fatigue and tiredness) complaints. Participants consisted of 44 women and 20 men with a mean age of 54.7 years. These individuals were randomly assigned to one of four groups receiving 80 mg (30 mg *Ginkgo* plus 50 mg *P. ginseng*), 160 mg (60 mg *Ginkgo* plus 100 mg *P. ginseng*) or 320 mg (120 mg *Ginkgo* plus 200 mg *P.ginseng*) of the combination twice daily, or placebo. Assessments consisted of the Cognitive Drug Research Cognitive Performance (CDR) tests, Bond-Lader Visual Analogue Scales, Vienna Determination Unit Emotional Overload Test, heart rates during cycle ergometry, and various questionnaires including the SCL-90-R Symptom Checklist. These evaluations were performed on days 1, 30, and 90. On day 90 at 1 hour post-morning dosing, dose-related improvements were observed on the CDR test, with the 320-mg dose being significantly superior to placebo. However, these effects were reversed 6 hours after an additional dose.

Recently, a series of placebo-controlled double-blind balanced crossover studies has demonstrated enhancement of cognitive performance following single doses of *P. ginseng* (standardized extract G115) in young healthy humans. The most consistent finding is of improved memory performance following G115 alone and in combination with both *Ginkgo biloba*[29] and guarana (*Paullinia cupana*).[30] *P. ginseng* at a dose of 200 mg also significantly improved the speed of information retrieval, attention and arithmetical performance, significantly shortened the latency of the P300 component of auditory evoked potentials and faster responses on an attentional task 90 minutes following 400 mg of G115.[29,30] Furthermore, *P. ginseng* enhanced performance of a mental arithmetic task, ameliorated the increase in subjective feelings of mental fatigue experienced by participants during the later stages of the sustained, cognitively demanding task performance, and improved the accuracy of performing the Rapid Visual Information Processing task (RVIP).[31,32]

The mechanisms by which P. ginseng might modulate human cognitive performance are not well understood, but they may involve several central and peripheral physiological effects that are potentially relevant to human cognitive performance. These include effects on the cardiovascular system, platelet aggregation, the hypothalamic-pituitary-adrenal system, neurotransmission, and nitric oxide synthesis.[29] It has been known that fluctuations in levels of circulating blood glucose can modulate cognitive performance. Cognitive impairment has been demonstrated as a result of both hypoglycemia and lowered but supra-hypoglycaemic glucose levels. Several recent studies suggest that *P. ginseng* may have gluco-regulatory properties and *P. ginseng* has been reported to promote the transport of glucose, by an unknown mechanism, into active cells and thus facilitating metabolism in task-sensitive structures (i.e., leading to improved behavioral performance). Furthermore, administration of *P. ginseng* was found to result in improved behavioral performance concomitant with reduced blood glucose levels. Therefore, it is possible that ginseng exerts its beneficial cognition-enhancing effects via some unknown gluco-regulatory mechanism.[32]

F. Effects on Quality of Life or Well-Being

To date, most studies investigating the efficacy of *P. ginseng* have focused on clinical outcomes, with quality-of-life evaluations occurring only occasionally as a secondary endpoint. However, many consumers perceived taking *P. ginseng* to increase vitality and improve overall health and quality of life.

Coleman et al.[9] reviewed human trials published between 1966 and 2002. Nine human trials were located, eight of which were placebo controlled. Four studies investigated effects of standardized *P. ginseng* alone, while five included additional vitamins and minerals. The amount of *P. ginseng* administered ranged from 80 to 400 mg and the duration of trials was 2 to 9 months. Patient populations examined included postmenopausal women, type II diabetics, patients with age-associated memory impairment, and healthy volunteers of various ages and stress levels. Several quality-of-life measures were used, ranging from widely accepted or standardized core instruments to self-rating questionnaires. Nearly every study evaluated demonstrated some degree of improvement in quality of life. Benefits were evident within instrument summary component scores. There is no evidence suggesting any advantage of using ginseng doses > 200 mg. Studies evaluating 80- and 200-mg doses appeared to confer a similar degree of moderate improvement in summary component scores. Similarly, the presence or absence of vitamins and minerals did not result in added benefit. There did not appear to be a substantial difference between the responses of the various populations studied with respect to effects on quality of life.

A recent randomized double-blind placebo-controlled trial investigated the effects of ginseng on quality of life. Fifty-three patients diagnosed with cancer were randomly given ginseng (3000 mg/d) or placebo for 12 weeks. Quality of life was assessed using the World Health Organization Quality of Life Assessment-Bref (WHOQOL-BREF) and the General Health Questionnaire-12 (GHQ-12). At the end of 12 weeks, the "psychological domain" score of the WHOQOL-BREF was significantly improved in patients taking ginseng, compared with placebo. The GHQ-12 total score was also significantly more improved in patients treated with ginseng than in those with placebo. No significant adverse events were observed in both groups. Authors concluded that ginseng was found to be beneficial in improving some aspects of mental and physical functioning after 12 weeks' ingestion.[33]

Similar outcome was also reported in an epidemiological study with 1,455 breast cancer patients. Information on ginseng (roots or preparations) use before cancer diagnosis was collected at baseline. Survivors' ginseng use after cancer diagnosis was obtained at the follow-up survey and was correlated to General Quality of Life Inventory-74 (QOL) conducted at the same time. Approximately 27% of study participants were regular ginseng users before cancer diagnosis. Compared with patients who never used ginseng, regular users had a significantly reduced risk of death. Ginseng use after cancer diagnosis was positively associated with QOL scores, with the strongest effect in the psychological and social well-being domains. Additionally, QOL improved as cumulative ginseng use increased.[34]

G. Toxicity, Safety, and Drug Interactions

The toxicological profile of *P. ginseng* indicates it to be of rather low acute oral toxicity (LD_{50} > 5000 mg/kg for rats and mice, approximating 200 mg ginsenoside/kg). No toxicological effects were identified in mini pigs at a dose of 2000 mg/kg (80 mg ginsenoside/kg). As concluded from a 90-day dog study and in reproduction studies in rats and mice, 15 mg/kg (~ 0.6 mg ginsenoside/kg) was without effect. No effect was seen in rats administered 4000 mg/kg (160 mg ginsenoside/kg) for 20 days. There was no mutagenic activity observed in the *Salmonella typhimurium* TM677 system with the use of ginseng in the presence or absence of metabolic activation. The no observed-adverse-effect level (NOAEL) in rodents is likely within the range of 50 to 100 mg ginsenoside/kg.[19]

Humans have consumed *P. ginseng* for millennia. There are no confirmed reports of adverse reactions in humans attributed to ginseng alone. In a number of reports, ginseng was identified as one of a number of substances involved (including adulterants), although no report could unequivocally identify ginseng as the causative agent. Importantly, no consistent symptomology or findings have been attributed to, or identified as being associated with, ginseng consumption. Ginseng extracts standardized at a concentration of 4 mg ginsenosides/100 mg capsule and given at a dose of up to 114 μg ginsenoside/kg have not resulted in untoward effects when administered to humans for periods of up to12 weeks.[19]

Furthermore, interpretation of documented adverse effects and drug interactions can be difficult because of the variety of available ginseng formulations, and the exact amount of ginseng in these products may not be identified. Generally, *P. ginseng* is well tolerated, and its side effects are mild and reversible. Associated side effects include nausea, diarrhea, insomnia, headaches, hypertension, and vaginal bleeding. However, the exact incidence of those side effects is unknown, but seems to be low.[10,35]

Recently, several case reports describe interactions between *P. ginseng* and prescription drugs. It is speculated that drug interactions with prescription drugs may be due secondary to interactions with cytochrome P-450 enzyme system, interference with drug metabolism, or hematopoiesis. The cytochrome P-450 enzyme system is responsible for the oxidative metabolism of the majority of drugs and xenobiotics. The inhibition or interference with P-450 activities may result in clinically significant *P. ginseng*–drug interactions. There are several human studies investigating effects of *P. ginseng, P. ginseng* extracts, or naturally occurring ginsenosides on P450 activities. Those studies found that *P. ginseng* may have no or little effects on P-450 activities or effects on P-450 enzyme system, which are not likely to be clinically relevant. However, a recent clinical trial in healthy subjects showed that *P. ginseng* diminished the urine excretion rate of S-7-hydroxywarfarin, the metabolite from S-warfarin. Therefore, the use of *P. ginseng* should be avoided in patients on warfarin therapy.[36,37]

H. Recommended Dose

Most published human studies have used a standardized *P. ginseng* extract at a dose of 200 mg daily. Standardization extracts usually are recommended to contain 1.5% to 7% of ginsenosides. Other sources recommend 0.5 to 2 grams of dry root daily, equivalent to 200 to 600 mg of extract. For continuous administration, the equivalent of 1 gram of dry root should not be exceeded. Low quality products may be contaminated or contain no active components or ginsenosides at all and consumer should be advised to obtain products from reputable sources.[10,35]

I. Future Research Needs

For multiple reasons, it is difficult to reach a defensible conclusion as to whether *P. ginseng* is able to enhance physical and mental performance in humans. First, there are multiple different types of ginseng containing many different active compounds. Second, products contain varying amounts of these active compounds, and there seems to be lack of standardization of dosing. Furthermore, most studies have not been reproducible and yielded varying results. To avoid future methodological flaws and produce reproducible results, researchers need to: (a) assay the products they are using independently and confirm the source and amount of the substance employed; (b) confirm compliance of the user; (c) design randomized and placebo-controlled studies; and (d) calculate statistical power prior to the initiation of the studies and require at least the minimum sample size.

Areas of interest for future research also include the mechanisms of action in terms of performance enhancement and cognitive function augmentation, effects on nonathletes or people on recreational exercise, and the antistress effect with people of various stress levels.

J. Summary

P. ginseng supplements may enhance physical and mental performance if taken long enough and at sufficient doses. Ginseng may exert greater benefits for untrained or older (> 40 y) subjects. Ginseng does not appear to exert any acute effects on physical performance. In general, ginseng supplements are safe, although individual variability exists and potentiation with stimulants such as caffeine may occur.

III. *ELEUTHEROCOCCUS SENTICOSUS*

A. Introduction

Eleutherococcus senticosus (E. senticosus), previously also known as Siberian ginseng, is a thorny shrub that grows in the Russian far east and northern regions of Korea, Japan, and China. Although it belongs to the *Araliaceae* family, *E. senticosus* is completely different from *P. ginseng.* It is believed that *E. senticosus* is referred to as Siberian ginseng because it was first exported from Siberia in the Soviet era. In 1950s, wild *P. ginseng* was very scarce in the Soviet Union as well as in Korea. Recognizing that it takes a very long time (over 6 years) to cultivate high-quality *P. ginseng*, Soviet scientists turned their attention to the *Araliaceae* family and identifying an alternative and plentiful plant source that would have similar pharmacological activity and "tonic" properties. As it turns out, *E. senticosus* is the only species that grows in the territories of the former USSR and has a habit and gross morphology somewhat similar to *P. ginseng*, with "adaptogen" properties.[38]

E. senticosus is primarily used as an adaptogen that could induce antifatigue or antistress effects and enhance stamina and physical performance. In addition, this plant may also have immunomodulatory effects.[39]

E. senticosus contains a unique array of biologically active constituents. The eleutherosides have been given the most attention and are believed responsible for the proposed adaptogenic activity. Most commercially available extracts have been standardized according to their content of eleutheroside B (syringin 4-β-D-glucoside) and eleutheroside E (syringaresinol 4, 4'-O-β-D-diglucoside). Other components with reported biological activities include sesamin, β-sitosterol, hedarasaponin B, and isofraxidin as well as various flavonoids and hydroxycinnamates.[38,40]

B. Adaptogen

Originally, an adaptogen is defined as a substance that can increase body "nonspecific" resistance to counteract adverse physical, chemical, or biological stressors and challenges.[40] More recently, an adaptogen has been defined as a compound that increases the ability of an organism to adapt to environmental factors and to avoid damage from such factors.[41] It is believed that administration of adaptogens allows the body to pre-adapt itself to be more capable of responding appropriately when diverse demands are eventually placed on it. When a stressful situation occurs, an adaptogen generates a degree of adaptation (or nonspecific resistance) that allows the body to handle the stressful situation in a more resourceful manner.[42]

It is suggested that adaptogens are mainly associated with their effects on the neuroendocrine-immunologic axis, which is considered to play a key role in the stress system. A well-trained athlete responds to stress stimuli with a mildly increased activity in the hypothalamic-pituitary axis (HPA), as opposed to a pronounced increase in HPA activity in an untrained individual. Similarly, adaptogens counteract the stress through modulating the biosynthesis of eicosanoids, which include prostaglandins E_2 and F_2, 5-hydroxyeicosatetraenoic acid (5-HETE), 12-HETE, and leukotriene B_4. In addition, they may also regulate the blood levels of arachidonic acid. Furthermore, adaptogens may stimulate the formation of endogenous "messenger" substances such as catecholamines, prostagladins, cytokines, nitric oxide, and platelet-activating factor, which in turn activate other factors that may counteract stress.[43]

P. ginseng, *E. senticosus*, and *R. rosea* are considered plant adaptogens. *E. senticosus* and *R. rosea* contain relatively high amounts of phenolic compounds, particularly phenylpropane or phenylethane derivatives. These compounds are structurally related to the catecholamines and it is assumed that *E. senticosus* and *R. rosea* counteract stress through the central nervous system. On the other hand, *P. ginseng* contains relatively large amounts of tetracyclic triterpenes, which are structurally similar to corticosteroids. It is believed to counteract stress through HPA axis.[42]

C. Anti-Stress/Anti-Fatigue Effects of *E. senticosus*

In his review of the Russian scientific literature, Farnsworth et al.[44] noted that a single dose of 4 ml 33% *E. senticosus* ethanolic extract given to five male skiers 1–1.5 hours before a 20–50 kilometer race increased skiers' resistance to hypoxemia and enhanced their ability to adapt to increased exercise demands.

In a double-blind study, 45 healthy volunteers were randomized to receive *E. senticosus*or or placebo for 30 days. Participants were subject to the Stroop Colour-Word (Stroop CW) test to assess their stress response, along with heart rate and blood pressure, before and after treatment. Unlike those in the placebo group, those who received *E. senticosus* had a 40% reduction in heart rate response to the Stroop CW stressor. Moreover, in female subjects, the use of *E. senticosus* accounted for a 60% reduction in systolic blood pressure response to the cognitive challenge test. The authors concluded that *E. senticosus* might be helpful for stress adaptation.[45]

Another randomized double-blind controlled trial involving 96 patients diagnosed with idiopathic chronic fatigue evaluated the effectiveness of an *E. senticosus* extract. The extract was standardized to contain 2.24 mg eleutherosides per four 500-mg capsules (daily dose). Forty-nine subjects received the *E. senticosus* extract and 47 received a placebo. At the end of 2 months, subjects with mild-to-moderate fatigue demonstrated statistically significant improvement in Rand Vitality Index (RVI) scores compared with placebo. In addition, when subjects in the placebo group were given *E. senticosus* extract, the RVI was also improved after 2 months' ingestion of the extract.[46]

A recent randomized double-blind controlled study investigated the effects of *E. senticosus* on the quality of life. Twenty elderly people with unspecific fatigue and asthenia were given *E. senticosus* extract, 300 mg/d, or placebo. The quality of life was measured by using SF-36V2 (a validated general health status questionnaire). At the end of the 4 weeks of treatment, subjects treated with *E. senticosus* had significantly higher scores in social functioning scales. No adverse events were observed in either group. Authors concluded that *E. senticosus* was safe and effective in improving the quality of life, especially with regard to mental health and social functioning.[47]

Finally, a double-blind placebo-controlled randomized study[48] showed that Chisan (a standardized fixed combination of extracts of *Rhodiola rosea, Schisandra chinensis, Turcz. Baill., and E. senticosus*) was effective in speeding up the recovery process and improving quality of life in patients suffering from acute nonspecific pneumonia. Sixty patients undergoing antibody treatment participated in the study. Thirty of the patients received Chisan twice daily, while another 30 patients were given a placebo. The primary outcomes were the duration of antibiotic treatment, mental performance measured by a psychometric test, and the self-evaluation of QOL. The mean duration of antibody treatment was 2 days shorter in patients treated with Chisan than in those in the placebo group. The Chisan group also had significantly higher scores in all QOL parameters (physical, psychological, social, and ecological) than those in placebo. The authors concluded that adjuvant therapy with Chisan had a positive effect on the recovery of patients by reducing the duration of the illness, increasing mental performance during the rehabilitation period, and improving their QOL.

D. Effects on Physical Performance

Originally identified and developed by Russian scientists, virtually all of the early work (from the 1960s to the 1980s) of the effects of *E. senticosus* on physical performance was published in foreign journals, symposia proceedings, and books, mostly in Russian, but some in German and Chinese. A summary of the early work in Russia with weight lifters, wrestlers, gymnasts, and truck drivers suggested that *E. senticosus* improved general mental and physical health, increased work capacity, and decreased fatigue.[49]

Asano et al.[50] reported a performance-enhancing effect of *E.senticosus* in single-blind, crossover study. Two milliliters of *E. senticosus* ethanol extract (each milliliter of ethanol extract contained 0.53 mg of eleutheroside B and 0.12 mg of eleutheroside D) or its placebo was given to six athletes, once in the morning and again in the evening for 8 consecutive days. Compared with controls, athletes who received *E. senticosus* extract had significant increases in overall work performance, including maximal oxygen uptake ($p<0.01$), oxygen pulse ($p<0.025$), total work capacity ($p<0.005$), and exhaustion time ($p<0.005$). The *E. senticosus* group experienced a 23.3% increase in total work capacity and a 16.3% increase in exhaustion time compared with only a 7.5% and 5.4% increase in respective placebo values ($p<0.05$).

A randomized double-blind placebo-controlled crossover study[51] evaluated effects of *E. senticosus, P. ginseng*, and a placebo on maximal oxygen uptake, heart rate recovery, and muscle strength. Thirty athletes were randomly assigned to three groups. Subjects were administered randomly *E. senticosus* powder (1000 mg/day), *P. ginseng*, or a placebo for 6 weeks. At the end of the study, *E. senticosus* significantly increased pectoral and quadriceps strength by 13% and 15%, respectively. Results of this study suggest that *E.senticosus* improves muscle strength. Furthermore, a recent study with 50 subjects[52] compared the effects of ethanol extracts (35%) of *E. senticosus* and Echinacea. Participants were given either *E. senticosus* extract (25 drops) or Echinacea extract (40 drops) three times daily. A significant improvement in maximal oxygen uptake ($VO_{2\ max}$) was observed.

However, Dowling et al.[53] showed that administering 3.4 mL of an *E. senticosus* extract (30%–34% ethanol extract containing eleutherosides B and E) failed to improve exhaustion time, heart rate, lactate production, ventilation equivalent for oxygen, oxygen consumption, ratings of perceived exertion, and respiratory exchange ratio. At the end of the study, the authors noted that the statistical power for measured indices ranged from 0.16 to 0.52, which casts great doubt on the ability of this study to detect any significant changes if they were present.

Recently, several other studies also found no effects of Endurox™ (800–1200 mg/day) on fat oxidation, lactate production, heart rate, or physical performance. Endurox™ is a product containing leaves of Ciwujia (*Acanthopanax senticosus*).[54–56] Most human studies with positive outcomes used the root of *E. senticosus* or its extract standardized to contain eleutheroside, not leaves of Ciwujia. In addition, none of the above studies, which reported no beneficial effects of Endurox™, identified the existence of eleutherosides and verified the content of Endurox™ through appropriate chemical analysis. Furthermore, it has been demonstrated that active components in *E. senticosus* preparations are highly variable. The total eleutheroside concentration varied 43-fold in the *E. senticosus* powder and >200 fold in the liquid extract.[21]

E. Toxicity, Safety and Drug Interactions

The oral LD_{50} of the 33% ethanolic extract is estimated to be 14.5 g/kg. The extract is not considered to be teratogenic in mice at 10 mg/kg.[39]

One case report indicated oral use of *E. senticosus* concomitantly with digoxin might result in dangerously high blood levels of digoxin. However, no digoxin or digitoxin contamination was found with samples of the Siberian ginseng capsules. No analysis was carried out to determine whether the capsules did in fact contain Siberian ginseng.[91] In addition, a study in mice demonstrated no digoxin like immnoreactivity of E. senticosus when measured by five separation serum digoxin assays.[39]

An *in vitro* study using isolated cDNA-expressed human liver microsomes indicated that the *E. senticosus* extract did not inhibit the activity of human CYP3A4.[39] A recent human study demonstrated standardized extracts of *E. senticosus* at generally recommended dosages did not significantly alter the metabolism of medications dependent on the cytochrome hepato-detoxification pathways, CYP3A4 or CYP2D6.[57]

F. Future Research Needs

Recognizing the great variation of active components in herbal products, Wolsko et al.[58] investigated and characterized the content of an herbal supplement used in recent published randomized controlled trials between January 1, 2000, and February 9,

2004. Of 81 randomized controlled trials, 12 (15%) reported performing tests to quantify actual contents, and three (4%) provided adequate data to compare actual with expected content values of at least one chemical constituent. In those three studies, actual content varied between 80% and 113% of expected values. Lack of documented characterization of the herbal supplements used in published randomized controlled trials detracts from the value of what were otherwise well-designed clinical trials. Results from randomized controlled trials with poor-quality supplements not only add little value, but also may create confusion on the true benefits of herbal supplements.

Therefore, future studies for effects of *E. senticosus* must use robust experimental protocols. Investigators must ensure the identity, purity, quality, and composition of the testing material being evaluated. It would make sense to recommend that the products being used be assayed by an independent group and that the source and amount of the substance employed be conformed.

Ciwujianosides (from leaf of Ciwujia) and eleutherosides (from root of *E. senticosus)* are chemically distinct. As ciwujianosides and eleutherosides may be derived from the same plant, they should not be used interchangeably and their respective effects should be evaluated separately. To date, the minimum dose of *E. senticosus* (ciwujianosides and eleutherosides) to produce biological effects remains unknown. It would be important in future studies to determine the dose needed.

Research is also needed to determine the effects and possible mechanisms of action of *E. senticosus* on muscular strength, physical capacity, and quality of life.

G. Summary and Recommended Dose

Given the paucity of human studies and the inadequate verification of the potency of the product used in the studies, it is very difficult to reach a conclusion regarding the effects of *E. senticosus* on physical performance. Adequately controlled studies with sufficient statistical power and consistent identity and intake of eleutherosides are needed. It appears that *E. senticosus* may possess some antistress or antifatigue properties. It may generate a degree of adaptation (or non-specific resistance) that allows the body to handle the stressful situation (heavy exercise or illness) in a more resourceful manner. In adults, the recommended dosage for the 33% ethanolic root extract is 10 mL three times daily, the root powder 2–3 g/d, and extracts standardized to eleutheroside B and E, 300-400 mg/d.

III. *RHODIOLA ROSEA*

A. Introduction

Rhodiola rosea (R. rosea) is a perennial plant from the *Crassulaceae* family. It grows at high altitudes in the mountain and arctic regions of Europe and Asia. Also known as "golden root" or "Arctic root," *R. rosea* has been used for centuries in folk medicine to increase physical endurance and work productivity; increase resistance to high-altitude sickness; treat mental fatigue, cold and flu; and to stimulate the central nervous system.[59]

R. rosea contains many phytochemicals including phenylpropanoids (rosavin, rosin, rosarin), phenylethanol derivatives (salidrosides/rhodioloside and tyrosol), monoterpernes (rosiridol and rosaridin), and flavonoids (rodiolin, rodionin, rodiosin, and acetylrhodalgin).[40] Phenylpropanoids (rosavin, rosin, and rosarin) are considered to be specific to *R.rosea*.[60] In most reported human studies, *R. rosea* extracts were standardized to contain 3% rosavin and 0.8%–1% salidroside.[59]

R. rosea has been intensively studied in Russia and Scandinavia for more than 35 years. It is classified as an adaptogen due to its ability to increase resistance to a variety of chemical, biological, and physical stressors via cardioprotection and central nervous system enhancement.[40] Similar to other plant adaptogens investigated by Russian researchers, such as *Eleutherococcus senticosus* (Siberian ginseng) and *Panax ginseng* (Asian ginseng), extracts of this plant produce favorable changes in a variety of diverse areas of physiological functions, including neurotransmitter levels, central nervous system activity, and cardiovascular function.[61]

B. Effects on Fatigue and Mental Performance

R. rosea is used by the aborigines of Siberia to prevent fatigue and general disinclination to work.[40] The effects of a single dose of *R. rosea* extract on mental performance was investigated in 85 healthy volunteers using Anfimov's table (an instrument to obtain numerical data comparing the quality and quantity of performance). Each subject was asked to complete the test twice, before and one hour after the treatment (*R. rosea* extract or placebo). Compared with placebo, subjects treated with *R. rosea* extract considerably reduced the number of errors. Doses of 5–10 drops were found to be the most effective, reducing the number of errors by an average of 46%.[42]

Spasov et al.[62] investigated the effects of the SHR-5 (a standardized *R. rosea* extract containing 3.6% rosavin and 1.6% salidroside) on male medical students during a stressful examination period. Forty students were randomized to receive either 50 mg SHR-5 or placebo twice daily for a period of 20 days. Physical and mental performance was assessed before and after the period through a series of objective tests and subjective questionnaires. The students receiving the SHR-5 extract showed significant improvements in physical fitness, psychomotor function, mental performance, and general well-being. They were also reported to have significant reductions in mental fatigue, improved sleep patterns, a reduced need for sleep, greater mood stability, and a greater motivation to study. In addition, the average examination scores were higher in students receiving SHR-5 extract as compared with placebo (3.47 vs. 3.20).

Darbinyan et al.[63] evaluated the effect of daily administration of SHR-5 extract (a standardized extract of *R. rosea,* 170 mg/d) on mental performance and fatigue in 56 healthy physicians during night duty. The effects were measured by a series of tests associated with thinking, short-term memory, calculation, concentration, and speed of audiovisual perception. A Fatigue Index was calculated using scores of these parameters. These parameters were then measured before and after night duty during three periods of 2 weeks each: (1) a test period of SHR-5 or placebo tablet daily; (2) a washout period; and (3) a third period of placebo or SHR-5 tablet daily, in a double-blind crossover fashion. A significant improvement in Fatigue Index scores was observed after 2 weeks of taking SHR-5 extract. The researchers concluded that SHR-5 extract possessed a clear antifatigue effect without any reported adverse reactions or side effects.

Recently, Shevtsov et al.[64] completed a randomized double-blind placebo controlled study with four control groups (2 treatments, placebo, and untreated). The study was to investigate effects of a single dose (two or three capsules) of SHR-5 (a standardized extract of *R. rosea*,180 mg/capsule containing 4.5 mg salidroside) on the capacity for mental (psychometric tests) work against a background of fatigue and stress. Results from 161 cadets showed that both doses of the extract produced statistically significant antifatigue effects measured by the Total Antifatigue Index (a measurement of amount of work per unit of time and quality of work). It also revealed significant beneficial effects on pulse pressure, compared with the placebo.

The antifatigue property of *R. rosea* has been attributed primarily to its ability to influence levels and activities of biogenic monoamines such as serotonin, dopamine, and norepinephrine in the cerebral cortex, brain stem, and hypothalamus. Several Russian studies reported that *R. rosea* may facilitate transport of neurotransmitters in the brain. In addition, *R. rosea* has been shown to stimulate the synthesis, transport, and receptor activity of monoamines and opioid receptor and peptides such as β-endorphins. It has been suggested that increased levels of some brain neurotransmitters such as β-endorphins could lead to an improvement in mental or cognitive functions (thinking, analyzing, evaluating, calculating, and planning). Other neurotransmitters such as acetylcholine may improve memory function via pathways ascending from the memory storage systems of the limbic systems to various area of the cerebral cortex. Agents that block acetylcholine suppress the activities of these ascending pathways and interfere with memory. *R. rosea* reverses this blockade. Furthermore, *R. rosea* may also prevent or ameliorate some age-related deterioration of these neural systems.[59]

C. Effects on Physical Performance

A number of studies have shown that *R. rosea* may increase physical capacity and shorten the recovery time after intensive exercise.[59] In his study with male medical students, Spasov et al.[62] found that the SHR-5- (*R. rosea* extract) treated group was able to achieve 980 ± 40 kgm/min versus 920 ± 52 kgm/min in placebo during PWC-170 (physical working capacity) ergometry tests. In addition, investigators also observed a significantly faster decrease in heart rate following the test in the SHR-5 group than in the placebo.

De Bock et al.[65] completed a double blind placebo-controlled randomized two-phase study investigating the effects of immediate and 4-week intakes of *R. rosea* extract on physical capacity, muscle strength, speed of limb movement, reaction time, and attention. Phase I was a crossover study to determine the immediate effects of *R. rosea* administration. Twenty-four men and women participated in the Phase I study. Participants took either 200 mg of *R. rosea* extract (standardized to contain 3% rosavin and 1% salidroside) or placebo. Arm movement speed, aural and visual reaction times, the ability to sustain attention, muscle strength, and exercise endurance capacity were measured 1 hour after ingestion (it works). After a 5-day washout period, participants switched the treatment regimens and repeated the measurements performed before the crossover period. Phase II was to investigate effects of 4 weeks of *R. rosea* intake. Twelve participants were assigned to receive either 100 mg twice daily of *R. rosea* extract or placebo for 4 weeks. At the beginning and end of the 4 weeks, participants went through the same crossover session as in Phase I and its effect on physical performance was measured.

During Phase I, *R. rosea* significantly increased the amount of time that the participants were able to exercise before becoming fatigued. The participants taking *R. rosea* were able to exercise about 3% longer than those taking placebo. In addition, *R. rosea* also increased oxygen uptake and CO_2 output at peak exercise with no impact on peak lactate concentration. However, the effects were not observed in Phase II. Furthermore, no significant difference in muscle strength, speed of arm movement, reaction times, and sustained attention were observed between the *R. rosea* and placebo groups during both phases of the study. The authors speculated that the rosavin and salidroside (active component) in *R. rosea* extract might be able to stimulate the activity of monoamines, opioid receptor or peptides, and endorphin, which might offset the discomfort and pain induced by intensive endurance exercise. However, this effect on the central nervous system may be transient and its effects on muscle strength and/or physical performance may be limited.[65]

In contrast to the positive results reported by Spasoval et al.[62] and DeBock et al.,[65] Earnest et al.[66] found no effect of a commercial herbal-based formula Optygen™ (each three capsules contain 1000 mg of Cordyceps, 300 mg *R. rosea* root, and 800 mg of proprietary blend) on physical performance in amateur cyclists. Nine cyclists in the treatment group ingested 6 capsules/d for 4 days (600 mg of *R. rosea* root) followed by 3 capsules/d (300 mg *R. rosea* root) for 11 days, while the placebo group (8 subjects) ingested an equivalent placebo. The results showed no significant differences between groups on peak VO_2, peak heart rate, peak output, and time to exhaustion. A similar study by Colson et al.[67] also found no differences in muscle tissue oxygen saturation, VO_{2max}, and time to exhaustion between a group of cyclists (4 subjects) who took Optygen™ for 13 days compared with a placebo group (4 subjects). The discrepancy of these results compared with other studies with positive outcomes might be due to the variations of products used in the studies. In those studies, Optygen™ was not analyzed independently for its potency, which is necessary prior to the study. Furthermore, both studies had fewer than 20 subjects each, which might have limited statistical power to detect potential significances between groups.

D. Antioxidant and Antistress Effects

Like many herbal products, *R. rosea* has antioxidant properties due to its phytochemcical constituents, which include flavonoids, phenylpropanpoids, and proanthocyanidins.[68] Abidov et al.[69] examined effects of *R. rosea* extracts on blood levels of inflammatory C-reactive (CRP) protein and creatinine kinase (CK) in healthy untrained volunteers before and after exhausting exercise. CRP and CK are markers of inflammation and muscle damage, and are normally elevated after exercise in proportion to the amount of activity and muscle injury. Thirty-six healthy untrained volunteers were divided into three groups after initial test of VO_{2max}, weight, body fat, and blood CRP and CK levels.

Group 1 (n = 12) received 340 mg of RHODAX™ (a preparation containing 30 mg of *R. rosea* extract) twice daily (morning and evening), while group 2 (n = 12) received placebo for 30 days prior to and 6 days after exhausting cycling exercise. Group 3 (n = 12) served as the control. It was found that exhausting cycling exercise significantly increased blood CRP and CK levels in all volunteers. However, this increase was significantly less in people receiving RHODAX (group 1). On the 5th day after exhausting cycling exercise, blood CRP levels remained high in groups 2 and 3, while they were lowered to initial levels in group 1. The authors concluded that long-term treatment of RHODAX inhibited the increase in CRP induced by exhausting cycling exercise, indicating that RHODAX may possess anti-inflammatory effects.

Wing et al.[68] investigated the effects of *R. rosea* on blood oxygen and oxidative stress levels. Fifteen volunteers received three separate 60-minute hypoxic exposures by breathing 13.6% oxygen at an ambient barometric pressure of 633 mm Hg (simulating the partial pressure of oxygen at 4600 m elevation). Each subject received, in random order, treatments of a 7-day supply of placebo or *R. rosea* capsule (1788 mg of *R. rosea*). Arterialized capillary blood oxygen samples (PcO_2) were measured at baseline, 30, and 60 minutes after exposure. Blood lipid peroxides and urinary malondialdehyde were measured for levels of oxidative stress. It was found that *R. rosea* supplement decreased blood lipid peroxidation (oxidative stress) induced by hypoxia. However, it did not improve blood oxygen levels. The antioxidant characteristics of *R. rosea* could be one of the mechanisms on physical performance, because growing evidence indicates that free radicals are responsible for exercise-induced protein oxidation and contribute to muscle fatigue.[70]

E. Toxicity, Safety, and Drug Interactions

R. rosea extract has a very low level toxicity. The LD_{50} (the lethal dose at which 50% of animals die) in the rat is 3.36 g/kg. The equivalent dosage in a 70-kg man would be 235 g. Since the usual clinical doses are 0.2–0.6 g/day, there is a huge margin of safety.[59]

Data from clinical trials suggest that *R. rosea* extract is safe to use with no or few reported side effects.[63,65] Some individuals, particularly those who tend to be anxious, may feel overly activated, jittery, or agitated. If this occurs, a smaller dose with very gradual increases may be needed. *R. rosea* should be taken early during the day, as it may interfere with sleep or cause vivid dreams during the first several days of use. This herb does not appear to interact with other medication, though it may have additive effects with stimulants. It is advised not to take this herb with prescription medication.[59]

F. Future Research Needs

It appears that whether *R. rosea* possesses some ability to enhance physical performance remains unclear. The dosages, populations, and intensities of exercise under which it may work are still ambiguous. More well-controlled human studies are needed to determine if such effects truly exist. Furthermore, since research attempting to elucidate the underlying mechanisms of *R. rosea* is limited, more studies are needed to investigate whether the key constituents (rosavin and salidroside) in *R. rosea* extract can stimulate endorphin action during exercise, either by enhancing endorphin secretion or by increasing sensitivity of the central nervous system to endorphin.

G. Summary and Recommended Dose

Given the current evidence described above, *R. rosea* appears to be able to relieve mental stress and fatigue, improve mental performance, and resist free radical damage induced by exercise or other stress. To obtain an observed beneficial effect of *R. rosea*, a daily dose of 360–600 mg *R. rosea* extract standardized for 1% rosavin, 180–300 mg of an extract standardized for 2% rosavin, or 100–170 mg of an extract standardized for 3.6% rosavin is suggested. At this time, it remains unclear whether *R. rosea* possesses some ability to enhance physical performance. More well-controlled studies are needed.

IV. *ECHINACEA*

A. Introduction

Echinacea, a perennial herb found in eastern and central United States and southern Canada, is commonly known as the purple coneflower. Of nine species of *Echinacea*, three are of medicinal interest (*E. angustifolia, E. purpurea, and E. pallida*). Medicinal use of this herb began with the Native Americans' using it for a variety of conditions including wounds, insect bites, infections, toothache, joint pain, and as an antidote for rattlesnake bites. At the end of the 19th century, *Echinacea* was employed as a cold and flu remedy, and as an anti-infective until the advent of modern antibiotics. During the 20th century, U.S. interest in *Echinacea* waned until the 1980s, when consumer interest in *Echinacea* as an immune stimulant and as a remedy for upper respiratory infections (URIs), including influenza and the common cold, was renewed.[71,72]

More than 800 *Echinacea* preparations are commercially available in tablet, extract, fresh juice, tincture, and tea formulations. The chemical properties of these preparations may differ according to the species, plant parts (flower, stem, roots, leaves, or whole plants) used, time of harvest, geographical location, method of extraction (fresh pressed juice, infusion, tincture in alcohol, water, or combination), and the presence of other plant extracts.[73] By extract type, 50% alcohol/water tincture is considered as the most potent immune stimulant.[74]

All three species of *Echinacea* contain water-soluble polysaccharides, a lipophilic fraction (alkamides, polyacetylenes), caffeoyl conjugates (echinacosides, chicoric acid, caffeic acid), and flavonoids.[73] Cichoric acid is found consistently in all parts of *E. purpurea* while echinacosides are commonly found in *E. pallida* and *E. angustifolia*.[75] To date, it remains unclear if it is one, a few, or the combined effect of these constituents (mainly alkamides, echinacosides, chicoric acid, and polysaccharides) that induce immune-stimulation.[73]

B. Efficacy in Treating and Preventing Upper Respiratory Infections

The German Commission E, World Health Organization (WHO), and the Canadian Natural Health Product Directorate have advocated *Echinacea* use for the common cold. There have been a number of clinical trials of *Echinacea* in treating or preventing upper respiratory infection (URI) symptoms in adults. Quite a few studies suggest that *Echinacea* may be effective in lessening the severity and shortening the duration of the common cold when taken early during the illness.[73] An early systematic (Cochrane) review and its update summarized 16 randomized clinical trials of *Echinacea* for upper respiratory tract infection and concluded that there is some evidence that preparations based on the aerial, or above-ground, part from *Echinacea* (particularly *E. purpurea*) might be efficacious for the early treatment of colds in adults, but results are not fully consistent. Beneficial effects of other *Echinacea* preparations for preventive purposes might exist but have not been shown in independently replicated, rigorous randomized trials.[76,77]

Schoop et al.[78] analyzed three rhinovirus inoculation studies investigating the prophylactic effects of standardized *Echinacea* extracts to determine whether the results obtained in those studies were a consequence of efficacy or of sample size. Based on their analysis, the likelihood of experiencing a clinical cold was 55% higher with placebo than with *Echinacea*. The absolute difference in total symptom scores between groups was -1.96. The authors concluded that standardized extracts of *Echinacea* were effective in the prevention of symptoms of the common cold after clinical inoculation, compared with placebo. Furthermore, in a recent meta-analysis,[73] 14 clinical trials were analyzed to determine the effect of *Echinacea* on the incidence and duration of the common cold. Echinacea was found to decrease the odds of developing the common cold by 58% and the duration of a cold by 1.4 days. Compared with the previous systematic (Cochrane) review,[76,77] this investigation included studies that used experimental rhinovirus or that combined *Echinacea* with other nutraceutical ingredients. Current published evidence supports the benefit of *Echinacea* in decreasing the incidence and duration of the common cold.

C. Mechanisms of Action

Echinacea is widely promoted for its ability to "boost" the immune system. Researchers demonstrated that *Echinacea* can modulate production of specific cytokines from human and rodent macrophages and peripheral blood mononuclear cells *in vitro* and *in vivo*. It may stimulate proliferation of peripheral blood mononuclear cells (PBMC), increase the number of circulating lymphocytes and monocytes, and increase the percentage of spleen NK cells.[74]

E. purpurea and *E. angustifolia* appear to activate nonspecific cellular and humoral immunity and the complement system. Polysaccharides from *E. purpurea* have been shown *in vitro* to preferentially stimulate the mononuclear immune system and release of interleukin-1 (IL-1). Similarly, in *in vitro* studies, arabinogalactans from *E. purpurea* have been observed to induce a dose-dependent release of tumor necrosis factor-alpha (TNF-α) from peritoneal macrophages. Furthermore, glycoproteins (arabinogalactan-proteins) from *E. pallida* have been reported to have immunomodulatory effects by stimulating immunoglobulin M (IgM) production and proliferation of lymphocytes.[79]

D. Immune Modulation in Athletes

Although consumption of products containing *Echinacea* is widespread among athletes, research examining its effects on exercise-induced changes in immune function is limited. In a double-blind placebo-controlled study,[80] the effect of a daily oral pretreatment for 28 days with pressed juice of *E. purpurea* was investigated in 42 triathletes before and after a sprint triathlon. A sub-group of athletes was also treated with magnesium as a reference for supplementation with a micronutrient important for optimal muscular function. The most important finding was that during the 28-day pretreatment period, none of the athletes in the *Echinacea* group fell ill, compared with three individuals in the magnesium group and four in the placebo group who became ill. Pretreatment with *Echinacea* appeared to reduce the release of soluble IL-2 receptor before and after the race and increased the exercise-induced rise in IL-6.

Another study[81] investigated the effects of *E. purpurea* on mucosal immunity and the incidence and duration of URI. Thirty-two athletes completed an exercise protocol known to affect mucosal immunity. Saliva was collected prior to and 5 minutes after completion of exercise testing. Subjects then took either a placebo or *Echinacea* supplement for 4 weeks and the testing procedure was repeated. Each time, s-IgA concentrations and saliva flow rate were measured and the secretion rate of s-IgA was calculated. In addition, standard logs indicating symptoms of upper respiratory infection (URI) were completed throughout the study. Both groups demonstrated significant exercise-induced reductions in s-IgA and the secretion rate of s-IgA at the beginning of the study. Following the 4-week intervention, only the control group experienced the post-intervention decrease in s-IgA and the secretion rate of s-IgA. Furthermore, while there was no significant difference in the number of URIs between groups, the reported duration was significantly shorter in *Echinacea* groups (3.4 days vs. 8.6 days). The results suggest that *Echinacea* may attenuate the mucosal immune suppression known to occur with intense exercise and reduce the duration of URIs that subjects incur.

E. Toxicity, Safety, and Drug Interactions

Adverse effects of *Echinacea* preparations seem rare. Those reported have generally been uncommon and minor, mainly abdominal upset, nausea, and dizziness. Anaphylaxis, asthma exacerbation, and angioedema have been reported in isolated cases. Persons with a history of allergy to any plant in the daisy family (including ragweed, marigold, and chrysanthemum) may be at risk of allergic reaction to *Echinacea*.[35,71] Two studies found no evidence of adverse pregnancy outcomes after *Echinacea* consumption (it works).[35,72]

No significant herb–drug interactions with *Echinacea* have been reported. Based on *in vitro* studies, *Echinacea* may be a mild inhibitor of the cytochrome P450 3A4 enzyme complex system. This inhibition tends to increase levels of drugs metabolized by this system, such as itraconazole (Sporanox), fexofenadine (Allegra), and lovastatin (Mevacor). Although no such interaction has been reported in humans, it is probably advisable to use *Echinacea* with caution in patients who are taking these medications. Theoretically, the immune-stimulating properties of *Echinacea* might interfere with the use of immunosuppressive medications in patients with autoimmune disease. However, it has not been documented in animals or humans.[71]

F. Recommended Dose

The most commonly used preparation in the United States is a liquid extract of *E. purpurea* root; typical dosing of such a preparation would be 3 mL every 3 to 4 hours for the first 1 to 2 days of upper respiratory illness, then three times daily for the subsequent week. Patients who are using an *Echinacea* tea (made from *E. angustifolia* or *E. purpurea* root) will need to take higher dosages, typically 6 to 8 oz. four times daily for the first 2 days, titrating down to once or twice daily on days 3 to 7.[35,72]

G. Future Research Needs

Systematic analysis of current evidence in the literature suggests that *Echinacea* has a benefit in decreasing the incidence and duration of the common cold. However, large-scale randomized prospective studies controlling for variables such as species, part of plant used, quality of preparation, and dosages of *Echinacea*, method of cold induction, and outcome measurement are needed. Furthermore, active components (alkamides, echinacosides, chicoric acid, and polysaccharides) in *Echinacea* are essential for the immune modulating effects. Future research could standardize active component levels in the product and test them in human clinical trials.

H. Summary

Current evidence suggests that *E. purpurea* may decrease the symptoms and severity of the common cold and may also decrease the number of colds when taken prophylactically. *E. pallida* root extracts may decrease the duration of symptoms of the common cold. Clinical data on *E. angustifolia* remains contradictory, and thus has not been recommended by the German Commission E. The most commonly used preparation in the United States is a liquid extract of *E. purpurea* root; typical dosing of such a preparation would be 3 mL every 3 to 4 hours for the first 1 to 2 days of upper respiratory illness, then three times daily for the subsequent week.

V. *EPHEDRA*

A. Introduction

Ephedra species, also know as *Ma Huang*, are plants indigenous to China, Pakistan, and northwestern India. It has been used for over 5,000 years to treat bronchial asthma and URIs. Although some 40 species are known worldwide, its effects are attributable to the contents of ephedrine and related alkaloids found primarily in the species of Chinese origin (*Ephedra sinica*). Historically, *E. sinica* has generally been consumed in the form of an invigorating tea or infusion with beneficial effects on respiration.[82,83]

Most recently, *Ephedra* in pill form, which is not comparable with traditional use, has been promoted for weight reduction and as a performance enhancer in body building and other sports. Dietary supplements containing *Ephedra* typically contain no more than 25 mg of ephedrine alkaloids per unit dose and it is recommended that one take no more than 100 mg total ephedrine alkaloids (four units) daily.[11] However, due to safety concerns, in April 2004, the Food and Drug Administration (FDA) officially banned buying or selling Ephedra-containing dietary supplements in the United States.[83]

B. Mechanisms of Action

Ephedra contains several alkaloids, including ephedrine, as well as smaller amounts of pseudoephedrine, phenylpropanolamine, methylephedrine, methylpseudoephedrine, and norpseudoephedrine.[84] Ephedrine and pseudoephedrine are classified as sympathomimetic alkaloids because they directly stimulate the sympathetic, or "fight or flight," nervous system. These alkaloids are structurally similar to amphetamines and have direct α- and β-agonistic properties and catecholamine-releasing actions. Ephedrine alkaloids also function as indirect adrenoreceptor agonists. Thus, they augment the availability and action of the natural neurotransmitter norepinephrine in the brain and in the heart. Furthermore, ephedrine mediates its effects via circulating epinephrine and is a bronchial dilator that has been used in the treatment of asthma.[82] Like other stimulants, ingestion of ephedrine or pseudoephedrine will lead to various physiologic responses, including vasoconstriction, bronchodilation, and increases in blood pressure, heart rate, cardiac contractile force, and automaticity.[84]

Although ephedrine and its alkaloids are considered to contribute to its biological effects, *Ephedra* may not have the same physiological effect as the pure ephedrine. A study reported that it took longer for the ephedrine to reach peak levels in the plasma (approximately 4 hours) when ingested in the form of *Ephedra*.[85] However, another study showed that ephedrine from three commercial products containing *Ephedra* had the same absorption kinetics as those following ingestion of a 25-mg synthetic ephedrine capsule.[86]

C. Effects on Physical Performance

Ephedra-containing supplements are popular among athletes. A recent survey revealed that about half of the athletes surveyed (48.5%) reported having used *Ephedra* at least once to improve athletic performance. Additionally, 17.4% reported using pseudoephedrine to improve performance in the 30 days prior to survey administration. The majority of athletes began use prior to college.[87] However, research investigating the effects of *Ephedra* or ephedrine and performance in an athletic population is limited.

A systematic review[88] located eight published controlled trials investigating the effects of synthetic ephedrine on athletic performance. However, no trial assessed the effects of herbal *Ephedra* on athletic performance. Six trials reported that neither caffeine nor ephedrine alone had significant effects on parameters of exercise performance such as oxygen consumption, time to exhaustion, or carbon dioxide production, but the combination of ephedrine and caffeine consistently demonstrated a 20% to 30% increase in performance.

D. Toxicity, Safety, and Drug Interactions

Because of its direct sympathomimetic effects, ephedrine can increase heart rate, contractility, cardiac output, and peripheral resistance. Thus, increases in both heart rate and blood pressure are common observations after ephedrine ingestion. This may also be true for *Ephedra*, when used chronically and in sustained high doses (> 100 mg/day), especially when overdosed. Although these effects are not serious in most users, the consequences can be severe in those with underlying heart disease, hypertension, or diabetes, and those sensitive to ephedrine. Most common side effects are nervousness, anxiety, heart palpitations, headaches, nausea, hyperthermia, hypertension, and cardiac arrhythmias, while more serious side effects include seizures, severe hypertension, arrhythmias, psychosis, hepatitis, stroke, myocardial injury, and intracranial hemorrhage.[11,82]

Numerous case reports have documented adverse effects in persons using *Ephedra*. In the largest published case series, Haller and Benowitz [89] reviewed 140 adverse event reports involving *Ephedra* that were submitted to the FDA. They concluded that 43 were definitely or probably related to *Ephedra* and another 44 were possibly related. In well controlled clinical trials, where subject recruitment and health status is screened and confined to healthy individuals, ephedrine or *Ephedra* are associated with, on average, 2 to 4 times the risk for developing psychiatric symptoms, autonomic symptoms, upper GI symptoms, and heart palpitations.[88] Compared with other herbal supplements, products containing *Ephedra* were responsible for 64% of the adverse reactions reported to the Toxic Event Surveillance Systems of the American Association of Poison Control Centers.[84]

E. Future Research Needs

In April 2005, just 1 year after FDA's ban of buying or selling *Ephedra*-containing dietary supplements in the United States, a federal judge ruled against the FDA ban stating that *Ephedra* was wrongly being regulated by the FDA as a drug and not a food. This ruling in effect allows once again buying and selling of supplements containing *Ephedra*. Since then, Internet sales of supplements containing *Ephedra* have started, though it has not yet returned to major retail markets. It is important to determine the prevalence of use in the United States after the over-ruling of the FDA ban, and *Ephedra*'s use in other athletic populations. Furthermore, a proper study to assess the possible association of *Ephedra* or ephedrine consumption and the occurrence of serious adverse events is also needed, because continued analysis of case reports cannot substitute for a properly designed study to assess causality.

F. Summary

Although *Ephedra*-containing supplements are popular among athletes, the use of those products may expose the users to unacceptable health risks relative to undefined or unknown benefits on performance. It is recommended not to use *Ephedra*-containing products as stimulants to enhance physical performance.

VI. CONCLUSIONS

During the past decade, herbal supplements have gained in popularity and acceptance among athletes and people who exercise regularly. The most frequently cited reasons for supplement use were to increase energy, prevent illness, and enhance physical performance.

To date, much of the knowledge concerning the efficacy of herbal supplements in athletes and people who exercise regularly is mainly based on traditional use, identities of ingredients, and personal recommendations (family member/friends, fellow athletes, trainer, coaches, and healthcare professionals). Among commonly used herbal supplements, quite a few well-controlled research studies suggest that *P. ginseng*, *R. rosea*, and *Echinacea* may be effective in the enhancement of physical and mental performance, relief of mental stress, and decrease of symptoms and severity of the common colds, if taken long enough and at sufficient doses. Moreover, greater benefits may be observed for untrained or older (>40 y) subjects.

It has long been known that commercial herbal supplements may vary greatly in terms of their purity, strength, and composition. This is because there are large variations in materials used and manufacturing practice, which may include variations in plant species, plant sources, part of the plant used, years of growth, season of harvest, and methods of processing. Therefore, supplement users should keep themselves informed regarding ingredients, product labels, recommended daily doses, and quality of products.

The following are suggestions to follow in selecting good quality herbal supplements. One should choose:

- A product composed of correct plant species and parts
- A product that is manufactured using proper processing methods

- A product labeled with a description of appropriate levels of active components
- A product that has been verified independently for its label claims
- A product that has established its efficacy through well-controlled human studies

REFERENCES

1. Eisenberg, D. M. , Davis, R. B. , Ettner, S. L. , Appel, S. , Wilkey, S. , Rompay, M. V., and Kessler, R. C., Trends in alternative medicine use in the United States, 1990–1997: Results of a follow-up national survey. *JAMA*. 280, 1569–1575, 1998.
2. Kelly, J. P., Kaufman. D. W., Kelley, K., Rosenberg, L., Anderson, T. E., and Mitchell, A. A., Recent trends in use of herbal and other natural products. *Arch. Intern. Med.* 165, 281–286, 2005.
3. Ziegler, P. J., Nelson, J. A., and Jonnalagadda, S. S., Use of dietary supplements by elite figure skaters. *Int. J. Sport Nutr. Exerc. Metab*. 13, 266–276, 2003.
4. Herbold, N., Visconti, B., Frates, S., and Bandini, L., Traditional and nontraditional supplement use by collegiate female varsity athletes. *Int. J. Sport Nutr. Exerc. Metab.* 14, 586–593, 2004.
5. Froiland, K., Koszewski, W., Hingst, J., and Kopecky, L., Nutritional supplement use among college athletes and their sources of information. *Int. J. Sport Nutr. Exerc. Metab.* 14, 104–120, 2004.
6. Morrison, L. J., Gizis, F., and Shorter, B., Prevalent use of dietary supplements among people who exercise at a commercial gym. *Int. J. Sport Nutr. Exerc. Metab.* 14, 481–492, 2004.
7. Bahrke, M. S. and Morgan, W. P., Evaluation of the ergogenic properties of ginseng: An update. *Sports Med.* 29, 113–133, 2000.
8. Zhu, S., Zou, K., Fushim, H., Cai, S., and Komatsu, K., Comparative study on triterpene saponins of ginseng drugs. *Planta Med.* 70, 666–677, 2004.
9. Coleman, C. I., Hebert, J. H., and Reddy P., The effects of Panax ginseng on quality of life. *J. Clin. Pharm. Ther*. 28, 5–15, 2003.
10. Kiefer, D. and Pantuso, T., *Panax ginseng. Am. Fam. Physician*, 68, 1539–1542, 2003.
11. Bucci, L., Selected herbals and human exercise performance. *Am. J. Clin. Nutr.,* 72, 624S–636S, 2000.
12. Chuang, W. C., Wu, H. K., Sheu, S. J., Chiou, S. H., Chang, H. C., and Chen, Y. P., A comparative study on commercial sample of ginseng radix. *Plant Med.* 61, 459–465, 1995.
13. Reynolds, L. B., Effects of drying on chemical and physical characteristics of American ginseng. *J. Herbs Spices Med. Plants,* 6, 9–21,1998.
14. Kim, W. Y., Kim, J. M., Han, S. B., Lee, S. K., Kim N. D., Park, M. K., et al., Steaming of ginseng at high temperature enhances biological activity. *J. Nat. Prod.*, 63, 1702–1704, 2000.
15. Vogler, B. K., Pittler, M. H., and Ernst, E., The efficacy of ginseng: A systematic review of randomized clinical trials. *Eur. J. Clin. Pharmacol.* 55, 567–575, 1999.
16. Krochmal, R., Hardy, M., Bowerman, S., Lu, Q. Y., Wang, H. J., Elashoff, R. M., and Heber, D., Phytochemical assays of commercial botanical dietary supplements. *eCAM* 1, 305–313, 2004.
17. Ma, Y. C., Zhu, J., Benkrima, L., Luo, M., Sun, L., Sain, S. and Kont, K., Plaut–Carcasson Y. Y., A comparative evaluation of ginsenosides in commercial ginseng products and tissue culture samples using HPLC. *J. Herbs Spices Med. Plants* 3, 41–50, 1995.

18. Wang, X., Sakuman, T., Asafu-Adjaye, E., and Shiu G. K., Determination of ginsenosides in plant extracts from *Panax ginseng* and *Panax quinquefolius* L. by LC/MS/MS. *Anal. Chem.* 71,1579–1584, 1999.
19. Carabin, I. G., Burdock, G. A., and Chris, C., Safety assessment of Panax ginseng. *Int. J. Toxicol.* 19, 293–301, 2000.
20. Cui, J., Garie, M., Eneroth, P., and Bjorkhem, I., What do commercial ginseng preparations contain? *Lancet* 344, 134, 1994.
21. Harkey, M. R., Henderson, G. L., Gershwin, M. E., Stern, J. S., and Hackman, R. M., Variability in commercial ginseng products: An analysis of 25 preparations. *Am. J. Clin. Nutr.* 73, 1101–1106, 2001.
22. Tachikawa, E. and Kudo, K., Proof of the mysterious efficacy of ginseng: Basic and clinical trials: Suppression of adrenal medullary function in vitro by ginseng. *J. Pharmcol. Sci.* 95, 140–144, 2004.
23. Han, M., Sha, X., Wu, Y., and Fang, X., Oral absorption of ginsenoside Rb_1 using *in vitro* and *in vivo* models. *Plant Med.* 71, 398–404, 2005.
24. Tawab, M. A., Bahr, U., Karas, M., Wurglics, M., and Schubert-Zsilavecz, M., Degradation of ginsenosides in humans after oral administration. *Drug Met. Dispos.* 31, 1065–1071, 2003.
25. Ziemba, A. W., Chmura, J., Kaciuba-Uscilko, H., Nazar, K., Wisnik, P. and Gawronski, W., Ginseng treatment improves psychomotor performance at rest and during graded exercise in young athletes. *Int. J. Sport Nutr.* 4, 371–377, 1999.
26. Kim, S. H., Park, K. S., Chang, M. J., and Sung, J. H., Effects of Panax ginseng extract on exercise-induced oxidative stress. *J. Sports Med. Phys. Fitness.* 45, 178–182, 2005.
27. Rogers, M. E., Bohlken, R. M., Beets, M. W., Hammer, S. B., Ziegenfuss, T. N., and Šarabon, N., Effects of creatine, ginseng, and astragalus supplementation on strength, body composition, mood, and blood lipids during strength training in older adults. *J. Sport Sci. Med.* 5, 60–69, 2006.
28. Wesnes, K. A., Faleni R. A., Hefting N. R., Hoogsteen, G., Houben J. J. G., Jenkins, E., et al., The cognitive, subjective, and physical effects of Ginkgo biloba/Panax ginseng combination in healthy volunteers with neurasthenic complaints. *Psychopharmacol. Bull.* 33, 677–683, 1997.
29. Kennedy, D. O. and Scholey, A. B., Ginseng: Potential for the enhancement of cognitive performance and mood. *Pharmacol. Biochem. Behav.* 75, 687–700, 2003.
30. Kennedy, D. O., Haskell, C. F., Wesnes, K. A., and Scholey, A. B., Improved cognitive performance in humans volunteers following administration of guarana (*Paulinia cupana*) extract: Comparison and interaction with *Panax ginseng*. *Pharmacol. Biochem. Behav.* 79, 401–411, 2004.
31. Reay, J. L., Kennedy, D. O., and Scholey, A. B., Single doses of panax ginseng (G115) reduce blood glucose levels and improve cognitive performance during sustained mental activity. *J. Psychopharmacol. 19,* 357–365, 2005.
32. Reay, J. L., Kennedy, D. O., and Scholey, A. B., Effects of *Panax ginseng*, consumed with and without glucose, on blood glucose levels and cognitive performance during sustained "mentally demanding" tasks. *J. Psychopharmacol.* 20, 771–781, 2006.
33. Kim, J. H., Park, C. Y., and Lee, S. J., Effects of sun ginseng on subjective quality of life in cancer patients: A double-blind, placebo-controlled pilot trial. *J. Clin. Pharm. Ther.* 31, 331–334, 2006.
34. Cui, Y., Shu, X. O., Gao, Y. T., Cai, H., Tao, M. H., and Zheng, W., Association of ginseng use with survival and quality of life among breast cancer patients. *Am. J. Epidemiol.* 163, 645–653, 2006.
35. Ernst, E., The risk–benefit profile of commonly used herbal therapies: Ginkgo, St. John's Wort, Ginseng, Echinacea, Saw Palmetto, and Kava. *Ann. Intern. Med.* 136, 42–53, 2002.

36. Gurley, B. J., Gardner, S. F., Hubbard, M. A., Williams, K., Gentry, W. B., Cui, Y., and Ang, C. Y. W., Clinical assessment of botanical supplementation on cytochrome P450 phenotypes in the elderly: St. John's wort, garlic oil, *Panax ginseng*, and *Ginkgo biloba. Drugs Aging* 22, 525–539, 2005.
37. Liu, Y., Zhang, J. W., Li, W., Ma, H., Sun, J., Deng, M. C., and Yang, L., Ginsenoside metabolites, rather than naturally occurring ginsenosides, lead to inhibition of human cytochrome P450 enzymes. *Toxicol. Sci.* 91, 356–364, 2006.
38. Davydov, M. and Krikorian, A. D., *Eleutherococcus senticosus* (Rupr. & Maxim.) Maxim. (Araliaceae) as an adaptogen: A closer look. *J. Ethnopharmacol.* 72, 345–393, 2000.
39. Monograph., *Eleutherococcus senticosus. Altern. Med. Rev.* 11, 151–155, 2006.
40. Wagner, H., Horr, H., and Winterhoff, H., Plant adaptogens. *Phytomedicine* 1, 63–76, 1994.
41. Panossian, A., Wikman, G. and Wagner, H., Plant adaptogens III. Earlier and more recent aspects and concepts on their mode of actions. *Phytomedicine* 6, 287–300, 1999.
42. Panossian, A. and Wagner, H., Stimulating effect of adaptogens: an overview with particular reference to their efficacy following single dose administration. *Phytother. Res.* 19, 819–838, 2005.
43. Panossian, A., Adaptogens: tonic herbs for fatigue and stress. *Alt. Comp. Ther.* 9, 327–332, 2003.
44. Farnsworth, N. R., Kinghorn, A. D., Soejarto, D. D., and Waller, D. P., Siberian ginseng (*Eleutherococcus senticosus*): Current status as an adaptogen. in *Economic and Medicinal Plant Research Vol 1,* Wagner, H., Hikino, H. and Farnsworth, N. R., Eds. Academic Press, New York, NY, 155–215, 1985.
45. Facchinetti, F., Neri, I., and Tarabusi, M., *Eleutherococcus senticosus* reduces cardiovascular response in healthy subjects: A randomized, placebo-controlled trial. *Stress Health* 18, 11–17, 2002.
46. Hartz, A. J., Bentler, S., Noyes, R., Hoehns, J., Logemann, C., Sinift, S., et al., Randomized controlled trial of Siberian ginseng for chronic fatigue. *Psychol. Med.*, 34, 51–61, 2004.
47. Cicero, A. F., Derosa, G., Brillante, R., Bernardi, R., Nascetti, S., and Gaddi, A., Effects of Siberian ginseng (*Eleutherococcus senticosus* maxim.) on elderly quality of life: A randomized clinical trial. *Arch. Gerontol. Geriatr. Suppl.* 9, 69–73, 2004.
48. Narimanian, M., Badalyan, M., Panosyan, V., Gabrielyan, E., Panossian, A., Wikman, G. and Wagner, H., Impact of Chisan (ADAPT–232) on the quality-of-life and its efficacy as an adjuvant in the treatment of acute non-specific pneumonia. *Phytomedicine* 12, 723–729, 2005.
49. Walker, M., Adaptogens: Nature's answer to stress. *Townsend Lett. Doc.*, July, 751–755, 1994.
50. Asano, K., Takahashi, T., Miyashita, M., Matsuzaka, A., Muramatsu, S., Kuboyama, M., et al., Effect of *Eleutheroccocus senticosus* extract on human physical working capacity. *Planta Med.* 52, 175–177, 1986.
51. McNaughton, L., Egan, G., and Caelli, G., A comparison of Chinese and Russian ginseng as ergogenic aids to improve various facets of physical fitness. *Int. Clin. Nutr. Rev.* 9, 32–35, 1989.
52. Szolomicki, S., Samochowiec, L., Wojcicki, J., and Drozdzik, M., The influence of active components of *Eleutherococcus senticosus* on cellular defense and physical fitness in man. *Phytotherapy Res.* 14, 30–35, 2000.
53. Dowling, E. A., Redondo, D. R., Branch, J. D., Jones, S., McNabb, G., and Williams, M. H., Effect of *Eleutherococcus senticosus* on submaximal and maximal exercise performance. *Med. Sci. Sports Exerc.* 28, 482–489, 1996.

54. Cheuvront, S. N., Moffatt, R. J., Biggerstaff, K. D., Bearden, S., and McDonough, P., Effect of ENDUROX™ on metabolic responses to submaximal exercise. *Int. J. Sport Nutr.* 9, 434–442, 1999.
55. Plowman, S. A., Dustman, K., Walicek, H., Corless, C., and Ehlers, G., The effects of ENDUROX™ on the physiological responses to stair-stepping exercise. *Res. Q. Exerc. Sport* 70, 385–388, 1999.
56. Eschbach, L. C., Webster, M. J., Boyd, J. C. and McArthur, P. D., and Evetovich, T. K., The effect of Siberian Ginseng (*Eleutherococcus senticosus*) on substrate utilization and performance during prolonged cycling. *Int. J. Sport Nutr. Exerc. Metab.* 10, 444–451, 2000.
57. Donovan, J. L., DeVane, L., Chavin, K. D., Taylor, R. M., and Markowitz, J. S., Siberian ginseng (*Eleutherococcus senticosus*) effects on CYP2D6 and CYP3A4 activity in normal volunteers. *Drug Met. Dis.* 31, 519–522, 2003.
58. Wolsko, P. M., Solondz, D. K., Phillips, R. S., Schachter, S. C., and Eisenberg, D. M., Lack of herbal supplement characterization in published randomized controlled trials. *Am. J. Med.* 118, 1087–1093, 2005.
59. Brown, R. P., Gerbarg, P. L., and Ramazanov, Z., *Rhodiola rosea*: A phytomedicinal overview. *HerbalGram,* 56, 40–52, 2002.
60. Ganzera, M., Yayla, Y., and Khan, I. A., Analysis of the marker compounds of *Rhodioloa rosea* L (Golden Root) by reversed phase high performance liquid chromatography. *Chem. Pharm. Bull. (Tokyo)*, 49, 465–467, 2001.
61. Kelly, G. S., *Rhodiola rosea*: A possible plant adaptogen. *Altern. Med. Rev.* 6, 293–302, 2001.
62. Spasov, A. A., Wikman, G. K., Mandrikov, V. B., Mironova, I. A., and Neumoni, V. V., A double–blind, placebo–controlled pilot study of the stimulating and adaptogenic effect of *Rhodiola rosea* SHR–5 extract on the fatigue of students caused by stress during an examination period with a repeated low-dose regimen. *Phytomedicine* 7, 85–89, 2000.
63. Darbinyan, V., Kteyan, A., Panossian, A., Gabrielyan, E., Wikman, G., and Wagner, H., *Rhodiola rosea* in stress induced fatigue—A double blind cross-over study of a standardized extract SHR-5 with a repeated low-dose regimen on the mental performance of healthy physicians during night duty. *Phytomedicine,* 7, 365–371, 2000.
64. Shevtsov, V. A., Zholus, B. I., Shervarly, V. I., Vol'skij, V. B., Korovin, Y. P., Khristich, M. P., et al., A randomized trial of two different doses of a SHR–5 Rhodiola rosea extract versus placebo and control of capacity for mental work. *Phytomedicine.* 10, 95–105, 2003.
65. De Bock, K., Eijnde, B. O., Ramaekers, M., and Hespel, P., Acute Rhodiola rosea intake can improve endurance exercise performance. *Int. J. Sport Nutr. Exerc. Metab.* 14, 298–307, 2004.
66. Earnest, C. P., Morss, G. M., Wyatt, F., Jordan, A. N., Colson, S., Church, T. S., et al., Effects of a commercial herbal-based formula on exercise performance in cyclists. *Med. Sci. Sports Exerc.* 36, 504–509, 2004.
67. Colson, S. N., Wyatt, F. B., Johnston, D. L., Autrey, L. D., FitzGerald, Y. L., and Earnest, C. P., Cordyceps sinensis- and Rhodiola rosea-based supplementation in male cyclists and its effect on muscle tissue oxygen saturation. *J. Strength Cond. Res.* 19, 358–63, 2005.
68. Wing, S. L., Askew, E. W., Luetkemeier, M. J., Ryujin, D. T., Kamimori, G. H., and Grissom, C. K., Lack of effect of Rhodiola or oxygenated water supplementation on hypoxemia and oxidative stress. *Wilderness Environ. Med.* 14, 9–16, 2003.
69. Abidov, M., Grachev, S., Seifulla, R. D., and Ziegenfuss, T. N, Extract of Rhodiola rosea radix reduces the level of C-reactive protein and creatinine kinase in the blood. *Bull. Exp. Biol. Med.* 138, 63–64, 2004.
70. Powers, S. K., DeRuisseau, K. C., Quindry, J., and Hamilton, K. L., Dietary antioxidants and exercise. *J. Sports Sci.* 22, 81–94, 2004.

71. Kligler, B., Echinacea. *Am. Fam. Physician* 67, 77–80, 83, 2003.
72. Perri, D., Dugoua, J. J., Mills, E., and Koren, G., Safety and efficacy of echinacea (*Echinacea angustifolia, E. purpurea* and *E. pallida*) during pregnancy and lactation. *Can. J. Clin. Pharmacol.* 13, 262–267, 2006.
73. Shah, S. A., Sander, S., White, C. M., Rinaldi, M., and Coleman, C. I., Evaluation of echinacea for the prevention and treatment of the common cold: A meta-analysis. *Lancet Infect. Dis.* 7, 473–480, 2007.
74. Senchina, D. S., McCann, D. A., Aspc, J. M., Johnson, J. A., Cunnick, J. E., Kaisere, M. S., and Kohuta, M. L., Changes in immunomodulatory properties of *Echinacea* spp. root infusions and tinctures stored at 4°C for four days. *Clin. Chim. Acta* 355, 67–82, 2005.
75. Gilroy C. M., Steiner, J. F., Byers, T., Shapiro, H., and Georgian, W., Echinacea and truth in labeling. *Arch. Intern. Med.* 163, 699–704, 2003.
76. Melchart, D., Linde, K., Fischer, P., and Kaesmayr, J., Echinacea for preventing and treating the common cold. *Cochrane Database Syst. Rev.* 2000; (2):CD000530.
77. Linde, K., Barrett, B., Wolkart, K., Bauer, R., and Melchart, D., Echinacea for preventing and treating the common cold. *Cochrane Database Syst Rev.* Issue 1, Art. No. CD000530, last substantive update Nov 8, 2005.
78. Schoop, R., Klein, P., Suter, A. and Johnston, S. L., Echinacea in the prevention of induced rhinovirus colds: A meta-analysis. *Clin. Ther.* 28, 174–183, 2006.
79. Roxas, M. and Jurenka, J., Colds and Influenza: A review of diagnosis and conventional, botanical, and nutritional considerations. *Altern. Med. Rev.* 12, 25–48, 2007.
80. Berg, A., Northoff, H., and Konig, D., Influence of Echinacin (E31) treatment on the exercise-induced immune response in athletes. *J. Clin. Res.* 1, 367–380, 1998.
81. Hall, H., Fahlman, M. M., and Engels, H. J., Echinacea purpurea and mucosal immunity. *Int. J. Sports Med.* 28, 792–797, 2007.
82. Power, M. E., Ephedra and its application to sport performance: Another concern for the athletic trainer? *J. Athlet. Train.* 36, 420–424, 2001.
83. Stahl, C. E., Borlongan, C. V., Szerlip, H., and Szerlip, M., No pain, no gain—Exercise-induced rhabdomyolysis associated with the performance enhancer herbal supplement ephedra. *Med. Sci. Monit.* 12, CS81–84, 2006.
84. Bent, S., Tiedt, T. N, Odden, M. C., and Shlipak, M. G., The relative safety of ephedra compared with other herbal products. *Ann. Intern. Med.* 138, 468–471, 2003.
85. White, L. M., Gardner, S. F., Gurley, B. J., Marx, M. A., Wang, P. L., and Estes, M., Pharmacokinetics and cardiovascular effects of ma-huang (Ephedra sinica) in normotensive adults. *J. Clin. Pharmacol.* 37, 116–122, 1997.
86. Gurley, B. J., Gardner, S. F., White, L. M., and Wang, P. L., Ephedrine pharmacokinetics after the ingestion of nutritional supplements containing *Ephedra sinica* (ma huang). *Ther. Drug Monit.* 20, 439–445, 1998.
87. Bents, R. T. and Marsh, E., Patterns of Ephedra and other stimulant use in collegiate hockey athletes. *Int. J. Sport Nutr. Exerc. Metab.* 16, 636–643, 2006.
88. Shekelle, P. G., Hardy, M. L., Morton, S. C., Maglione, M., Mojica, W. A., Suttorp, M. K., et al., Efficacy and safety of ephedra and ephedrine for weight loss and athletic performance. *JAMA* 289, 1537–1545, 2003.
89. Haller, C. A. and Benowitz, N. L., Adverse cardiovascular and central nervous system events associated with dietary supplements containing Ephedra alkaloids. *N. Eng. J. Med.* 343, 1833–1838, 2000.
90. Odani, T., Tanizawa, H., and Takino, Y., Studies on the absorption, distribution, excretion and metabolism of ginseng saponins. II. The absorption, distribution and excretion of ginsenoside Rg1 in the rat. *Chem. Pharm. Bull.* 31, 292–298,1983.
91. McRae, S. Elevated serum digoxin levels in a patient taking digoxin and Siberian ginseng. *CMAJ*, 155, 293–295, 1996.

Section VII

Recreational Activities

14 Endurance Training

Shawn R. Simonson and
Catherine G. Ratzin-Jackson

CONTENTS

I. INTRODUCTION

The numerous benefits of physical activity range from improvements in bone mineral density to ameliorating the effects of aging (Table 14.1). Not only are physically active individuals healthier, but they are also happier, live longer, sleep better, experience less pain, and have more energy and better day-to-day function. Many of these benefits can be attributed to simply increasing the amount of moderate physical activity in one's day and to increasing the amount of activity that works the heart, blood vessels, and lungs—the cardiovascular and respiratory systems. This type of physical activity has many names that mean the same thing: cardiovascular, cardiorespiratory, aerobic, and endurance activity are all longer duration, rhythmic activities that use large muscle masses and require the utilization of oxygen to break down nutrients to produce energy.

II. ENDURANCE EXERCISE DEFINED

Physical activity is any bodily movement produced by skeletal muscle that results in an expenditure of energy.[1] The definition of exercise is more specific; it is planned,

TABLE 14.1

Benefits Associated with Regular Physical Activity[3,4,91,93]

Energy expenditure	Improved balance
Improved cardiovascular function	Improved fat utilization
Improved glucose (sugar) utilization	Improved immunity
Improved lipid (cholesterol, triglycerides) profile	Improved mood
Improved sleep	Improved strength
Improved weight management	Increased bone mineral density (weight bearing)
Increased energy	Reduced back pain
Reduced blood pressure	Reduced bone/joint problems
Reduced cancer	Reduced falls
Slows aging	

structured, repetitive, and purposeful physical activity for the sake of keeping the body in a healthy state or improving performance.[2] Taking it a step further—conditioning is frequent and regular exercise with the intent of improving fitness, and training is the improvement of fitness in preparation for a sport or athletic competition. Physical fitness comprises all of the components that allow physical activity and includes considerations of muscle strength and endurance, bone integrity, flexibility, body composition, metabolic fitness (resistance to disease and the ability to provide energy), skill, balance, reaction time, and cardiorespiratory fitness.[1–3] Muscular endurance, bone integrity, flexibility, body composition, metabolic fitness, skill, balance, and cardiorespiratory fitness can all be improved through endurance exercise.

Endurance exercise goes by many names that all mean the same thing: cardiovascular, cardiorespiratory, aerobic, and endurance exercise or activity. Aerobic activity is any rhythmic movement that continuously uses large muscle groups over a period of time, increases heart rate and energy expenditure, and requires primarily oxygen for energy production—such as walking, jogging, cycling, aerobics, and swimming.[2,4] Rhythmic movement is the repeated alternating of muscle contraction and relaxation as in walking or pedaling a bicycle. The large muscle groups can be those of the upper body, as used in the crawl swim stroke, those of the lower extremities, as in running, or those of both the upper and lower extremities, as in rowing. Oxygen utilization for energy production refers to cellular processes used to break down carbohydrates, fats, and protein into energy used to generate movement.

For enhanced clarity it is important to understand the basic principles of the production of energy. Humans have to convert all three energy substrates, carbohydrates, fats, and proteins, into a common high-energy molecule to generate movement. The common high-energy molecule is adenosine triphosphate (ATP), an adenosine molecule with three inorganic phosphate groups attached. Energy is liberated for movement when the phosphate groups are cleaved from ATP. Not a lot of ATP is stored in human cells, so there must be a mechanism to rapidly replenish the ATP that has lost a phosphate molecule and become adenosine diphosphate (ADP). Three metabolic pathways supply ATP for movement. All three of these are always functioning, but their relative contribution to the energy supply is determined by exercise duration and intensity.

The first energy pathway is often termed the phosphagen system in that it uses the limited stored ATP and creatine phosphate (CP) to fuel initial and high-intensity movements. Stored ATP is used to initiate movement; however, the amount of ATP available is only enough to do just that—initiate movement. There is another high-energy storage molecule available to rapidly replenish the used ATP and that is CP. Creatine phosphate gives up its phosphate group to ATP so that ATP can continue to fuel the activity. However, humans cannot store a lot of CP, so this system can supply energy only for a matter of seconds—perhaps up to 10 seconds—and depends on the intensity of the movement.

As ATP is used and the phosphagen system starts up, the second metabolic pathway has already been initiated. Termed glycolysis, this provides energy to continue the movement and is somewhat slower than the phosphagen system. Notice that no mention was made of the three energy substrates in the phosphagen system. Glycolysis is the first, in which a more efficient energy source is used. Here, glucose (a simple sugar used by animals for energy) or glycogen (a chain of glucose molecules strung together for storage) is rapidly broken down to release energy that can be transferred to ADP and form ATP, which can be used in muscle contraction. This breakdown splits the glucose molecule into two equal elements that are eventually converted to pyruvate. At the beginning of movement and when exercise is very intense, the two pyruvate molecules are converted to lactate, which can be shuttled out of the cell and allow activity to continue. This system produces quite a bit of energy very rapidly, but only for a short time—up to 2 min—again, depending on intensity.

As ATP is used and glycolysis continues to produce pyruvate, the third system begins to function at higher levels. This third system is termed aerobic or oxidative metabolism because oxygen is required to release the energy, which occurs in the mitochondria, cellular organelles sometimes termed the powerhouse of the cell. The two pyruvate molecules, instead of being converted to lactate, enter Kreb's cycle (also called the tricarboxylic acid (TCA) or citric acid cycle) and then the electron transport system or chain to be broken down to carbon dioxide and water. The electrons and protons given off during Kreb's cycle move through the cascade of the electron transport chain and this results in the formation of ATP and water. It is the formation of water that requires oxygen as the final hydrogen and electron acceptor. One important fact about this third system is that pyruvate is not the only substrate that can be used for the liberation of energy. Fats and proteins can be broken down into subunits that can be used in this oxidative system to replenish ATP. This system is slower, but can provide ATP for an extended period of time—as long as there is energy available. Thus, this third system—the aerobic or oxidative system—is the energy system used to fuel endurance activity.

III. BENEFITS OF ENDURANCE ACTIVITY

The population of the United States shows high rates of chronic, degenerative, hypokinetic (sedentary lifestyle) diseases. Insufficient physical activity can lead to poorer health in as little as 6 months (Table 14.2).[5] Regular participation in endurance

TABLE14.2

Effects of Six Months of Continued Physical Inactivity[5]

Decreased insulin sensitivity
Decreased time to fatigue
Increased abdominal fat
Increased body weight
Increased fasting insulin
Increased LDL cholesterol
Increased visceral fat
Increased waist circumference
Increased waist to hip ratio

activity improves many aspects of health and physical function. These range from combating heart disease to increasing one's ability to perform the myriad activities of daily living to the impressive feats of endurance observed in athletic competition.

The leading cause of death in the United States is heart disease. It has been every year since 1900—with the exception of 1918 when there was an influenza pandemic. In addition, four of the top five leading causes of death in persons 65 and older, with the exception of cancer, are directly related to the deterioration of the cardiovascular and respiratory systems (Table 14.3). Three of these five—heart disease, stroke, and chronic obstructive pulmonary disease (COPD)—are related to cardiovascular disease (CVD).[6] Cardiovascular disease includes over 20 diseases of the heart and blood vessels, including hypertension and stroke. Considerable progress has been made in the last decades in reducing the overall percentage of deaths due to CVD, yet the vast numbers and costs still remain: 25.6 million (8.6% of the U.S. adult population) are diagnosed with heart disease and it is estimated that 100 million (37% of the adult population) have two or more risk factors for CVD.[7] This costs the United States $258 billion per year and results in 4.2 million hospitalizations and 652,486 deaths (27%) per year.[7,8]

Cardiovascular complications are also the cause of death for 67% of those with diabetes. Diabetes affects an estimated 20.8 million Americans (7% of the adult population); 14.6 million of these have been diagnosed while about 6.2 million people have undiagnosed diabetes. This is a growing issue and it is anticipated that there will be an annual increase of 1.5 million adult cases. Diabetes is the third most expensive medical condition in that it costs $132 billion per year in the United States and is the primary cause of blindness, lower-limb amputation, kidney disease, and nerve damage.[9]

Cancer, the number two cause of death, is also the second most costly at 10.8 million diagnosed cases (3.6% of the U.S. adult population) with 1,444,920 new diagnoses per year—and the rate is expected to double by 2060. This costs an estimated $219.2 billion per year and results in 553,888 deaths per year.[10]

The fourth most expensive medical condition in the United States is arthritis, with 46 million (15.5% of the adult population) experiencing some form of it. It is

TABLE 14.3

Fifteen Leading Causes of Death for 2004[8]

Rank	Cause of death	Number	Percent of total deaths
	All causes	2,397,615	100.0
1	Diseases of heart	652,486	27.2
2	Malignant neoplasms	553,888	23.1
3	Cerebrovascular diseases	150,074	6.3
4	Chronic lower respiratory diseases	121,987	5.1
5	Accidents (unintentional injuries)	112,012	4.7
6	Diabetes mellitus	73,138	3.1
7	Alzheimer's disease	65,965	2.8
8	Influenza and pneumonia	59,664	2.5
9	Nephritis, nephrotic syndrome and nephrosis	42,480	1.8
10	Septicemia	33,373	1.4
11	Intentional self–harm (suicide)	32,439	1.4
12	Chronic liver disease and cirrhosis	27,013	1.1
13	Essential (primary) hypertension and hypertensive renal disease	23,076	1.0
14	Parkinson's disease	17,989	0.8
15	Assault (homicide)	17,357	0.7
	All other causes (Residual)	414,674	17.3

predicted that 67 million people will be afflicted by 2030. Arthritis costs $128 billion per year and is one of the most common causes of limited physical activity. It results in 36 million outpatient visits, 750,000 hospitalizations, and 9,500 deaths per year.[11]

Overweight and obesity is the fifth most costly medical condition in the United States Approximately 66% of U.S. adults are overweight and 32.9% are obese. This has increased from 15.0% in 1980. This condition costs $117 billion per year and increases the potential for developing CVD, dyslipidemia, gallbladder disease, hypertension, osteoarthritis, sleep apnea and respiratory problems, stroke, type 2 diabetes, and some cancers, and contributes to 224,092 deaths per year.[12]

Associated with CVD, type 2 diabetes, and body weight is a clustering of risk factors termed metabolic syndrome (MetS). There are various definitions of the syndrome, but the most accepted—because of its ease of use in clinical management—was proposed by the National Cholesterol Education Program.[13] An individual may be classified as having MetS if he or she has three or more of the following risk factors: abdominal obesity, increased triglycerides, decreased HDL-C cholesterol, increased blood pressure or increased fasting glucose due to insulin resistance.[13] It is estimated that 47 million adults in the United States (21.8% of the population) have MetS. The prevalence increases with age from 6.7% among those 20 through 29 years to 43.5% of those 60 through 69 years of age.[14]

Yet another issue associated with aging is the loss of bone mass. Bone density begins to decline 0.5–1.0 % per year after women enter their late 20s and this accelerates to about 6.5% after menopause.[15] Men also experience this bone loss beginning in their mid 30s. Osteoporosis occurs when bone density is more than 2.5 standard deviations below the mean bone density for young adults—a history or fractures need not be present.[16] Ten million Americans have osteoporosis and an additional 34 million have the primary risk factor of low bone density. Fifty percent of women and 25% of men over age 50 will have an osteoporosis-related fracture at some time. Osteoporosis costs exceed $14 billion per year and results in more than 1.5 million fractures per year.[17]

Becoming older is "not necessarily to be beset with numerous and complex physical disabilities"[19] (p. 1214), but it does result in the decline of many of the body's systems and this decline leads to a reduced ability to carry out the activities of daily living (ADL), an increase in the risk for falls and associated injuries, and may contribute to the increase in depression seen in older adults.[18–20] The age-associated decline in cardiovascular function also is due to several factors and includes maximal heart rate decreasing 6 to 10 beats per min (bpm) per decade which is usually a loss of 1 heartbeat per min per year. Older adults also tend to have reduced stroke volumes and reduced blood volume and oxygen carrying capacity.[21–23] Exercise capacity also declines with age as maximal oxygen consumption ($\dot{V}O_{2max}$) decreases 5–15% per decade, endurance times decrease, and strength declines with the age-associated loss of muscle mass.[19,22,24]

What do CVD, cancer, diabetes, arthritis, overweight/obesity, MetS, osteoporosis, and aging all have in common? They can be successfully treated, prevented, or improved with physical activity—particularly endurance activity. Lifestyle and behavior compose the majority of modifiable risks for these diseases.[25] Major risk factors are exercise deficiency or sedentary lifestyle, smoking, and poor diet.[13] The diseases and early death mostly attributable to these three unhealthy lifestyle choices constitute a major health problem in this country.

The decline in physical activity levels as people age usually has the most impact.[26] Thus, remaining physically active, or adding physical activity into one's lifestyle, can prevent, delay, or reduce the progression of many of the diseases that primarily afflict older individuals.

- The decline in cardiovascular function is slowed and much less pronounced in individuals who exercise aerobically.[13,27]
- COPD lung function is improved and the deterioration slowed with physical activity.[28]
- Colon and breast cancer rates are lower in those who exercise regularly.[29]
- Those who are physically active are 63–65% less likely to develop diabetes.[30]
- A properly designed and adhered to physical activity program can help preserve or restore the range of motion and flexibility around arthritic joints.[31]
- Weight gain can be prevented with sufficient physical activity.[27]
- Endurance exercise has a positive effect on all five of the MetS risk factors and can prevent the development of this syndrome.[13,32]

- Bone loss can be slowed with regular exercise.[15,33]
- Age-associated declines in function are prevented with exercise.[19,34]

Hence, prevention and cure are found in appropriate exercise and it is one of the principal first-line lifestyle changes recommended for the slowing or reversal of age-related declines in health and losses of function.[5,13,30,32]

A. Physiological Basic for the Adaptations to Endurance Exercise

How does endurance activity bring about all the aforementioned changes? Exercise at the physiological level affects the basic functioning and adaptations that occur within the muscle, endocrine, nervous, and cardiovascular systems. Even if one is older, changes in a positive direction can usually be seen even if a chronic condition has already developed.

First, the amount of change, or the level of adaptation, is proportional to the volume of exercise or caloric expenditure (energy output). The greater number of calories burned during physical activity, the greater the adaptation and the greater the protective effect against developing chronic health problems and early death.[1, 4, 5, 15, 26, 35–39] This is true up to a point; exercise caloric expenditure beyond 6000—10000 Calories/week (60—100 miles running or 14—26 miles swimming) does not appear to provide any additional conditioning effect.[40] This is not to say that prolonged exercise is necessary, as exercise volume and caloric expenditure are not only functions of the duration of exercise, but also of the frequency and intensity of exercise; however, higher levels of energy expenditure are associated with more dramatic adaptations.[1] Actually, more intense period of activity interspersed with less intense periods within the same exercise session—also known as interval training—increases the rate and amount of adaptation that occurs in response to endurance exercise.[40, 41] Does this mean that if all were to do the perfect amount of aerobic interval activity that everyone will become great endurance athletes? Unfortunately no; each will only improve within their genetic potential and that potential can be highly variable.[42] However, most have a long way to go before reaching their aerobic performance maximum.

It appears that the level of adaptation is still proportional to caloric expenditure in older adults and that this holds true for those with chronic conditions.[30,36,37,43–47] The magnitude of the physiological changes appears to be similar between older and younger individuals; however, the rate of change may be slower in older adults.[27,34,47–50] Also, as found in the general population, interval exercise is an effective conditioning protocol for the elderly and those with chronic conditions and will increase the rate and amount of adaptation that occurs in response to endurance exercise.[51] Interval training may not just be beneficial, but also necessary for someone of lower initial fitness or who has peripheral vascular disease or intermittent claudication.[52] In addition, more intense aerobic activity, more weekly accumulated aerobic activity, and longer duration sessions may eventually lead to reductions in risk for chronic conditions and decrease utilization of antidiabetic, antihypertensive, and LDL cholesterol-lowering medication.[26,30,37,46] Older adults can still create significant physiological adaptations and move from a sedentary lifestyle to that of a much healthier person who is more capable of performing ADLs or even competing in athletics.

Many of the earliest adaptations to endurance activity occur in the nervous system. Coordination of neural recruitment improves so that movements become more fluid and efficient. This entails inhibiting antagonistic muscles, stimulating synergistic muscles, and reducing inhibition to the working muscles. The neuromuscular junction, the point where the nerve communicates with the muscle also changes as the surface area increases and becomes more compact and symmetrical, thus enhancing communication between the systems.

Changes in muscle also occur as endurance training continues. Muscle cells are referred to as muscle fibers and there are changes within the fibers themselves. Oxygen availability and utilization become more important than force generation, so the muscle fiber size and aerobic capacity change with aerobic conditioning. Those who are very sedentary may see an increase in fiber size when they start to exercise; however, more often the fibers may actually get smaller to reduce the distance that oxygen must travel to get from the fiber surface—where the blood vessels are located—to the mitochondria. This is especially true for type IIx muscle fibers—those that are used for generating faster and stronger contractions. There are two types of type IIx muscle fibers: IIa, those that have higher aerobic and glycolytic capacities; and type IIb, those that have lower aerobic capacity and a greater fast glycolytic and force generation capacity. Aerobic conditioning may result in a conversion of IIb fibers to IIa to improve the muscle's ability to use oxygen. However, there does not seem to be a fiber type conversion of type IIx to type I, the most efficient aerobic fibers, with aerobic conditioning. This fiber type conversion is related to the type of myosin and myosin ATPase within the contractile apparatus.

Actin and myosin are the contractile proteins with each muscle fiber. Calcium is released from the sarcoplasmic reticulum (a network of channels and storage sites) when a signal arrives telling the muscle to contract. This calcium allows myosin to bind to actin. Myosin then undergoes a conformational change and pulls the actin along its length. ATP is then consumed and myosin releases actin and returns to its original position. This process is repeated as long as calcium and ATP are present. ATPase is the enzyme that catalyzes the breakdown of ATP. ATPase can have different isoforms; they do they same job, but have a slightly different composition, or shape, and rates of action. There are also different isoforms of myosin. The type of myosin and myosin ATPase isoforms relate to how quickly the myosin can cross-bridge cycle and what type of fiber the cell is. First, calcium release and transport by the sarcoplasmic reticulum is increased by aerobic conditioning. Second, myosin ATPase is altered to a slower form, both within the working muscle and the working heart, by aerobic conditioning. And third, the myosin isoforms are altered from IIb to IIa by aerobic conditioning.

The ability to use oxygen to produce energy increases due to aerobic conditioning. Recall that the second energy system used is glycolysis—the efficiency of this energy system in providing rapid energy actually decreases while the efficiency at providing slower energy improves. Activity of lactate dehydrogenase, the enzyme that catalyzes the conversion of pyruvate to lactate, decreases by 20% with aerobic conditioning. However, this does not hurt performance, as the aerobic enzyme quantity and activity increase significantly. Hexokinase activity, the enzyme that adds a phosphate to glucose so that it can be broken down in glycolysis, increases from 2.4 activity units in unconditioned individuals to 2.9 in moderately conditioned and to 4.2 in elite endurance athletes.[53] Activity of citrate synthetase, one of the first enzymes in the mitochondrial pathway, increases from 28 activity units in the unconditioned individual to 37 in the moderately conditioned and 78 in the elite endurance athlete.[53] Enzymes that catalyze the use of lipids as an energy source also become more active; palmityl Co-A (an intermediate in the utilization of fatty acids to produce energy in the mitochondria) oxidation activity is increased by 30% as a result of endurance training. This results in an increased ability to use lipid as an energy source and the sparing of muscle glycogen at submaximal workloads. These increases in enzyme activity are occurring as the amount of mitochondria is also increasing.

Given enough aerobic conditioning, the muscle fibers can become so efficient at producing energy via aerobic metabolism that the energy pathway is not a limiting factor in exercise. Rather, substrate, or fuel, availability becomes limiting in endurance activity. In addition to increasing lipid catabolism, another adaptation is to increase the amount of substrate available within the muscle. Aerobically conditioned muscles can double the amount of internally stored glycogen, while triglyceride storage near the mitochondria also increases. These adaptations occur only in type I fibers at lower exercise intensities, but can occur in type II fibers with high-intensity aerobic intervals.

Yet another aerobic conditioning response to increase the fuel supply available for oxidation is the increase in glucose uptake by muscle fibers. At rest the muscle fibers take up little glucose and this obviously increases with exercise onset. Glucose does not simply diffuse across the cell membrane (sarcolemma), rather is transported across the sarcolemma by specific transporters (GLUT). The number (density) of GLUT on a cell's surface indicates the amount and speed with which glucose can be taken up. GLUT4 is the most studied of these glucose transporters. It actually resides inside the cell membrane when not in use. The hormone insulin controls glucose uptake. Increased blood sugar causes an increase in insulin secretion from the β-cells of the Islets of Langerhans in the pancreas. Insulin then is carried through the blood to act on GLUT4 to cause it move from inside the cell membrane to the outside where it can bind with glucose and transport the glucose into the cell for utilization. In type 1 diabetes this signal is absent and in type 2 diabetes the sensitivity of this signal is greatly reduced; thus leading to an inability to clear blood glucose and to make glucose available within the cells for energy production. The ability to synthesize glycogen, and thus store glucose in the muscle, also appears to be impaired in type 2 diabetes.[54]

Insulin is not the only signal that can cause GLUT4 to migrate from within the sarcolemma to without. Exercise causes the GLUT4 complex to migrate to the fiber surface and increase glucose uptake *independent of insulin*. Because their energy demands are higher, type I fibers have a greater GLUT4 density within their sarcolemma and a greater potential for glucose uptake. So, aerobic activity increases insulin independent glucose uptake and utilization. However, this is not where this story ends, as GLUT4 density responds to aerobic conditioning. When the energy demands of the muscle fiber are repeatedly increased through regular aerobic exercise, the density of GLUT4 also increases to enhance the amount and speed of glucose uptake during exercise. This not only benefits endurance performance, but glucose regulation in general. The physical activity-induced enhancement of insulin-dependent glucose uptake improves management of blood glucose and can reduce the need for diabetes medications.[46]

Insulin sensitivity decreases with age; however, regular participation in physical activity results in improved insulin sensitivity and muscle glycogen synthesis in individuals without diabetes and those with type 2 diabetes.[36,50,54,55] In addition, postprandial, blood glucose was lower in those who exercised regularly and this may be due to increased insulin secretion after a meal.[55] The liver may also reduce its glucose production, thus reducing its contribution to blood glucose levels.[55] The evidence is not conclusive for a dose response between blood glucose control and exercise, but when walking distance exceeds 35 km (21.9 miles) per week, physical activity-induced enhancement of insulin-dependent glucose uptake reduces the incidence of diabetes, improves management of blood glucose, and reduces the need for diabetes medications.[46, 56]

Not only does muscle have an improved ability to utilize oxygen, glucose, and lipid, it has an increased ability to extract oxygen from the blood and transport it from the periphery of the fiber to the mitochondria. Myoglobin, a heme iron-containing molecule similar to hemoglobin, aids in the transport and storage of oxygen within the muscle fiber. In addition, given enough exercise stimuli, muscles that periodically experience insufficient oxygen supply, through aerobic exercise will grow more blood vessels (angiogenesis). Angiogenesis increases the number of blood vessels per muscle fiber from 1.2 capillaries/fiber in the unconditioned to 1.4 capillaries per fiber in moderately conditioned and 3.2 capillaries/fiber in elite endurance athletes.[53] This results in an increase from 290 capillaries/mm^2 of muscle in unconditioned individuals to 350 capillaries/mm^2 in moderately conditioned and 460 capillaries/mm^2 in elite endurance athletes.[53] These changes in energy utilization and oxygen delivery lead to the muscle's extracting a greater amount of oxygen from the blood, expressed as the arteriovenous oxygen (a-vO_2) difference: from a maximal value of 14.5 mmol/100 mL in the untrained individual to 15.2 mmol/100 mL in the moderately conditioned and 16.4 mmol/100 mL in elite endurance athletes.[53] Thus, the muscle has an improved aerobic capacity in that the ability to extract oxygen from the blood and use it in the production of energy to sustain activity is increased. The a-vO_2 difference declines with aging; however, regular aerobic activity leads to improvements in the a-vO_2 difference in older adults and those with chronic condition, such as CAD.[23,52] This indicates that the muscle is undergoing at least some of the same adaptations seen in younger exercisers.

Recall that with the initiation of exercise and the maintenance of high-intensity exercise there is some lactate production during the utilization of glucose to form ATP. Much of the lactate produced during activity is transported out of the muscle fiber so that it does not limit the fiber's ability to continue to generate energy. This leads to accumulation of lactate in the blood—at first linearly and then nonlinearly. The inflection point at which lactate accumulate changes from linear to nonlinear is termed the lactate threshold.[57] Because the amount of lactate produced at a given submaximal exercise intensity is lower, the point at which blood lactate increases is delayed.[58] Aerobic conditioning enhances oxidation and results in the production of less lactate. But, as with other adaptations to aerobic exercise, there is more. Not only is lactate production slowed, but lactate clearance is also improved. Lactate clearance can be enhanced in several ways. The liver and kidneys can take up lactate and reverse the process of converting pyruvate to lactate and combine two pyruvate to re-form glucose. This glucose can then be used as an energy source. The lactate can also be used as an energy source by other cells. Type I muscle fibers and the muscle cells of the heart can take up lactate and utilize it as an energy source. The red blood cells also utilize lactate to produce energy. And, as one might expect, the ability of these tissues to utilize lactate as an energy source is increased by aerobic conditioning.

Endurance conditioning has not only local effects within the muscle, but cardiovascular effects as well. Blood pressure is one such factor that is modified by regular aerobic activity. Blood pressure is made up of two components: systolic and diastolic blood pressure. Systolic blood pressure is the pressure exerted by the contracting heart pushing the blood through the circulatory system and is the higher number. Diastolic blood pressure is the resting pressure maintained in the blood vessels as the heart is filling and is the lower number. Resting systolic blood pressure declines with aerobic conditioning, particularly for those who have elevated blood pressure; by 2.6 mmHg in normotensive vs. 7.4 mmHg in hypertensives.[59] The maximum value achieved during maximal exercise does not appear to change. The resting diastolic blood pressure also decreases as a result of aerobic conditioning; by 1.8 mmHg in normotensive and 5.8 mmHg in hypertensive.[59] However, different from the systolic pressure, diastolic blood pressure also decreases during maximal exercise. The decreased resting systolic blood pressure indicates that the heart is not working as hard to move blood through the circulation and reduces the potential for heart disease. The decreased diastolic blood pressure also reduces the work that the heart must do as it reduces the resistance to blood flow. A lower diastolic pressure is also beneficial to the blood vessels themselves and is associated with a lower incidence of vascular diseases, i.e., plaque and clot formation. A reduced diastolic blood pressure is beneficial in yet another manner—the perfused tissues experience a reduced pressure and can prolong their effectiveness, i.e., the kidneys remain healthier when diastolic blood pressure is within an appropriate range.

Regular aerobic activity reduces the onset of hypertension, with those having greater exercise capacity experiencing lower risk for developing hypertension.[37,47,56,60] Physical activity is also a key component of first line therapy for hypertension.[47,61] Hypertensive patients experience a greater decline in resting blood pressure than do normotensive; systolic decreases by an average of 7.4 mmHg and diastolic by an average of 5.8 mmHg.[47,49,59] Antihypertensive medication use also declines and this is proportional to the amount of physical activity performed.[46] In addition, those with hypertension who participate in regular aerobic activity have lower mortality rates than those with hypertension who are inactive.[60]

The endurance-conditioned heart does not have to work as hard as the unconditioned heart for more reasons than just reduced blood pressure. Heart rate (HR), expressed as the number of beats per min, is also improved by endurance conditioning. Resting HR declines with endurance conditioning from an average of 70 beats per min (BPM) to 40 bpm or lower in those who are very well trained. This lower resting HR translates to a lower working HR at the same absolute exercise intensity; meaning that the individual can do more and derive more benefit at the same exercise HR. Resting and submaximal HR are lower, but maximum HR does not appear to change as a result of endurance conditioning; however, the age-associated decline in maximum HR appears to be slowed by a lifetime of aerobic activity. Not only is the resting HR lower, but HR recovery rate, a measure of fitness, is also improved; HR returns to resting values much faster in the conditioned individual and recovery may be a better indicator of aerobic fitness than actual HR.

The rate-pressure product (HR x systolic blood pressure) can be used to predict when angina pectoris, the chest pain associated with an ischemic heart, will occur in an exercise bout in that the chest pain tends to occur at the same rate-pressure product from session to session.[62] Aerobic conditioning reduces the HR and systolic blood pressure; thus, the rate-pressure product, at the same absolute exercise intensity and this serves to delay or eliminate angina pectoris.[62, 63] This exercise-induced improvement in work capacity is on the order of the same magnitude as that seen with sublingual nitroglycerin.[62] Exercise and functional capacity are also increased as the symptom-limited heart rate increases in those with congestive heart failure.[63]

If the blood pressure is lower and the heart is beating slower, does this mean that blood flow to the tissues is compromised? Not at all. One factor that aids the decline in these two values is the increase in stroke volume (SV). Stroke volume is the amount of blood ejected from the heart with each beat. It is the difference between the volume of blood in the heart at the end of diastole (end diastolic volume, EDV) and the volume of blood in the heart at the end of systole (end systolic volume, ESV): SV = EDV – ESV. A resting SV of 64 mL in the unconditioned individual can increase to 82 mL with moderate conditioning and be 127 mL in elite endurance athletes. Maximal SV increases similarly from 122 mL in the unconditioned to 142 mL in the moderately conditioned and 201 mL in elite endurance athletes.[53]

The increase in SV is due to multiple factors. Quite simply, the heart becomes larger, increasing from an average size of 750 mL in the unconditioned individual to 823 mL in the moderately conditioned individual, and 1250 mL in the highly conditioned individual.[53] This increase is partially due to an increase in the size of the ventricles, particularly the left ventricle—the side that pumps blood to the body. So a larger heart can move a larger volume of blood with one contraction; this adaptation does not occur in all individuals who exercise aerobically. However, when the adaptation does occur, not only is the heart larger, but more blood is entering it as blood volume has also increased.[21] Blood volume increases from 4.8 L in the unconditioned individual to 5.2 L in the moderately conditioned person and 6.1 L in the elite endurance athlete.[53] Increased blood volume leads to increased SV via the Frank-Starling mechanism. This is related to preload or the stretch shortening cycle of muscle in that a muscle that is stretched will generate greater contraction strength. Thus, a heart that has filled with more blood due to increased blood volume will generate a more forceful contraction to increase the SV.

Stroke volume declines as one ages; however, the hearts of those with many of the varieties of cardiac disease still utilize the Frank-Starling mechanism to increase contraction in response to an increased preload.[22,23] Thus, the conditioning response of increasing the SV also occurs in those with cardiovascular disease.[52] In the aged, just as in the young, total blood volume is proportional to physical activity levels.[21]

It has been stated that blood volume increases with aerobic conditioning. Blood is generally made up of two components, liquid and solid. The liquid portion, plasma, is largely water. The solid portion is made up of red and white blood cells and platelets. Red blood cells are primarily responsible for transporting oxygen from the lungs to the tissues, but are also involved in transporting carbon dioxide from the cells to the lungs and in metabolizing lactate. The oxygen-transporting molecule within the red blood cell is hemoglobin. The absolute amount of hemoglobin is increased as a result of endurance conditioning. The absolute number of red blood cells is also increased as a result of endurance conditioning. This increase in hemoglobin and red blood cells leads to an increased ability to transport oxygen and carbon dioxide, as well as clear lactate. Blood plasma also increases in response to endurance conditioning. However, the increase in plasma volume is greater than the increase in red blood cells so the hematocrit, the percentage of blood made up of solid constituents, may decrease in the aerobically conditioned individual. A lower hematocrit indicates that blood is more fluid, or less viscous. Viscosity is a fluid's resistance to flow. A lower viscosity indicates a lower resistance to flow, meaning an easier passage through the blood vessels, thus a reduced need to generate force by the heart and reduced blood pressure.

The heart is bigger, has more blood to pump, and becomes more efficient via endurance conditioning. Contractility is improved with aerobic conditioning. Contractility is the ability of the cardiac muscle fiber to contract at a given muscle length. Improved contractility means that the fiber can generate a greater contraction when all else remains the same. Increased contractility leads to a greater SV with each beat of the heart. Ejection fraction (EF) is the proportion of the EDV that becomes SV: EF = SV/EDV or (EDV – ESV)/EDV. The EF increases with aerobic conditioning. A typical healthy EF is around 55% at rest; during exercise this can increase to 73%—81% in the conditioned individual.

While HR is decreased and SV is increased, cardiac output ($\dot{Q}$) at rest remains the same. Cardiac output is equal to stroke volume multiplied by heart rate: $\dot{Q}$ (L/min) = SV × HR. Resting $\dot{Q}$ does not change with aerobic conditioning; thus, the decrease in HR and increase in SV do equalize. However, since maximal HR does not change and SV increases with conditioning, there will be changes during maximal exercise. An increased maximal $\dot{Q}$ from 22.3 L/min in the unconditioned individual to 25.8 L/min with moderate conditioning and 34.9 L/min in elite endurance athletes.[53] As HR and SV have declined with age, so does $\dot{Q}$.[23] And, just as HR and SV improve with aerobic conditioning so does $\dot{Q}$ in the aged.[23]

Aerobic conditioning also improves blood distribution. Blood flow to the upper lungs improves and leads to increased perfusion of the lungs and a greater surface area of blood to pick up oxygen and dispose of carbon dioxide. Blood flow to the working muscles is also improved with aerobic conditioning. This is due to increased vasodilation within the muscles. This contributes to the reduced blood pressure as wider blood vessels offer less resistance to blood flow. It also results in greater oxygen delivery to working muscles. Angiogenesis also serves to increase blood flow to the muscle. This process does not appear to occur in the healthy heart in response to aerobic conditioning, but does in the diseased heart. This development of collateral circulation in response to aerobic activity can improve blood flow to damaged regions of the heart. The conditioning-induced improved blood flow results in the improved exchange of gases, heat, fuel, and metabolites. This does not require long-term conditioning as a 15% increase in local blood flow has been observed at 8 weeks of aerobic conditioning. Thus, the muscle tissue can use more oxygen to generate energy and the cardiovascular system can deliver more oxygen to that working muscle.

The ability to uptake and utilize oxygen is termed oxygen consumption ($\dot{V}O_2$) and the maximal amount of oxygen that an individual can utilize during maximal exercise is the $\dot{V}O_{2max}$. Oxygen uptake and oxygen utilization are improved so $\dot{V}O_2$ also responds to aerobic conditioning. $\dot{V}O_2$ at rest is slightly decreased or unchanged. At submaximal workloads the $\dot{V}O_2$ is decreased and $\dot{V}O_{2max}$ can be increased by 5–30%, depending on the genetic potential of the individual and how all of the aforementioned adaptations occur. This increase seems to occur over the first 18 months of conditioning and further improvements in performance arise from improved mechanical and metabolic efficiency.

Due to the increases in the a-vO_2 difference and stroke volume, $\dot{V}O_{2max}$ (or peak in those who are symptom limited) increases 10–60% ($\bar{x} \approx 20\%$) in the aged and those with coronary artery disease (CAD).[23,27,48,52,63–65] In addition, this trainability does not appear to be limited by a history of myocardial infarction or coronary artery bypass surgery.[65] A higher $\dot{V}O_{2max}$ is proving to be of protective benefit against developing chronic hypokinetic disease.[32,37,66]

We have discussed how aerobic conditioning improves muscle and cardiovascular function to enhance endurance performance. It has also been pointed out that these changes can occur with regular moderate exercise and can be further enhanced at higher levels of conditioning. But oxygen utilization (the muscle) and oxygen delivery (the cardiovascular system) are not all we should consider. What about getting more oxygen into the lungs? How does aerobic conditioning alter pulmonary function? Pulmonary function does not seem to change much as a result of aerobic conditioning. Resting respiratory rate does decline some from 14 breaths per min in untrained individuals to 12 in moderately trained and 11 breaths per min in elite endurance athletes.[53] Respiratory rate during maximal exercise does also increase from 42 breaths per min in untrained individuals to 47 in moderately trained and 59 breaths per min in elite endurance athletes.[53] This results in increased maximal voluntary ventilation. Tidal volume, the amount of air moved with each respiration, is unchanged at rest and slightly increased during maximal exercise from 2.8 L in untrained individuals to 3.1 L in both moderately trained and elite endurance athletes.[53] Thus, there are small changes in the pulmonary system, but the majority of improvement in oxygen uptake, delivery, and utilization occur within the cardiovascular and muscular systems (see Table 14.4).

Recall the brief discussion of insulin's regulating blood glucose. Insulin is a hormone, the chemical messenger of the endocrine system. And, like all other systems, the endocrine system is affected by endurance conditioning. The purpose of the endocrine system is to regulate the internal environment and maintain homeostasis. Exercise perturbs homeostasis by reducing blood glucose. The initiation of exercise increases the muscle's removal of glucose from the blood and the reduction in blood glucose causes a release of the catecholamines, epinephrine and norepinephrine,

TABLE 14.4

Benefits of Regular Physical Activity for the Well Population[3,4,91,93]

Organ/System	Aerobic
Blood and Blood Vessels	Increases hemoglobin. Improves and maintains blood vessel compliance. Reduces build–up of plaque.
Bones	Increases density of stressed bones. Most effective when activities are weight bearing.
Connective Tissue	Strengthens and maintains tendons and ligaments. Can improve range of motion if fully utilized during activity.
Coordination and Balance	Improves.
Gastrointestinal	Improves gastric motility and reduces incidence of inflammatory disorders and cancer.
Heart	Improves compliance, efficiency, and recovery more than other movement types.
Immune	Improves immunosurveillance and reduces infectious episodes.
Lungs	Improves compliance and efficiency.
Metabolism	Increased during activity and recovery. Can lead to weight loss.
Mood	Improves.
Muscle	Improves endurance and may improve strength in the low fit.
Nervous System	Improves cognitive function. Improves coordination of neural signals and movement.
Thermoregulation	Improved in that sweating begins earlier and is more efficient.

and cortisol—to help bring blood glucose back up. The liver and kidneys respond to reduced blood glucose and the catecholamines by supplying additional glucose to maintain blood concentration and may actually elevate the blood glucose concentration above resting. The catecholamines also inhibit the secretion of insulin by the pancreas and reduce glucose uptake by nonworking tissues.

Aerobic conditioning generally reduces endocrine response to a submaximal exercise bout and increases the endocrine response to a maximal exercise bout. The reduction in insulin is decreased and blood glucose is better maintained. Blood glucose maintenance is also aided by the increased lipid utilization and creation of new glucose by the liver and kidneys. Aerobic training may also reduce the amount of testosterone and this may need to be monitored in those with low testosterone levels. However, the endocrine response overall is positive.

B. Effects of Endurance Exercise on Osteoporosis, Arthritis, and Cancer

Osteoporosis is a syndrome in which minerals are lost from bone, thus making it more prone to fractures. Bone loss can be reduced by participating in weight-bearing exercise that mechanically loads the bones and increases bone strength; however, the evidence for increasing bone mass via physical activity is inconclusive.[15,17,33,67] Walking, jogging, stair climbing, dancing, and aerobics are all examples of weight-bearing aerobic exercise that have the potential to maintain bone density. There are caveats, however: the total amount of physical activity, as determined by intensity, duration, and frequency, must be relatively high (for example—daily 2-hr moderate to vigorous walk) to result in improvements in bone density from exercise alone—loading benefits only those bones stressed by higher-intensity activities—and adequate caloric and calcium intake must be maintained.[1,33,67]

Aerobic activity also serves to increase collagen metabolism. Collagen is the primary protein in connective tissues: tendons, ligament, fascia, and cartilage. Damaged fibrils are replaced more rapidly and in a stronger orientation with regular aerobic activity. This leads to a stronger, healthier fibril without a net gain in the amount of connective tissue. Weight-bearing forces and complete movement throughout the range of motion seem essential to maintain connective tissue viability. Moderate aerobic exercise seems adequate for increasing cartilage thickness, while there is no evidence that strenuous exercise causes degenerative joint disease.[67] This bodes well for those who suffer from arthritis. Physical activity can be one of the most effective tools for the management of the pain and inflammation of both rheumatoid and osteoarthritis and this has led the American College of Rheumatology to state that *... appropriate exercise is very important.*[68]

The benefits of physical activity particular to those with arthritis are the same as those in the general population. However, some of these benefits are of greater relevance to individuals managing their arthritis. Regular participation in physical activity improves joint range of motion and reduces stiffness.[68] A well-designed program also increases joint stability.[1,68] This, in turn, decreases small-joint damage and bone loss. Physical activity does not increase pain or the progression of the disease; rather it aids pain management by reducing both physical and psychological pain.[31,67] In addition, the weight management benefits of regular endurance activity also reduce arthritis-related symptoms.

Physical activity reduces the incidence and mortality of all-site cancers.[29] There is an inverse dose relationship between colon and breast cancers and physical activity, in that those who are the most active have the lowest risk for these two cancers; however, this relationship has not been observed in other site-specific types of cancer.[29] It is thought that this protective effect arises, in part, from the improved cardiorespiratory, endocrine, immune, and bowel functions that result from the regular participation in physical activity as well as the increased energy expenditure and the enhanced ability of cells to repair themselves.[29]

C. Endurance Exercise and Risk Factor Reduction

There is some inconsistency in the individual study methodologies and chosen classification systems of activity; however, the evidence is clear that physical inactivity is a causative factor in the development of CVD, and that endurance activity reduces the incidence of CAD.[1,69] The rate of CAD (a subset of CVD and commonly called atherosclerotic cardiovascular disease) are half those of sedentary persons with a dose response of decreased incidence of CVD with increased activity levels, at both work and leisure.[56,69,70] In addition, it appears that up to 22% of all hypertension, 20% of all CVD-related deaths, and 15–43% of strokes could be prevented simply by individuals' meeting the recommended amount of physical activity.[37,39,43] Aerobic conditioning also serves as a protective and therapeutic mechanism regardless of overweight or obesity. That is, those who are more physically active are less likely to develop, and are more likely to improve, chronic conditions than someone of similar weight and body composition who is inactive.[32,36,37,39,66,71] While it has been conclusively demonstrated that the incidence of CAD is reduced with aerobic exercise, this type of physical activity also reduces almost all of the known risk factors for CAD and CVD.

The most recent list of risk factors for heart disease published by the American Heart Association includes the modifiable risk factors of diabetes, abnormal lipid levels, hypertension, obesity and overweight, physical inactivity, and tobacco use; high levels of stress and high alcohol consumption can also contribute.[72] Hypertension is in itself a risk factor for developing CVD and the risk doubles for each 20/10 mmHg resting blood pressure is above 115/75 mmHg.[61] As stated, these are all modifiable risk factors in that changing individual behaviors can reduce their impact on the heart. Endurance exercise is known to reduce risk in all of the modifiable risk factors.[73] Examples of non-modifiable risk factors include heredity, male gender, and aging.[72]

When risk factors and hypokinetic diseases are considered collectively and individually it becomes clear that endurance exercise is associated with a reduction of risk.[30,60] Abnormal lipid levels are improved by appropriate exercise interventions as it has been shown to increase high-density lipoprotein-cholesterol (HDL-C) levels and reduce triglyceride and low-density lipoprotein-cholesterol (LDL-C) concentrations in both ideal-weight, overweight, and obese exercisers.[27,48,71, 4–78] The magnitude of the changes in LDL, HDL, and triglyceride levels appears to be related to the magnitude of the decreases in the waist-to-hip ratio, body weight, and to increases in $\dot{V}O_{2max}$.[48,71,74] The magnitude of the changes in LDL and triglyceride levels also appears to be related to initial cholesterol levels in that those with the highest pre-exercise levels experienced the greatest declines in LDL and triglyceride values due to aerobic conditioning; thus, having the greatest effect on those with the greatest risk.[49,74] A reduction in the total cholesterol or elevation in HDL results in a more favorable total-C to HDL-C ratio that leads to a reduced risk for CVD.[27] The dose responsiveness of this leads a decline in the need for LDL cholesterol-lowering medications when walking distance exceeds 35 km (21.9 miles) per week.[46] Hypertension is affected by endurance exercise to such an extent that mildly hypertensive individuals may not need drug therapy.[59]

It has been found that hypertension and elevated triglycerides not only contribute to the development of heart disease, but also to the development of type 2 diabetes.[66] Physical activity reduces hypertension, insulin resistance, and other factors related to diabetes.[36,50] In addition, those with diabetes are more than twice as likely to develop arthritis than those without.[79] As physical activity has been shown to be beneficial in the treatment of both these chronic conditions, it would appear that aerobic activity may be more relevant for those with diabetes. Not only has it been shown that aerobic conditioning is beneficial when diabetes has already been diagnosed, but it is also clear that exercise can be used in the prevention of type 2 diabetes in at-risk individuals.[30,54,55,66,80] While the exact mechanism is unclear, the exercise becomes the medicine and is related to the response to each individual exercise session.

Increased physical activity, particularly aerobic conditioning, is also related to weight loss and its maintenance, as reported by the National Weight Control

Registry.[81] Regular aerobic activity reduces body weight, body fat, and the age associated weight gain.[27,35,38,65,82] A reduced body weight is associated with reductions in the risks for, and complications from, arthritis, diabetes, insulin resistance, hypertension, hyperlipidemia, and MetS.[13,30,31,36,48,52,71,75,78] The reduction in waist circumference, an indicator of intra-abdominal fat and a risk factor for MetS, is dose dependent in that the more aerobic activity one does, the greater the reduction in waist size and CAD risk.[38]

While few physically active people smoke cigarettes, exercise provides a protective effect to those who do and it also improves smoking cessation.[39,83,84] Exercisers who add health education to their workouts tend to achieve a higher rate of continuous abstinence at the end of exercise interventions than do controls.[84] This appears to hold true for those exercising after a myocardial infarction as well and has a reciprocal positive feedback effect in that those who quit smoking also have a greater adherence to exercise in the long term.[83] This effect may be prolonged as the rate of continuous abstinence was shown to be twice as high as controls a year later.[85]

Regular aerobic activity has also been demonstrated to improve quality of life, reduce depression, and improve cognitive function.[31,44,64,86] All of these improvements—from the local muscle to the cardiovascular to the psychological—combine to improve older individuals' functional capacity and ability to carry out their activities of daily living.[27,31,48,52,63,86–89] This includes those with chronic conditions and results in the delay of disability (see Table 14.5).[89]

IV. RECOMMENDATIONS FOR TYPES AND AMOUNTS OF PHYSICAL ACTIVITY IN OLDER ADULTS

Health, weight management, and well-being are improved with regular physical activity and reduced sedentary activity. Benefits can be seen with as little exercise energy expenditure as 1000 kilocalories per week, or the equivalent of walking 8 miles per week.[1,5,80] One caveat must accompany this—individual variability can make the minimum amount of physical activity greater or smaller; there must be some level of personal investigation to determine what works for each individual.[5] The recommended minimum for health is 30 min of moderate-intensity physical activity (beyond the activities of daily living and work) on most days of the week.[26,60,87,90] A joint report from the American College of Sports Medicine (ACSM) and the American Heart Association further refines this recommendation to 30 min of moderate aerobic activity on 5 days a week, 20 min of vigorous aerobic activity on 3 days a week, or a combination of the two with 30 min of moderate activity 2 days a week and vigorous activity for 20 min on 2 other days of the week.[26] The 30 min of moderate-intensity aerobic activity do not have to be completed continuously. This can be broken up into shorter bouts lasting 10 min or more.[26] The ACSM also recommends that the moderate to vigorous activity be weight bearing 3–5 days a week to help maintain bone density.[15] However, evidence suggests that faithfulness to high-intensity programs may be less than to that of moderate-intensity programs; thus, if an individual will not continue to perform a high-intensity program, perhaps a moderate-intensity program would be more beneficial for long-term adherence.[4]

TABLE 14.5

Benefits of Physical Activity for Those with Chronic Conditions [3,4,18,91,93]

Condition	Benefits
Arthritis and Other Rheumatic Disorders	Increases joint strength
	Increases muscle strength
	Reduces incidence and severity of inflammatory episodes and pain
Asthma	Reduces severity and frequency of exacerbations
	A warm and humid environment (indoor pools) elicits fewer exacerbations
	Environmental allergens should be avoided or accounted for
Cardiovascular Disease and Hypertension	Reduces blood pressure
	Increases vascular compliance
	Reduces LDL
	Reduces triglycerides
	Increases HDL
	Strengthens the heart, increases ejection fraction and efficiency
	Decreases stress
	Stimulates angiogenesis
	Collaterals (natural bypasses) are stimulated by exercise and can greatly improve the circulation to the heart and the rest of the body
	Better functional capacity with activities of daily living
	May lead to reversal of cardiovascular disease
Chronic Obstructive Pulmonary Disease	Increases oxygen carrying capacity
	Improves circulation
	Strengthens breathing muscles
Diabetes	Increases insulin sensitivity and enhances non–insulin dependent glucose uptake
	Increases utilization of glucose
	Decreases body fat, which also leads to improved insulin sensitivity
	Reduces HbA1c
	The previous four improvements can result in lower doses, or elimination, of medications
	Safety precautions regarding hypoglycemia should be incorporated
Metabolic Syndrome	Increases insulin sensitivity and enhances non–insulin dependent glucose uptake
	Increases utilization of glucose
	Decreases body fat, which also leads to improved insulin sensitivity
	Reduce blood pressure
	Reduce LDL
	Reduce triglycerides
	Increase HDL
	Strengthens the heart, increases ejection fraction and efficiency
	Decreases stress

Recommendations from the American Heart Association and the ACSM have been updated for both adults in general and for older adults specifically in order to improve and maintain health.[26] For healthy adults aged 18 to 65 it is recommended that moderate-intensity aerobic or endurance exercise be performed for a minimum of 30 min 5 days each week. An example of moderate-intensity exercise would be a brisk walk, which elevates heart rate noticeably. It does not have to be done all at once and can be accomplished in 10-min bouts to an accumulated time of 30 min on the exercise day. If exercise intensity is increased and becomes vigorous, it can be performed for a minimum of 20 min 3 days each week. Examples of vigorous-intensity exercise would be jogging, which elevates breathing pattern and shows a substantial increase in heart rate. Both types of exercise can be combined in a week such that moderate exercise could be done 2 days of the week for 30 min, while 2 other days of the week vigorous exercise can be performed for 20 min. The recommendation is also made that muscular strength and endurance activities should be performed for a minimum of 2 days per week using 8–10 exercises per session. Exceeding these minimum recommended amounts of physical activity will further reduce risk for chronic diseases, reduce weight gain, and improve health.[26]

There is some concern that these recommendations might not be appropriate for older adults or those with some of the chronic conditions discussed previously; however, the ACSM, the American Heart Association, and the Joint National Committee on the Prevention, Detection, Evaluation, and Treatment of High Blood Pressure make the same recommendation for these populations.[15, 45, 47, 51, 61, 80] The aforementioned recommendations were further reviewed and modified by a panel of scientists for healthy adults equal to or over the age of 65 and for adults between the ages of 50 and 64 with known clinically significant conditions or functional limitations.[45] The latter group, who would have conditions that would affect their ability to move, overall fitness, or physical activity, might use suggested modifications. Moderate- and vigorous-intensity exercise is described in terms of effort on a scale of 1–10. With 0 as sitting and maximum effort defined as 10, moderate exercise would be given a 5–6 as it increases heart rate and breathing. Vigorous exercise would be given a 7 or 8 with larger increases in heart and breathing. Since fitness levels vary widely in older group, which is categorized as the most unfit segment of the population, moderate and vigorous intensity will be different for different individuals. The recommendations for muscular strength and endurance exercise should also be followed with modifications. The resistance or weight used should allow for 10–15 repetitions for muscular endurance. Muscular strength development should increase the resistance and decrease the repetitions. The same scale is used as in aerobic conditioning: 5–6 is classified as moderate and 7 or 8 is classified as vigorous. In addition, those who are concerned about the potential complications associated with higher-intensity exercise should consult with their physician and undertake moderate-intensity exercise for longer durations.[4]

It is further recommended that older adults incorporate flexibility exercises at least 2 days each week for at least 10 min each session. It is also suggested that, because of the high incidence of injury from falls in this population, balance exercises should be performed. If chronic conditions prohibit following the recommendations completely, any type of regular physical activity is encouraged in order to avoid becoming sedentary. A gradual approach is recommended and it is imperative that a plan be developed incorporating the previously mentioned suggestions.[45]

V. GENERAL TRAINING PRINCIPLES

Many people see improvement when they first start a physical activity program, but they soon find that their progress slows and they reach a plateau. They stop losing weight, their waist size does not go down, or their strength stops increasing. When these things happen, it is usually because the "OPS principles" are not being met. The OPS principles are three basic rules that must be considered if a person is going to improve fitness and lose weight. OPS stands for Overload, Progression, and Specificity.

Overload simply means that in order to improve fitness or to lose weight, one must do more than is the norm.[91] In other words; one must overload the system. This does not mean to start running marathons tomorrow. This means that one simply needs to increase physical activity. There is improvement only if physical activity is an increase over what is regularly done on a daily basis. This can apply to walking, resistance training, or any other movement type. The exercise stimulus has to be greater than what is experienced during the activities of daily living if there is to be a conditioning response. This is where discomfort comes in—some discomfort indicates that an overload is occurring and the individual is on track, but pain is not appropriate.

Progression is related to overload. If there is an increase in the amount of physical activity performed, the body will adapt and eventually get used to that new level of activity. It will no longer be an overload. So individuals must increase what they are doing to continue to have an overload.[91] They must progress. The body is much like the mind in that if one continues to do the same thing for a long time, the mind and body get bored and quit improving. The idea is to gradually, or progressively, increase physical activity as the body adapts to the new demands. This increase can be in intensity, time (duration), or frequency. It is generally safer to increase only one of these three at once. As time goes by, one can and should work harder.

Specificity refers to what is improved. For example, if people walk, their legs, lungs, and heart will get stronger, but their arms will not. Only the movements, muscles, organs, and bones that are stressed during physical activity improve.[91] This is what athletes refer to when they talk about getting into "playing shape." They may have spent the off-season staying fit, but they must use the pre-season to specifically prepare for their game. Some examples: to increase strength, one must do some form of resistance training. To improve stair-climbing, movements that place similar demands on the body as stair climbing must be performed. Specificity is why even someone in great shape can still get sore when he or she does a new and different activity.

Another component of physical activity and the specificity of conditioning is reversibility. Use it or lose it, as the saying goes. The body is truly quite efficient. Maintaining muscle mass (including heart mass), bone density, red blood cells, etc., costs energy. If the body perceives that these are not necessary, it will eliminate the excess to reduce the amount of work that must be done to maintain the body. In other words, if one does not keep using newly conditioned muscles, bones, etc., the body will decondition in an effort to conserve energy and reduce metabolic rate, and all gains will be lost.[15,92]

VI. GENERAL STEPS TO START AN ENDURANCE EXERCISE PROGRAM

Based on suggestions made by the Strategic Health Initiative on Aging of the ACSM,[90] there are five simple steps to begin an endurance exercise program:

1. Determine location.
2. Determine intensity.
3. Determine duration.
4. Determine frequency.
5. Insure safety.

Once these choices are made, it is recommended that older adults begin their programs by considering frequency first, then increasing duration, and then intensity.

First, individuals should determine where they will exercise. Will this be at home, outdoors, at a health club, or somewhere else? The decision as to where to exercise is contingent upon what type of endurance activity will be done. This decision should be based on what is available. What does the individual have the skill to do? What does the individual like to do? What can the individual do within appropriate medical limitations? What will the individual do?

It becomes obvious that some level of self-assessment is necessary to find the activity that will be initiated and that can be maintained. It is also appropriate to check with a physician to determine any potential limitations on physical activity and a pharmacist regarding any interactions or complications between medications and exercise; for example, one needs to consider whether any prescribed medications might affect heart rate or function or blood pressure. An exercise physiologist or ACSM or National Strength and Conditioning Association (NSCA) personal trainer can provide assistance in determining what activities are appropriate within pertinent medical limitations. The choices are numerous and include walking, jogging, or running outdoors, or indoors on a treadmill; stair-stepping or climbing; bicycle riding or ergometry; swimming or water aerobics; aerobics, dance, or kickboxing; rowing indoors or out—again, anything that rhythmically uses large muscles over an extended time.

The key to choosing an activity is to find one that will be enjoyed, is realistic for the individual, and will meet his or her needs. Some activities will involve impact—jumping or pounding—that can lead to injury, especially if these are new to the individual. A base level of conditioning should be attained before beginning impact-type activities and even then they should slowly be added into the fitness routine. One of the best predictors for whether someone will stick with a new exercise program is convenience. The less convenient, the less likely that it will be done. People will be more successful if they choose activities that will fit into their current lifestyle. The number one predictor of how often people will attend a fitness center or gym is simply how close that facility is to their home. Cost can also be a prohibitive factor. It does not have to be. No- or low-cost options can be explored. There are also many activities that require a considerable amount of skill that may be discouraging to some. Starting with activities that require little or no skill is generally better. Those who wish to pursue activities requiring high levels of skill should choose activities requiring less skill while they learn the new skills required for their activity. Some discomfort is normal—and even desired—to create the conditioning effect. Pain, however, is not. Those participating in sedentary activities for long periods of time should get up every 30 min to keep the metabolism elevated and to reduce the potential for the complications associated with long-term inactivity. This will also help reduce the onset and severity of delayed onset muscle soreness.

Another consideration in determining where and what will be done is the equipment needed. Equipment should be of good quality, as poor or poorly fit equipment can lead to injuries and decreased enjoyment. For example, if walking outdoors is chosen, the only piece of equipment one needs is a good pair of walking shoes, while bicycling should include a solid, reliable bicycle.

Older adults might consider some other modifications. Walking is perhaps the safest way to begin an endurance exercise program. Cycle ergonometry should be chosen over machines such as stair steppers because of balance considerations. Machines for the development of muscular endurance and muscular strength are safer than free weights, but do not improve balance and coordination as much. Exercises that can be performed sitting are safer than those performed standing, but do not help maintain bone mineral density or improve balance and coordination as much. Isometric exercises, those where a contraction is held against a stationary resistance, should be avoided because of the increased pressures within the cardiovascular system. The exercises should initially be relatively simple. People also tend to better adhere to exercise programs if there is a social component to the activity, such as a class or group program. Thus, finding an activity that encourages interacting with others improves the potential for success.

The next step is to become familiar with the concept of intensity of exercise. Intensity is how hard one works and is a measure of the effort required to complete the exercise.[1] The intensity at which people exercise will depend upon their goals. The intensity necessary to improve health is less than that necessary to improve fitness, which is generally less than that required to improve performance.[4] Moderate-intensity exercise can be used to improve health and manage weight. Heavier activity is necessary to improve health and promote weight loss. Vigorous activity is then required to improve athletic performance.

It is important to monitor exercise intensity to aid in goal achievement and to obtain maximum benefit. This can be done by monitoring heart rate, using a scale of perceived exertion, or the talk test. The talk test is based on the ability to speak while exercising and ranges from being able to carry on a conversation (mild to moderate activity) to being unable to talk (extremely hard activity). The most accurate objective measure for aerobic exercise that does not require extensive equipment is heart rate. Relative intensity is measured as a percentage of the maximal heart rate (HR_{max}, estimate = 220 – age) or a percentage of the heart rate reserve (HRR = $HR_{max} - HR_{rest}$). Maximum, or peak, heart rate can be determined by the aforementioned estimate or during a stress test. Individuals with CVD and congestive heart failure (CHF) will work at a percentage of their symptom-limited HR_{peak}.[52] This is the peak heart rate achieved during the physician-supervised stress test prior to any detectable symptoms of cardiac distress. Rating of perceived exertion (RPE) is a subjective, personal estimate as to how hard an individual is working. The talk test is based on the ability to talk while exercising. Individuals should also judge how they feel; pain and an inability to speak while exercising are indications that the exercise is too vigorous (Table 14.6).

Using Table 14.6 and the goals of the individual, recommended intensities are:

1. For weight loss: Heart Rate: 50–75% of HR_{max} (35–65% of HRR); RPE: 11–14; Talk Test: Able to converse in complete sentences; light sweat.
2. For fitness and improved health: Heart Rate: 60–85% of HR_{max} (55–75% of HRR); RPE: 12–16; Talk Test: Able to converse in complete sentences, with pauses for breathing; moderate to heavy sweat.
3. For performance: Heart Rate: ≥75% of HR_{max} (≥65% of HRR); RPE: 15 +; Talk Test: Able to talk in short sentences to unable to speak; heavy sweat.

Notice that the exercise intensity to improve health is moderate or above.[34] As mentioned previously, novice exercisers should start at the lower end and progress to higher intensities as their exercise tolerance and fitness improves.[52]

It is neither advisable nor really possible to immediately start exercising at the prescribed intensity.[4,50] There should be at least a 5-min warm-up period and each exercise bout should start slowly to allow the cardiovascular and muscular systems to prepare and to elevate body temperature. At the end of the exercise bout a 5–10 min cool-down should then be completed to slow down the cardiovascular and muscles systems and bring down body temperature. Flexibility exercises may be included in the cool-down.

The duration of the exercise session should be considered.[1] The U.S. Surgeon General and the Centers for Disease Control and Prevention recommend a minimum of 30 min daily.[3,87,93] For aerobic exercise:[91] (1) weight loss: 60 min, (2) fitness: 30 min, and (3) performance: event specific. Novice exercisers should start with shorter times and progress to longer-duration activities as their exercise tolerance and fitness improves.[52] If one has not exercised for a long period of time the length of the exercise bout should probably be no more than 5 min. The objective then is to gradually extend this until one is comfortably exercising for 20 min. As time continues to go by and conditioning occurs, the exercise time can be extended to the ideal of 30–60 min. Remember that the exercise does not have to occur in one continuous bout. Bouts of exercise spaced throughout the day can be just as effective in improving health, as long as the total amount of activity adds up to 30 min. Warm-up and cool-down times are not generally included in the calculation of duration, as they should not be within the target intensity.[52]

The frequency of exercise should be decided. Frequency is the number of exercise sessions that occur in a given period (generally a week for this discussion).[1] A minimum of 3 days per week, up to every day of the week is recommended.[26,60,87,90] However, different exercise types require various recovery times and are optimally improved at different frequencies and aerobic exercise—walking, jogging, swimming, and bicycling—should be done 3–7 days per week.[87,93] It may be wise for the novice exerciser to start with 3 non-consecutive days.[52] Cross training is recommended if aerobic activity is going to be performed on a daily basis. Cross training

TABLE 14.6

Intensity monitoring[1]

RPE	Meaning	Description	Talk Test	% HR_{max} (HR_{peak})	% HRR	Examples
6	No exertion at all					
7.5	Extremely light					
9	Very light	Walking slowly at a comfortable pace		< 50	< 20	
10—11	Light		Sing	50—63	20—39	Walking, Gardening, Stretching
12—13	Somewhat hard	**Moderate** A little challenging, but okay to continue	Talk in sentences	64—76	40—59	Swimming, Lawn Mowing, Bicycling
14—16	Hard (heavy)	Vigorous	Talk in short sentences	77—93	60—84	Brisk walking, Jogging, Moving Furniture
17	Very hard	Very strenuovus. A person can still continue, but must really push themselves. It feels very heavy, and the person is very tired				Running, Bicycling (hills), Swimming (laps)
19	Extremely hard	Extremely strenuous	Unable to talk	≥94	≥85	
20	Maximal exertion			100%	100%	

is simply doing different activities so that the muscles, bones, and energy systems are utilized in different ways.[91]

The final consideration should be safety. Older adults and those with chronic conditions should start any new exercise program with a visit to their primary care physician.[47,94] Exercise is appropriate for these populations, but the physician can provide guidelines and help identify any special needs that might exist.

Safety concerns continue once the exercise program begins. Any angina (chest pain), increased breathlessness (as opposed to increased respirations), sudden weight gain, leg swelling, or increased difficulty in managing blood sugar should be reported to a physician immediately.[51] Older adults generally have less total body water than younger and should pay particular attention to hydration, even in the winter months. People do lose more water to sweat during the heat of summer months and staying hydrated is important for health at this time. But, dehydration can also be an issue during the winter months, when the air is dryer and more water can be lost via respiration and through the skin. Appropriate clothing is also important. Good shoes can help prevent or alleviate many foot, ankle, knee, hip, and even back problems. Clothing that traps or releases heat appropriately can also make physical activity more comfortable and safe. Alternate forms of activity should be found during weather extremes. A cell phone, personal identification, and medic alert identification are all appropriate safety precautions. Warming up and cooling down make exercise more effective, comfortable, and safe. Stretching afterward can also prove beneficial for improving flexibility. (Table 14.7)

Older adults may have special needs that necessitate modifying the exercise prescription. Some general recommendations for special populations are made here, but consultation with a physician, exercise physiologist, or ACSM- or NSCA-certified personal trainer is strongly encouraged. Special considerations may exist, such as increased vigilance in foot care for those with diabetes.[50] Individuals with chronic

TABLE 14.7

Ensuring Safe Participation in Physical Activity[4,93,94]

Check with Physician	Individuals with known cardiac, pulmonary, or metabolic diseases, an unstable medical condition, or injury should consult with a physician before starting a new exercise program.
Drink Fluids	Insure adequate water intake during all seasons
Wear Appropriate Clothing	Good shoes and socks
	Appropriate to air temperature
	Breathable to allow sweat management
Safety Devices	Carry appropriate safety devices
	Cell phone, personal identification, medic alert, etc.
Warm Up and Cool Down	Gradually increase and reduce exercise intensity
	Stretch

conditions have often become sedentary as well.[80] This makes it difficult to meet the recommended exercise criteria. But something has to be done to improve fitness. Thus, it is recommended that the individual start with what he or she can do. This may be initially limited to just a few seconds of light exercise followed by a few min of rest and then followed by another period of activity. The idea is to start with what is possible and gradually build up to the recommended frequency, intensity, and time. Recall as well that the total exercise time does not have to be continuous. Multiple shorter-duration sessions can be used throughout the day to add up to the recommended total time.[51]

Medications may limit exercise capacity and responsiveness of the body to the increased stress of exercise. Again, consulting with a knowledgeable physician, pharmacist, exercise physiologist, or ACSM- or NSCA-certified personal trainer is strongly encouraged. Vasodilators, such as ACE inhibitors, hydralazine, and digoxin can complicate exercise by lowering blood pressure to the point to dizziness and syncope.[51] Beta adrenergic blockers reduce exercise capacity by reducing HR_{rest} and the responsiveness of heart rate to physical activity.[52] Insulin or sulfonylurea therapy can alter the exercise-induced mobilization of glucose, fats, and proteins and may result in ketoacidosis or hypoglycemia.[50]

There has been some concern expressed that increasing physical activity can actually be an increase in risk itself. Data support an increase in the rate of activity-related injuries, but a decrease in nonactivity-related injuries.[26] The risk for activity-related injuries increases with the intensity of the exercise, but remains very low.[26] The risk for a cardiovascular event's occurring does also increase during physical activity; however, the risk declines as one becomes more accustomed to physical activity and the risk of being inactive is much greater than that of being active.[26,95] Individuals who are concerned about the risks associated with physical activity should consult with their physician prior to participation (Table 14.8 and Table 14.9).

Recall that interval training—periods of higher-intensity work followed by periods of lower-intensity recovery exercise—results in greater adaptation. Aerobic intervals need to be long enough to engage the oxidative energy systems and not so intense as to shift completely into the fast glycolytic and phosphagen energy systems. Thus, the intervals are generally 3 min or longer (but can be shorter if more intense) and the duration of recovery generally declines as the work period gets longer, for example if the work interval is intense enough to last only 3 min, the recovery might be 9 min; however, if the work interval is less intense and lasts 6 min, the recovery might also last 6 min (Table 14.10).

VII. NUTRITIONAL CONSIDERATIONS

The digestive system changes in several ways as one becomes older. Digestion slows down and it takes the stomach longer to empty. This can lead to a loss of appetite, less frequent eating and reduced energy intake. Loss of appetite can also be related to a decreased sense of taste. The stomach itself often produces less hydrochloric acid and digestive enzymes, which can lead to the development of intolerances of once-enjoyed acidic foods such as citrus fruits and tomatoes.

TABLE 14.8

Aerobic Conditioning Principles[26]

	Moderate Only		Vigorous Only		Combined
Frequency	5 times per week		3 times per week		2/wk & 2/wk
Intensity	Moderate: Talk Test: can speak normally	or	Vigorous: Talk Test: can talk in short sentences	or	Moderate & Vigorous
Time	30 min		20 min		30 min & 20 min
Type	Walking, jogging, aerobics, swimming, water exercise, bicycling, rowing, etc.				

TABLE 14.9

Conditioning Recommendations

	Novice	Trained
Frequency	3—5 d/wk	5—7 d/wk
Intensity (of maximum heart rate)	60%	70—90%
Duration	15 min	≥ 60 min

The absorption of many vitamins and minerals also changes. Research has shown decreased absorption of the fat-soluble vitamins A, D, and E and the water-soluble B complexes. Calcium absorption also decreases (increasing the potential for the development of osteoporosis) and this is exacerbated as the incidence of lactose intolerance increases and the consumption of dairy products declines. Decreased absorption of zinc is associated with poor twilight vision and poor stress tolerance. Decreased absorption of iron, cobalt, and vitamin B_{12} may lead to low levels that are associated with anemia. Reduced chromium absorption may lead to low levels that promote glucose tolerance. This is exacerbated by the previously discussed elevation of blood glucose in older adults as the insulin response becomes blunted over time.

Protein deficiencies in older populations are common and are due to complex causes. Part of the problem may be due to the high cost of protein for individuals on fixed incomes. Protein is also harder to digest and food preferences may change to those that are more easily tolerated. The loss of taste may be associated with a loss of interest in eating. Sedentary lifestyle itself is associated with lowered appetite. Most of the aforementioned difficulties show improvements with exercise.

There are some nutritional concerns when endurance activity is added to one's routine. Recall that energy is supplied by muscle and liver glycogen, blood glucose, free fatty acids, and some amino acids as well. At low exercise intensities, the majority of energy is supplied via lipid metabolism, and up to 60% of lipid comes from within muscle. The reliance on carbohydrates increases as intensity increases. As exercise continues and carbohydrate stores are depleted, lipid and amino acid metabolism

TABLE 14.10

Interval Conditioning

Duration	Work:Recovery
1—3 min	1:3—1:4
≥ 3 min	1:1—1:3

become greater. This low-carbohydrate status (low glycogen stores) reduces exercise performance and increases fatigue. Thus, the question arises as to how to maintain optimum carbohydrate status. This relates to nutrition, the food consumed.

Pre-exercise nutrition is really where the most difference is made and it is dependent on the individual's goals and medical concerns. A consultation and assessment with a physician or registered dietician may be required or prudent to insure that any special needs are identified and met. The general dietary recommendation for the average person to consume 55–60% (6–10 g/kg body mass) of daily caloric intake from carbohydrates applies to older adults. For those who regularly participate in endurance activities at the higher end of the physical activity recommendations it is encouraged that they increase their carbohydrate intake to 65–70% of their dietary calories. The majority of these should come from complex sources that also have a higher micronutrient density. Twenty to 25% of calories should then come from fats and oils, with unsaturated oils making up the majority of these. The remaining 10–15% of calories is then derived from protein. At the same time, one wants to insure adequate micronutrient intake and remain hydrated.

Carbohydrate energy stores are generally enough to sustain activity for approximately 2 hours. There is generally no benefit to performance of enhancing muscular carbohydrate stores, called carbohydrate loading, if the exercise duration is less than 90 min and if the diet is adequate. Older adults generally do not exceed this exercise duration. However, ingesting carbohydrate during longer bouts of exercise can improve performance. The objective is to take in approximately 45–60 g/hour. Simple carbohydrates are easier to digest and get into the bloodstream faster and can be via solid or liquid forms. For a liquid glucose source the optimum solution is approximately a 6% solution (6 g of carbohydrate/100 mL of water). A benefit of this is that it also provides fluid to maintain hydration. Solid carbohydrate supplements require that water be ingested at the same time; some find that solid foods during exercise can result in greater gastric distress. In either event, if carbohydrate is to be ingested during exercise, it is good to gradually add it in so that one understands how the body will probably react to the supplement.

Maintaining proper hydration during exercise is of particular concern for older adults as they are more prone to dehydration. Intense exercise during extreme heat or humidity can result in the loss of 2–3 L/hour. This will lead to dehydration and subsequent heat injury. Thus, a rehydration beverage should be consumed and the loss of more than 2% of body weight during activity avoided.[96,97] Most do not replace lost body water with commercial beverages any better than with plain water, although there is some interesting data suggesting that beverages containing sodium citrate or glycerol may enhance water uptake.[97] Individuals on fluid restriction due to medical conditions should consult with a physician, pharmacist, dietician, exercise physiologist, or ACSM- or NSCA-certified personal trainer.

Rehydration after exercise is also key. The objective is to replace lost body water. There are several ways to monitor adequate hydration and rehydration. Any weight lost during exercise is due to water loss, thus consuming an equal amount of water (1 gallon equals approximately 8.3 pounds) would replenish this.[50,96,97] Assuming no metabolic disorders (i.e., diabetes) the quantity and quality of urine can also provide a rough measure of hydration.[96,97] If there are large amounts of light-colored and relatively odorless urine then hydration is probably adequate; however, dark and odiferous urine may be an indication that hydration is inadequate.

The diet after exercise is also important in that glycogen synthesis is maximal immediately after exercise. Optimum intake, again assuming no metabolic disorders, is 0.7 g carbohydrate/kg body mass. Here the high-glycemic foods (simple sugars) are absorbed more quickly and make their way to the fatigued muscles faster. Adding protein to the post-exercise meal increases glycogen synthesis. The optimum carbohydrate to protein ration is 4:1 and can be found in skim chocolate milk.

A. Ergogenic Aids

Finally, the topic of nutritional ergogenic (work-enhancing) aids is frequently brought up related to endurance exercise. An excellent and thorough treatment can be found in the book *Nutritional Ergogenic Aids* edited by Wolinsky and Driskell (ch. 25, pp 470–472).[98] These regimens should be used for long-term endurance exercise performance. The most effective aids are sports drinks, carbohydrates, and caffeine. Sports drinks with added electrolytes and carbohydrates consumed before, during, and after endurance exercise have the benefit of enhancing the activity along with the added positive effect of reducing high rates of body water loss and its consequences. Limited enhancement has been seen with antioxidants under specific environmental conditions such as altitude. Data also suggest that carnitine salts and coenzyme Q_{10} supplementation improve exercise performance in those with CVD. Those with iron deficiencies will improve performance with appropriate iron supplementation. However, consultation with a physician, dietician, or pharmacist is recommended to ensure that the use of ergogenic aids is not contrary to treatment plans, medications, or restrictions appropriate for the management of chronic health conditions.

VII. CONCLUSIONS

Regular exercise makes the greatest contribution to good health and long life when compared with other interventions. Exercise, the most effective preventive medicine, could be compared to the legendary Fountain of Youth.[99] The return exceeds the investment. Researchers at the Cooper Institute have shown that for each min of exercise one gains 8–9 min of life. This equates to an approximate extension in lifespan of about 7 years when compared with a sedentary counterpart.

The volume, or dose, of physical activity can be determined by combining the frequency, duration, and intensity of physical activity and is directly proportional to the total energy expenditure due to physical activity.[1] Greater benefits can be achieved with greater volume—a higher dose—of physical activity.[1,4,26,35–38,43,45,46,82] This dose response can be found in weight management and loss; the recommendation is for approximately 60 min of moderate to vigorous activity (again, beyond the activities of daily living and work) on most days of the week, while weight maintenance may require 60–90 min of daily moderate-intensity physical activity.[82] The incidence and mortality of cardiovascular and CAD demonstrates an inverse dose response in that the greater the dose of physical activity, the lower the incidence of heart disease.[1,56,69] Improvements in blood pressure do not appear to be dose dependent and moderate activity of the recommended quantity and intensity appears to be sufficient; however, more recent evidence indicates that the incidence of hypertension decreases and a decline in antihypertensive medication use occurs proportional to the amount of physical activity undertaken.[46,56,60] The incidence of colon cancer also demonstrates an inverse relationship to the dose of physical activity.[1] Moderate physical activity improves blood glucose control for those with diabetes, and the probability of developing type 2 diabetes declines with increasing volume of physical activity as do the potential cardiovascular complications associated with type 2 diabetes.[1,56] There also appears to be a dose response of bone density to physical activity.[100] This dose-response relationship does not exist only for fitness and chronic conditions, but also in the ability to perform activities of daily living related to the amount of physical activity.[1]

Given that there appears to be a dose response of most of the age-associated declines in function and increases in incidence of chronic conditions, one might believe that running a marathon tomorrow is essential. This is neither realistic for the vast majority of the population, nor necessary. The evidence that, within reason, more is generally better, should also not discourage the non-active individual from starting—something is better than nothing and everyone must start somewhere. Thus, the general recommendations for someone who is planning to start a new aerobic conditioning program are to: (1) start with an activity without a lot of impact on the joints, (2) start slow, (3) do more net physical activity than was being done before, (4) progress gradually, (5) be patient, and (6) be consistent.[45]

REFERENCES

1. Kesaniemi, Y. A., Danforth, E., Jr., Jensen, M. D., Kopelman, P. G., Lefebvre, P., Reeder, B. A., Dose–response issues concerning physical activity and health: An evidence-based symposium, *Med. Sci. Sports Exerc.* 33(6s), S351–8, 2001.
2. Howley, E. T., Type of activity: Resistance, aerobic and leisure versus occupational physical activity, *Med. Sci. Sports Exerc.* 33(6s), S364–9, 2001.
3. Corbin, C. B., Welk, G. J., Lindsey, R., Corbin, W. R., *Concepts of Fitness and Wellness: A Comprehensive Lifestyle Approach*, 5 ed., McGraw-Hill, New York, NY, 2004.
4. Pollock, M. L., Gaesser, G. A., Butcher, J. D., Despres, J. -P., Dishman, R. K., Franklin, B. A., Garber, C. E., The recommended quantity and quality of exercise for developing and maintaining cardiorespiratory and muscular fitness, and flexibility in healthy adults, *Med. Sci. Sports Exerc.* 30(6), 975–91, 1998.

5. Slentz, C. A., Houmard, J. A., Kraus, W. E., Modest exercise prevents the progressive disease associated with physical inactivity, *Exerc. Sport Sci. Rev.* 35(1), 18–23, 2007.
6. Sahyoun, N. R., Lentzner, H., Hoyert, D., Robinson, K. N., *Trends in Causes of Death among the Elderly*; National Center for Health Statistics, Atlanta, GA, 2001, 1–10.
7. Centers for Disease Control and Prevention, Heart Disease Fact Sheet, 2008. http://www.cdc.gov/DHDSP/library/fs_heart_disease.htm.
8. Minono, A. M., Heron, M. P., Murphy, S. L., Kochanek, K. D., *Deaths: Final data for 2004*, National Vital Statistics System: August 21, 2007, 2007; 120.
9. National Diabetes Fact Sheet: General Information and National Estimates on Diabetes in the United States, 2005. http://apps.nccd.cdc.gov/DDTSTRS/FactSheet.aspx. (March 11, 2008).
10. United States Cancer Statistics: 2004 Incidence and Mortality. http://apps.nccd.cdc.gov/uscs/ (March 11, 2008).
11. Centers for Disease Control and Prevention, Targeting Arthritis: Improving Quality of Life for More than 46 Million Americans 2008, 2008. http://www.cdc.gov/nccdphp/publications/AAG/arthritis_text.htm#1.
12. Overweight and Obesity. http://www.cdc.gov/nccdphp/dnpa/obesity/index.htm. (March 4, 2008).
13. Third Report of the National Cholesterol Education Program (NCEP) Expert Panel on detection, Evaluation, and Treatment of High Blood Cholesterol in Adults (Adult Treatment Panel III) Final Report. *Circulation* 106, 3143–421, 2002.
14. Ford, E. S., Giles, W. H., Dietz, W. H., Prevalence of the metabolic syndrome among US adults: Findings from the third National Health and Nutrition Examination survey, *JAMA* 287, 356–9, 2002.
15. Kohrt, W. M., Bloomfield, S. A., Little, K., Nelson, M. E., Yingling, V. R., Physical activity and bone health. *Med. Sci. Sports Exerc.* 36(11), 1985–96, 2004.
16. Kanis, K., McKay, H., Kannus, P., Bailey, D., Wark, J., Bennel, K., The diagnosis of osteoporosis. *J. Bone Min. Res.* 9, 1137–41, 1994.
17. Osteoporosis Overview, http://www.niams.nih.gov/Health_Info/Bone/Osteoporosis/default.asp (April 28, 2008),
18. American Geriatrics Society, British Geriatrics Society, and American Academy of Orthopaedic Surgeons Panel on Falls Prevention, Guideline for the prevention of falls in older persons, *J. Am. Geriatric Soc.* 49, 664–72, 2001.
19. Jette, A. M., Branch, L. G., The Framingham disability study: II—Physical disability among the aging, *Am. J. Public Health* 71(11), 1211–6, 1981.
20. Branch, L. G., Jette, A. M., The Framingham Disability Study: I. Social disability among the aging, *Am. J. Public Health* 71(11), 1202–10, 1981.
21. Davy, K. P., Seals, D. R., Total blood volume in healthy young and older men, J. *Appl. Physiol,* 76, 2059–2062, 1994.
22. Fleg, J. L., O'Connor, F., Gerstenblith, G., Becker, L. C., Clulow, J., Schulman, S. P., Lakkatta, E., Impact of age on the cardiovascular response to dynamic upright exercise in healthy men and women, *J. Appl. Physiol.* 78(3), 890–900, 1995.
23. Ogawa, T., Spina, R. J., Martin, W. H., III, Kohrt, W. M., Schechtman, K. B., Holloszy, J. O., Ehsani, A. A., Effects of aging, sex, and physical training on cardiovascular response to exercise, *Circulation* 86(2), 494–503, 1992.
24. Heath, G., Hagberg, J. M., Ehsani, A. A., Holloszy, J. O., A physiological comparison of young and older endurance athletes, *J. Appl. Physiol.* 51, 634–40, 1981.
25. McGinnis, J. M., The public health burden of a sedentary lifestyle, *Med. Sci. Sports Exerc.* 24, S196–200, 1992.

26. Haskell, W. H., Lee, I.-M., Pate, R. R., Powell, K. E., Blair, S. N., Franklin, B. A., Macera, C. A., et al., Physical activity and public health: Updated recommendation for adults from the American College of Sports Medicine and the American Heart Association. *Med. Sci. Sports Exerc.* 39(8), 1423–34, 2007.
27. Lavie, C. J., Milani, R. V., Littman, A. B., Benefits of cardiac rehabilitation and exercise training in secondary coronary prevention in the elderly, *J. Am. Coll. Cardiol.* 22, 678–83, 1993.
28. Exercise and Keep Active, http://www.lungusa.org/site/apps/nlnet/content3.aspx?c=dvLUK9O0E&b=2060053&content_id={5431F32F–CB92–4D32–A7CE–C8C0801EAD2F}¬oc=1 (Sept. 24, 2008).
29. Thune, I., Furberg, A.-S., Physical activity and cancer risk: Dose–response and cancer, all sites and site-specific, *Med. Sci. Sports Exerc.* 33(6S), S530–50, 2001.
30. Laaksonen, D. E., Lindstrom, J., Lakka, T. A., Eriksson, J. G., Niskanen, L., Wikstrom, K., et al., Physical activity in the prevention of type 2 diabetes: the Finnish Diabetes Prevention study. *Diabetes* 54(1), 158–65, 2005.
31. Penninx, B. W. J. H., Messier, S. P., Rejeski, W. J., Williamson, J. D., DiBari, M., Cavazzini, C., et al., Physical exercise and the prevention of disability in activities of daily living in older persons with osteoarthritis, *Arch. Intern. Med.* 161(19), 2309–16, 2001.
32. LaMonte, M. J., Barlow, C. E., Jurca, R., Kampert, J. B., Church, T. S., Blair, S. N., Cardiorespiratory fitness is inversely associated with the incidence of metabolic syndrome: A prospective study of men and women, *Circulation* 112, 505–12, 2005.
33. Prince, R. L., Smith, M., Dick, I. M., Price, R. I., Webb, P. G., Henderson, K., Harris, M. M., Prevention of postmenopausal osteoporosis: A comparative study of exercise, calcium supplementation, and hormone-replacement therapy, *New Engl. J. Med.* 325(17), 1189–95, 1991.
34. Mazzeo, R. S., Cavanagh, P., Evans, W. J., Fiatarone, M. A., Hagberg, J. M., McAuley, E., Startzell, J., Exercise and physical activity for older adults, *Med. Sci. Sports Exerc.* 30(6), 992–1008, 1998.
35. Williams, P. T., Nonlinear relationships between weekly walking distance and adiposity in 27,596 women, *Med. Sci. Sports Exerc.* 37(11), 1893–901, 2005.
36. Mayer-Davis, E. J., D'Agostino, R. D., Karter, A. J., Haffner, S. M., Rewers, M. J., Saad, M., Bergman, R. N., Intensity and amount of physical activity in relation to insulin sensitivity: The insulin resistance atherosclerosis study, *JAMA* 279(9), 669–74, 1998.
37. Barlow, C. E., LaMonte, M. J., FitzGerald, S. J., Kampert, J. B., Perrin, J. L., Blair, S. N., Cardiorespiratory fitness is an independent predictor of hypertension incidence among initially normotensive healthy women, *Am. J. Epidemiol.* 163(2), 142–50, 2005.
38. Williams, P. T., Thompson, P. D., Dose-dependent effects of training and detraining on weight in 6406 runners during 7.4 years, *Obesity (Silver Spring)* 14(11), 1975–84, 2006.
39. Farrell, S. W., Kampert, J. B., Kohl, H. W., III, Barlow, C. E., Macera, C. A., Paffenbarger, R. S., et al., Influence of cardiorespiratory fitness levels and other predictors on cardiovascular disease mortality in men, *Med. Sci. Sports Exerc.* 30(6), 899–905, 1998
40. Wilmore, J. H., Costill, D. L., *Training for sport and activity: The physiological basis of the conditioning process*, 3 ed., Human Kinetics Publishers, Champaign, IL, 1988, 420.
41. Gibala, M. J., McGee, S. L., Metabolic adaptations to short-term high-intensity interval training: A little pain for a lot of gain? *Exerc. Sport Sci. Rev.* 36(2), 58–63, 2008.
42. Bouchard, C., Rankinen, T., Individual differences in response to regular physical activity, *Med. Sci. Sports Exerc.* 33(6s), S446–51, 2001.

43. Wendel-Vos, G. C. W., Schuit, A. J. ; Feskens, E. J. M. ; Boshuizen, H. C., Verschuren, W. M. M., Saris, W. H. M., Kromhout, D., Physical activity and stroke: A meta-analysis of observational data, *Intern. J. Epidemiol.* 33(4), 787–98, 2004.
44. Weuve, J., Kang, J. H., Manson, J. E., Breteler, M. M. B., Ware, J. H., Grodstein, F., Physical activity, including walking, and cognitive function in older women, *JAMA* 292(12), 1454–61, 2004. .
45. Nelson, M. E., Rejeski, W. J., Blair, S. N., Duncan, P. W., Judge, J. O., King, A. C., et al., Physical activity and public health in older adults: Recommendation from the American College of Sports Medicine and the American Heart Association, *Med. Sci. Sports Exerc.* 39(8), 1435–45, 2007.
46. Williams, P. T., Reduced diabetic, hypertensive, and cholesterol medication use with walking, *Med. Sci. Sports Exerc.* 40(3), 433–43, 2008.
47. Pescatello, L. S., Franklin, B. A., Fagard, R. H., Farquhar, W. B., Kelley, G. A., Ray, C. A., Exercise and hypertension, *Med. Sci. Sports Exerc.* 36(3), 533–53, 2004.
48. King, A. C., Haskell, W. L., Young, D. R., Oka, R. K., Stefanick, M. L., Long-term effects of varying intensities and formats of physical activity on participation rates, fitness, and lipoproteins in men and women aged 50 to 65 years, *Circulation* 91, 2596–2604, 1995.
49. Wilmore, J. H., Dose-response: Variation with age, sex, and health status, *Med. Sci. Sports Exerc.* 33(6s), S622–34, 2001.
50. Zinman, B., Ruderman, N., Campaigne, B. N., Devlin, J. T., Schneider, S. H., ADA/ACSM joint statement: diabetes mellitus and exercise, *Med. Sci. Sports Exerc.* 29(12), 1–6, 1997.
51. Clark, J. R., Sherman, C., Congestive heart failure: Training for a better life, *Physician Sportsmed.* 26(8), 49,53–6, 1998.
52. van Camp, S. P., Cantwell, J. D., Fletcher, G. F., Smith, L. K., Thompson, P. D., Exercise for patients with coronary artery disease, *Med. Sci. Sports Exerc.* 26(3), i–v, 1994.
53. Kraemer, W. J., Physiological adaptations to anaerobic and aerobic endurance training, In *Essentials of strength training and conditioning*, 2 ed., Baechle, T. R., Earle, R. W., Eds., Human Kinetics Publisher, Champaign, IL, 2000; 137–68.
54. Perseghin, G., Price, T. B., Petersen, K. F., Roden, M., Cline, G. W., Gerow, K., et al., Increased glucose transport-phosphorylation and muscle glycogen synthesis after exercise training in insulin-resistant subjects, *New Engl. J. Med.* 335, 1357–62, 1996.
55. Kelley, D. E., Goodpaster, B. H., Effects of exercise on glucose homeostasis in type 2 diabetes mellitus, *Med. Sci. Sports Exerc.* 33(6s), S495–S501, 2001.
56. Williams, P. T., Vigorous exercise, fitness, and incident hypertension, high cholesterol, and diabetes, *Med. Sci. Sports Exerc.* 40(6), 998–1006, 2008.
57. Brooks, G. A., Fahey, T. D., Baldwin, K. M., *Exercise physiology: Human bioenergetics and its implications*, 4 ed., McGraw-Hill, New York, 2005; p. 876.
58. Londeree, B. R., Effect of training on lactate/ventilatory thresholds: a meta-analysis, *Med. Sci. Sports Exerc.* 29(6), 837–43, 1997.
59. Fagard, R. H., Exercise characteristics and the blood pressure response to dynamic physical training, *Med. Sci. Sports Exerc.* 33(6s), S484–92, 2001.
60. Hagberg, J. M., Blair, S. N., Ehasani, A. A., Gordon, N. F., Kaplan, N., Tipton, C. M., Zambraski, E. J., Physical activity, physical fitness, and hypertension. *Med. Sci. Sports Exerc.* 25(10), i–x, 1993.
61. Chobanian, A. V., Bakris, G. L., Black, H. R., Cushman, W. C., Green, L. A., Izzo, J. L., et al., The seventh report of the joint national committee on prevention, detection, evaluation, and treatment of high blood pressure, *JAMA* 289(19), 2560–72, 2003.

62. Clausen, J. P., Trap-Jensen, J., Heart rate and arterial blood pressure during exercise in patients with angina pectoris: Effects of training and nitroglycerin, *Circulation* 53(3), 436–42, 1976.
63. Keteyian, S. J., Levine, A. B., Brawner, C. A., Kataoka, T., Rogers, F. J., Schairer, J. R., et al., Exercise training in patients with heart failure, *Ann. Internal Med.* 124, 1051–7, 1996.
64. Thompson, P. D., The benefits and risks of exercise training in patients with chronic coronary artery disease, *JAMA* 259(10), 1537–40, 1988.
65. Hartung, G. H., Rangel, R., Exercise training in post–myocardial infarction patients: comparison of results with high risk coronary and post–bypass patients, *Arch. Phys. Med. Rehabilitation* 62, 147–50, 1981.
66. Wei, M., Gibbons, L. W., Mitchell, T. L., Kampert, J. B., Lee, C. D., Blair, S. N., The association between cardiorespiratory fitness and impaired fasting glucose and type 2 diabetes mellitus in men, *Ann. Internal Med.* 130(2), 89–96, 1999.
67. Vuori, I. M., Dose-response of physical activity and low back pain, osteoarthritis, and osteoporosis, *Med. Sci. Sports Exerc.* 33(6s), S551–86, 2001.
68. American College of Rheumatology, Exercise and arthritis, http://www.rheumatology.org/public/factsheets/exercise_new.asp (February 15, 2008).
69. Kohl, H. W., III, Physical activity and cardiovascular disease: Evidence for a dose response, *Med. Sci. Sports Exerc.* 33(6s), S472–83, 2001.
70. Lee, C. D., Blair, S. N., Cardiorespiratory fitness and stroke mortality in men, *Med. Sci. Sports Exerc.* 34, 592–5, 2002.
71. Williams, P. T., Health effects resulting from exercise versus those from body fat loss. *Med. Sci. Sports Exerc.* 33(6s), S611–21, 2001.
72. American Heart Association, Risk factors and coronary heart disease, http://www.americanheart.org/presenter.jhtml?identifier=4726 (May 22, 2008),
73. Thompson, P. D., Buchner, D., Pina, I. L., Balady, G. J., Williams, M. A., Marcus, B. H., et al., Exercise and physical activity in the prevention and treatment of atherosclerotic cardiovascular disease: AHA Scientific Statement, *Circulation* 107, 3109–16, 2003.
74. Lokey, E. A., Tran, Z. V., Effects of exercise training on serum lipid and lipoprotein concentrations in women: A meta-analysis, *Intern. J. Sports Med.* 10(6), 424–9, 1989.
75. Kelley, G. A., Kelley, K. S., Tran, Z. V., Aerobic exercise, lipids and lipoproteins in overweight and obese adults: A meta-analysis of randomized controlled trials, *Intern. J. Obesity* 29, 881–93, 2005.
76. Leon, A. S., Sanchez, O. A., Response of blood lipids to exercise training alone or combined with dietary intervention, *Med. Sci. Sports Exerc.* 33(6s), S502–15, 2001.
77. Kelley, G. A., Kelley, K. S., Tran, Z. V., Walking, lipids, and lipoproteins: A meta-analysis of randomized controlled trials, *Prev. Med.* 38, 651–61, 2004.
78. Tran, Z. V., Weltman, A., Differential effects of exercise on serum lipid and lipoprotein levels seen with changes in body weight, *JAMA* 254(7), 919–24, 1985.
79. Arthritis as a potential barrier to physical activity among adults with diabetes—United States, 2005 and 2007, *Morbidity and Mortality Weekly Report* 57(18), 486–9, Centers for Disease Control and Prevention, Atlanta, GA, 2008.
80. Albright, A., Franz, M., Hornsby, G., Kriska, A., Marrero, D., Ulrich, I., Verity, L. S., Exercise and type 2 diabetes, *Med. Sci. Sports Exerc.* 32(7), 1345–60, 2000.
81. Wing, R. R., Hill, J. O., Successful weight loss maintenance, *Ann. Rev. Nutr.* 21, 323–41, 2001.
82. Jakicic, J. M., Clark, K., Coleman, E., Donnelly, J. E., Foreyt, J., Melanson, E., et al., Appropriate intervention strategies for weight loss and prevention of weight regain in adults, *Med. Sci. Sports Exerc.* 33(12), 2145–56, 2001.

83. Taylor, C. B., Houston-Miller, N., Haskell, W. L., Debusk, R. F., Smoking cessation after acute myocardial infarction: The effects of exercise training, *Addictive Behav.* 13(4), 331–5, 1988.
84. Ussher, M. H., West, R., Taylor, A. H., McEwen, A., Exercise interventions for smoking cessations, *Cochrane Database Systematic Rev.* 3, (CD002295), 2000.
85. Marcus, B. H., Albrecht, A. E., King, T. K., Parisi, A. F., Pinto, B. M., Roberts, M., et al., The efficacy of exercise as an aid for smoking cessation in women: A randomized controlled trial, *Archi. Intern. Med.* 159, 1229–34, 1999.
86. Taylor, C. B., Sallis, J. F., Needle, R., The relation of physical activity and exercise to mental health, *Public Health Reports* 100(2), 195–202, 1985.
87. Are there special recommendations for older adults? http://www.cdc.gov/nccdphp/dnpa/physical/everyone/recommendations/older_adults.htm (May 5, 2008).
88. Squires, R. W., Lavie, C. J., Brandt, T. R., Gau, G. T., Bailey, K. R., Cardiac rehabilitation in patients with severe ischemic left ventricular dysfunction, *Mayo Clinic Proc.* 1987, 62, (11), 997–1002, 2001.
89. Spirduso, W. W., Cronin, D. L., Exercise dose–response effects on quality of life and independent living in older adults. *Med. Sci. Sports Exerc.* 33(6s), S598–S608.
90. Pate, R. R., Pratt, M., Blair, S. N., Physical activity and public health in older adults: Recommendations from the Centers for Disease Control and Prevention and the American College of Sports Medicine, *JAMA* 273, 402–7, 1995.
91. Baechle, T. R., Earle, R. W., *Essentials of strength training and conditioning,* 2 ed., Human Kinetics Publisher, Champaign, IL, 2000, p. 658.
92. McArdle, W. D., Katch, F. I., Katch, V. L., *Exercise physiology: Energy, nutrition, and human performance*, 3 ed., Lea and Febiger, Philadelphia, PA, 1991.
93. Physical Activity and Health: A report of the Surgeon General, Centers for Disease Control and Prevention, President's Council on Physical Fitness and Sport, 1996.
94. Whaley, M. H., Brubaker, P. H., Otto, R. M., *ACSM's guidelines for exercise testing and prescription,* 7 ed., Lippincott Williams and Wilkins, Philadelphia, PA, 2006, p. 366.
95. Thompson, P. D., Franklin, B. A., Balady, G. J., Blair, S. N., Corrado, D., Estes, M., III, et al., Exercise and acute cardiovascular events: Placing the risks into perspective, *Med. Sci. Sports Exerc.* 39(5), 886–97, 2007.
96. Sawka, M. N., Burke, L. M., Eichner, E. R., Maughan, R. J., Montain, S. J., Stachenfeld, N. S., Exercise and fluid replacement, *Med. Sci. Sports Exerc.* 39(2), 377–90, 2007.
97. Casa, D. J., Armstrong, L. E., Hillman, S. K., Montain, S. J., Reiff, R. V., Rich, B. S. E., et al., National Athletic Trainers' Association position statement: Fluid replacement for athletes, *J. Athletic Training* 35(2), 212–24, 2000.
98. Wolinsky, I., Driskell, J. A., *Nutritional ergogenic aids,* CRC Press, Boca Raton, FL, 2004, p. 520.
99. Shaw, J., The deadliest sin, *Harvard Mag.* 106(4), 36–43, 98–9, 2004.
100. Shephard, R. J., Absolute versus relative intensity of physical activity in a dose–response context, *Med. Sci. Sports Exerc.* 33(6s), S400–18, 2001.

15 Resistance Training

Robert J. Moffatt, Jacob M. Wilson, and Tait Lawrence

CONTENTS

I. INTRODUCTION

In the 20th century the United States experienced a 57% increase in lifespan (from 49.2 to 76.5 years).[1] With continued growth, per annum life expectancy is projected to rise to approximately 80–84 years of age in women and men respectively by the year 2050.[1] With the average college graduate obtaining his or her degree by age 25 and reaching retirement by 65, it is during the midlife (30–60) portion of these longer lifespans that an individual may have the greatest opportunity to make an impact on society.[2,3] During these working years many will perform physically demanding jobs that have been correlated to various measures of strength.[4] Data suggests that middle-aged (35–57) individuals in physically demanding jobs demonstrate progressive worry about their usefulness in society.[5]

Extensive interviews with middle-aged carpenters revealed emerging themes related to concern over their aging body, its relation to declines in strength and accompanying feeling of uselessness.[5] Engineers who were interviewed revealed consistent thoughts about countering age by keeping their body in shape as a mechanism to tackle stress.[5] For these middle-aged individuals, optimizing strength becomes a necessity. Musculoskeletal strength is also important for those with less physically demanding jobs who enjoy recreational and sports-related activities. There are strong associations between musculoskeletal strength and performance in soccer,[6] football,[7] softball,[8] sprinting,[6] rock climbing,[9] and even hiking.[10] Thus, musculoskeletal strength is important for maintaining physically demanding job excellence, countering feelings of uselessness, and experiencing high performance in enjoyable recreational activities.

For the scientist studying the aging process, midlife becomes particularly important as this period serves as a link between young and old adulthood, that, in the latter, is associated with an accelerated loss of muscle tissue and strength. This loss is associated with a greater likelihood of disability and functional impairment in the activities of daily living,[11,12] incidence of falls,[11–14] insulin resistance,[13] and hip fractures.[14] Each of these factors appears to contribute to a projected doubling of 65-year-olds using nursing homes by 2020.[1] As individuals aged 65 years or older increase from 13% to 20% of the population from 2000 to 2030,[1] a paralleled two to six billion dollar increase in hip fracture expenditures is projected to occur.[1] Yet, there is strong evidence that individuals who strength train throughout midlife can maintain extreme levels of function into old age. Thus, an understanding of factors that can optimize musculoskeletal morphology and strength throughout midlife becomes imperative for performance both during peak working years and to prepare the individual to optimize function throughout old age. The purpose of this chapter will therefore be to focus on optimizing muscle tissue size and anaerobic components of musculoskeletal performance through strength training and how these principles can be applied to the middle-aged individual. Because muscle tissue is highly sensitive to nutritional status,[15] we will also provide an extensive analysis of research characterizing how nutrition can interact with load manipulation to maximize musculoskeletal performance in midlife.

The chapter is divided into five sections: (1) Characteristic changes in muscle tissue across age spans, (2) hypertrophy and functional responses of muscle tissue to resistance training across age spans, (3) additional health benefits of resistance training (4) strength training principles, (5) and nutritional augmentation of musculoskeletal performance.

II. DEFINING STRENGTH TRAINING

Before discussing changes in muscle tissue and how strength training can influence musculoskeletal performance, it is important to first define key variables that will be utilized throughout the chapter. The term "strength" can be defined simply for our purposes as a measure of the task-specific application of muscular force. Two principle categories of strength have bearing on this discussion: maximal strength and strength endurance. Maximal strength is best described as the maximal muscular force that can be applied to a task by a given individual. Strength endurance is the ability of an individual to preserve muscular force application over repeated bouts of a particular task. Another term related to strength and also very important to our discussion is "power," that is a measure of work rate and is closely related to the rate at which muscular force can be applied to a given task.

Both strength and power are largely determined by the interplay of two principal factors, neural and musculoskeletal. Examples of neural factors that may affect the expression of strength or power are: neuromuscular function, motor unit recruitment, arousal level, and the skill set of the individual. Some examples of musculoskeletal factors would be: the size and metabolic characteristics of muscle tissue, the location of muscular attachments, and the mechanical properties of the joints involved. Some of these factors cannot readily be modified by training (i.e., muscular attachment, joint shape) and others are beyond the scope of this discussion (i.e., skill set), the focus will be kept to those factors that can be easily modified with a basic strength-training program.

The terms "strength training" or "resistance training" can be used interchangeably within the text, and it should be understood that unless otherwise specified these terms are referring to progressive resistance exercise (PRE). PRE is a training scheme that utilizes musculoskeletal loading, such as weight lifting, that is increased in intensity or volume incrementally over time to improve strength and increase muscle mass. Power training is a specific type of PRE that makes use of explosive and ballistic movements to improve both the musculoskeletal and neural factors that affect power output.

III. CHARACTERISTIC CHANGES IN MUSCLE TISSUE WITH AGING

A great deal of data on the characteristics of muscle tissue changes across the life span was provided by Lexal et al.,[16] who investigated the total number, size, and proportion of different fiber types in whole *vastus lateralis* muscle in 15- to 83-year-old men. Results indicated that muscle mass peaked at approximately 25 years of age and began to decline thereafter. Of importance to middle-aged individuals is the finding that a moderate 10% loss of muscle size occurred from age 25 to 50. From age 50 to 80 a further dramatic 30% loss of muscle tissue was found that was mainly attributed to a 35% decrease in fiber number. Because motor units remain relatively stable in number up to age 60,[17] it can be inferred that overall atrophy in middle-aged individuals is explained largely by changes in protein balance[15] and a small loss of muscle fibers prior to age 60.[16] Age-related muscle tissue atrophy appears to occur in type II muscle fibers with little or no changes occurring in type I fiber cross-sectional area (CSA).[18] For example, Coggan and colleagues[18] found that type IIX fibers were 22% and 30% smaller respectively compared with 13% and 24% smaller in IIA fibers in aged men and women respectively. These findings are further supported by data that demonstrates an age-related decrement in myosin heavy chain (MHC) IIa and IIX mRNA, with no change occurring in type I MHC messenger ribonucleic acid (mRNA).[20] Muscle tissue loss in men and women occurs similarly when utilizing whole lean mass indices,[18,20] while an analysis within fast twitch fiber types indicates more pronounced atrophy in elderly women than in elderly men.[16]

In summary, current research suggests that muscle tissue size peaks at approximately 25 years of age and decreases by 10% by age 50.[21] Thereafter, an accelerated loss of muscle ranging from 0.5 to 1.0% in cross-sectional studies[17] to 1.4% annually in longitudinal studies[15] occurs. Because motor units remain relatively stable in number up to age 60, it can be inferred that overall atrophy is explained largely by changes in protein balance in middle-aged individuals.[16] Protein balance and nutritional strategies to enhance protein balance will be discussed later in this chapter. The repercussions of losses in muscle tissue size relate to changes in strength and power, each of which will be discussed in depth subsequently.

IV. CHANGES IN ABSOLUTE AND RELATIVE STRENGTH

Data indicate that, after 74 years of age, 30% of men and an astonishing 66% of women in the United States are incapable of lifting objectsweighing more than 4.5 kg.[22] The following section will characterize changes in strength with increasing age, as well as possible mechanisms behind these changes. Larsson et al.,[23] in an extensive cross-sectional analysis of both isometric and dynamic strength in 114 sedentary men aged 11 to 70 years of age, found that strength rose up to 30 years of age, was maintained through age 50, and progressively declined thereafter. These findings were supported by Vandervoort and McComas,[24] who found no significant relationship between normalized strength and age from young to middle-aged (20–52 yr) subjects ($r = 0.043$), with a significant negative relationship occurring for subjects aged 60–100 years of age ($r = -0.604$), though studies have indicated strength can begin to decline as early as age 40.[25] Larsson's[23] findings are generally supported across protocols,[32,33] occurring in a similar manner across genders when normalized for either fat-free mass or muscle mass,[21] or when CSA is plotted against age.[25] Data from cross-sectional studies indicate an 8–15% loss of strength after the age of 50 per decade,[21,23,25,26] while longitudinal data indicate even higher rates ranging from 1.4–5% per annum.[27–32]

While a number of factors may contribute to losses in strength, longitudinal data indicate that 90% of the variance in decrements are explained by changes in CSA such that a decrease of 1 cm^2 in CSA of a given muscle is associated with a 2.68 N • m decrease in strength.[30] In addition to absolute strength changes, there is also a change in relative strength. Relative strength is expressed as strength per unit whole muscle CSA,[33] as well as through direct force transduction in isolated muscle fibers.[30] At the whole muscle level, changes in relative strength are at least partially attributed to a reduction in functional motor units, as illustrated by Stalberg and Fawcett[34] who found a 25% reduction in functional motor units after the age of 60. Other changes may be related to an increase in fat and connective tissue with age,[35] as well as atrophy of type II fibers that demonstrate up to a 1.8 times greater intrinsic force than type I fibers.[33] Strength losses at the single muscle fiber level appear to be related to a progressive impairment in excitation contraction coupling processes and therefore a reduced formation of actin myosin cross bridges.[30]

In summary, strength reaches its apex at age 30, is maintained throughout the majority of midlife, and begins to decline in the final one third of midlife (50–60) years to old age at an accelerated rate. For the middle-aged individual, this would suggest that the capacity to perform in activities that require strength as discussed in the introduction should be relatively similar to the young. However, near the latter part of middle-aged years, individuals will need to rely heavily on interventions that prevent strength loss. These strategies are related to mechanical loading and its interaction with nutrition, and will be discussed shortly.

V. CHANGES IN POWER AND VELOCITY WITH AGE

Power, a function of work done over time, is strongly associated with activities of daily living such as climbing a flight of stairs,[36–38] and in sport activities.[36] Decrements in power due to aging appear to take place earlier (30–40 yr) than for strength (50 yr) in both women and men.[37] An extensive analysis of 335 healthy men ranging from 22–88 years of age revealed a near 10% loss of cycle ergometer power per decade.[37] However, when each decade was evaluated as a single unit, declines in power were found to accelerate following age 60 such that power declined per annum by 1.03% from the sixth to seventh decade, 1.42% from the seventh to eighth and 2.36% from the eighth to ninth decade. Declines in force only partly explain losses in power.[38,39] This is illustrated by Skelton et al.[38] who found that isometric strength and leg extensor power decreased over the age range of 65–89 years in elderly men (N = 50) and women (N = 50) at a rate of 1–2% per year and 3.5% per year, respectively (see Figure 15.1).

Velocity loss also appears to partly explain power decrements. As data from Kostka[37] suggested, a 10% loss in cycling power was explained by a loss of thigh

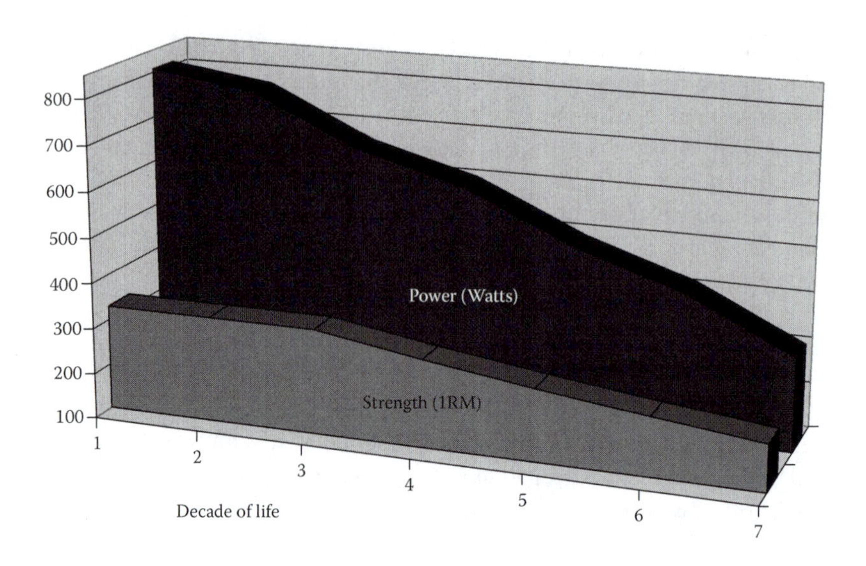

FIGURE 15.1 Strength and Power loss in a typical sedentary male across the lifespan. Strength example estimated from median data taken from: Frontera, W. R. et al. (1991); Kallman, D. A., Plato, C. C. and Tobin, J. D. (1990); Larsson, L., Grimby, G., and Karlsson, J. (1979); Lindle, R. S. et al. (1997). Power data from Kostka, T. (2005).

muscle mass (4.1% decline per decade) and maximal velocity (6.6% decline per decade).

Prior to age 60 selective atrophy of fast twitch muscle fibers[18] appears to partly mediate changes in velocity. However, selective deinervation of fast twitch motor units[40] and accelerated excitation contraction uncoupling[41–43] increase in their role in velocity declines following middle age. Based on these findings, middle-aged individuals should focus on two components to maintain power: (1) strength and (2) velocity. Both of these components can be manipulated through resistance training.

VI. THE EFFECTS OF CHRONIC RESISTANCE TRAINING ON MUSCLE TISSUE SIZE AND FUNCTION ACROSS AGE GROUPS

A. Changes in Muscle Tissue and Strength

The capacity of individuals to increase muscle tissue and function in response to resistance training across the lifespan has been demonstrated in healthy and even frail institutionalized elderly (50–101 yrs) including increased CSA of trained muscle groups ranging from 2–12%,[44–49] with accompanying 7 to 36%[44–49] and 60 to 260%[50,51] elevations in isometric and dynamic strength respectively in mixed-gender studies. These findings suggest that the progressive loss of function and muscle tissue with aging may be in part due to lowered activity and loading.

One possible way to infer the effects of lifelong frequent loading patterns from both endurance and resistance training stimuli is through the use of masters-level athlete vs. sedentary and young athletic models.[48,52,53] In general, masters-level endurance athletes demonstrate a maintenance of relative force per unit CSA, but display similar characteristic absolute declines as sedentary controls in muscle tissue and function with age,[52] while masters-level resistance-trained athletes are able to maintain muscle mass and function similar to the young.[53] Klitgaard et al.[53] investigated the function and morphology of the knee extensors and elbow flexors in young (28 yr) and elderly (68-70 yr) participants classified as sedentary, endurance (swimmer and runners), and strength-trained. Both sedentary and endurance elderly participants demonstrated similar declines in knee extension (–44%), elbow flexion (–32%), speed of movement (–20–26%), and CSA of the elbow flexors (–20%) and knee extensors (24%). In contrast, the elderly strength-trained participants had values identical to young sedentary participants in maximal isometric torques, speed of movement, CSA, specific tension, and content of myosin isoforms in all muscle groups studied. Similarly age-matched middle-aged and elderly sprinters with regular weight training regimens have demonstrated greater force, power, and cross-sectional area in type I, IIa, and IIb fibers than sedentary controls.[54] These results appear to indicate that long-term high-intensity loading may blunt or reverse characteristic changes in muscle mass and performance with age (see Figure 15.2).

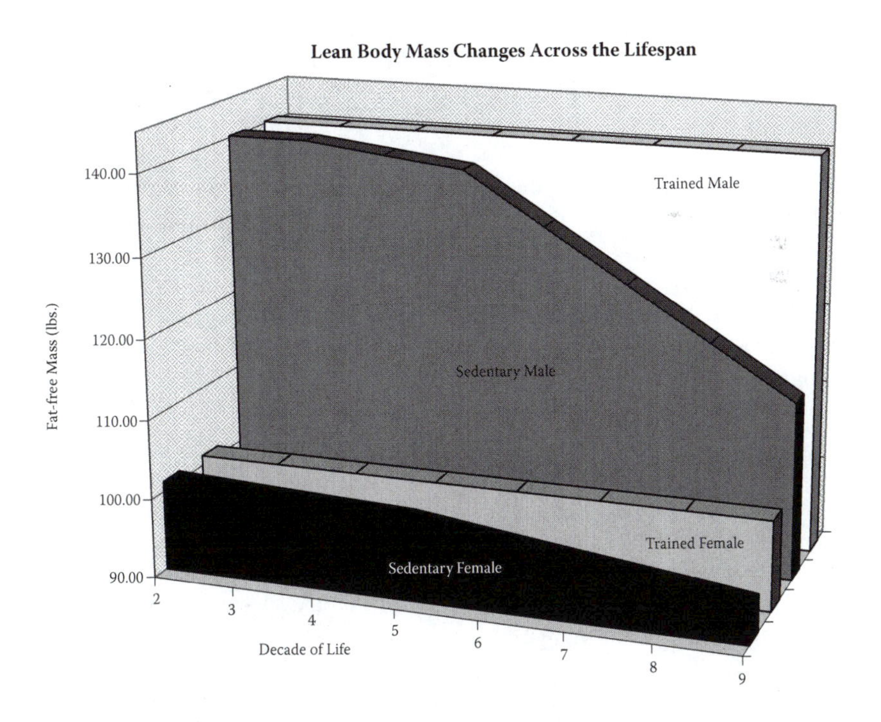

FIGURE 15.2 Example of typical changes in fat–free mass between sedentary and strength trained men and women based on median data from Guo, S. S. et. al. (1999), Kyle, U. G. et. al. (2001) & Klitgaard, H. (1990).

While a number of studies have compared young with elderly individuals' responses to chronic training, there is a general lack of data in the hypertrophic response that directly compares young and middle-aged individuals. What is known is that muscle mass only slightly decreases from age 25 to 50 yrs (10%), with no significant changes in strength.[16] These findings coupled with the knowledge that motor unit numbers remain relatively stable until the sixth decade[16] suggest that middle-aged individuals may gain similar size and functional outcomes in comparison with the young. This contention was recently supported in an 8-week split-body periodized resistance training program that investigated body composition in 24 college-aged (CA) (18–22 year) and 25 middle-aged (MA) males (35–50 year).[55] Participants trained their upper body and lower body twice per week using a variety of exercises with sets ranging from 3 to 6 for small to large body parts respectively. As with previous studies, no significant differences were observed in total lifting volume and lean body mass between groups, however, the middle-aged participants had significantly greater fat mass (CA: 10.8 ± 4.6 kg; MA: 16.8 ± 6.0) and body fat percentage (CA: 14.3 ± 5.1%; MA: 20.1 ± 5.5%) than CA individuals. Results indicated that both young and middle-aged participants gained lean body mass (LBM: 1 kg), with no differences between conditions. In addition, the middle-aged participants lost more fat mass and decreased body fat percentage to a greater extent than the young individuals. These findings suggest that over an 8-week period of time that age-associated gains in fat mass and body fat percentage can be attenuated and reversed by engaging in a periodized resistance training program. Future studies will need to investigate longer training periods (> 16 wk) as well as explore changes in strength and power in young versus middle-aged individuals.

In conclusion, data suggests that aging-associated losses in muscle and strength are at least partially due to decreased high-intensity loading as indicated by masters level athlete models. When analyzing direct resistance training studies, results strongly suggest that even the oldest old (>100 yr) can mount a functional and hypertrophy response. While data is limited, it appears that middle-aged individuals can increase cross-sectional area similar to CA males, at least following 8 weeks of training.

B. Elevations in Power in Response to Resistance Training

The capacity to increase power appears relatively stable with age in response to resistance training. Hakkinen et al.[56] investigated the effects of a combination of heavy- and "explosive"-strength training on the rate of force development over a 6-month period of time in middle-aged (40 yr) and elderly (70 yr.) men and women. Men and women increased leg extension rates of force development by approximately 30%, independent of age. Changes were paralleled by increased neural activation of agonist muscle groups with a concomitant decrease in antagonist muscle activity during the leg extension exercise. Similarly, Jozsi and colleagues[57] found similar increases in upper middle-aged/elderly (55–66 yr) and young (21–30) men and women in leg extension and arm pull power at a number of velocities following a traditional 12-week progressive resistance training protocol.

In conclusion, aging populations appear to maintain the capacity to elevate power output in response to progressive resistance training programs ranging from 3–6 months in duration.

C. Increases in Functionality in Response to Resistance Training

One primary concern, particularly for upper middle-aged individuals as they approach their elderly years, is a decrease in functionality. Resistance training in the elderly has been demonstrated to enhance performance in activities of daily living as indicated by increased gait speed,[49,58] stair-climbing power,[59] balance,[59] and total score on the Continuous Scale Physical Functional Performance test.[60] Data suggest that these changes are related to increased muscle tissue,[11,12] strength,[22] and power[61] implicating each component as essential for the individual wanting to maximize his or her functionality with aging. An analysis of how to maximize these variables is presented next.

VII. OPTIMIZING ACUTE TRAINING VARIABLES FOR ENDURANCE, HYPERTROPHY, STRENGTH, AND POWER

Optimal resistance training prescription begins by providing an individual with a needs analysis, or an analysis that takes into consideration the individual's goals, training experience, and age. Following, an individual must select a series of acute training variables to attain these goals. Acute training variables are factors that can be manipulated during a resistance training session. According to the American College of Sports Medicine (ACSM) acute training variables can be fractionated into (1) muscle action, (2) rest periods (3) load and volume, (4) repetition velocity, and finally (5) training frequency. The following sections will briefly discuss what research suggests optimizes the goals of (1) strength, (2) power, (3) hypertrophy, and (4) endurance. In general, these recommendations yield similar "relative results" regardless of age. For example, muscle tissue growth is optimized with hypertrophy-oriented routines compared with primarily strength and power routines in both young, middle-aged, and elderly participants.[65,66]

A. Strength and Power

Strength is a factor of both muscular hypertrophy and neurological tuning that optimizes force output. Muscle action refers to concentric, isometric, and eccentric loading.[62] Overall, selecting movements that combine eccentric and concentric muscle actions produce greater overall strength development than using either of them in isolation[63] and are more specific to general everyday actions such as running and jumping. In general, strength is optimized with 3–5 minute rest periods,[64,65] high loads ranging from one–eight repetitions, four sets for novice and moderately trained (1–2 yrs),[66] and eight for elite athletes,[67] a moderate lifting velocity,[68] and finally 2–3 training sessions per body part per week.[66,67] The rationale is to maximize work done per set within a heavy enough repetition range to stimulate neural firing patterns conducive to maximal force output. For example, 5- versus 1-minute rest periods have been demonstrated to produce an average of 6 repetitions per set compared to 4.5 repetitions per set respectively over 4 sets using 8 repetition maximum loads,[65] while Robinson et al.[64] found a 7% increase in squat performance when resting for 3 minutes compared with a 2% increase when resting for 30 seconds over a 12-week progressive resistance training program.

Power is a factor of both force and velocity. According to Kraemer and Ratamess,[69] two strategies can be incorporated to enhance power. For the force component, an individual can incorporate heavy loads (1–3 repetition maximal loads), while to enhance the velocity component, they can select lighter loads (30–60% of 1 repetition maximum [RM]). For the remaining variables, power is optimized with extended rest periods (5–8 min), an emphasis on explosiveness on repetitions performed with sets ranging from 3–5, and a frequency of three training sessions per week.[70]

B. Hypertrophy

Research suggests that hypertrophy is optimized with 1-minute rest periods,[71] 8–15 repetition maximum loads,[70] and training frequencies of 2–3 training sessions per week.[70] The rationale is to optimize anabolic hormone secretion, blood flow, and metabolites.[69] To illustrate, growth hormone increases 200-fold in 10 sets multiplied by 10 repetitions, as compared with 4.5 fold in 20 sets of 1-repetition maximum training. Moreover, Kramer et al.[71] found significant increases in growth hormone (GH) following 1-minute rest periods, with no significant increases found for 3 minutes of rest. In general, higher-volume protocols that utilize multiple sets (e.g 3 or more) over multiple exercises in both short (9–10 weeks)[72] and longer term (3–6 months)[21,49] training programs result in greater hypertrophy in men and women regardless of age than programs incorporating single sets over multiple exercises.[73] For example, 6 months of training consisting of 12 exercises performed at 1 set per exercise in 62 elderly men and women resulted in a 17% rise in strength with no changes in fat-free mass.[73] However, data from Brown et al.,[74] Fiatarone et al.[49] and Frontera et al.[75] utilizing multiple sets resulted in 48–113% increases in strength and 11–34% increases in whole muscle or single fiber CSA.

C. Endurance

An additional benefit to resistance training is the capacity to increase local muscular endurance. To optimize local muscular endurance research indicates that rest period lengths should be 30 seconds, with repetitions greater than or equal to 20, over multiple sets (e.g., 3–5 sets or greater).[70] Table 15.1 presents a summary of the training recommendations discussed above.

TABLE 15. 1

Recommended Resistance Regimes for Specific Goals

Goal	Load	Sessions per week	Reps, Sets	Movement speed	Rest period (min)
Strength	high	2–3	1–8, 4–8	moderate	3 to 5
Power	low/moderate	2–3	6–10, 3–5	fast	5 to 8
Hypertrophy	moderate	2–3	8–15, ≥3	moderate	≈1
Muscular endurance	low	2–3	≥20, 3–5	moderate	≈0. 5

VIII. ADDITIONAL HEALTH IMPLICATIONS OF STRENGTH TRAINING

A number of additional benefits are provided by strength training including its capacity to optimize body composition, lower cardiovascular risk factors, enhance bone density, and increase the psychological profile.

A. Aging and Body Composition

It has been mentioned previously that muscle mass (fat-free mass) tends to decline with age. Cross-sectional data indicate that muscle mass likely peaks during young adulthood to early middle age in men and women.[76] Longitudinal and cross-sectional data show that declines in fat-free mass (FFM) (per decade) are relatively small prior to the 6th decade in both men and women (0.4–0.7kg/decade in men, 0.1–0.3kg/decade in women).[76,77] After the 6th decade FFM is lost at an accelerated rate.[76,77]

Despite the tendency for a decline in muscle mass with age, fat mass gain is prominent throughout adulthood in industrialized nations.[78] Although it is not completely clear whether gains in fat mass continue throughout very old age, there is plentiful data that fat mass increases during middle age and may peak in elderly between 65 and 75 years of age.[76–79] Data indicate that fat mass increases by 2.1–3.7 kg/decade in men and 1.4–4.1 kg/decade in women prior to approximately 65 years of age.[76,77] Although fat mass may peak during old age, it is clear that increased adiposity during middle age years contributes significantly

One rationale for these changes is that a sufficient gain of fat mass throughout life appears necessary to offset or eliminate loss of FFM.[78] Additional fat mass provides a modicum of defense against loss of muscle mass via the additional muscular workload it provides; it has been previously estimated that approximately 2kg/decade gain of fat mass is necessary to offset age-related muscle loss.[80] This pattern is most likely to occur in industrialized nations where weight gain generally occurs gradually across the lifespan. It is also very common to see a loss of muscle mass with concomitant gain of fat mass across adulthood. This phenomenon can produce a relatively stable body weight over a long time, which can sometimes have the unfortunate effect of masking negative changes in body composition (see Figure 15.3).[79,81]

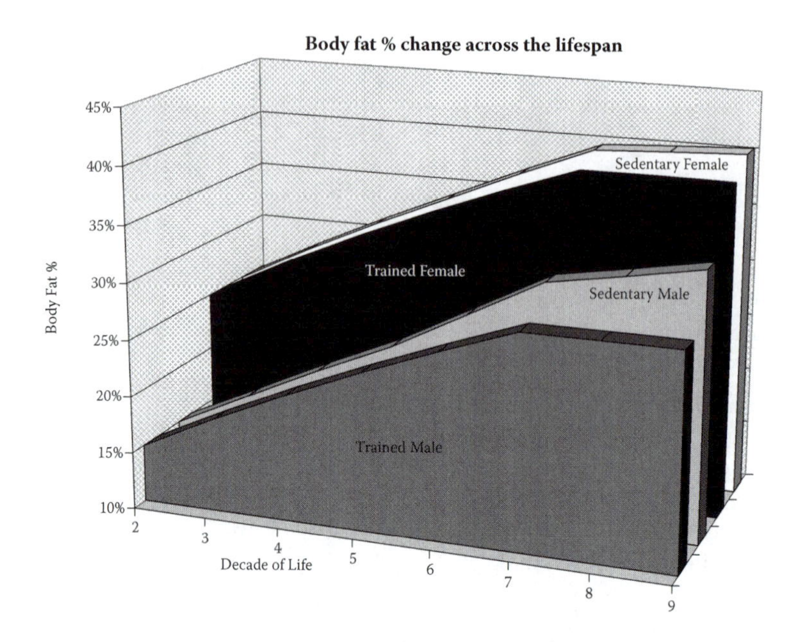

FIGURE 15.3 Example of estimated changes in body fat percentage between sedentary and strength trained men and women based on median data from Guo, S. S. et al. (1999), Kyle U. G. et al. (2001) & Klitgaard, H. (1990). Note: This is a simple illustration based on typical decreases in FFM and increases in FM across the lifespan; this example does not take into account the possible effect that maintenance of FFM may have on the accumulation of FM throughout life.

Strength training may potentially ameliorate the increasing contribution of fat mass to body composition with the aging process. Strength training has the potential to reduce body fat percentage through both an increase in lean mass and a decrease in fat mass, even in aging populations,[83–84] and lowers the necessity of increased fat mass to offset changes in muscle tissue. More detail will be provided later in the chapter regarding lean mass gain during middle and old age. The important idea is that the gain and preservation of lean mass via strength training can be an important tool in maintaining a healthy body composition across the lifespan.

B. Cardiovascular and Metabolic Considerations

During middle age the threat of cardiovascular disease or diabetes becomes very real for adults in industrialized nations. Heart disease, stroke, and diabetes are among the top ten killers in the United States.[85] Heart disease is the third leading cause of death overall; however, by middle age it jumps to number one.[85] Exercise is an important tool for reducing the risk of developing these lifestyle diseases. Much of the focus has been on cardiovascular exercise; however, strength training plays a role as well.

It has already been mentioned that strength training may be beneficial in improving body composition, that it may reduce risk by combating obesity. Strength training may also reduce risk via other mechanisms. Meta-analysis reveals a significant reduction in resting blood pressure (–3.2 mmHg SBP and –3.5 mmHg

DBP) as a consequence of strength training.[86] There is also well documented data demonstrating that strength training improves glucose control and insulin sensitivity in diabetics.[87–89] The mechanisms behind these changes appear to be related to increased muscle tissue mass, as well as increasing insulin signaling action. Data from our lab suggests that resistance training may lower risk of atherosclerosis through positively affecting the lipid profile. Specifically, we found that high-volume resistance training increased high density lipoprotein-cholesterol (HDL-C) by 11% 24 hours post exercise, while depressing plasma triglyceride concentrations.[90] In an additional study we found that individuals who chronically resistance train and did not take steroids had higher HDL-C than controls.[91]

In conclusion, strength training can produce a reduction in risk factors for cardiovascular disease, stroke, and diabetes via both direct and indirect means. Strength training may improve blood pressure, glucose control, and insulin sensitivity directly, while combating obesity and poor blood lipids by favorably affecting body composition.

C. Strength Training and Bone Density

Cross-sectional data has demonstrated that resistance-trained individuals have greater regional bone mineral density (BMD) than either endurance or untrained individuals.[92–96] The data obtained in prospective and experimental design studies generally supports the conclusions drawn from cross-sectional data. Several studies have indicated that regional BMD can be either maintained or increased significantly via strength training intervention.[73,97–103] Improvement in total BMD is rarely demonstrated as a consequence of strength training, however, significant improvement in key weight bearing regions, such as the hip, femur, and lumbar spine have been shown repeatedly.[73,97–103]

Postmenopausal women are at a high risk of osteoporosis and associated fractures due to a lack of estrogen, which exerts a protective effect on bone density. Strength training has been shown to improve regional BMD even in postmenopausal women when combined with calcium supplementation and may still maintain BMD without supplementation.[99,103]

In conclusion, the prevailing data suggests that strength training is beneficial for both the improvement and maintenance of BMD throughout the aging process in both men and women.

D. Miscellaneous Benefits

Strength training has been shown to improve mood and reduce anxiety throughout one's lifespan.[104–107] Strength training may also be useful for reducing pain and dysfunction associated with conditions such as osteoarthritis, rheumatoid arthritis, and chronic neck pain.[108–113]

IX. NUTRITION AND SUPPLEMENTATION FOR OPTIMAL TRAINING

A. Energy Balance

The total energy expenditure (TEE) of a person is the sum of three components of metabolism: resting metabolic rate (RMR), activity-induced energy expenditure (AEE), and diet-induced energy expenditure (DEE). RMR is the sum total of all the energy expended for the maintenance of basic physiological processes necessary for survival, RMR is the largest portion of TEE, composing approximately 65–75%.[114] RMR is largely determined by fat-free mass (FFM), approximately 63% of inter-individual variance in RMR is explained by differences in FFM.[115] DEE is the energy cost involved with the digestion and absorption of nutrients, generally making up about 10% of calories consumed.[116,117] AEE is by far the most variable of the three components of TEE, average AEE is about 25–35% of TEE, it may however be more than double these values in highly trained athletes.[117]

To maintain a steady body weight, one's TEE must be equal to caloric intake (CI) over the long term. The relationship between TEE and CI is known as "energy balance"; any deviation from equality between TEE and CI results in either a positive or negative energy balance. A long-term positive energy balance will result in increased body mass, while long-term negative energy balance will have the opposite effect. Depending on certain modifying factors (i.e., exercise, diet composition, genetics) the mass lost or gained during periods of energy imbalance may be FFM, fat mass or both.

B. Caloric Needs for Middle-Aged Athletes

Several methods are available for accurately measuring caloric needs in adults; however, these methods are generally expensive, time consuming, and inconvenient. Caloric needs can be estimated without expensive laboratory equipment. Several equations exist for this purpose, and, while such methods are not totally accurate, they are generally acceptable for use as a rough guideline regarding appropriate energy intake. One common equation for predicting resting energy expenditure is the Harris-Benedict equation.[118]

For women:

$$\text{REE (kcal/d)} = 655 + 9.5\ (\text{weight in kg}) + 1.9\ (\text{height in cm}) - 4.7\ (\text{age in y})$$

For men:

$$\text{REE (kcal/d)} = 66 + 13.8\ (\text{weight in kg}) + 5.0\ (\text{height in cm}) - 6.8\ (\text{age in y})$$

The REE from the Harris-Benedict equation can be multiplied by an activity factor obtained from a physical activity questionnaire; the result is an estimation of TEE. It appears that this method of calculating TEE has an acceptable accuracy up to an activity factor of approximately 1.7; higher activity factors may produce an overestimation of caloric needs.[119]

Another simple method of determining caloric needs is based on the metabolic equivalent (MET). One MET is equal to an individual's metabolic rate at rest (approximately 1 kcal/kg/hr). The MET value of various physical activities is included in many exercise and nutrition texts, as well as on the World Wide Web. Using this method, TEE can be calculated by multiplying the MET value of normal daily activities (including rest, sleep, and exercise) with the time engaged in these activities. It should be noted that recent research has demonstrated that MET values may overestimate resting metabolism by approximately 20% while underestimating exercise values by a similar amount in an obese population.[120]

The use of equations to determine caloric needs can provide a starting point for attempts at regulating energy balance, however, validation of whether the desired energy balance is actually being achieved can be done only by monitoring changes in body mass and body composition.

An understanding of energy balance (or imbalance) is very useful but does not provide a complete picture of nutritional status in an athlete. Not only is energy balance important, but equally important to the success of the athlete is an understanding of how each macronutrient within the diet affects body composition, exercise, and recovery. A discussion of each of the major macronutrients and how they are involved in performance, specifically in regard to strength training, can be found in the next section.

C. Protein Intake with Aging

The amount of protein ingested in a given day should reflect the general goal of individuals as well as their current exercise regimen. These goals include increased muscle tissue and decreased fat mass, as well as a host of performance variables ranging from extreme endurance to extreme strength outcomes. This section will emphasize protein intake as it concerns general needs with aging, as well as optimizing protein intake beyond need-based criteria and toward a more optimal body composition and performance-based structure.

Current recommended protein requirements for adult men and women across age spans include a 0.75 g * kg-1d recommendation by the World Health Organization (WHO) and a similar 0.8 g * kg-1d by the Food and Nutrition Board of US National Research Council (NRC).[121] However, expert panelists from WHO and NRC [(121)] have indicated that these recommendations are based primarily on young populations, due to a general lack of research in middle-aged and elderly populations. To date, the gold standard procedure for analyzing protein requirements has been the nitrogen balance technique, which suggests that an individual's protein needs are met when the amount of nitrogen consumed is equal to the amount of nitrogen excreted or lost (zero nitrogen balance).[122] The technique is founded on the principle that approximately 16% of any given protein is composed of nitrogen. By knowing the difference between the amount of nitrogen consumed (0.16 daily protein intake) and excreted (e.g. urinary, feces, and insensible nitrogen excretion) a scientist can determine whether a population's protein needs have been met.

While studies in middle-aged individuals are lacking, they have recently increased in elderly populations. Prior to work that will be discussed shortly from Campbell and colleagues,[121] the small number of studies conducted in the elderly were conflicting in that contrasting studies support both higher[123] and lower[124] than recommended daily allowance (RDA) protein intakes. According to Campbell et al., conflicting results were an artifact of differing equations to calculate nitrogen balance, and the measurement of participants under varying metabolic states. Campbell et al. therefore reanalyzed these past studies accounting for varying methodologies and combined the recalculated data with a more current study of 12 adults aged 56 to 80 years of age. Results were much greater than what had been calculated for young individuals (1.14 g * kg-1d). More recently, Campbell and colleagues[125] validated their data using the Accommodation/Adaptation paradigm. Contextually, adaptation can be defined as a steady state change in protein metabolism in response to a change in protein intake that at minimum does not compromise physiological function and may enhance physiological function. In contrast, accommodation takes place via non-steady state metabolic changes in response to a decreased protein intake that occurs to conserve protein but only through compromise or loss in physiological function. To assess these processes nitrogen balance is taken beyond the normal 2 week assessment periods to more longitudinal time frames. In this context, Campbell et al. conducted a 14-week nitrogen balance and body composition study in 10 healthy, ambulatory men and women, aged 55 to 77 years consuming the RDA for protein daily. Results indicated that nitrogen excretion continued to decrease from weeks 2 to 14 (21%), suggesting that the body had not yet reached steady state by the 14th week. These decreases in nitrogen extraction were strongly correlated ($r = 0.83$) with decreased mid-thigh muscle area that had an average –1.7 cm loss, suggesting that the RDA leads to metabolic accommodation characterized by a loss of muscle tissue.[125] Further research from Thalacker-Mercer[126] and colleagues found that sub RDA protein intake was associated with upregulation of transcripts related to the negative control of proliferation, and downregulation of transcripts associated with satellite cell proliferation and myosin light and heavy chain formation.

While these studies were not conducted in middle-aged participants, they do indicate that there is a progressive increase in protein needs with aging that is critical to address, considering data from Rousset et al.,[127] which suggests that protein intake is inversely proportional to age such that 50% of individuals past middle ages consume less than Campbell et al. recommendations,[121] while 25% of men and women consume less than 0.86 and 0.81 g * kg-1d of protein respectively.[127] Considering that, prior to 60, changes in protein balance explain a large variance in changes in muscle tissue, it is possible that progressive inclines in protein needs explain these differences. In fact, as will be discussed shortly, favorable changes in body composition are found with increasing protein intakes.

D. Protein Consumption with General Body Composition

With aging there is a progressive loss in muscle tissue coupled to a steady increase in fat mass such that body fat doubles from the second to fifth decade of life.[128,129] Body fat reportedly continues to increase at a rate of approximately 7.5% per decade until old age.[79] These changes are paralleled by a progressive increase in insulin resistance that favors an increased ratio of fat mass to protein mass. Research by Layman and colleagues[130–132] has strongly suggested that these changes, at in least part, result from the ratio of carbohydrates to protein in the general population's diet. According to Dietary Reference Intakes (DRI) criteria, a nutrient imposes risks to an individual when provided in inadequate or excessive amounts. Between these extremes lies an intake sufficient to prevent deficiencies (RDA), with an upper limit reached prior to experiencing adverse events. Laymen et al.[130–132] suggest that the optimal range for nutrient intake can be found between the RDA and upper limit (UL). For example, the range sufficient to maintain nitrogen balance with the branched chain amino acid leucine has been calculated to range from 1–4 grams daily,[133] while the intake that maximizes its additional anabolic and metabolic effects has been demonstrated to be as high as 12 grams daily.[134] Additional metabolic roles include signaling effects for increased and decreased protein synthesis and degradation respectively,[135,136] and participation in glucose homeostasis, and insulin function.[130–132] When leucine is given at RDA levels, its metabolic effects are minimized, while data from nitrogen balance studies suggest that its structural role is maintained. Current standard recommendations allow for a 3.5 to 1.0 ratio of carbohydrates to protein,[137] which, according to the DRI scale, provides the minimal level of protein consumption (RDA) while maximizing carbohydrates' upper range in excess of metabolic needs.[130] An analysis of the literature demonstrates that this type of ratio impairs glycemic control, causes sustained hyperinsulemia after food absorption, reduces fasting blood glucose levels,[130,132] impairs fat oxidation due to increased inhibition of carnitine transferase,[138,139] stimulates greater hunger, and can lead to increases in blood triglyceride levels.[138,139]

To determine the effects of maximizing the metabolic effects of protein while minimizing carbohydrate to account for general needs, Layman et al.[130,132] investigated the effects 16 weeks of a general exercise program combined with a diet with a ratio of carbohydrates to protein of <1.4 or 3.5 on measures of body composition in middle-aged female adults (45–56 yr). Both diets were designed to induce a caloric deficit of 500 calories daily. In the <.4 ratio condition, participants consumed carbohydrates, fats, and proteins at percentages of 40%, 30%, and 30% respectively, while the 3.5 condition received these nutrients at percentages of 55%, 30%, and 15% respectively. Results demonstrated that fat loss was nearly double in the high protein condition relative to the high carbohydrate condition (19.4 vs. 12.3 pounds), while lean tissue loss was more than double in the high carbohydrate group (–0.9 vs. 2.7).

Further analysis of a 10-week study in middle-aged women demonstrated that a higher protein diet resulted in greater insulin sensitivity as determined by fasting and absorptive plasma insulin and glucose concentrations.[132] The rationale for greater fat loss, increased insulin control, and a higher percentage of LBM maintained in the high protein conditions were a lower efficiency of protein metabolism relative to carbohydrate metabolism, slower digestion rates in the high protein meals resulting in lower insulin levels, and a greater anabolic stimulus for protein synthesis through essential amino acid provision.

In summary, data suggest that aging is associated with a progressive loss of muscle tissue with paralleled increases in adipose tissue deposition. Standard recommendations that maximize dietary carbohydrate consumption (e.g. 3.5 to 1 ratio of carbohydrates to protein) result in impaired fat metabolism, greater losses of LBM, and insulin resistance. In contrast, when dietary carbohydrates are lowered to a threshold that meets general metabolic needs while increasing protein to maximize the anabolic and glucose homeostasis effects of amino acids (e.g. < 1.5 to 1 ratio of carbohydrates to protein) results in increased fat loss, maintenance of LBM, higher satiety, lower post absorptive insulin levels, and decreased plasma triglyceride levels.[130–132] It seems logical therefore that a relatively higher protein intake may help offset typical increased body fat mass and decreased LBM from young to middle-aged individuals.

E. Protein Requirements for Resistance Trained Individuals

Unfortunately, resistance-training protein-requirement studies using the nitrogen balance technique have been constrained to populations under the age of 25.[140–142] Early research was conducted by Tarnopolsky and colleagues,[142] who demonstrated that experienced bodybuilders (> 3 yrs experience) training for three 75-minute weight training sessions were calculated to need 1.2 g * kg-1d of protein. Further research by the same researchers[141] and Lemon et al.[140] in beginner to novice resistance-trained individuals found protein needs ranged from 1.4 to 1.7 g * kg-1d. The rationale for lower protein needs in experienced athletes relative to novice is that resistance training may enhance the efficiency of amino acid utilization for protein synthesis, thus lowering overall protein needs.[143,144]

While nitrogen balance studies generalize from acute measures and assume they apply to chronic measures, a number of studies have investigated the effects of higher protein intakes on body composition in both young and elderly participants. In young individuals, Falvo and colleagues[(145)] found that a high-protein diet (2.00 g·kg-1·day-1) resulted in greater 1-RM squat increases (23.6 ± 13.6 kg vs. 9.09 ± 11.86 kg) than a low-protein group (1.24 g·kg-1·day-1). These results have also generalized to the elderly population. Specifically, Meredith et al.[146] demonstrated that a 560-calorie high-protein supplement increased mid thigh muscle area to a greater extent than a non supplemented group when combined with resistance training in a population of healthy elderly men (61 to 72 yr). The supplemented group consumed 118 ± 10 vs. 72 ± 11 g * kg-1d of protein compared with the non supplemented group. Changes in mid thigh muscle area were correlated with both a change in energy (r = 0.7) and protein (r = 0.63) intake during the 12-week program, suggesting that a high-protein supplement can enhance muscle tissue accretion in healthy elderly participants consuming near the RDA in energy and protein.

In general, extensive critical reviews suggest a range of protein requirements ranging from 1.2 to 2.0 g * kg-1d of protein.[144,147–150] While more studies of nitrogen balance in the middle-aged population need to be conducted, a progressively increasing need for protein suggests that this population would predictably need, at minimum, similar daily protein intakes as calculated for young individuals while engaging in a resistance-training regimen.

F. Protein Quality and Resistance Training

The quality of a protein is generally defined as the capacity of the protein source to deliver essential amino acids (EAAs) to the individual.[151] Generally, meat-based products contain a greater content of EAAs than vegetable-based proteins. The quality of protein intake appears to be an important variable across lifespan. For example, Phillips et al.[152] had young participants consume one of three drinks immediately and 1 hour after exercise. The drinks consisted of 500 ml of milk (18.2 grams of protein),an isonitrogenous and isoenergetic soy protein mixture, or a maltodextrin energy control condition. While soy is considered a complete protein, it contains a lower percentage of EAAs than milk, particularly in the amino acid methionine. After 12 weeks of resistance training, it was found that the milk consumption condition gained significantly greater lean muscle mass than the energy control, while there were no significant differences between the energy control and soy protein conditions.

These effects have been extended in the aging populations. Specifically, Campbell et al.[153] investigated the effects of an omnivorous diet compared with a lactoovovegetarian diet on muscle strength and size in upper middle-aged to elderly males (51–69 yr) participating in a 12-week strength training program. No differences were found in energy or macronutrient content. The omnivorous diet increased LBM by 2.4 kg, and decreased body fat by 1.4%. In contrast, the lactoovovegetarian diet resulted in a slight loss of LBM and an increase in body fat percentage.

A number of mechanisms may explain these results. First, evidence clearly demonstrates that protein balance increases proportionally to extracellular levels of EAAs.[154] Therefore, diets higher in EAA content would be predicted to elicit an overall greater stimulus on protein balance. A second explanation concerns the efficiency of EAA uptake by splanchnic tissue relative to non-essential amino acids (NEAAs). Splanchnic uptake accounts for up to a 90% extraction rate of individual amino acids,[155] effectively reducing their availability with peripheral tissues.[155] Branched chain amino acids (BCAAs) are generally highest in animal-based products.[156] For example, milk protein contains 120% more BCAAs than soy protein. Branched chain amino acids are unique in their ability to escape splanchnic uptake. As an illustration, after consumption of beef, more than half of the amino acids released from splanchnic tissues are BCAAs, even though beef is composed of only 20% BCAAs.[157] A further analysis of the total activity of branched chain aminotransferase and branched-chain alpha-keto acid dehydrogenase, the enzymes responsible for the first two steps in BCAA degradation, indicates that more than 50% of the capacity to degrade BCAAs lies within skeletal muscle tissue, with the liver accounting for only 20% of degradative capacity. These findings suggest that of the 20 amino acids, BCAAs have the greatest opportunity to interact with peripheral tissues, making them perfect candidates to regulate both the structure and function of skeletal muscle tissue.[158,159] Still further, of the nine EAAs, only the BCAA leucine is able to stimulate protein synthesis by itself.[136] Therefore, protein sources with lower EAAs, and particularly BCAA content, will be taken up by splanchnic tissues with greater efficiency than protein with higher content of these EEAs. To illustrate, Martinez et al.[160] found that a legume-based diet caused severe atrophy of the gastrocnemius muscle compared with a casein-based diet in rats. These findings were attributed to lowered muscular protein synthesis in the legume-based condition, with a subsequent higher rate of liver protein synthesis.

In conclusion, evidence suggests that the EAA content of a diet affects protein accretion across the age span. Because meat-based diets are higher in EAA content, middle-aged individuals are suggested to consume a diet rich in lean sources of meat-based products, or to supplement with an essential amino acid supplement.

G. Timing of Protein Intake

A final variable concerns the timing of protein consumption relative to exercise. In a landmark study, Esmarck and colleagues[161] found that a protein supplement was able to enhance mean fiber area and CSA of the *vastus lateralis* and *quadriceps femoris* in a population of elderly adults, while delaying the supplement 2 hours showed no change. These results suggest that protein supplementation is optimized when administered immediately following exercise as opposed to delaying intake. These results have been generalized from young (25 yr) to middle-aged (41 yr) individuals who demonstrate greater protein accretion when administered an amino acid-rich supplement immediately as compared with a delayed (3 h) condition.[162] A possible rationale for these findings is the greater blood flow to skeletal muscle tissue following exercise than at rest.[163] For example, Biolo et al.[163] found greater blood flow (64.5%), protein synthesis (291% vs. 141%), and amino acid transport (30–100%) following exercise relative to at rest.

H. Protein Intake to Combat Progressive Anabolic Resistance with Aging

During the course of a 24-hour period, human beings cycle through a flux of absorptive (following feeding) and postabsorptive (fasting) states. It is during absorptive periods that individuals generally enter into a state of net muscle tissue accretion, while during fasting conditions, the inverse is true. From age 25 to 50, the 10% loss of muscle tissue appears to be driven at least partly by changes in protein turnover such that net protein balance or the difference between skeletal muscle protein synthesis and breakdown would be predicted to favor a slow but continual state of net breakdown in middle-aged men and women.

As suggested, there are two time points when protein balance can differ in middle-aged compared with young individuals. During postabsorbtive periods, data suggests that there are no differences in protein balance in free-living elderly (70 yr) compared with young (28 yr) individuals.[15] However, differences do exist after feeding. Specifically, Katsanos and colleagues[164] demonstrated blunted protein synthesis in the elderly (–40%) relative to the young in response to a smaller bolus of EAAs (6.7 grams). This lowered sensitivity of aging muscle tissue to rising concentrations of EAAs has often been termed anabolic resistance and appears to be related to lower resting concentrations of key factors responsible for enhancing translation initiation, as well as a blunted capacity to activate these factors.[165] More recently, Katsanos et al.[166] investigated the effects of enriching an EAA mixture with leucine on muscle protein metabolism in elderly and young individuals. Briefly, of the 20 amino acids, only the 9 EAAs have been demonstrated to stimulate protein synthesis.[154] Of these, only leucine has been demonstrated to increase protein synthesis when administered alone.[136] To test the effects of enriching leucine on protein balance, Katsanos[166] divided young (mean age, 30) and elderly (mean age, 67) men and women into two equal groups (N = 10 per group) in that subjects either received a mixture of 6.7 grams of EAAs containing 26% leucine (1.7 grams) as is found in whey protein, or 46% leucine (2.7 grams). Results indicated increased protein synthesis to both the 26% and 46% mixture in the young with no differences between the two. In contrast, no increases in protein synthesis were found in the elderly in response to the 26% leucine condition, while the 46% mixture was able to stimulate protein synthesis to the same extent as both young conditions, suggesting that decreased leucine sensitivity at least partly explains anabolic resistance in the elderly. Similar results have been found in aging rats who failed to suppress protein degradation with normal feeding but regained the capacity following leucine enrichment.[167]

Data also suggest that if a serving of amino acids is high enough then no differences exist in young versus elderly participants. This was illustrated by Paddon-Jones et al.,[168] who administered 15 grams of essential amino acids (EAAs) to young (34 ± 4 yr) and elderly (67 ± 2 yr) individuals. Results indicated no differences between age groups in the net anabolic effect of the amino acid bolus. While it is uncertain when anabolic resistance begins to notably surface in middle-aged populations, recent data from Smymons et al.[169] found that middle-aged individuals were able to fully stimulate protein synthesis with 4 ounces of lean beef, which represents 30 grams of protein, 10 grams of EAAs and 1.9 grams of leucine.

In conclusion, data suggest a progressive desensitization of muscle tissue to amino acid feedings with age that may partly explain the 10% loss of LMB from young to middle-aged populations. While the extent of anabolic resistance has not yet been investigated in middle-aged individuals, recent studies suggest that they can fully stimulate protein synthesis with a serving of 4 ounces of lean protein, 30 grams of protein or 10–15 grams of essential amino acids per meal.

I. Carbohydrates

Carbohydrate (CHO) provides a major source of fuel for the human body with the central nervous system relying almost exclusively on it. An estimated 300–500 g of glycogen is stored in skeletal muscle, the liver stores approximately 60–100 g and an additional 15–20 g of CHO can be found in the form of blood glucose.[170] During moderate exercise, skeletal muscle uses a greater proportion of CHO than any other substrate. CHO is available within the blood as glucose and stored within the muscle and liver as glycogen. If CHO were the only substrate available for exercise, the body's CHO stores would provide only enough fuel for a 20-mile run.[170]

Because the store of CHO within the body is so limited, it would be logical to assume that during prolonged exercise the availability of CHO as fuel might be a limiting factor for performance. For this reason, the vast majority of exercise studies have involved endurance exercise as opposed to resistance training. The amount of CHO used during exercise is primarily related to the intensity of the exercise, therefore appreciable CHO depletion occurs only at moderate- and high-intensity exercise.[171,172] The CHO consumed during exercise comes from the utilization of both blood glucose and muscle glycogen; as intensity increases, the proportion of CHO from muscle glycogen also increases.[171,172]

Resistance training is a high-intensity form of exercise, although intermittent in nature, thus CHO utilization during this type of exercise is also expected to be high. Because resistance training is intermittent and the actual volume of calories expended is small in relation to aerobic training, it was thought that CHO availability was not an issue. Resistance exercise does not appear to provide sufficient taxation of CHO stores to produce a drop in blood glucose under normal circumstances.[173,174] However, resistance exercise has been shown to produce rapid reduction of muscle glycogen stores.[173,175] Decreased performance after glycogen depletion in high-intensity intermittent exercise and strength has been reported in several studies, but is not always observed.[176–179]

There is little information about the effect of CHO depletion specifically regarding resistance training. One study demonstrated a significant decrease in the number of squats performed after CHO depletion, interestingly, there was no reduction in the number of isokinetic knee extensions performed under the same conditions.[180] Because of the wide variety of protocols used in the above studies and because fatigue is a multifactorial phenomenon, it is difficult to generalize the effect of glycogen depletion on resistance exercise. There is also very little research regarding the affect of CHO supplementation prior to or during resistance training on subsequent exercise performance. The small amount of data available is equivocal.[181,182] It would appear that while resistance training and similar exercise may rapidly reduce muscle glycogen stores, it probably does not represent an important source of fatigue, and CHO supplementation prior to or during exercise in unnecessary.

The repletion of muscle glycogen after resistance exercise may be of importance in producing a quicker recovery and maintaining higher intensity during subsequent sessions. It has been previously demonstrated that heavy exercise over several days without adequate CHO intake decreases muscle glycogen content.[183] The rate of muscle glycogen repletion can be enhanced if CHO is consumed after aerobic exercise, especially when consumed immediately post-exercise.[184–186] At least one study has demonstrated that the rate of glycogen repletion is also increased when CHO is ingested immediately after resistance training.[187]

CHO supplementation after resistance exercise may have additional benefits beyond glycogen repletion. CHO supplementation after a bout of resistance exercise increases muscle protein synthesis while concurrently reducing muscle protein catabolism versus placebo, thus producing an improved environment for muscle growth.[188] CHO or CHO + protein supplementation produces an increase in insulin levels post-exercise; it may also produce a decrease in cortisol and a transient increase in growth hormone levels.[189] Increases in insulin and growth hormone promote anabolism, while a decrease in cortisol will limit catabolism.

The RDI of CHO for athletes is similar to the recommendations for the general public, approximately 55–60% of daily caloric intake or 6–10 g/kg of bodyweight.[190] This intake of CHO should be able to maintain glycogen stores for individuals performing resistance training, provided that the overall caloric intake is sufficient.

In conclusion, it is unlikely that individuals performing resistance training require additional carbohydrate supplementation beyond the recommended daily intake;

however, the timing of CHO intake may have significance. Consumption of ≥1g of CHO per kilogram of body weight during recovery may help to optimize glycogen storage and protein synthesis.

J. Lipids

Lipids are essential for a variety of physiological processes, as cellular components and as a source of fuel. The ACSM advocates that athletes follow the same general guidelines for fat consumption that are provided for the general population—approximately 20–25% of daily calorie consumption should be in the form of fats.[190]

There is little if any evidence that lipid supplementation is of any value to resistance exercise or adaptations to resistance exercise. Lipids provide little energy for muscular work during intense exercise such as resistance exercise; it has been demonstrated that the respiratory exchange ratio (RER) is significantly elevated above resting levels throughout a bout of resistance exercise.[191,192] An elevated RER is indicative of greater reliance on CHO for fuel; it has been estimated that CHO and high energy phospate stores provide nearly 100% of energy used during the work portion of strength exercise.[193] Lipids do provide a significant energy source for recovery from resistance exercise, lipid oxidation may be elevated above resting levels for up to 24 hours post-exercise.[194–197] It has also been demonstrated that a resistance exercise session can increase fat metabolism during a subsequent endurance exercise session, provided the rest between is of short duration.[198] An increase in fat metabolism post-exercise and during subsequent exercise has no real value for training purposes, but may have relevance regarding issues of weight management and body composition.

In conclusion, individuals should follow the recommended dietary guidelines concerning fat consumption. There is no evidence that fat supplementation improves performance or significantly contributes as fuel for resistance exercise; however, fat oxidation may be significantly increased during recovery. Finally, while increased fat[15] consumption is unlikely to improve strength performance and may contribute to gain of fat mass; fat consumption below recommended levels can have undesirable effects on both health and performance.

X. ERGOGENIC AIDS FOR STRENGTH TRAINING

A. Creatine Supplementation

Creatine has become one of the most well studied athletic supplements in history, hundreds of studies have been conducted on its ergogenic effects.

Creatine is a compound formed within the human body from arginine, glycine, and methionine; creatine is synthesized primarily within the liver and can also be obtained from the diet in meat sources.[199] Creatine is stored predominantly within muscle tissue and is a major contributor to anaerobic energy production as the compound phosphocreatine (Pcr) via the following pathway: PCr + ADP + H <---creatine kinase---> Creatine + ATP.[200] Theoretically, a higher muscular concentration of creatine will provide a greater capacity for anaerobic energy production and may have other effects on cellular metabolic processes.

It would appear that the theoretical role of increased muscle creatine actually does translate to improved anaerobic performance in humans. Meta-analysis of studies show that creatine supplementation alone produces improvement in anaerobic exercise performance and that effect size is greater in exercise sessions lasting less than 30s (ES 0.24 ± 0.02) than in those lasting between 30–150s (ES 0.19 ± 0.05); no significant effect size was found for exercise lasting greater than 150s.[201] The same analysis revealed that creatine supplementation produced a greater improvement in repeated bout exercise than in single bout exercise.[201] Another meta-analysis that investigated the effect of creatine supplementation combined with resistance training on strength gains demonstrated an even larger effect size (ES 0.36).[199] There is also evidence that creatine supplementation produces modest increases in lean body mass versus placebo, both alone or in conjunction with resistance training.[199,201]

Currently, it is theorized that creatine supplementation provides improvements in performance and strength primarily through two mechanisms: an acute effect of creatine loading on anaerobic/force capabilities and a permissive effect of creatine by allowing an increase in training volume.[202] There is evidence to support these theories. Arciero et al.[203] compared strength gains in groups using creatine supplementation. One group performed 4 weeks' resistance training and the other performed none. The results demonstrated that maximal bench press and leg press increased 8% and 16%, respectively, in the group using creatine without training and 18% and 42%, respectively, in the group using creatine and resistance training.[203] This information indicates that nearly half of the strength improvements in the training group could be attributed to the acute effects of creatine supplementation. Syrotuik et al. demonstrated that when training volume was matched between a placebo and creatine supplementation group the advantage normally provided by creatine supplementation was abolished at the end of the training period.[204]

The increases in training intensity and volume that may accompany creatine supplementation can also help explain the increases in lean body mass; however, there is also evidence that creatine supplementation alone produces increases in body water, myosin heavy chain expression, and other pro-myogenic factors.[203,205,206]

Creatine supplementation has been shown to improve both the decreased muscle mass and decreased strength associated with aging, whether alone or in combination with resistance training. Some data indicate that the muscle concentration of creatine and phosphocreatine resynthesis rate may be reduced with age; these values may have a more profound improvement after supplementation in middle-aged versus young men.[207]

In conclusion, creatine supplementation may aid the development of strength and lean body mass in conjunction with resistance training. In addition, it appears that aged athletes may receive a larger relative increase in muscle creatine levels with supplementation. This information taken together suggests that creatine supplementation may be a valuable ergogenic aid for middle-aged athletes attempting to improve or maintain muscle mass and strength.

B. BETA-HYDROXY-BETA-METHYLBUTYRATE SUPPLEMENTATION

Oral administration of the leucine metabolite Beta-Hydroxy-Beta-Methyl-Butyrate (HMB) has been strongly associated with increased strength, LBM and decreased fat mass in young (20 yr) to middle-aged (40 yr) individuals when combined with exercising conditions.[208–211] HMB has also been demonstrated to have clinical benefit in a number of muscle wasting/cachectic conditions including cancer[212] and limb immobilization.[213] The mechanisms of action of HMB appear directly relevant to aging populations. For example, HMB has been demonstrated in numerous studies to lower muscular protein degradation as measured by 3-methylhistadine techniques (3-MH),[210] as well as expression and activity of the ubiquitin-proteolytic pathway in cachectic models.[212] Moreover HMB administration prior to exercise has lowered serum levels of creatine kinase,[210,214] lactate dehydrogenase,[215] urine urea nitrogen and plasma urea,[209] as well as decreased levels of visual analog scale-determined muscular soreness.[214] These indirect measures of lowered muscle tissue damage suggest that HMB has a substantial capacity to strengthen the integrity of the sarcolema, that may enhance the regenerative capacity of aging muscle tissue.

While current research in elderly populations consuming HMB is not extensive, it generally provides support for HMB as an agent to hinder skeletal muscle wasting, while enhancing recovery during periods of stress. Following an 8-week resistance-training program Vukovich et al.[216] found a greater decrease in body fat percentage (–.66 vs. –.03%), as well as larger gains in lower (13 vs. 7%) and upper (13 vs. 11%) body strength in untrained elderly men consuming HMB compared with a placebo. Flakoll and colleagues[217] found that arginine, lysine, and HMB compared with a placebo during 12 weeks independent of training resulted in greater increases in limb circumference, leg and handgrip strength, and 24-hour measured rates of protein synthesis in 50 elderly women (76.6 yr). Panton et al.[218] examined the effects of 3 grams of HMB supplementation on strength and functionality in elderly males and females (70 yr). While measures of strength were not increased, these researchers did find an increase in "get up and go" performance.

Currently, studies have found HMB in both humans consuming 3–6 grams daily[63,92–94] and animals consuming variable dosages[11,30,95–98] to be extremely safe. For example, no adverse effects have been seen in animals consuming HMB up to 5000 mg•kg-1•day-1 for a period of 1 to 16 weeks.[219] For a 200-pound man, that would be approximately 450 g of HMB per day. HMB may also decrease cardiovascular risk factors including lowered total cholesterol (5.8%), decreased systolic blood pressure (4.4 mm Hg), and lowered LDL-C (7.3%).[220]

The current recommended dosage for HMB is 3 grams a day. This is based on the finding that in young individuals, increasing HMB from 1.5 to 3 grams increases strength and LBM, while doses over 3 grams per day does not have an effect. Unfortunately, the optimal dosage for middle-aged and elderly individuals is not currently known. However, with a greater potentiality for muscle damage with aging it may be that greater dosages are needed to obtain an optimal response.

C. Changes in Androgen Levels with Age and Possible Exercise and Supplementation Interventions

Testosterone has received a great deal of attention as a partial mechanism explaining changes in muscle tissue with age. For example, free testosterone in middle-aged to elderly individuals is negatively associated with BMI and fat mass,[221,222] while it is positively correlated to muscle strength in men from 20 to 90 years of age.[223,224] Ultimately, the severity of losses in muscle tissue and function with age are correlated to declines in testosterone levels.[225] Inoue et al.[226] found that training-induced muscle hypertrophy was inhibited by pharmacologic blockade of testosterone-specific cellular receptor. Testosterone's collective mechanisms of action appear to be related to direct stimulation of protein synthesis,[227] an increase in local muscular and circulating IGF-1 release,[228] and by its capacity to antagonize the catabolic hormone cortisol.[229]

As with other steroids, testosterone is modified from cholesterol, and is found in the interstitial cells of Leydig in the testes in males, and primarily in the adrenal glands in females. In general, testosterone peaks at age 25 to 30 yrs with a range of 300 ng/dl to 1200 ng/dl.[230] Data suggest that testosterone starts to decline at middle age at a rate of 0.8 and 2% of total and free testosterone per annum respectively.[231] The mechanisms of testosterone decrease appear to be related to decreased testicular volume,[232] an increase in sex hormone binding globulin that would lower free testosterone,[233] and a decrease in *zona reticularis* cells in the adrenal glands.[234] Data clearly suggest that these changes are not simply an artifact of age, but also of environment.[235] Epidemiological evidence suggests that testosterone levels may decrease with increasing insulin resistance, polypharmacy, smoking, drinking, and chronic illness.[235] For example, individuals who ceased smoking had a 9% lower decline in testosterone than those who continued to smoke in middle to elderly years, while general indicators of good health (lack of obesity, low frequency of drinking) added 10–15% in testosterone levels in elderly individuals.[235]

D. Effects of Resistance Training on Testosterine Levels in Middle-Aged Individuals

A number of studies have been conducted on the acute and chronic effects of resistance training on testosterone levels in middle-aged individuals. In general, testosterone increases are similar between young and middle-aged individuals subsequent to power and hypertrophy style resistance training.[236] Intriguingly, after 6 months of training, middle-aged and even elderly men, but not women, are able to increase their capacity to increase testosterone acutely following resistance training.[233] While resting levels of testosterone may increase in young individuals following chronic training,[237] this has not yet been demonstrated in middle-aged or elderly participants.[233] However, 16 weeks of training did result in lower resting cortisol levels, thus increasing the ratio of testosterone to cortisol, resulting in a greater anabolic milieu for net protein synthesis.[238] In general, acute increases in testosterone are highest during multiple set, moderate intensity (8–12 repetitions) training regimens.[239,240]

E. Dehydroepiandrosterone Supplementation

Dehydroepiandrosterone (DHEA) secreted from the adrenal glands can be converted to androstenedione that is converted to testosterone. DHEA represents the largest depot of circulating androgens in the body and, like testosterone, peaks in the 20s, and declines by 80% by age 75.[241] A number of studies have investigated the efficacy of DHEA supplementation in aging populations. Morales et al.[242,243] has analyzed the effects of DHEA in upper middle-aged (50 yr) to elderly men and found that 6 months of 100 mg of DHEA supplementation independent of training resulted in greater perceived physical and psychological well being, increased plasma IGF-I levels, a decline in fat mass, and increased knee and back extension muscle strength. Studies administering 50 mg of DHEA without training have not agreed with these results, suggesting that a minimum of 100 mg are needed. In contrast, recent data demonstrated that 50 mg of DHEA combined with resistance training resulted in greater muscle mass and strength gains relative to control.[241] The proposed mechanisms of DHEA action consist of its capacity to be converted to testosterone, and to block the actions of cortisol.[243, 242]

XI. CONCLUSIONS

In summary, while aging is associated with declines in muscle tissue size and strength, a number of ergogenic aids may possibly attenuate these changes. This section discussed findings strongly suggesting that creatine, HMB, and DHEA supplementation can enhance the development of strength and lean body mass in middle-aged and elderly populations.

REFERENCES

1. Kuczmarski, R. J., Ogden, C. I., Gummer-Strawn, L. M., Flegal, K. M., Guo, S. S., Wei, R., et al., CDC growth charts: United States. Advance data from vital and health statistics, *National Center for Health Statistics,* 314, 2000.
2. US Census Bureau, Current Population Survey 2005, http://www.census.gov/Press–Release/www/releases/archives/education/007660.html. Accessed February 26, 2008.
3. Social Security Administration, Normal Retirement Age 2005. http://www.ssa.gov/OACT/ProgData/nra.html. Accessed February 26, 2008.
4. Rhea, M. R., Alvar, B. A., and Gray, R., Physical fitness and job performance of firefighters, *J. Strength Cond. Res.* 18, 348–52, 2004.
5. Wandel, M. and Roos, G., Age perceptions and physical activity among middle-aged men in three occupational groups, *Soc. Sci. Med.* 62, 3024–34, 2006.
6. Wisloff, U., Castagna, C., Helgerud, J., Jones, R., and Hoff, J., Strong correlation of maximal squat strength with sprint performance and vertical jump height in elite soccer players, *Br. J. Sports Med.* 38, 285–8, 2004.
7. Newman, M. A., Tarpenning, K. M., and Marino, F. E., Relationships between isokinetic knee strength, single-sprint performance, and repeated-sprint ability in football players, *J. Strength Cond. Res.* 18, 867–72, 2004.
8. Wilk, K. E., Andrews, J. R., Arrigo, C. A., Keirns, M. A., and Erber, D. J., The strength characteristics of internal and external rotator muscles in professional baseball pitchers, *Am. J. Sports Med.* 21, 61–6, 1993.

9. Giles, L. V., Rhodes, E. C., and Taunton, J. E., The physiology of rock climbing, *Sports Med.* 36, 529–45, 2006.
10. Tan, B., Aziz, A. R., Spurway, N. C., Toh, C., Mackie, H., Xie, W., et al., Indicators of maximal hiking performance in Laser sailors, *Eur. J. Appl. Physiol.* 98, 169–76, 2006.
11. Avlund, K., Schroll, M., Davidsen, M., Lovborg, B., and Rantanen, T., Maximal isometric muscle strength and functional ability in daily activities among 75-year-old men and women, *Scand. J. Med. Sci. Sports* 4, 32–40, 1994.
12. Janssen, I., Heymsfield, S. B., and Ross, R., Low relative skeletal muscle mass (sarcopenia) in older persons is associated with functional impairment and physical disability, *J. Am. Geriatr. Soc.* 50, 889–96, 2002.
13. Dela, F. and Kjaer, M., Resistance training, insulin sensitivity and muscle function in the elderly, *Essays Biochem.* 42, 75–88, 2006.
14. Langlois, J. A., Visser, M., Davidovic, L. S., Maggi, S., Li, G., and Harris, T. B., Hip fracture risk in older white men is associated with change in body weight from age 50 years to old age, *Arch. Intern. Med.* 158, 990–6, 1998.
15. Volpi, E., Sheffield-Moore, M., Rasmussen, B. B., and Wolfe, R. R., Basal muscle amino acid kinetics and protein synthesis in healthy young and older men, *JAMA.* 286, 1206–12, 2001.
16. Lexell, J., Taylor, C. C., and Sjostrom, M., What is the cause of the ageing atrophy? Total number, size and proportion of different fiber types studied in whole vastus lateralis muscle from 15- to 83-year-old men, *J. Neurol. Sci.* 84, 275–94, 1988.
17. McComas, A. J., Invited review: Motor unit estimation: Methods, results, and present status, *Muscle Nerve.* 14, 585–97, 1991.
18. Coggan, A. R., Spina, R. J., King, D. S., Rogers, M. A., Brown, M., Nemeth, P. M., and Holloszy, J. O., Histochemical and enzymatic comparison of the gastrocnemius muscle of young and elderly men and women, *J. Gerontol.* 47, B71–6, 1992.
19. Balagopal, P., Schimke, J. C., Ades, P., Adey, D., and Nair, K. S., Age effect on transcript levels and synthesis rate of muscle MHC and response to resistance exercise, *Am. J. Physiol. Endocrinol. Metab.* 280, E203–8, 2001.
20. Petrella, J. K., Kim, J. S., Tuggle, S. C., Hall, S. R., and Bamman, M. M., Age differences in knee extension power, contractile velocity, and fatigability, *J. Appl. Physiol.* 98, 211–20, 2005.
21. Frontera, W. R., Hughes, V. A., Lutz, K. J., and Evans, W. J., A cross-sectional study of muscle strength and mass in 45- to 78-yr-old men and women, *J. Appl. Physiol.* 71, 644–50, 1991.
22. Jette, A. M. and Branch, L. G., The Framingham Disability Study: II. Physical disability among the aging, *Am. J. Public Health* 71, 1211–6, 1981.
23. Larsson, L., Grimby, G., and Karlsson, J., Muscle strength and speed of movement in relation to age and muscle morphology, *J. Appl. Physiol.* 46, 451–6, 1979.
24. Vandervoort, A. A. and McComas, A. J., Contractile changes in opposing muscles of the human ankle joint with aging, *J. Appl. Physiol.* 61, 361–7, 1986.
25. Lindle, R. S., Metter, E. J., Lynch, N. A., Fleg, J. L., Fozard, J. L., Tobin, J., et al., Age and gender comparisons of muscle strength in 654 women and men aged 20–93 yr, *J. Appl. Physiol.* 83, 1581–7, 1997.
26. Kallman, D. A., Plato, C. C., and Tobin, J. D., The role of muscle loss in the age-related decline of grip strength: Cross-sectional and longitudinal perspectives, *J. Gerontol.* 45, M82–8, 1990.
27. Aniansson, A., Grimby, G., and Hedberg, M., Compensatory muscle fiber hypertrophy in elderly men, *J. Appl. Physiol.* 73, 812–6, 1992.

28. Aniansson, A., Hedberg, M., Henning, G. B., and Grimby, G., Muscle morphology, enzymatic activity, and muscle strength in elderly men: A follow–up study, *Muscle Nerve* 9, 585–91, 1986.
29. Aniansson, A., Sperling, L., Rundgren, A., and Lehnberg, E., Muscle function in 75-year-old men and women. A longitudinal study, *Scand. J. Rehabil. Med. Suppl.* 9, 92–102, 1983.
30. Frontera, W. R., Suh, D., Krivickas, L. S., Hughes, V. A., Goldstein, R., and Roubenoff, R., Skeletal muscle fiber quality in older men and women, *Am. J. Physiol. Cell Physiol.* 279, C611–8, 2000.
31. Rantanen, T., Masaki, K., Foley, D., Izmirlian, G., White, L., and Guralnik, J. M., Grip strength changes over 27 yr. in Japanese-American men, *J. Appl. Physiol.* 85, 2047–53, 1998.
32. Winegard, K. J., Hicks, A. L., Sale, D. G., and Vandervoort, A. A., A 12-year follow-up study of ankle muscle function in older adults, *J. Gerontol. Series A Biol. Sci. Med. Sci.* 51, B202–7, 1996.
33. Narici, M. V., Bordini, M., and Cerretelli, P., Effect of aging on human adductor pollicis muscle function, *J. Appl. Physiol.* 71, 1277–81, 1991.
34. Stalberg, E., and Fawcett, P. R., Macro EMG in healthy subjects of different ages, *J. Neurol. Neurosurg. Psychiatry* 45, 870–8, 1982.
35. Macaluso, A. and De Vito, G., Muscle strength, power and adaptations to resistance training in older people, *Eur. J. Appl. Physiol.* 91, 450–72, 2004.
36. Hopkins, W. G., Hawley, J. A., and Burke, L. M., Design and analysis of research on sport performance enhancement, *Med. Sci. Sports Exerc.* 31, 472–85, 1999.
37. Kostka, T., Quadriceps maximal power and optimal shortening velocity in 335 men aged 23–88 years, *Eur. J. Appl. Physiol.* 95, 140–5, 2005.
38. Skelton, D. A., Greig, C. A., Davies, J. M., and Young, A., Strength, power and related functional ability of healthy people aged 65–89 years, *Age Ageing* 23, 371–7, 1994.
39. Ferretti, G., Narici, M. V., Binzoni, T., Gariod, L., Le Bas, J. F., Reutenauer, H., and Cerretelli, P., Determinants of peak muscle power: Effects of age and physical conditioning, *Eur. J. Appl. Physiol. Occup. Physiol.* 68, 111–5, 1994.
40. Vaillancourt, D. E., Larsson, L., and Newell, K. M., Effects of aging on force variability, single motor unit discharge patterns, and the structure of 10, 20, and 40 Hz EMG activity, *Neurobiol. Aging* 24, 25–35, 2003.
41. Delbono, O., Calcium current activation and charge movement in denervated mammalian skeletal muscle fibres, *J. Physiol.* 451, 187–203, 1992.
42. Delbono, O., O'Rourke, K. S., and Ettinger, W. H., Excitation-calcium release uncoupling in aged single human skeletal muscle fibers, *J. Membr. Biol.* 148, 211–22, 1995.
43. Payne, A. M. and Delbono, O., Neurogenesis of excitation-contraction uncoupling in aging skeletal muscle, *Exerc. Sport Sci. Rev.* 32, 36–40, 2004.
44. Welle, S., Totterman, S., and Thornton, C., Effect of age on muscle hypertrophy induced by resistance training, *J. Gerontol. Series A Biol. Sci. Med. Sci.* 51, M270–5, 1996.
45. Jones, D. A. and Rutherford, O. M., Human muscle strength training: The effects of three different regimens and the nature of the resultant changes, *J. Physiol.* 391, 1–11, 1987.
46. Young, A., Stokes, M., Round, J. M., and Edwards, R. H., The effect of high-resistance training on the strength and cross-sectional area of the human quadriceps, *Eur. J. Clin. Invest.* 13, 411–7, 1983.

47. Reeves, N. D., Narici, M. V., and Maganaris, C. N., In vivo human muscle structure and function: Adaptations to resistance training in old age, *Exp. Physiol.* 89, 675–89, 2004.
48. Harridge, S. D., Kryger, A., and Stensgaard, A., Knee extensor strength, activation, and size in very elderly people following strength training, *Muscle Nerve* 22, 831–9, 1999.
49. Fiatarone, M. A., Marks, E. C., Ryan, N. D., Meredith, C. N., Lipsitz, L. A., and Evans, W. J., High-intensity strength training in nonagenarians: Effects on skeletal muscle, *JAMA*. 263, 3029–34, 1990.
50. Pyka, G., Lindenberger, E., Charette, S., and Marcus, R., Muscle strength and fiber adaptations to a year-long resistance training program in elderly men and women, *J. Gerontol.* 49, M22–7, 1994.
51. Singh, M. A., Ding, W., Manfredi, T. J., Solares, G. S., O'Neill, E. F., Clements, K. M., et al., Insulin-like growth factor I in skeletal muscle after weight-lifting exercise in frail elders, *Am. J. Physiol.* 277, E135–43, 1999.
52. Alway, S. E., Coggan, A. R., Sproul, M. S., Abduljalil, A. M., and Robitaille, P. M., Muscle torque in young and older untrained and endurance-trained men, *J. Gerontol. Series A Biol. Sci. Med. Sci.* 51, B195–201, 1996.
53. Klitgaard, H., Mantoni, M., Schiaffino, S., Ausoni, S., Gorza, L., Laurent-Winter, C., et al., Function, morphology and protein expression of ageing skeletal muscle: A cross-sectional study of elderly men with different training backgrounds, *Acta Physiol. Scand.* 140, 41–54, 1990.
54. Korhonen, M. T., Cristea, A., Alen, M., Hakkinen, K., Sipila, S., Mero, A., et al., Aging, muscle fiber type, and contractile function in sprint-trained athletes, *J. Appl. Physiol.* 101, 906–17, 2006.
55. Campbell, B. , Kerksick, C., Wilborn, C., Rasmussen, C., Greenwood, M., and Kreider, R., Body composition changes following an eight-week split-body periodized resistance training program in college-aged and middle-aged males, *J. Strength Conditioning Res.* 20, E–30, 2006.
56. Hakkinen, K., Newton, R U., Gordon, S E., McCormick, M., Volek, J S., Nindl, B C., et al., Changes in muscle morphology, electromyographic activity, and force production characteristics during progressive strength training in young and older men, *J. Gerontol. Series A Biol. Sci. Med. Sci.* 53, B415–23, 1998.
57. Jozsi, A. C., Campbell, W. W., Joseph, L., Davey, S. L., and Evans, W. J., Changes in power with resistance training in older and younger men and women, *J. Gerontol. Series A Biol. Sci. Med. Sci.* 54, M591–6, 1999.
58. Sipila, S., Viitasalo, J., Era, P., and Suominen, H., Muscle strength in male athletes aged 70–81 years and a population sample, *Eur. J. Appl. Physiol. Occup. Physiol.* 63, 399–403, 1991.
59. Fiatarone, M. A., O'Neill, E. F., Ryan, N. D., Clements, K. M., Solares, G. R., et al., Exercise training and nutritional supplementation for physical frailty in very elderly people, *N. Engl. J. Med.* 330, 1769–75, 1994.
60. Miszko, T. A., Cress, M. E., Slade, J. M., Covey, C. J., Agrawal, S. K., and Doerr, C. E., Effect of strength and power training on physical function in community-dwelling older adults, *J. Gerontol. Series A Biol. Sci. Med. Sci.* 58, 171–5, 2003.
61. Skelton, D. A., Kennedy, J., and Rutherford, O. M., Explosive power and asymmetry in leg muscle function in frequent fallers and non-fallers aged over 65, *Age Ageing* 31, 119–25, 2002.
62. Kraemer, W. J., Adams, K., Cafarelli, E., Dudley, G. A., Dooly, C., Feigenbaum, M. S., et al., American College of Sports Medicine position stand. Progression models in resistance training for healthy adults, *Med. Sci. Sports Exerc.* 34, 364–80, 2002.

63. Colliander, E. B. and Tesch, P. A., Effects of eccentric and concentric muscle actions in resistance training, *Acta Physiol. Scand.* 140, 31–9, 1990.
64. Robinson, J. M., Stone, M. H., Johnson, R. L., Penland, C. M., Warren, B. J., and Lewis, David, Effects of different weight training exercise/rest intervals on strength, power, and high intensity exercise endurance, *J. Strength Cond. Res.* 9, 216–221, 1995.
65. Rahimi, R., Effects of different rest intervals on the exercise volume completed during squat bouts, *J. Sport Sci. Med.* 4, 361–366, 2005.
66. Rhea, M. R., Alvar, B. A., Burkett, L. N., and Ball, S. D., A meta-analysis to determine the dose response for strength development, *Med. Sci. Sports Exerc.* 35, 456–64, 2003.
67. Peterson, M. D., Rhea, M. R., and Alvar, B. A., Maximizing strength development in athletes: A meta-analysis to determine the dose–response relationship, *J. Strength Cond. Res.* 18, 377–82, 2004.
68. Kanehisa, H. and Miyashita, M., Specificity of velocity in strength training, *Eur. J. Appl. Physiol. Occup. Physiol.* 52, 104–6, 1983.
69. Kraemer, W. J. and Ratamess, N. A., Fundamentals of resistance training: Progression and exercise prescription, *Med. Sci. Sports Exerc.* 36, 674–88, 2004.
70. Bird, S. P., Tarpenning, K. M., and Marino, F. E., Designing resistance training programmes to enhance muscular fitness: A review of the acute programme variables, *Sports Med.* 35, 841–51, 2005.
71. Kraemer, W. J., Marchitelli, L., Gordon, S. E., Harman, E., Dziados, J. E., Mello, R., et al., Hormonal and growth factor responses to heavy resistance exercise protocols, *J. Appl. Physiol.* 69, 1442–50, 1990.
72. Tracy, B. L., Ivey, F. M., Hurlbut, D., Martel, G. F., Lemmer, J. T., Siegel, E. L., et al., Muscle quality. II. Effects of strength training in 65- to 75-yr-old men and women, *J. Appl. Physiol.* 86, 195–201, 1999.
73. Vincent, K. R. and Braith, R. W., Resistance exercise and bone turnover in elderly men and women, *Med. Sci. Sports Exerc.* 34, 17–23, 2002.
74. Brown, A. B., McCartney, N., and Sale, D. G., Positive adaptations to weight-lifting training in the elderly, *J. Appl. Physiol.* 69, 1725–33, 1990.
75. Frontera, W. R., Meredith, C. N., O'Reilly, K. P., Knuttgen, H. G., and Evans, W. J., Strength conditioning in older men: Skeletal muscle hypertrophy and improved function, *J. Appl. Physiol.* 64, 1038–44, 1988.
76. Kyle, U. G., Genton, L., Hans, D., Karsegard, L., Slosman, D. O., and Pichard, C., Age-related differences in fat-free mass, skeletal muscle, body cell mass and fat mass between 18 and 94 years, *Eur. J. Clin. Nutr.* 55, 663–72, 2001.
77. Guo, S. S., Zeller, C., Chumlea, W. C., and Siervogel, R. M., Aging, body composition, and lifestyle: The Fels Longitudinal Study, *Am. J. Clin. Nutr.* 70, 405–11, 1999.
78. Schutz, Y., Kyle, U. U., and Pichard, C., Fat-free mass index and fat mass index percentiles in Caucasians aged 18–98 y, *Int. J. Obes. Relat. Metab. Disord.* 26, 953–60, 2002.
79. Hughes, V. A., Frontera, W. R., Roubenoff, R., Evans, W. J., and Singh, M. A., Longitudinal changes in body composition in older men and women: Role of body weight change and physical activity, *Am. J. Clin. Nutr.* 76, 473–81, 2002.
80. Forbes, G. B., Exercise and lean weight: The influence of body weight, *Nutr. Rev.* 50, 157–61, 1992.
81. Forbes, G. B., Longitudinal changes in adult body composition: Influence of body weight, *Appl. Radiat. Isot.* 49, 571–3, 1998.
82. Joseph, L. J., Davey, S. L., Evans, W. J., and Campbell, W. W., Differential effect of resistance training on the body composition and lipoprotein-lipid profile in older men and women, *Metabolism* 48, 1474–80, 1999.

83. Campbell, W. W., Crim, M. C., Young, V. R., and Evans, W. J., Increased energy requirements and changes in body composition with resistance training in older adults, *Am. J. Clin. Nutr.* 60, 167–75, 1994.
84. Binder, E. F., Yarasheski, K. E., Steger-May, K., Sinacore, D. R., Brown, M., Schechtman, K. B., and Holloszy, J. O., Effects of progressive resistance training on body composition in frail older adults: Results of a randomized, controlled trial, *J. Gerontol. Series A Biol. Sci. Med. Sci.* 60, 1425–31, 2005.
85. Adams, G. R., Hather, B. M., and Dudley, G. A., Effect of short-term unweighting on human skeletal muscle strength and size, *Aviation Space Environ. Med.* 65, 1116–21, 1994.
86. Cornelissen, V. A. and Fagard, R. H., Effect of resistance training on resting blood pressure: A meta-analysis of randomized controlled trials, *J. Hypertens.* 23, 251–9, 2005.
87. Fenicchia, L. M., Kanaley, J. A., Azevedo, J. L., Jr., Miller, C. S., Weinstock, R. S., Carhart, R. L., and Ploutz-Snyder, L. L., Influence of resistance exercise training on glucose control in women with type 2 diabetes, *Metabolism* 53, 284–9, 2004.
88. Snowling, N. J. and Hopkins, W. G., Effects of different modes of exercise training on glucose control and risk factors for complications in type 2 diabetic patients: A meta-analysis, *Diabetes Care* 29, 2518–27, 2006.
89. Ibañez, J., Izquierdo, M., Argüelles, I., Forga, L., Larrión, J. L., García-Unciti, M., et al., Twice-weekly progressive resistance training decreases abdominal fat and improves insulin sensitivity in older men with type 2 diabetes, *Diabetes Care* 28, 662–7, 2005.
90. Wallace, M. B., Moffatt, R. J., Haymes, E. M., and Green, N. R., Acute effects of resistance exercise on parameters of lipoprotein metabolism, *Med. Sci. Sports Exerc.* 23, 199–204, 1991.
91. Moffatt, R. J. , Wallace, B. M., and Sady, S. P., Effects of anabolic steroids on lipoprotein profiles of female weight lifters, *Physician Sports Med.* 18, 106–115, 1989.
92. Heinonen, A., Oja, P., Kannus, P., Sievanen, H., Manttari, A., and Vuori, I., Bone mineral density of female athletes in different sports, *Bone Miner.* 23, 1–14, 1993.
93. Heinrich, C. H., Going, S. B., Pamenter, R. W., Perry, C. D., Boyden, T. W., and Lohman, T. G., Bone mineral content of cyclically menstruating female resistance and endurance trained athletes, *Med. Sci. Sports Exerc.* 22, 558–63, 1990.
94. Davee, A. M., Rosen, C. J., and Adler, R. A., Exercise patterns and trabecular bone density in college women, *J. Bone Miner. Res.* 5, 245–50, 1990.
95. Tsuzuku, S., Ikegami, Y., and Yabe, K., Effects of high-intensity resistance training on bone mineral density in young male powerlifters, *Calcif. Tissue Int.* 63, 283–6, 1998.
96. Colletti, L. A., Edwards, J., Gordon, L., Shary, J., and Bell, N. H., The effects of muscle-building exercise on bone mineral density of the radius, spine, and hip in young men, *Calcif. Tissue Int.* 45, 12–4, 1989.
97. Braith, R. W., Mills, R. M., Welsch, M. A., Keller, J. W., and Pollock, M. L., Resistance exercise training restores bone mineral density in heart transplant recipients, *J. Am. Coll. Cardiol.* 28, 1471–7, 1996.
98. Menkes, A., Mazel, S., Redmond, R. A., Koffler, K., Libanati, C. R., Gundberg, C. M., et al., Strength training increases regional bone mineral density and bone remodeling in middle-aged and older men, *J. Appl. Physiol.* 74, 2478–84, 1993.
99. Nelson, M. E., Fiatarone, M. A., Morganti, C. M., Trice, I., Greenberg, R. A., and Evans, W. J., Effects of high-intensity strength training on multiple risk factors for osteoporotic fractures: A randomized controlled trial, *JAMA.* 272, 1909–14, 1994.

100. Snow-Harter, C., Bouxsein, M. L., Lewis, B. T., Carter, D. R., and Marcus, R., Effects of resistance and endurance exercise on bone mineral status of young women: A randomized exercise intervention trial, *J. Bone Miner. Res.* 7, 761–9, 1992.
101. Maddalozzo, G. F. and Snow, C. M., High intensity resistance training: Effects on bone in older men and women, *Calcif. Tissue Int.* 66, 399–404, 2000.
102. Lohman, T., Going, S., Pamenter, R., Hall, M., Boyden, T., Houtkooper, L., et al., Effects of resistance training on regional and total bone mineral density in premenopausal women: A randomized prospective study, *J. Bone Miner. Res.* 10, 1015–24, 1995.
103. Kerr, D., Ackland, T., Maslen, B., Morton, A., and Prince, R., Resistance training over 2 years increases bone mass in calcium-replete postmenopausal women, *J. Bone Miner. Res.* 16, 175–81, 2001.
104. McLafferty, C. L., Jr., Wetzstein, C. J., and Hunter, G. R., Resistance training is associated with improved mood in healthy older adults, *Percept. Mot. Skills* 98(3) Pt 1, 947–57, 2004.
105. Tsutsumi, T., Don, B. M., Zaichkowsky, L. D., and Delizonna, L. L., Physical fitness and psychological benefits of strength training in community dwelling older adults, *Appl. Human Sci.* 16, 257–66, 1997.
106. Hale, B. S. and Raglin, J. S., State anxiety responses to acute resistance training and step aerobic exercise across eight weeks of training, *J. Sports Med. Phys. Fitness* 42, 108–12, 2002.
107. Tsutsumi, T., Don, B. M., Zaichkowsky, L. D., Takenaka, K., Oka, K., and Ohno, T., Comparison of high and moderate intensity of strength training on mood and anxiety in older adults, *Percept. Mot. Skills* 87(3) Pt 1, 1003–11, 1998.
108. Berg, H. E., Berggren, G., and Tesch, P. A., Dynamic neck strength training effect on pain and function, *Arch. Phys. Med. Rehabil.* 75, 661–5, 1994.
109. Schilke, J. M., Johnson, G. O., Housh, T. J., and O'Dell, J. R., Effects of muscle-strength training on the functional status of patients with osteoarthritis of the knee joint, *Nurs. Res.* 45, 68–72, 1996.
110. Rall, L. C., Meydani, S. N., Kehayias, J. J., Dawson-Hughes, B., and Roubenoff, R., The effect of progressive resistance training in rheumatoid arthritis: Increased strength without changes in energy balance or body composition, *Arthritis Rheum.* 39, 415–26, 1996.
111. Rogers, M. W., and Wilder, F. V., The effects of strength training among persons with hand osteoarthritis: A two-year follow-up study, *J. Hand Ther.* 20, 244–9; quiz 250, 2007.
112. Mikesky, A. E., Mazzuca, S. A., Brandt, K. D., Perkins, S. M., Damush, T., and Lane, K. A., Effects of strength training on the incidence and progression of knee osteoarthritis, *Arthritis Rheum.* 55, 690–9, 2006.
113. Ylinen, J J., Takala, E. P., Nykänen, M. J., Kautiainen, H. J., Häkkinen, A. H., and Airaksinen, O. V., Effects of twelve-month strength training subsequent to twelve-month stretching exercise in treatment of chronic neck pain, *J. Strength Cond. Res.* 20, 304–8, 2006.
114. Poehlman, E. T. and Melby, C., Resistance training and energy balance, *Int. J. Sport Nutr.* 8, 143–59, 1998.
115. Johnstone, A. M., Murison, S. D., Duncan, J. S., Rance, K. A., and Speakman, J. R., Factors influencing variation in basal metabolic rate include fat-free mass, fat mass, age, and circulating thyroxine but not sex, circulating leptin, or triiodothyronine, *Am. J. Clin. Nutr.* 82, 941–8, 2005.
116. D'Alessio, D. A., Kavle, E. C., Mozzoli, M. A., Smalley, K. J., Polansky, M., Kendrick, Z. V., et al., Thermic effect of food in lean and obese men, *J. Clin. Invest.* 81, 1781–9, 1988.

117. Westerterp, K. R., Alterations in energy balance with exercise, *Am. J. Clin. Nutr.* 68, 970S–974S, 1998.
118. Harris, J. and Benedict, F. A, Biometric study of basal metabolism in man., *Carnegie Institution*, 1919.
119. Lin, P. H., Proschan, M. A., Bray, G. A., Fernandez, C. P., Hoben, K., Most-Windhauser, M., et al., Estimation of energy requirements in a controlled feeding trial, *Am. J. Clin. Nutr.* 77, 639–45, 2003.
120. Byrne, N. M., Hills, A. P., Hunter, G. R., Weinsier, R. L., and Schutz, Y., Metabolic equivalent: One size does not fit all, *J. Appl. Physiol.* 99, 1112–9, 2005.
121. Campbell, W. W., Crim, M. C., Dallal, G. E., Young, V. R., and Evans, W., Increased protein requirements in elderly people: New data and retrospective reassessments, *Am. J. Clin. Nutr.* 60, 501–9, 1994.
122. FAO/WHO/UNU, Energy and Protein Requirements, *Technical Report Series,* 1989.
123. Gersovitz, M., Motil, K., Munro, H. N., Scrimshaw, N. S., and Young, V. R., Human protein requirements: Assessment of the adequacy of the current Recommended Dietary Allowance for dietary protein in elderly men and women, *Am. J. Clin. Nutr.* 35, 6–14, 1982.
124. Zanni, E., Calloway, D. H., and Zezulka, A. Y., Protein requirements of elderly men, *J. Nutr.* 109, 513–24, 1979.
125. Campbell, W. W., Trappe, T. A., Wolfe, R. R., and Evans, W. J., The recommended dietary allowance for protein may not be adequate for older people to maintain skeletal muscle, *J. Gerontol. Series A Biol. Sci. Med. Sci.* 56, M373–80, 2001.
126. Thalacker-Mercer, A. E., Fleet, J. C., Craig, B. A., Carnell, N. S., and Campbell, W. W., Inadequate protein intake affects skeletal muscle transcript profiles in older humans, *Am. J. Clin. Nutr.* 85, 1344–52, 2007.
127. Rousset, S., Patureau Mirand, P., Brandolini, M., Martin, J. F., and Boirie, Y., Daily protein intakes and eating patterns in young and elderly French, *Br. J. Nutr.* 90, 1107–15, 2003.
128. Perissinotto, E., Pisent, C., Sergi, G., and Grigoletto, F., Anthropometric measurements in the elderly: Age and gender differences, *Br. J. Nutr.* 87, 177–86, 2002.
129. Roberts, S. B., and Dallal, G. E., Effects of age on energy balance, *Am. J. Clin. Nutr.* 68, 975S–979S, 1998.
130. Layman, D. K., The role of leucine in weight loss diets and glucose homeostasis, *J. Nutr.* 133, 261S–267S, 2003.
131. Layman, D. K., and Baum, J. I., Dietary protein impact on glycemic control during weight loss, *J. Nutr.* 134, 968S–73S, 2004.
132. Layman, D. K., Shiue, H., Sather, C., Erickson, D. J., and Baum, J., Increased dietary protein modifies glucose and insulin homeostasis in adult women during weight loss, *J. Nutr.* 133, 405–10, 2003.
133. FAO/WHO/UNU, Energy and protein requirements: Report of joint FAO/WHO/UNU expert consultation, *WHO Tech. Pep. Ser.* 724, 1–206., 1988.
134. el-Khoury, A. E., Fukagawa, N. K., Sanchez, M., Tsay, R. H., Gleason, R. E., Chapman, T. E., and Young, V. R., The 24-h pattern and rate of leucine oxidation, with particular reference to tracer estimates of leucine requirements in healthy adults, *Am. J. Clin. Nutr.* 59, 1012–20, 1994.
135. Norton, L. E., and Layman, D. K., Leucine regulates translation initiation of protein synthesis in skeletal muscle after exercise, *J. Nutr.* 136, 533S–537S, 2006.
136. Garlick, P. J., The role of leucine in the regulation of protein metabolism, *J. Nutr.* 135, 1553S–6S, 2005.

137. Krauss, R. M., Eckel, R. H., Howard, B., Appel, L. J., Daniels, S. R., Deckelbaum, R. J., et al., AHA Dietary Guidelines: revision 2000: A statement for healthcare professionals from the Nutrition Committee of the American Heart Association, *Circulation* 102, 2284–99, 2000.
138. Sidossis, L. S., Mittendorfer, B., Walser, E., Chinkes, D., and Wolfe, R. R., Hyperglycemia-induced inhibition of splanchnic fatty acid oxidation increases hepatic triacylglycerol secretion, *Am. J. Physiol.* 275, E798–805, 1998.
139. Sidossis, L. S., Mittendorfer, B., Chinkes, D., Walser, E., and Wolfe, R. R., Effect of hyperglycemia-hyperinsulinemia on whole body and regional fatty acid metabolism, *Am. J. Physiol.* 276, E427–34, 1999.
140. Lemon, P. W., Tarnopolsky, M. A., MacDougall, J. D., and Atkinson, S. A., Protein requirements and muscle mass/strength changes during intensive training in novice bodybuilders, *J. Appl. Physiol.* 73, 767–75, 1992.
141. Tarnopolsky, M. A., Atkinson, S. A., MacDougall, J. D., Chesley, A., Phillips, S., and Schwarcz, H. P., Evaluation of protein requirements for trained strength athletes, *J. Appl. Physiol.* 73, 1986–95, 1992.
142. Tarnopolsky, M. A., MacDougall, J. D., and Atkinson, S. A., Influence of protein intake and training status on nitrogen balance and lean body mass, *J. Appl. Physiol.* 64, 187–93, 1988.
143. Campbell, W. W., Crim, M. C., Young, V. R., Joseph, L. J., and Evans, W. J., Effects of resistance training and dietary protein intake on protein metabolism in older adults, *Am. J. Physiol.* 268, E1143–53, 1995.
144. Wilson, J., and Wilson, G. J., Contemporary issues in protein requirements and consumption for resistance trained athletes, *JISSN* 3, 7–27, 2006.
145. Falvo, M. J., Hoffman, J. R. , Ratamess, N. A., and Kang, J, Effect of protein supplementation during a 6 month strength and conditioning program on muscular strength, *Med. Sci. Sports Exercise* 37, Suppl 45, 2005.
146. Meredith, C. N., Frontera, W. R., O'Reilly, K. P., and Evans, W. J., Body composition in elderly men: Effect of dietary modification during strength training, *J. Am. Geriatr. Soc.* 40, 155–62, 1992.
147. Lemon, P. W., Effect of exercise on protein requirements, *J. Sports Sci.* 9 Spec No, 53–70, 1991.
148. Lemon, P. W., Is increased dietary protein necessary or beneficial for individuals with a physically active lifestyle? *Nutr. Rev.* 54, S169–75, 1996.
149. Lemon, P. W., Beyond the zone: protein needs of active individuals, *J. Am. Coll. Nutr.* 19, 513S–521S, 2000.
150. Lemon, P. W. and Proctor, D. N., Protein intake and athletic performance, *Sports Med.* 12, 313–25, 1991.
151. Tome, D. and Bos, C., Dietary protein and nitrogen utilization, *J. Nutr.* 130, 1868S–73S, 2000.
152. Phillips, S. M., Protein requirements and supplementation in strength sports, *Nutrition* 20, 689–95, 2004.
153. Campbell, W. W., Barton, M. L., Jr., Cyr-Campbell, D., Davey, S. L., Beard, J. L., Parise, G., and Evans, W. J., Effects of an omnivorous diet compared with a lactoovovegetarian diet on resistance-training-induced changes in body composition and skeletal muscle in older men, *Am. J. Clin. Nutr.* 70, 1032–9, 1999.
154. Bohe, J., Low, A., Wolfe, R. R., and Rennie, M. J., Human muscle protein synthesis is modulated by extracellular, not intramuscular amino acid availability: A dose–response study, *J. Physiol.* 552, 315–24, 2003.

155. Tipton, K. D., Gurkin, B. E., Matin, S., and Wolfe, R. R., Nonessential amino acids are not necessary to stimulate net muscle protein synthesis in healthy volunteers, *J. Nutr. Biochem.* 10, 89–95, 1999.
156. Bos, C., Metges, C. C., Gaudichon, C., Petzke, K. J., Pueyo, M. E., Morens, C., et al., Postprandial kinetics of dietary amino acids are the main determinant of their metabolism after soy or milk protein ingestion in humans, *J. Nutr.* 133, 1308–15, 2003.
157. Wahren, J., Felig, P. and Hagenfeldt, L., Effect of protein ingestion on splanchnic and leg metabolism in normal man and in patients with diabetes mellitus, *J. Clin. Invest.* 57, 987–99, 1976.
158. Brosnan, J. T. and Brosnan, M. E., Branched-chain amino acids: Enzyme and substrate regulation, *J. Nutr.* 136, 207S–11S, 2006.
159. Hargreaves, M. H. and Snow, R., Amino acids and endurance exercise, *Int. J. Sport Nutr. Exerc. Metab.* 11, 133–45, 2001.
160. Martinez, J. A., Goena, M., Santidrian, S., and Larralde, J., Response of muscle, liver and whole-body protein turnover to two different sources of protein in growing rats, *Ann. Nutr. Metab.* 31, 146–53, 1987.
161. Esmarck, B., Andersen, J. L., Olsen, S., Richter, E. A., Mizuno, M., and Kjaer, M., Timing of postexercise protein intake is important for muscle hypertrophy with resistance training in elderly humans, *J. Physiol.* 535, 301–11, 2001.
162. Levenhagen, D. K., Gresham, J. D., Carlson, M. G., Maron, D. J., Borel, M. J., and Flakoll, P. J., Postexercise nutrient intake timing in humans is critical to recovery of leg glucose and protein homeostasis, *Am. J. Physiol. Endocrinol. Metab.* 280, E982–93, 2001.
163. Biolo, G., Maggi, S. P., Williams, B. D., Tipton, K. D., and Wolfe, R. R., Increased rates of muscle protein turnover and amino acid transport after resistance exercise in humans, *Am. J. Physiol.* 268, E514–20, 1995.
164. Katsanos, C. S., Kobayashi, H., Sheffield-Moore, M., Aarsland, A., and Wolfe, R. R., Aging is associated with diminished accretion of muscle proteins after the ingestion of a small bolus of essential amino acids, *Am. J. Clin. Nutr.* 82, 1065–73, 2005.
165. Cuthbertson, D., Smith, K., Babraj, J., Leese, G., Waddell, T., Atherton, P., et al., Anabolic signaling deficits underlie amino acid resistance of wasting, aging muscle, *FASEB J.* 19, 422–4, 2005.
166. Katsanos, C. S., Kobayashi, H., Sheffield-Moore, M., Aarsland, A., and Wolfe, R R., A high proportion of leucine is required for optimal stimulation of the rate of muscle protein synthesis by essential amino acids in the elderly, *Am. J. Physiol. Endocrinol Metab.* 291, E381–7, 2006.
167. Combaret, L., Dardevet, D., Rieu, I., Pouch, M. N., Bechet, D., Taillandier, D., et al., A leucine-supplemented diet restores the defective postprandial inhibition of proteasome–dependent proteolysis in aged rat skeletal muscle, *J. Physiol.* 569, 489–99, 2005.
168. Paddon-Jones, D., Sheffield-Moore, M., Zhang, X. J., Volpi, E., Wolf, S. E., Aarsland, A., et al., Amino acid ingestion improves muscle protein synthesis in the young and elderly, *Am. J. Physiol. Endocrinol. Metab.* 286, E321–8, 2004.
169. Symons, T. B., Schutzler, S. E., Cocke, T. L., Chinkes, D. L., Wolfe, R. R., and Paddon-Jones, D., Aging does not impair the anabolic response to a protein-rich meal, *Am. J. Clin. Nutr.* 86, 451–6, 2007.
170. Ivy, J. L., Role of carbohydrate in physical activity, *Clinics in sports medicine* 18, 469–84, Jul 1999.
171. Romijn, J. A., Coyle, E. F., Sidossis, L. S., Gastaldelli, A., Horowitz, J. F., Endert, E., and Wolfe, R. R., Regulation of endogenous fat and carbohydrate metabolism in relation to exercise intensity and duration, *Am. J. Physiol.* 265, E380–91, Sep 1993.

172. Romijn, J. A., Coyle, E. F., Sidossis, L. S., Rosenblatt, J., and Wolfe, R. R., Substrate metabolism during different exercise intensities in endurance-trained women, *J. Applied Physiol.,* Bethesda, MD, 1985, 88, 1707–14, May 2000.
173. Robergs, R. A., Pearson, D. R., Costill, D. L., Fink, W. J., Pascoe, D. D., Benedict, M. A., et al., Muscle glycogenolysis during differing intensities of weight-resistance exercise, *J. Appl. Physiol.* 70, 1700–6, 1991.
174. Keul, J., Haralambie, G., Bruder, M., and Gottstein, H. J., The effect of weight lifting exercise on heart rate and metabolism in experienced weight lifters, *Med. Sci. Sports* 10, 13–5, 1978.
175. Tesch, P. A., Colliander, E. B., and Kaiser, P., Muscle metabolism during intense, heavy–resistance exercise, *Eur. J. Appl. Physiol. Occup. Physiol.* 55, 362–6, 1986.
176. Balsom, P. D., Gaitanos, G. C., Soderlund, K., and Ekblom, B, High-intensity exercise and muscle glycogen availability in humans, *Acta physiologica Scandinavica* 165, 337–45, Apr 1999.
177. Jacobs, I., Kaiser, P., and Tesch, P., Muscle strength and fatigue after selective glycogen depletion in human skeletal muscle fibers, *Eur. J. Appl. Physiol. Occup. Physiol.* 46, 47–53, 1981.
178. Rockwell, M. S., Rankin, J. W., and Dixon, H., Effects of muscle glycogen on performance of repeated sprints and mechanisms of fatigue, *Intern. J. Sport Nutr. Exerc. Metab.* 13, 1–14, Mar 2003.
179. Symons, J. D. and Jacobs, I., High-intensity exercise performance is not impaired by low intramuscular glycogen, *Med. Sci. Sports Exerc.* 21, 550–7, Oct 1989.
180. Leveritt, M. and Abernethy, P. J., Effects of carbohydrate restriction on strength performance. *J. Strength Cond. Res.* 13, 52–57, February 1999.
181. Conley, M. S. and Stone, M. H., Carbohydrate ingestion/supplementation or resistance exercise and training, *Sports Med.* 21, 7–17, Jan 1996.
182. Lambert, C. P., Flynn, M. G., Boone, J. B., Michaud, T. J., and Rodriguez-Zayas, J., Effects of carbohydrate feeding on multiple-bout resistance exercise, *J. Applied Sport Sc. Res.* 5, 192–197, Nov 1991.
183. Sherman, W. M., Doyle, J. A., Lamb, D. R., and Strauss, R. H., Dietary carbohydrate, muscle glycogen, and exercise performance during 7 d of training, *Am. J. Clin. Nutr.* 57, 27–31, Jan 1993.
184. van Loon, L. J., Saris, W. H., Kruijshoop, M., and Wagenmakers, A. J., Maximizing postexercise muscle glycogen synthesis: Carbohydrate supplementation and the application of amino acid or protein hydrolysate mixtures, *Am. J. Clin. Nutr.* 72, 106–11, Jul 2000.
185. Ivy, J. L., Lee, M. C., Brozinick, J. T., and Reed, M. J., Muscle glycogen storage after different amounts of carbohydrate ingestion, *J. Appl. Physiol.,* Bethesda, Md., 1985, 65, 2018–23, Nov 1988.
186. Ivy, J. L., Katz, A. L., Cutler, C. L., Sherman, W. M., and Coyle, E. F., Muscle glycogen synthesis after exercise: Effect of time of carbohydrate ingestion, *J. Appl. Physiol.,* Bethesda, Md., 1985, 64, 1480–5, Apr 1988.
187. Pascoe, D. D., Costill, D. L., Fink, W. J., Robergs, R. A., and Zachwieja, J. J., Glycogen resynthesis in skeletal muscle following resistive exercise, *Med. Sci. Sports Exerc.* 25, 349–54, 1993.
188. Roy, B. D., Tarnopolsky, M. A., MacDougall, J. D., Fowles, J., and Yarasheski, K. E., Effect of glucose supplement timing on protein metabolism after resistance training, *J. Appl. Physiol.,* Bethesda, Md., 1985, 82, 1882–8, Jun 1997.
189. Chandler, R. M., Byrne, H. K., Patterson, J. G., and Ivy, J. L., Dietary supplements affect the anabolic hormones after weight-training exercise, *J. Appl. Physiol.* 76, 839–45, 1994.

190. Manore, M. M., Butterfield, G. E., and Barr, S. I., Nutrition and Athletic Performance, http://www. acsm–msse.org/pt/pt–core/template–journal/msse/media/1200.pdf, 2000.
191. Ratamess, N. A., Falvo, M. J., Mangine, G. T., Hoffman, J. R., Faigenbaum, A. D., and Kang, J., The effect of rest interval length on metabolic responses to the bench press exercise, *Eur. J. Applied Physiol.* 100, 1–17, May 2007.
192. Thornton, M. K. and Potteiger, J. A., Effects of resistance exercise bouts of different intensities but equal work on EPOC, *Med. Sci. Sports Exerc.* 34, 715–22, Apr 2002.
193. Lambert, C. P. and Flynn, M. G., Fatigue during high-intensity intermittent exercise: Application to bodybuilding, *Sports Med. (Auckland, N. Z.)*. 32, 511–22, 2002.
194. Binzen, C. A., Swan, P. D., and Manore, M. M., Postexercise oxygen consumption and substrate use after resistance exercise in women, *Med. Sci. Sports Exer.,* 33, 932–8, Jun 2001.
195. Jamurtas, A. Z., Koutedakis, Y., Paschalis, V., Tofas, T., Yfanti, C., Tsiokanos, A., et al., The effects of a single bout of exercise on resting energy expenditure and respiratory exchange ratio, *Eur. J. Appl. Physiol.* 92, 393–8, Aug 2004.
196. Melby, C., Scholl, C., Edwards, G., and Bullough, R., Effect of acute resistance exercise on postexercise energy expenditure and resting metabolic rate, *J. Appl. Physiol.* 75, 1847–53, Oct 1993.
197. Osterberg, K. L. and Melby, C. L., Effect of acute resistance exercise on postexercise oxygen consumption and resting metabolic rate in young women, *Intern. J. Sport Nutr. Exerc. Metab.* 10, 71–81, Mar 2000.
198. Goto, K., Ishii, N., Sugihara, S., Yoshioka, T., and Takamatsu, Kaoru, Effects of resistance exercise on lipolysis during subsequent submaximal exercise, *Med. Sci. Sports Exerc.* 39, 308–15, Feb 2007.
199. Nissen, S. L. and Sharp, R. L., Effect of dietary supplements on lean mass and strength gains with resistance exercise: A meta-analysis, *J. Appl. Physiol.* 94, 651–9, Feb 2003.
200. Tarnopolsky, M. A., Potential benefits of creatine monohydrate supplementation in the elderly, *Curr. Op. Clin. Nutr. Metab. Care* 3, 497–502, Nov 2000.
201. Branch, J. David, Effect of creatine supplementation on body composition and performance: A meta-analysis, *Intern. J. Sport Nutr. Exerc. Metab.* 13, 198–226, Jun 2003.
202. Volek, Jeff S. and Rawson, Eric S., Scientific basis and practical aspects of creatine supplementation for athletes, *Nutrition*, 20, 609–14, 2004.
203. Arciero, P. J., Hannibal, N. S., 3rd, Nindl, B. C., Gentile, C. L., Hamed, J., and Vukovich, M. D., Comparison of creatine ingestion and resistance training on energy expenditure and limb blood flow, *Metabolism,* 50, 1429–34, 2001.
204. Syrotuik, D., Bell, G., Burnham, R., Sim, L., Calvert, R., and MacLean, I., Absolute and relative strength performance following creatine monohydrate supplementation combined with periodized resistance training, *J. Strength Cond. Res.* 14, 182–190, 2000.
205. Willoughby, D. S. and Rosene, J., Effects of oral creatine and resistance training on myosin heavy chain expression, *Med. Sci. Sports Exerc.* 33, 1674–81, 2001.
206. Willoughby, D. S. and Rosene, J. M., Effects of oral creatine and resistance training on myogenic regulatory factor expression, *Med. Sci. Sports Exerc.* 35, 923–9, 2003.
207. Smith, S. A., Montain, S. J., Matott, R. P., Zientara, G. P., Jolesz, F. A., and Fielding, R. A., Creatine supplementation and age influence muscle metabolism during exercise, *J. Appl. Physiol.* 85, 1349–56, 1998.
208. Gallagher, P. M., Carrithers, J. A., Godard, M. P., Schulze, K. E., and Trappe, S. W., Beta–hydroxy–beta–methylbutyrate ingestion, Part I: Effects on strength and fat-free mass, *Med. Sci. Sports Exerc.* 32, 2109–15, 2000.

209. Jowko, E., Ostaszewski, P., Jank, M., Sacharuk, J., Zieniewicz, A., Wilczak, J., and Nissen, S., Creatine and beta-hydroxy-beta-methylbutyrate (HMB) additively increase lean body mass and muscle strength during a weight-training program, *Nutrition* 17, 558–66, 2001.
210. Nissen, S., Sharp, R., Ray, M., Rathmacher, J. A., Rice, D., Fuller, J. C., Jr., et al., Effect of leucine metabolite beta-hydroxy-beta-methylbutyrate on muscle metabolism during resistance-exercise training, *J. Appl. Physiol.* 81, 2095–104, 1996.
211. Panton, L. B., Rathmacher, J. A., Baier, S., and Nissen, S., Nutritional supplementation of the leucine metabolite beta-hydroxy-beta-methylbutyrate (HMB) during resistance training, *Nutrition* 16, 734–9, 2000.
212. Smith, H. J., Mukerji, P., and Tisdale, M. J., Attenuation of proteasome-induced proteolysis in skeletal muscle by beta-hydroxy-beta-methylbutyrate in cancer-induced muscle loss, *Cancer Res.* 65, 277–83, 2005.
213. Soares, J. M. C., Póvoas, S., Neuparth, M J., and Duarte, J A. , The effects of beta-hydroxy-beta-methylbuturate (HMB) on muscle atrophy induced by immobilization, *Med. Sci. Sports Exerc.* 33, supp 140, 2001.
214. van Someren, K. A., Edwards, A. J., and Howatson, G., Supplementation with beta-hydroxy-beta-methylbutyrate (HMB) and alpha-ketoisocaproic acid (KIC) reduces signs and symptoms of exercise-induced muscle damage in man, *Int. J. Sport Nutr. Exerc. Metab.* 15, 413–24, 2005.
215. Knitter, A. E., Panton, L., Rathmacher, J. A., Petersen, A., and Sharp, R., Effects of beta-hydroxy-beta-methylbutyrate on muscle damage after a prolonged run, *J. Appl. Physiol.* 89, 1340–4, 2000.
216. Vukovich, M. D., Stubbs, N. B., and Bohlken, R. M., Body composition in 70-year-old adults responds to dietary beta-hydroxy-beta-methylbutyrate similarly to that of young adults, *J. Nutr.* 131, 2049–52, 2001.
217. Flakoll, P., Sharp, R., Baier, S., Levenhagen, D., Carr, C., and Nissen, S., Effect of beta-hydroxy-beta-methylbutyrate, arginine, and lysine supplementation on strength, functionality, body composition, and protein metabolism in elderly women, *Nutrition* 20, 445–51, 2004.
218. Panton, L., Rathmacher, J., Fuller, J., Gammon, J., Cannon, L., Stettler, S., and Nissen, S, Effect of β-hydroxy-β-methylbutyrate and resistance training on strength and functional ability in the elderly, *Med. Sci. Sports Exerc.* 30, suppl. 194, 1998.
219. Nissen, S., Morrical, D., and J. C. Fuller, Jr., The effects of the leucine catabolite β-hydroxy-β-methylbuyrate on the growth and health of growing lambs, *J. Anim. Sci.* 77, 234, 1994.
220. Nissen, S., Sharp, R. L., Panton, L., Vukovich, M., Trappe, S., and Fuller, J. C., Jr., beta-hydroxy-beta-methylbutyrate (HMB) supplementation in humans is safe and may decrease cardiovascular risk factors, *J. Nutr.* 130, 1937–45, 2000.
221. Vermeulen, A., Ageing, hormones, body composition, metabolic effects, *World J. Urol.* 20, 23–7, 2002.
222. Vermeulen, A., Goemaere, S., and Kaufman, J. M., Testosterone, body composition and aging, *J. Endocrinol Invest.* 22, 110–6, 1999.
223. van den Beld, A. W., de Jong, F. H., Grobbee, D. E., Pols, H. A., and Lamberts, S. W., Measures of bioavailable serum testosterone and estradiol and their relationships with muscle strength, bone density, and body composition in elderly men, *J. Clin. Endocrinol Metab.* 85, 3276–82, 2000.
224. Roy, T. A., Blackman, M. R., Harman, S. M., Tobin, J. D., Schrager, M., and Metter, E. J., Interrelationships of serum testosterone and free testosterone index with FFM and strength in aging men, *Am. J. Physiol. Endocrinol Metab.* 283, E284–94, 2002.

225. Abbasi, A. A., Drinka, P. J., Mattson, D. E., and Rudman, D., Low circulating levels of insulin-like growth factors and testosterone in chronically institutionalized elderly men, *J. Am. Geriatr Soc.* 41, 975–82, 1993.
226. Inoue, K., Yamasaki, S., Fushiki, T., Okada, Y., and Sugimoto, E., Androgen receptor antagonist suppresses exercise–induced hypertrophy of skeletal muscle, *Eur. J. Appl. Physiol. Occ. Physiol.* . 69, 88–91, 1994.
227. Urban, R. J., Bodenburg, Y. H., Gilkinson, C., Foxworth, J., Coggan, A. R., Wolfe, R. R., and Ferrando, A., Testosterone administration to elderly men increases skeletal muscle strength and protein synthesis, *Am. J. Physiol.* 269, E820–E826, 1995.
228. Lewis, M. I., Horvitz, G. D., Clemmons, D. R., and Fournier, M., Role of IGF-I and IGF-binding proteins within diaphragm muscle in modulating the effects of nandrolone, *Am. J. Physiol Endocrinol Metab.* 282, E483–90, 2002.
229. Van Balkom, R. H., Dekhuijzen, P. N., Folgering, H. T., Veerkamp, J. H., Van Moerkerk, H. T., Fransen, J. A., and Van Herwaarden, C. L., Anabolic steroids in part reverse glucocorticoid-induced alterations in rat diaphragm, *J. Appl. Physiol.* 84, 1492–9, 1998.
230. Bhasin, S., Testosterone supplementation for aging-associated sarcopenia, *J. Gerontol. Series A Biol. Sci. Med. Sci.* 58, 1002–8, 2003.
231. Feldman, H. A., Longcope, C., Derby, C. A., Johannes, C. B., Araujo, A. B., Coviello, A. D., et al., Age trends in the level of serum testosterone and other hormones in middle-aged men: Longitudinal results from the Massachusetts male aging study, *J. Clin. Endocrinol Metab.* 87, 589–98, 2002.
232. Zirkin, B. R. and Chen, H., Regulation of Leydig cell steroidogenic function during aging, *Biol. Reprod.* 63, 977–81, 2000.
233. Hakkinen, K., Pakarinen, A., Kraemer, W. J., Newton, R. U., and Alen, M., Basal concentrations and acute responses of serum hormones and strength development during heavy resistance training in middle-aged and elderly men and women, *J. Gerontol. Series A Biol. Sci. Med. Sci.* 55, B95–105, 2000.
234. Laughlin, G. A. and Barrett-Connor, E., Sexual dimorphism in the influence of advanced aging on adrenal hormone levels: The Rancho Bernardo Study, *J. Clin. Endocrinol. Metab.* 85, 3561–8, 2000.
235. Travison, T. G., Araujo, A. B., Kupelian, V., O'Donnell, A. B., and McKinlay, J. B., The relative contributions of aging, health, and lifestyle factors to serum testosterone decline in men, *J. Clin. Endocrinol Metab.* 92, 549–55, 2007.
236. Hakkinen, K., and Pakarinen, A., Acute hormonal responses to heavy resistance exercise in men and women at different ages, *Int. J. Sports Med.* 16, 507–13, 1995.
237. Hakkinen, K., Pakarinen, A., Alen, M., Kauhanen, H., and Komi, P. V., Neuromuscular and hormonal adaptations in athletes to strength training in two years, *J Appl Physiol.* 65, 2406–12, 1988.
238. Kraemer, W. J., Hakkinen, K., Newton, R. U., Nindl, B. C., Volek, J. S., McCormick, M., et al., Effects of heavy resistance training on hormonal response patterns in younger vs. older men, *J. Appl. Physiol.* 87, 982–92, 1999.
239. Hakkinen, K. and Pakarinen, A., Acute hormonal responses to two different fatiguing heavy-resistance protocols in male athletes, *J. Appl. Physiol.* 74, 882–7, 1993.
240. Schwab, R., Johnson, G. O., Housh, T. J., Kinder, J. E., and Weir, J. P., Acute effects of different intensities of weight lifting on serum testosterone, *Med. Sci. Sports Exerc.* 25, 1381–5, 1993.
241. Villareal, D. T., and Holloszy, J. O., DHEA enhances effects of weight training on muscle mass and strength in elderly women and men, *Am. J. Physiol. Endocrinol Metab.* 291, E1003–8, 2006.

242. Morales, A. J., Haubrich, R. H., Hwang, J. Y., Asakura, H., and Yen, S. S., The effect of six months treatment with a 100 mg daily dose of dehydroepiandrosterone (DHEA) on circulating sex steroids, body composition and muscle strength in age-advanced men and women, *Clin. Endocrin.* 49, 421–32, 1998.
243. Morales, A. J., Nolan, J. J., Nelson, J. C., and Yen, S. S., Effects of replacement dose of dehydroepiandrosterone in men and women of advancing age, *J. Clin. Endocrinol. Metab.* 78, 1360–7, 1994.

Section VIII

Age-Related Disorders

16 Cardiovascular Issues

Susan Hazels Mitmesser

CONTENTS

I. INTRODUCTION

The term cardiovascular disease (CVD) includes hypertension, coronary heart disease (CHD), heart failure, and stroke. CVD is the leading cause of death and disability in the industrialized world for both men and women, regardless of race or ethnicity, accounting for up to 50% of all deaths annually.[1–4] Furthermore, it is estimated to remain the greatest cause of death worldwide through the year 2020.[5] Factors that contribute to CVD include a poor diet, physical inactivity, obesity, elevated blood pressure, diabetes, smoking, and low socioeconomic status.

There appears to be growing evidence that most cardiovascular disease is preventable. Long-term prospective studies identify populations with low levels of risk factors as having lifelong low levels of heart disease and stroke.[6,7] Moreover, the low levels of risk factors are related to a healthy lifestyle. For example, results from the Nurses Health Study indicate that maintaining a desirable body weight, eating a healthy diet, exercising regularly, not smoking, and consuming a moderate amount of alcohol could account for an 84% reduction in risk.[8] However, only 3% of the women studied could be placed in that category, indicating that the majority of causes of CVD are known and modifiable, but not necessarily adopted as a permanent lifestyle.

The economics of CVD is also becoming more and more apparent and a continual burden on society. Of the annual $666 billion in national health care costs, 30% are related to an inappropriate diet.[9] Extensive scientific evidence highlights the association between foods or eating patterns and health maintenance and chronic disease. Of the many disease states that cause metabolic, physiologic, and psychological trauma, five have a scientific-based connection to the diet: anemia, osteoporosis, heart disease, diabetes, and certain types of cancer, all of which often can begin to exhibit symptoms in the 40s, leaving the middle age an ideal time to actively monitor personal health closely. Risk factors for CVD, such as overweight, dyslipidemia, an unhealthy diet, elevated blood pressure, diabetes mellitus, elevated CVD markers, smoking, and low socioeconomic status, are detailed in the following section.

II. CARDIOVASCULAR DISEASE RISK FACTORS

A. Overweight

The prevalence of overweight and obesity has increased dramatically over the past 20 years and there appears to be no sign of this trend dwindling. A healthy body weight is currently defined as a body mass index (BMI) of 18.5 to 24.9 kg/m^2. Overweight is defined as a BMI of 25–29.9 kg/m^2, with obesity defined as a BMI of >30 kg/m^2. Recent research indicates that a higher BMI is associated with less favorable levels of glucose, low-density lipoprotein (LDL) cholesterol, high-density lipoprotein (HDL) cholesterol, triglycerides, and systolic and diastolic blood pressure.[10–12] It has been estimated that about one third of adults are overweight and an additional one third are obese.[13] The incidence of overweight individuals today appears to be highest in women. Thirty-seven percent of U.S. women age 25-40 years of age gain 5–15% of their body weight over a 10-year period.[14] As an independent risk factor for CVD, excess body weight has been linked to all of the following complications: hypertension, dyslipidemia, type 2 diabetes, ischemic heart disease, hypertensive heart disease, stroke, renal failure, peripheral vascular disease, retinopathy, osteoarthritis, breast cancer, depression, and polycystic ovary syndrome.[15] Furthermore, research indicates a linear relationship between body weight gain after 18 years of age and subsequent risk of developing CVD and diabetes.[16]

The cause of overweight and obesity is multifactorial; implicated factors include: increased portion sizes, easy access to inexpensive food, high calorie dense foods, and a sedentary lifestyle. On average, Americans gain weight throughout the early and middle adult years and this trend may continue through the sixth and seventh decade.[17–22] The presence of excessive subcutaneous and visceral adipose tissue could drive harmful changes in risk. Weight maintenance implies no change in body weight, however there can be an increase in the percentage of fat mass relative to lean mass, which can have an impact on CVD risk. Not only is the addition of body fat critical in the development of CVD, but the distribution of the added fat is also predictive of risk. Abdominal obesity, for example, is associated with a worsening of LDL cholesterol and insulin resistance.[23] Furthermore, the economics of obesity cannot be overlooked. Obese populations are more likely to be taking medications for diabetes, elevated cholesterol, and hypertension, all of which have a hefty price tag.[10]

B. Dyslipidemia

Elevated levels of total cholesterol, LDL cholesterol, and triglycerides, and low levels of HDL cholesterol have been associated with CHD, stroke, and peripheral vascular disease.[24–27] Numerous studies have identified the prevalence of abnormal cholesterol levels across different age and ethnic groups, indicating a higher percentage of the population's having higher levels as the population ages.[28–30]

1. Low-density Lipoprotein (LDL)

The major cholesterol-carrying lipoprotein particle in plasma, LDL, is primarily derived from lipoprotein particles made by the liver. The risk of developing CVD increases as levels of LDL increase.[31] LDL cholesterol levels are classified as optimal (<100 mg/dL), near optimal (100–129 mg/dL), borderline high (130–159 mg/dL), high (160–189 mg/dL), very high (>190 mg/dL).[31] Research indicated that 17% of non-Hispanic white women and 20% of non-Hispanic white men in the United States have LDL levels >160 mg/dL.[32] Similarly, 19% of non-Hispanic black women, 9% of non-Hispanic black men, 14% of Mexican American women, and 17% of Mexican American men have LDL cholesterol levels >160 mg/dL.[13]

Elevated LDL cholesterol levels are more predictive of coronary risk in men than in premenopausal women, due in part to lower levels of LDL cholesterol in premenopausal women than in middle-aged men.[24] However, this does not hold true for postmenopausal women, whose circulating LDL cholesterol increases due to declining levels of estrogen, whereas the LDL cholesterol levels of males around this same age begins to plateau.

2. High-density Lipoprotein (HDL)

HDL is another plasma lipid measure related to CVD risk that is affected by diet and body weight.[33] HDL directly protects against the development of atherosclerosis through the transport of cholesterol from peripheral tissues to the liver for subsequent metabolism or excretion. There is no specific goal for HDL cholesterol as there is for LDL cholesterol, but HDL cholesterol levels of <50 mg/dL in women and <40 mg/dL in men are one of the criteria for classifying metabolic syndrome.[31] Nongenetic factors that contribute to low HDL cholesterol levels are hyperglycemia, diabetes, hypertriglyceridemia, very low-fat diets (<15% energy from fat), and excess body weight.[33]

HDL cholesterol is an important predictor of CVD, perhaps more so in women than men.[25,26,34] The Lipid Research Clinics Prevalence Mortality Follow-up Study indicated an association of 0.025 mmol/L increase in HDL cholesterol with a 4.7% reduction in CVD mortality among women and a 3.7% reduction among men.[35] Similarly, in the Framingham Heart Study, a 0.025 mmol/L increase in HDL cholesterol level was associated with a 3% decrease in the incidence of CHD in women and a 2% decrease in men.[34]

3. Triglyceride

Diet and body weight also affect triglyceride levels, which are related to CVD risk. Similar to HDL cholesterol, there is no specific goal for triglyceride levels. However, levels >150 mg/dL are considered one of the criteria for the classification of metabolic syndrome.[31] The same nongenetic factors that contribute to HDL levels also contribute to triglyceride levels. Research indicates that high levels of triglycerides are a significant risk factor for CVD. Elevated triglyceride levels have been associated with a 37% increase in risk of CVD-related events in women and a 14% increase in men.[27] However, elevated triglycerides are often accompanied by other metabolic disorders that may predispose to CVD, making it difficult to assess the independent risk association with triglycerides.

C. Diet

All macronutrients (e.g., fat, protein, carbohydrate) can play a role in CVD risk to varying degrees. Factors that contribute to excess calorie intake are increased portion sizes, high-calorie foods, and easy access to plentiful inexpensive food. The effects of such factors and of individual nutrients and food groups on overweight and obesity (e.g., role of added sugar, fat, low fruit and vegetable consumption, high-fat dairy products, and lack of physical activity) have been and currently are being explored.

The primary quandary of an increase in fat consumption in the diet is that it can lead to obesity. The amount and type of fat in the diet can be an indicator of CVD risk. It has long been known that saturated fat intake can increase LDL cholesterol, which is a well-established risk factor of CVD.[36,37] It is not surprising that research can confirm that overweight individuals have higher total energy and total and saturated fat intakes than normal-weight individuals. Furthermore, the percentage of calories from fat and dietary cholesterol are also higher in overweight and obese individuals.[10]

Protein choices in the diet can directly affect and contribute to the overall amount of fat in the diet. Choosing lean protein sources over high-fat protein can decrease weight gain. In addition to fat and protein, carbohydrate has been linked to individual weight gain. The intake of sucrose, corn syrup, and high-fructose corn syrup increased from 13.1% of energy between 1977 to 1978 to 16.6% of energy between 1999 to 2002.[38,39] Research indicates that individuals who consume large amounts of beverages with added sugar tend to consume more calories and gain weight.[40,41] While an overconsumption of simple carbohydrate can cause weight gain, consuming complex carbohydrate rich in fiber can help maintain weight. Evidence supports fiber as having a cholesterol lowering effect.[42,43]

D. Elevated Blood Pressure

Blood pressure is a strong, independent, relevant risk factor for CVD. Normal is considered a systolic blood pressure of <120 mm Hg and a diastolic blood pressure of <80 mm Hg. Environmental factors that affect blood pressure include diet, physical inactivity, toxins, and psychosocial factors. The risk of CVD increases progressively throughout the range of blood pressure, including the prehypertensive range (systolic

BP of 120–139 mm Hg or diastolic BP of 80–89 mm Hg).[44] It has been estimated that the lifetime risk of developing hypertension approaches 90% for adults >50 years of age. National Health and Nutrition Examination Survey (NHANES) data indicate that 27% of American adults have hypertension (systolic BP >140 mm Hg, diastolic BP >90 mm Hg) and 31% are prehypertensive.[45] Dietary modifications that lower blood pressure are reduced salt intake, caloric intake that induces weight loss, moderation of alcohol consumption, increased potassium intake, and consumption of an overall healthy diet.[46]

E. Diabetes Mellitus

It has been well established that diabetes mellitus is an independent risk factor for the development of CVD.[47] While the prevalence of diabetes is higher in developed countries, developing countries are experiencing the greatest increase in this disease.[48] People with diabetes have a 2- to 4-fold greater risk of developing CVD than those without the disease.[49] Obese and overweight individuals have a greater risk of developing diabetes which, in turn, puts one at greater risk for developing CVD. Recent research found that those with a BMI of 18.5 to <25.0 kg/m^2 had smaller increases in glucose than those with a BMI greater than 25.0 kg/m^2.[10] Inferior clinical outcomes following myocardial infarction (MI), stroke, and percutaneous and surgical revascularization have been demonstrated in populations with diabetes compared with non-diabetic populations.[50–53] Women with diabetes may, in fact, be at greater risk for CVD than their male counterparts. There appears to be a unique interaction between women with diabetes and CVD, making them more vulnerable to endothelial dysfunction.[54] Huxley and colleagues found that women with diabetes had a 3.5-fold increase in CVD mortality compared with non-diabetic women, which was significantly higher than the risk association in men.[53]

F. Cardiovascular Risk Markers

Changes in certain cardiovascular markers, such as C-reactive protein, homocysteine, apolipoprotein E, fibrinogen, plasminogen activator inhibitor type 1, and lipoprotein (a) (Lp[a]), also appear to be linked to CVD risk. The inflammatory biomarker C-reactive protein has been shown to play an important role in the pathogenesis of CVD.[55–57] A quartile increase in C-reactive protein concentration can increase the risk of CVD by 50%.[56] In populations with established heart disease, high C-reactive protein levels have been associated with increased MI.[58]

Elevated homocysteine levels have also been associated with CVD. According to researchers, men and women with CHD have significantly higher homocysteine levels.[59–61] A 3 umol/L decrease in homocysteine level was associated with an 11% decrease in risk of ischemic heart disease.[62] Additionally, recent research implicates apolipoprotein E as a major modulator of total cholesterol and LDL cholesterol.[63–65] Results from the Framingham Offspring Study indicated that the association of apolipoprotein E with LDL cholesterol level is significantly greater in postmenopausal women than in men or premenopausal women.[65]

Numerous studies indicate that an increase in plasma fibrinogen is associated with an increased risk of MI and stroke.[66–68] Subjects having plasma fibrinogen levels in the highest third have a 2- to 3-fold higher risk of MI and stroke than those having fibrinogen levels in the lowest third.[69] Similarly, elevated levels of plasminogen activator inhibitor type-1 ($PAI\text{-}_I$) have shown a significant associated risk of MI; specifically, a 2-fold increase in risk has been identified.[68,70–73] Moreover, elevated levels of Lp(a) show a positive interaction with high LDL cholesterol levels, hypertension, hyperhomocysteinemia, and elevated fibrinogen concentrations.[74–76]

G. Smoking

Smoking is the number one preventable risk factor contributing to CVD morbidity and mortality.[77] Nearly 23% of U.S. adults smoke.[13] Worldwide, the highest prevalence of smoking for men is in Eastern Europe (rates exceed 60%) and women in Central Europe and parts of South America, while the lowest smoking prevalence for both genders is in African countries.[78] There appears to be a link among a high smoking prevalence and low-income households, low-status jobs or unemployment, single parents or divorce, and low levels of education.[79, 80] Generally, smoking and the risk of CVD appears to be the same across genders with the exception among women smokers taking oral contraceptives, where the risk of stroke is much greater.[81] Although smoking prevalence has steadily declined over the past decades, this trend does not appear until age 30–49 years.[82,83] The impact of smoking on CVD development includes endothelial dysfunction, lipid abnormalities, increased concentration of fibrinogen, and platelet aggregation.[84,85] Furthermore, the effects of smoking are the strongest determinant of high fibrinogen levels.[86]

H. Low Socioeconomic Status

The complexity of socioeconomic status is influenced by a combination of financial, employment, and education experiences. A negative relationship between CVD and socioeconomic status has been demonstrated in numerous studies throughout the world. Research shows that those in the lowest socioeconomic strata have the highest risk of cardiovascular events.[87,88] Low-income women and men have an increase in risk of CVD mortality of 61% and 29%, respectively.[89] Barriers to health care appear to contribute to the higher rate of CVD mortality; those with low income do not obtain health care as effectively as the more solvent.[90,91] Certain disease states and lifestyle risk factors are more prevalent in lower socioeconomic populations, such as diabetes, obesity, sedentary lifestyle, smoking, and hypertension.[92] Lower socioeconomic status has consistently been linked with lower levels of HDL cholesterol and apolipoprotein.[93] Furthermore, the influence of psychological and social behaviors on the development of heart disease are becoming more apparent.[94] People who experience depression are more likely to be women and are more likely to have low income.[95]

The reasons for such differences in socioeconomic status are complex and multifactorial. Diet and lifestyle changes as a means to reduce these disparities should be addressed. Specific diet and lifestyle messages and policies are desperately needed to reduce CVD health disparities.

III. IMPLICATIONS FOR THE MIDDLE AGED

Many factors contribute to the age effect on CVD risk. The risk of developing CVD increases with age, with atherosclerosis development beginning in youth. As age increases, glucose, triglycerides, and systolic blood pressure also increase over time.[10] Because of the high incidence of CVD events in middle-aged adults, even small improvements in risk factors (e.g., small reductions in BP, LDL cholesterol) will be of substantial benefit.[96,97]

A sedentary lifestyle is associated with older age. Most Americans gain weight as they pass from early to late adulthood.[17–22] Weight maintenance may be a more attainable goal than weight loss for some individuals. While the public health message remains that obesity and excess weight gain should be avoided in order to reduce CVD risk, it is beneficial to note that obese individuals who simply maintain their weight and not gain weight are, indeed, lowering their CVD risk.

LDL cholesterol levels tend to plateau in men while increasing in women between ages 40 and 60 years at an average rate of 0.05 mmol/L a year.[98] This increase in LDL cholesterol around menopause could be the result of advancing age and declining levels of estrogen, which result in downregulation of LDL receptors in the liver leading to decreased clearance of LDL cholesterol from the serum. Similarly, HDL cholesterol levels have been shown to decrease.[28] HDL cholesterol levels are 0.25 mmol/L higher in premenopausal women than in men, which may account for the lower incidence of CVD before age 50 in women compared to men.

Plasma fibrinogen levels increase with menopause, pregnancy, and with the use of oral contraceptives. However, hormone replacement therapy (HRT) may decrease circulating fibrinogen levels.[99, 100] Similarly, a few studies have indicated that premenopausal women have lower plasma PAI-1 than postmenopausal women. However, HRT has been shown to decrease plasma PAI-1.[101–103] Lp(a) levels tend to increase with age, which parallels other age-related increases such as LDL cholesterol and fibrinogen.[76]

IV. DECREASING YOUR RISK

In spite of all the major medical advancements, maintaining a healthy diet and lifestyle offers the greatest potential for reducing the risk of CVD in the general public. Healthy dietary patterns are associated with a considerably reduced risk of CVD.[104–106] Just as the risk of CVD is multifactorial, the solution must also be multifactorial. Therefore, rather than focusing on a single nutrient, the aim should be to improve the overall diet. In a recent study of 45–64-year-old adults, researchers found that obese participants who maintained their weight for 9 years had similar changes to their total LDL, HDL, triglycerides, and diastolic blood pressure to those of normal weight participants.[10] This indicates that maintaining weight may be another way to decrease risk of CVD if decreasing body weight is not achieved.

Many cardiovascular organizations, governing bodies, and policy makers have established guidelines and recommendations as a basis to detour the risk of CVD. The guide to the Primary Prevention of Cardiovascular Diseases was initially established in 1997 as a resource to healthcare professionals and their patients.[107] The intent was to complement the American Heart Association (AHA) /American College of Cardiology (ACC) Guidelines for Preventing Heart Attack and Death in Patients with Atherosclerotic Cardiovascular Disease.[108] Furthermore, the 2006 AHA diet and lifestyle goals for cardiovascular disease risk reduction are as follow: consume an overall healthy diet; aim for a healthy body weight; aim for recommended levels of LDL cholesterol, HDL cholesterol, and triglycerides; aim for a normal blood pressure; aim for a normal blood glucose level; be physically active; and avoid use of and exposure to tobacco products.[109]

A. Diet

Many dietary components have been linked to a cardiovascular benefit. Such dietary components include fiber, fish, and certain fats. Additionally, awareness of the calorie content of foods and beverages per portion consumed and portion size needs to be the focus to control overall calorie intake.[110] For that purpose, the 2006 AHA diet and lifestyle recommendations for CVD risk reduction are as follows:

- Balance calorie intake and physical activity to achieve or maintain a healthy body weight.
- Consume a diet rich in vegetables an fruits.
- Choose whole-grain, high-fiber foods.
- Consume fish, especially oily fish, at least twice a week.
- Limit intake of saturated fat to <7% of energy, *trans* fat to <1% of energy, and cholesterol to <300 mg per day by choosing lean meats and vegetable alternatives, selecting fat-free (skim), 1%, and low-fat dairy products, and minimizing intake of partially hydrogenated fats.
- Minimize intake of beverages and foods with added sugar.
- Choose prepared foods with little or no salt.
- If you consume alcohol, do so in moderation.
- When you eat food that is prepared outside of the home, follow the AHA diet and lifestyle recommendations.[109]

More attention is also required in order to make wise choices when food is eaten and prepared outside of the home due to the association between frequency of meal consumption at quick-serve restaurants and total energy intake, weight gain, and insulin resistance.[111]

Most fruits and vegetables are rich in nutrients, low in calories, and high in fiber. Whole-grain foods high in fiber have been associated with a decreased risk of CVD.[42] This association may be the result of dietary fiber's promoting satiety by slowing gastric emptying, which may lead to an overall decrease in calorie intake.[43,112] Specifically, research has indicated soluble fiber increased short-chain fatty acid synthesis, which reduces endogenous cholesterol production.[43] Short-term randomized trials[105,106,113] and longitudinal observational studies[114,115] have indicated diets rich in vegetables and fruits lower BP and improve other CVD risk factors. Equally as important is the method of preparation of fruits and vegetables. Cooking techniques that preserve nutrient and fiber content without adding unnecessary calories, saturated or *trans* fat, sugar, and salt are recommended by the AHA.[109] Moreover, protein from plant sources as a replacement of some carbohydrate and monounsaturated fat can further lower blood pressure.[106]

Research indicates that blood pressure can be improved by an overall healthy diet that consists of fruits, vegetables, low-fat dairy products, whole grains, poultry, fish, and nuts, and is reduced in fats, red meat, sweets, and sugar-containing beverages, which is consistent with the AHA recommendations. The AHA recommends that individuals consume a variety of fruits, vegetables, and whole grains; choose fat-free and low-fat dairy products, legumes, poultry, and lean meats; and eat oily fish at least twice a week.[109]

A range of 25%–35% of total calories from fat is recommended and endorsed by the AHA, Institute of Medicine, and the National Cholesterol Education Program.[109] The AHA recommends intakes of <7% of energy as saturated fat, <1% of energy as *trans* fat, and <300 mg cholesterol per day.[109] Diets low in saturated fats, *trans* fats, and cholesterol reduce the risk of CVD through their effects on LDL cholesterol levels.[116,117] Beginning January 2006, it became mandatory to list *trans* fat on the labels of foods, enabling consumers to more easily identify and limit their *trans* fat intake. The strongest dietary determinants of elevated LDL cholesterol concentrations are dietary saturated fatty acid and *trans* fatty acid intakes. While saturated fatty acids tend to increase LDL cholesterol levels, *trans* fatty acids have a slightly lower impact on LDL levels.[32] In the United States, the major sources of saturated fat and *trans* fat are animal fats (meat and dairy) and partially hydrogenated fats used in fried and baked products, respectively.

Oily fish is rich in omega-3 polyunsaturated fatty acids [eicosapentaenoic acid (EPA) and docosahexaenoic acid (DHA)]. Studies have indicated that two servings of oily fish per week are associated with a reduced risk of sudden death and death from coronary artery disease in adults.[118,119] Consuming high amounts of fish may, in turn, reduce the amount of foods higher in saturated and *trans* fatty acids consumed.

B. Exercise

To maintain physical and cardiovascular fitness, maintain a healthy weight, and sustain weight loss once achieved, regular physical activity is essential.[120] Regardless of body weight, a physically active lifestyle is necessary to reduce risk of CVD in all individuals.[121] It is estimated that 61% of U.S. adults do not engage in any regular physical activity.[13] Regular physical activity improves blood pressure, lipid profiles, and blood sugar (all of which are cardiovascular risk factors) and lowers the risk of developing other chronic diseases, such as type II diabetes, osteoporosis, obesity, depression, and cancer of the breast and colon.[122] Reducing caloric intake and increasing physical activity to achieve even a modest weight loss can decrease insulin resistance and improve glucose control and the concomitant metabolic abnormalities.[123]

The AHA recommends >30 minutes of physical activity most days of the week for all adults.[109] To lose or maintain weight, >60 minutes of activity most days of the week is recommended. Achieving a physically active lifestyle requires effective time management, with a focus on reducing sedentary activities such as watching television, surfing the Web, and playing computer games.

Once weight loss is achieved, regular daily physical activity has been shown to maintain body weight.[124] Many different weight loss programs have shown some success in reducing body weight in the short term, but little success in maintaining weight loss in the long term. Therefore, investigators are now developing and testing interventions designed specifically to promote weight maintenance.[125–128]

V. CONCLUSIONS

There is no disagreement that overconsumption of calories and a sedentary lifestyle is encouraged by the environment we live in. Experts agree that changes in the environment are a major driving force behind the obesity epidemic.[129] Thus far, it is evident that multiple factors are responsible for the obesity epidemic and that the optimal strategy to impede the epidemic will also be multifactorial.

Regardless of risk level, men and women should increase their consumption of dietary fiber, fruits, vegetables, whole grains, and fish, and decrease their consumption of saturated fat (<7% of energy), *trans*-fat (<1% of energy, cholesterol (<300 mg/d), and sodium (<2.3 g/d). Additionally, the cessation of smoking, an increase in physical activity, and maintaining or reducing body weight to a healthy level should be encouraged for the middle-aged population. Lifestyle modifications such as these can effectively control CVD risk factors and lower CVD risk.

Moreover, the economics of obesity cannot be overlooked. With the obese population's taking more medications for diabetes, hypertension, and elevated cholesterol, overall healthcare costs are directly affected. While obesity and overweight are not the only risk factors for CVD, they can directly or indirectly affect many of the other risk factors. Weight loss programs designed to maintain as well as decrease weight could prove to be beneficial. Governing bodies, nutrition policy makers, educators, and health care professionals need to work together to lessen the proportion of the population that is overweight and obese, which will inevitably affect CVD risk and overall health care cost.

REFERENCES

1. Vuori, I., Andersen, L., Cavill, N., Marti, B. and Sellier, P., Physical activity and cardiovascular disease prevention in the European Union, *The European Heart Network*. Brussels; 1999.
2. Yusuf, S., Reddy, S., Oumpuu, S. and Anand, S., Global burden of cardiovascular disease: Part II: variations in cardiovascular disease by specific ethnic groups and geographic regions and prevention strategies, *Clin. Cardiol.* 104, 2855–2864, 2001.
3. WHO. *Cardiovascular Disease Program: WHO CVD-Risk Management Package for Low- and Medium-Resource Settings*, WHO, Geneva, Switzerland, 2002.

4. American Heart Association/American Stroke Association. Heart Disease and Stroke Statistics. http://www.americanheart.org/downloadable/heart/1166712318459hs_statsinsidetext.pdf. Accessed 11/27/2007.
5. Murray, C. and Lopez, A., Alternative projections of mortality and disability by cause 1990–2020: Global burden of disease study, *Lancet* 349, 1498–1504, 1997.
6. Rosengren, A., Dotevall, A., and Eriksson, H., Optimal risk factors in the population: Prognosis, prevalence, and secular trends; data from Goteborg population studies, *Eur. Heart J.* 22, 136–44, 2001.
7. Stamker, J., Stamler, R., and Neaton, J., Low risk factor profile and long-term cardiovascular and noncardiovascular mortality and life expectancy: Findings from 5 large cohorts of young adult and middle-aged men and women, *JAMA* 282, 2012–8, 1999.
8. Stampfer, M., Hu, F., and Manson, J., Primary prevention of coronary heart disease in women through diet and lifestyle, *New Eng. J. Med.* 343, 16–22, 2000.
9. Bidlack, W., Interrelationships of food, nutrition, diet and health: The national association of state universities and land grant colleges white paper, *J. Am. Coll. Nutr.* 15, 422, 1996.
10. Truesdale, K., Stevens, J., and Cai, J., Nine-year changes in cardiovascular disease risk factors with weight maintenance in the atherosclerosis risk in communities cohort, *Am. J. Epidemiol.* 165, 890–900, 2007.
11. Truesdale, K., Stevens, J., and Lewis, C., Changes in risk factors for cardiovascular disease by baseline weight status in young adults who maintain or gain weight over 15 years: The CARDIA Study, *Int. J. Obes.* 30, 1397–1407, 2006.
12. Szklo, M., Chambless, L., and Folsom, A., Trends in plasma cholesterol levels in the Atherosclerosis Risk in Communities (ARIC) Study, *Prev. Med.* 30, 252–9, 2000.
13. American Heart Association. Heart Disease and Stroke Statistics—2005 Update, http://www.americanheart.org. Accessed 12/2007.
14. Williamson, D., Descriptive epidemiology of body weight and weight change in U. S. adults, *Am. Intern. Med.* 119, 646, 1993.
15. Pilote, L., Dasgupta, K., Guru, V., Humphries, J. M., Norris, C., et al., A comprehensive view of sex-specific issues related to cardiovascular disease, *CMAJ.* 176(6), S1–S44, 2007.
16. U. S. Department of Health and Human Services, National Institutes of Health, National Heart Lung and Blood Institute. Guidelines on overweight and obesity: electronic textbook.
17. Lewis, C., Jacobs, D., and McCreath, H., Weight gain continues in the 1990s: 10-year trends in weight and overweight from the CARDIA Study, *Am. J. Epidemiol.* 151, 1171–1181, 2000.
18. Juhaeri, S. J., Chambless, L., Hyroler, H. A., Rosamond, W., Nieto, F. J., Schreiner, P., et al., Associations between weight gain and incident hypertension in a bi-ethnic cohort: The Atherosclerosis Risk in Communities Study, *Int. J. Obes.* 26(1), 58–64, 2002.
19. Williamson, D., Kahn, H., and Remington, P., The 10-year incidence of overweight and major weight gain in U. S. adults, *Arch. Intern. Med.* 150, 655–672, 1990.
20. Sheehan, T., DuBrava, S., and DeChello, L, Fang, Z., Rates of weight change for black and white Americans over a twenty year period, *Int. J. Obes.* 27, 498–504, 2003.
21. McTigue, K., Garrett, J., and Popkin, B., The natural history of the development of obesity in a cohort of young U. S. adults between 1981 and 1998, *Ann. Intern. Med.* 136, 857–864, 2002.
22. He, Z. and Baker, D., Changes in weight among a nationally representative cohort of adults aged 51–61, 1992 to 2000, *Am. J. Prevent. Med.* 27, 8–15, 2004.
23. Soler, J., Folsom, A., and Kushi, L., Association of body fat distribution with plasma lipids, lipoproteins, apolipoproteins AI and B in postmenopausal women, *J. Clin. Epidemiol.* 41, 1075–1081, 1988.

24. Bass, K., Newschaffer, C., Klag, M., and Bush, T., Plasma lipoprotein levels as predictors of cardiovascular death in women, *Arch. Intern. Med.* 153(19), 2209–16, 1993.
25. Castelli, W., Epidemiology of triglycerides: A view from Framingham, *Am. J. Cardiol.* 70, 3H–9H, 1992.
26. Sharrett, A., Ballantyne, C., Coady S., Heiss, G., Sorlie, P. D., Catellier, D., and Patsch, W., Coronary heart disease prediction from lipoprotein cholesterol levels, triglycerides, lipoprotein(a), apolipoproteins A–I and B, and HDL density subfractions: The Atherosclerosis Risk in Communities (ARIC) Study, *Circulation.* 104(10), 1108–13, 2001.
27. Hokanson, J. and Austin, M., Plasma triglyceride level is a risk factor for cardiovascular disease independent of high-density lipoprotein cholesterol level: A meta-analysis of population-based prospective studies, *J. Cardio. Risk* 3, 213–19, 1996.
28. National Institutes of Health. National Cholesterol Education Program: ATP III guidelines at-a-glance quick desk reference, www.nhlbi.nih.gov/guidelines/cholesterol/atglance.pdf. Accessed 11/ 2007.
29. Centers for Disease Control and Prevention. Trends in cholesterol screening and awareness of high blood cholesterol—United States, 1991–2003, *MMWR Morb. Mortal. Wkly. Rep.* 54, 865–70, 2005.
30. Langille, D., Joffres, M., MacPherson, K., Andreou, P., Kirkland, S., and MacLean, D., Prevalence of risk factors for cardiovascular disease in Canadians 55 to 74 years of age: Results from the Canadian Heart Health Surveys, 1986–1992, *CMAJ.* 161(8 suppl), S3–S9, 1999.
31. Expert Panel on Detection E, and Treatment of High Blood Cholesterol in Adults. Executive summary of the third report of the National Cholesterol Education Program (NCEP) Expert Panel on Detection, Evaluation, and Treatment of High Blood Cholesterol in Adults (Adult Treatment Panel III), *JAMA* 285, 2486–97, 2001.
32. Lichtenstein, A., Ausman, L., Jalbert, S., and Schaefer, E., Effects of different forms of dietary hydrogenated fats on serum lipoprotein cholesterol levels, *New Engl. J. Med.* 340, 1933–40, 1999.
33. Wilson, P. and Grundy, S., The metabolic syndrome: A practical guide to origins and treatment, part II, *Circulation.* 108, 1537–1540, 2003.
34. Castelli, W., Anderson, K., Wilson, P., and Levy, D., Lipids and risk of coronary heart disease. The Framingham Study, *Ann. Epidemiol.* 2(1–2), 23–28, 1992.
35. Gordon, D., Probstfield, J., Garrison. R. J., Neaton, J. D., Castelli, W. P., et al., High-density lipoprotein cholesterol and cardiovascular disease. Four prospective American studies, *Circulation.* 79(1), 8–15, 1989.
36. Bass, K., Newschaffer, C., Klag, M., and Bush, T. L., Plasma lipoprotein levels as predictors of cardiovascular death in women, *Arch. Intern. Med.* 153, 2209–16, 1993.
37. Doll, R. and Peto, R., The causes of cancer: Quantitative estimates of avoidable risk of cancer in the United States today, *J. Natl. Cancer Inst.* 66, 1191, 1981.
38. Cook, A. and Friday, J. Pyramid Servings Intakes in the United States 1999–2002, 1 Day, Agricultural Research Service. Available at http://www.ars.usda.gov/Services/docs.htm?docid=85032005. Accessed 10/08/08.
39. Block, G., Foods contributing to energy intake in the U. S. : Data from NHANES III and NHANES 1999–2000, *J. Food Compos. Anal.* 17, 439–47, 2004.
40. Schulze, M., Manson, J., Ludwig, D., et al., Sugar-sweetened beverages, weight gain, and incidence of type 2 diabetes in young and middle-aged women, *JAMA* 292, 927–34, 2004.
41. Berkey, C., Rockett, H., Field, A., Gillman, M., and Colditz, G., Sugar-added beverages and adolescent weight change, *Obes. Res.* 12, 778–88, 2004.
42. Hu, F. and Willett, W., Optimal diets for prevention of coronary heart disease, *JAMA* 288, 2569–78, 2002.
43. Schneeman, B., Gastrointestinal physiology and functions, *Br. J. Nutr.* 88, S159–S163, 2002.

44. Lewington, S., Clarke, R., Qizilbash, N., Peto, R., and Collins, R., Prospective Studies Collaboration. Age-specific relevance of usual blood pressure to vascular mortality: A meta-analysis of individual data for one million adults in 61 prospective studies *Lance.* 360, 1903–13, 2002.
45. Wang, Y. and Wang Q., The prevalence of prehypertension and hypertension among U. S. adults according to the new joint national committee guidelines: New challenges of the old problem, *Arch. Intern. Med.* 164, 2126–34, 2004.
46. Appel, L., Brands, M., Daniels, S., Karanja, N., Elmer, P. J., and Sacks, F. M., Dietary approaches to prevent and treat hypertension. A scientific statement from the American Heart Association, *Hypertension* 47, 296–308, 2006.
47. Haffner, S., Lehto, S., Ronnemaa, T., Pyorala, K., and Laakso, M., Mortality from coronary heart disease in subjects with type 2 diabetes and in nondiabetic subjects with and without prior myocardial infarction, *New Engl. J. Med.* 339(4), 229–34, 1998.
48. British Heart Foundation. Estimated prevalence of diabetes and numbers of people with diabetes, 2003 and 2005, selected countries, the world. www.heartstats.org/temp/TABsp12.8spwebo6.xls . Accessed 11/2007.
49. Haffner, S., Epidemiology of insulin resistance and its relation to coronary artery disease, *Am. J. Cardiol.* 84, IIJ–4J, 1999.
50. Hu, F., Stampfer, M., Solomon, C., Liu, S., Willett, W. C., Speizer, F. E., et al., The impact of diabetes mellitus on mortality from all causes and coronary heart disease in women: 20 years of follow-up, *Arch. Intern. Med.* 161(14), 1717–23, 2001.
51. Graham, M., Ghali, W., Faris, P., Galbraith, D., Norris, C. M., and Knudtson, M. L., Sex differences in the prognostic importance of diabetes in patients with ischemic heart disease undergoing coronary angiography, *Diabetes Care* 26(11), 3142–47, 2003.
52. Lee, W., Cheung, A., Cape, D., and Zinman, B., Impact of diabetes on coronary artery disease in women and men: A meta-analysis of prospective studies, *Diabetes Care* 23(7), 962–68, 2000.
53. Huxley, R., Barzi, F., and Woodward, M., Excess risk of fatal coronary heart disease associated with diabetes in men and women: Meta-analysis of 27 prospective cohort studies, *Br. Med. J.* 332, 73–8, 2006.
54. Sowers, J., Insulin and insulin-like growth factors in normal and pathologic cardiovascular physiology, *Hypertension.* 29, 691–99,1997.
55. Ridker, P., Hennekens, C., Buring, J., and Rifai, N., C-reactive protein and other markers of inflammation in the prediction of cardiovascular disease in women, *New Engl. J. Med.* 342(12), 836–43, 2000.
56. Danesh, J., Wheeler, J., Hirschfield, G., Eda, S., Eiriksdottir, G., Rumley, A., et al., C-reactive protein and other circulating markers of inflammation in the prediction of coronary heart disease, *New Engl. J. Med.* 350(14), 1387–97, 2004.
57. Khor, L., Muhlestein, J., Carlquist, J., Horne, B. D., Bair, T. L., Maycock, C. A., and Anderson, J. L., Sex- and age-related differences in the prognostic value of C-reactive protein in patients with angiographic coronary artery disease, *Am. J. Med.* 117(9), 657–64, 2004.
58. Muhlestein, J., Horne, B., Carlquist, J., Madsen, T. E., Bair, T. L., Pearson, R. R., and Anderson, J. L., Cytomegalovirus seropositivity and C-reactive protein have independent and combined predictive value for mortality in patients with angiographically demonstrated coronary artery disease, *Circulation.* 102(16), 1917–23 ,2000.
59. Panagiotakos, D., Pitsavos, C., Zeimbekis, A., Chrysohoou, C. and Stefanadis, C., The association between lifestyle–related factors and plasma homocysteine levels in healthy individuals from the "ATTICA" Study, *Int. J. Cardiol.* 98(3), 471–77, 2005.
60. Dalery, K., Lussier-Cacan, S., Selhub, J., Davignon, J., Latour, Y., and Genest, J., Homocysteine and coronary artery disease in French Canadian subjects: Relation with vitamins B12, B6, pyridoxal phosphate, and folate, *Am. J. Cardiol.* 75(16), 1107–11,1995.

61. Eikelboom, J., Lonn, E., Genest, J., Hankey, G., and Yusuf, S., Homocyst(e)ine and cardiovascular disease: A critical review of the epidemiologic evidence, *Ann. Intern. Med.* 131(5), 363–75, 1999.
62. Homocysteine Studies Collaboration. Homocysteine and risk of ischemic heart disease and stroke: A meta-analysis, *JAMA* 88, 2015–22, 2002.
63. Srinivasan, S., Ehnholm, C., Elkasabany, A., and Berenson, G., Influence of apolipoprotein E polymorphism on serum lipids and lipoprotein changes from childhood to adulthood: The Bogalusa Heart Study, *Atherosclerosis.* 143(2), 435–43, 1999.
64. Ballantyne, C., Herd, J., Stein, E. et al., Apolipoprotein E genotypes and response of plasma lipids and progression–regression of coronary atherosclerosis to lipid-lowering drug therapy, *J. Am. Coll. Cardiol.* 36(5), 1572–78, 2000.
65. Schaefer, E., Lamon-Fava, S., Johnson, S., Ordovas, J. M., Schaefer, M. M., Castelli, W. P., and Wilson, P. W., Effects of gender and menopausal status on the association of apolipoprotein E phenotype with plasma lipoprotein levels. Results from the Framingham Offspring Study, *Arterioscler. Thromb.* 14(7), 1105–13, 1994.
66. Danesh, J., Collins, R., Appleby, P. and Peto, R., Association of fibrinogen, C-reactive protein, albumin, or leukocyte count with coronary heart disease: Meta-analyses of prospective studies, *JAMA* 279(18), 1477–82, 1998.
67. Maresca, G., Di Blasio, A., Marchioli, R., and Di Minno, G., Measuring plasma fibrinogen to predict stroke and myocardial infarction: An update, *Arterioscler. Thromb. Vasc. Biol.* 19(6), 1368–77, 1999.
68. Rajecki, M., Pajunen, P., Jousilahti, P., Rasi, V., Vahtera, E., and Salomaa, V., Hemostatic factors as predictors of stroke and cardiovascular diseases: the FINRISK '92 Hemostasis Study, *Blood Coagul. Fibrinolysis* 16(2), 119–24, 2005.
69. Voetsch, B. and Loscalzo, J., Genetics of thrombophilia: Impact on atherogenesis, *Curr. Opin. Lipidol.* 15, 129–43, 2004.
70. Thompson, S., Kienast, J., Pyke, S., Haverkate, F., and van de Loo, J. C. W., Hemostatic factors and the risk of myocardial infarction or sudden death in patients with angina pectoris. European Concerted Action on Thrombosis and Disabilities Angina Pectoris Study Group, *New Engl. J. Med.* 332(10), 635–41, 1995.
71. Hamsten, A., de Faire, U., Walldius, G., Dahlén, G., Szamosi, A., Landou, C. et al., Plasminogen activator inhibitor in plasma: risk factor for recurrent myocardial infarction, *Lancet.* 2, 3–9, 1987.
72. Scarabin, P., Aillaud, M., Amouyel, P., Evans, A., Luc, G., Ferrièras J., et al., Associations of fibrinogen, factor VII and PAI-1 with baseline findings among 10,500 male participants in a prospective study of myocardial infarction—the PRIME Study. Prospective Epidemiological Study of Myocardial Infarction, *Thromb. Haemost.* 80(5), 749–56, 1998.
73. Nordenhem, A., Leander, K., Hallqvist, J., de Faire, U., Sten-Linder, M., and Wiman, B., The complex between tPA and PAI-1: Risk factor for myocardial infarction as studied in the SHEEP project, *Thromb. Res.* 116(3), 223–32,2005.
74. Danesh, J., Collins, R., and Peto, R., Lipoprotein(a) and coronary heart disease. Meta-analysis of prospective studies, *Circulation.* 102, 1082–85, 2000.
75. Solfrizzi, V., Panza, F., Colacicco, A., Capurso, C., D'Introno, A., Torres, F., et al., Relation of lipoprotein(a) as coronary risk factor to type 2 diabetes mellitus and low-density lipoprotein cholesterol in patients ≥65 years of age (The Italian Longitudinal Study on Aging), *Am. J. Cardiol.* 89(7), 825–9, 2002.
76. LaRosa, J., Lipids and cardiovascular disease: do the findings and therapy apply equally to men and women? *Womens Health Issues* 2, 102–11, 1992.
77. Makomaski Illing, E. M., and Kaiserman, M. J., Mortality attributable to tobacco use in Canada and its regions, 1998. *Can. J. Public Health* 2004;95(1):38–44.
78. Mackay, J. and Eriksen, M., The tobacco atlas, www. who. int/tobacco/statistics/tobacco_atlas/en/. Accessed 11/ 2007.

79. Kirkland, S., Greaves, L., and Devichand, P., Gender differences in smoking and self reported indicators of health, *BMC Women's Health* 4, S7, 2004.
80. Watson, J., Scarinci, I., Klesges, R., Murray, D. M., Vander Weg, M., DeBon, M., et al., Relationships among smoking status, ethnicity, socioeconomic indicators, and lifestyle variables in a biracial sample of women, *Prev. Med.* 37(2), 138–47, 2003.
81. Richey Sharrett, A., Coady, S., Folsom, A., Couper, D., Heiss, G., Smoking and diabetes differ in their associations with subclinical atherosclerosis and coronary heart disease—the ARIC Study, *Atherosclerosis* 172(1), 143–9, 2004.
82. Health Canada. Canadian Tobacco Use Monitoring Survey (CTUMS), 2003, wave I. Summary of results, www. hc. sc. gc. ca/hl–vs/tobac–tabac/research–recherche/stat/ctums–esuc/2003/index_e. html. Accessed 11/ 2007.
83. Health Canada. Canadian Tobacco Use Monitoring Survey (CTUMS), 2002, wave I. Summary of results, www. hc. sc. gc. ca/hl–vs/tobac–tabac/research–recherche/stat/ctums–esuc/2002/index_e. html. Accessed 11/ 2007.
84. Bolego, C., Poli, A., and Paoletti, R., Smoking and gender, *Cardiovas. Res.* 53, 568–76, 2002.
85. Newby, D., Wright, R., Labinjoh, C., Ludlam, C. A., Fox, K. A. A., Boon, N. A. and David J. Webb, D. J., Endothelial dysfunction, impaired endogenous fibrinolysis, and cigarette smoking: a mechanism for arterial thrombosis and myocardial infarction, *Circulation* 99(11), 1411–15, 1999.
86. Vorster, H., Fibrinogen and women's health, *Thromb. Haemost.* 95, 137–54, 1999.
87. Hattersley, L., Trends in life expectancy by social class: An update, *Health Stat. Q.* 2, 16–24, 1999.
88. Winkleby, M. and Cubbin, C., Influence of individual and neighborhood socioeconomic status on mortality among black, Mexican-American and white women and men in the United States, *J. Epidemiol. Comm. Health* 57, 444–52, 2003.
89. Thurston, R., Kubzansky, L., Kawachi, I., and Berkman, L., Is the association between socioeconomic position and coronary heart disease stronger in women than in men? *Am. J. Epidemiol.* 162(1), 57–65, 2005.
90. Dunlop, S., Coyte, P., and McIsaac, W., Socio-economic status and the utilization of physicians' services: Results from the Canadian National Population Health Survey, *Soc. Sci. Med.* 51, 123–33, 2000.
91. Alter, D., Naylor, C., Austin, P., and Tu, J., Effects of socioeconomic status on access to invasive cardiac procedures and on mortality after acute myocardial infarction, *New Eng. J. Med.* 341(18), 1359–67, 1999.
92. Colhoun, H., Memingway, H., and Poulter, N., Socio-economic status and blood pressure: An overview analysis, *J. Hum. Hypertens.* 12, 91–110, 1998.
93. Brunner, E., Marmot, M., White, I., O'Brien, J. R., Etherington, M. D., Slavin, B. M., et al., Gender and employment grade differences in blood cholesterol, apolipoproteins and haemostatic factors in the Whitehall II study, *Atherosclerosis* 102(2), 195–207, 1993.
94. Yusuf, S., Hawken, S., Ounpuu, S., Dans, T., Avezum, A., Lanas, F., et al., Effect of potentially modifiable risk factors associated with myocardial infarction in 52 countries (the INTERHEART study): Case-control study, *Lancet* 364(9438), 937–52, 2004.
95. Inaba, A., Thoits, P., Ueno, K., Gove, W., Evenson, R., and Sloan, M., Depression in the United States and Japan: Gender, marital status, and SES patterns, *Soc. Sci. Med.* 61(11), 2280–92, 2005.
96. Mozaffarian, D., Longstreth, W., Lemaitre, R., Manolio, T. A., Kuller, L. H., Burke, G. L., and Siscovick, D. S., Fish consumption and stroke risk in elderly individuals: The cardiovascular health study, *Arch. Intern. Med.* 165, 200–6, 2005.
97. Klag, M., Whelton, P., and Appel, L., Effect of age on the efficacy of blood pressure treatment strategies, *Hypertension* 16, 700–5, 1990.

98. Johnson, C., Rifkind, B., Sempros, C., Carroll, M. D., Bachorik, P. S., Briefel, R. R., et al., Declining serum total cholesterol levels among U. S. adults. The National Health and Nutrition Examination Surveys, *JAMA* 269(23), 3002–8, 1993.
99. Voster, H., Jerling, J., Stevn, K., Badenhorst, C. J., Slazus, W., Venter, C. S., et al., Plasma fibrinogen of black South Africans: The BRISK study, *Public Health Nutr.* 1(3), 169–76, 1998.
100. Krobot, K., Hense, H., Cremer, P., Eberle, E., and Keil, U., Determinants of plasma fibrinogen: Relation to body weight, waist-to-hip ratio, smoking, alcohol, age, and sex. Results from the second MONICA Augsburg survey 1989–1990, *Arterioscler. Thromb.* 12 (7), 780–8, 1992.
101. Kohler, H. and Grant P. Plasminogen-activator inhibitor type I and coronary artery disease, *New Engl. J. Med.* 342, 1792–801, 2000.
102. Kroon, U., Silfverstolpe, G., and Tgborn, L., The effects of transdermal estradiol and oral conjugated estrogens on haemostasis variables, *Thromb. Haemost.* 71, 420–23, 1994.
103. Grancha, S., Estellés, A., Tormo, G., Falco, C., Gilabert, J., España, F. et al., Plasminogen activator inhibitor-1 (PAI-1) promoter 4G/5G genotype and increased PAI-1 circulating levels in postmenopausal women with coronary artery disease, *Thromb. Haemost.* 81(4), 516–21, 1999.
104. Knoops, K., de Groot, L., Kromhout, D., Perrin, A.-E., Moreiras-Varela, O., Menotti, A., and van Staveren, W. A., Mediterranean diet, lifestyle factors, and 10-year mortality in elderly European men and women: The HALE project, *JAMA* 292, 1433–9, 2004.
105. Appel, L., Moore, T., Obarzanek, E., Vollmer, W. M., Svetkey, L. P., et al., Clinical trial of the effects of dietary patterns on blood pressure. DASH Collaborative Research Group, *New Engl. J. Med.* 336, 1117–24, 1997.
106. Appel, L., Sacks, F., Carey, V., Obarzanek, E., Swain, J. F., et al., Effects of protein, monounsaturated fat, and carbohydrate intake on blood pressure and serum lipids: Results of the OmniHeart randomized trial, *JAMA* 294, 2455–64, 2005.
107. Grundy, S., Balady, G., and Criqui, M., Guide to primary prevention of cardiovascular diseases: A statement for healthcare professionals from the Task Force on Risk Reduction. American Heart Association Science Advisory and Coordinating Committee, *Circulation* 95, 2329–31, 1997.
108. Smith, S., Blair, S., and Bonow, R., AHA/ACC Scientific Statement: AHA/ACC guidelines for preventing heart attack and death in patients with atherosclerotic cardiovascular disease: 2001 update, *Circulation* 104, 1577–9, 2001.
109. Lichtenstein, A., Appel, L., Brands, M., Daniels, S., Franch, H. A., et al., Diet and Lifestyle recommendations revision 2006: A scientific statement from the American Heart Association Nutrition Committee, *Circulation* 114, 82–96, 2006.
110. Klein, S., Burke, L., Bray, G., Blair, S., Allison, D. B., Pi-Sunyer, X., et al., Clinical implications of obesity with specific focus on cardiovascular disease: A statement from professionals from the American Heart Association Council on Nutrition, Physical Activity, and Metabolism: Endorsed by the American College of Cardiology Foundation, *Circulation* 110, 2652–67, 2004.
111. Pereira, M., Kartashov, A., Ebbeling, C. B., Van Horn, L., Slattery, M. L., Jacobs, D. R. Jr., and Ludwig, D., Fast-food habits, weight gain, and insulin resistance (the CARDIA study): 15-year prospective analysis, *Lancet* 365, 36–42, 2005.
112. Pereira, M. and Ludwig, D., Dietary fiber and body-weight regulation. Observations and mechanisms, *Pediatr Clin. North Am.* 48, 969–80, 2001.
113. Obarzanek, E., Sacks, F., Vollmer, W., Bray, G. A., Miller, E. R., Effects on blood lipids of a blood pressure-lowering diet: The Dietary Approaches to Stop Hypertension (DASH) trial, *Am. J. Clin. Nutr.* 74, 80–9, 2001.
114. Bazzano, L., Serdula, M., and Liu, S., Dietary intake of fruits and vegetables and risk of cardiovascular disease, *Curr. Atheroscler. Rep.* 5, 492–9, 2003.

115. Hung, H.-C., Joshipura, K. J., Jiang, R., Hu, F. B., Hunter, D., et al., Fruit and vegetable intake and risk of major chronic disease, *J. Natl. Cancer Inst.* 96, 1577–84, 2004.
116. U. S. Department of Agriculture, Agriculture Research Service, Dietary Guidelines Advisory Committee. Report of the dietary guidelines advisory committee on the dietary guidelines for Americans, 2005.
117. Ascherio, A., Katan, M., Zock, P., Stampfer, M., and Willett, W., Trans fatty acids and coronary heart disease, *New Engl. J. Med.* 340, 1994–8, 1999.
118. Kris-Etherton, P., Harris, W., and Appel, L., American Heart Association, Nutrition Committee. Fish consumption, fish oil, omega-3 fatty acids, and cardiovascular disease, *Circulation* 106, 2747–57, 2002.
119. Wang, C., Harris, W. S., Chung, M., Lichtenstein, A. H., Balk, E. M., Kupelnick, B., et al., N-3 fatty acids from fish or fish-oil supplements, but not α-linolenic acid, benefit cardiovascular disease outcomes in primary and secondary-prevention studies: A systematic review, *Am. J. Clin. Nutr.* 84, 5–17, 2006.
120. Fogelholm, M. and Kukkonen-Harjula, K., Does physical activity prevent weight gain—A systematic review, *Obes. Res.* 1, 95–111, 2000.
121. Hill, J., Thompson, H., and Wyatt, H., Weight maintenance: What's missing? *J. Am. Diet. Assoc.* 105, S63–S66, 2005.
122. Maron, B. J., Chaitman, B. R., Ackerman, M. J., Bayés de Luna, A., Corrado, D., et al., Recommendations for physical activity and recreational sports participation for young patients with genetic cardiovascular disease, *Circulation* 109, 2807–16, 2004.
123. Knowler, W. C., Barrett-Connor, E., Fowler, S. E., Hamman, R. F., Lachin, J. M., Walker, E. A., and Nathan, D. M., Reduction in the incidence of type 2 diabetes with lifestyle intervention or metformin, *New Engl. J. Med.* 346, 393–403, 2002.
124. Wing, R. and Phelan, S., Long-term weight loss maintenance, *Am. J. Clin. Nutr.* 82, 222S–225S, 2005.
125. Harvey-Berino, J., Pintauro, S., and Buzzell, P., Does using the Internet facilitate the maintenance of weight loss? *Int. J. Obes. Relat. Metab. Discord.* 26, 1254–60, 2002.
126. Harvey-Berino, J., Pintauro, S., and Gold, E., The feasibility of using Internet support for the maintenance of weight loss, *Behav. Modif.* 26, 103–16, 2002.
127. Kovacs, E., Lejeune, M., and Nijs, I., Effects of green tea on weight maintenance after body-weight loss, *Br. J. Nutr.* 91, 431–7, 2004.
128. Borg, P., Kukkonen-Harjula, K., and Fogelholm, M., Effects of walking or resistance training on weight loss maintenance in obese, middle-aged men: A randomized trial, *Int. J. Obes. Relat. Metab. Discord.* 26, 676–83, 2002.
129. Hill, J., Wyatt, H., Reed, G., and Peters, J. , Obesity and the environment: where do we go from here? *Science.* 299, 853–5, 2003.

17 Cancer

Farid E. Ahmed

CONTENTS

I. INTRODUCTION

This chapter is intended to present in a balanced way the effect of diet (including modulation by sex, age, and race), environmental and occupational factors, physical activity, genetics and epigenetics, gene–environment interactions and immune response on cancers' development, progression, and prevention. More than 10 million people a year are diagnosed with cancer worldwide. With improvements in early detection and treatment, increasing numbers of patients can expect to live at least 5 years after they are diagnosed with cancer. These individuals will join the expanding number of cancer survivors estimated at about 25 million. Cancer is associated with several long-term health and psychological sequelae, and afflicted individuals are at greater risk of developing secondary malignant disease and other conditions such as cardiovascular disease (CVD), diabetes, and osteoporosis, compared with general age- and race-matched populations.[1] Patients with cancer are significantly more likely to die from noncancer causes than are the general population due to cancer treatment, genetic predisposition, or lifestyle factors.[2] Recent reviews and analyses[3,4] found that ~35% of worldwide cancer incidence can be attributed to unhealthy diets, alcohol drinking, smoking, certain infectious conditions, and related factors of obesity and physical inactivity, in addition to environmental and occupational carcinogens. Therefore, it is imperative to understand these factors and implement global interventions to slow this pandemic; otherwise, the incidence is bound to rise, especially in developing countries.[5]

The role of diet in cancer is a major public health issue.[6] Foods associated with a low risk of cancers such as colorectal, breast, prostate, pancreatic, and endometrial are those typically included in the so-called Mediterranean diet (MD), which is also associated with low mortality rates from CVD. Implementing such a diet would involve increasing the consumption of fruits, vegetables, cereals, whole grains, and fish, while reducing the intake of refined carbohydrates and red meat. In addition, olive oil, which is a typical aspect of the MD known for its high levels of monounsaturated fatty acids and as a good source of phytochemicals such as polyphenolic compounds, squalene, and α-tocopherol, should replace saturated fats and ω-3 fatty acids. It has also been inversely related to cancers of the colorectum and breast, and mainly of the upper digestive and respiratory tract systems. Fiber can bind bile acids, which produce carcinogenic metabolites, and fermented fiber produces volatile fatty acids that can protect against colon cancer. It has been hypothesized that the anticancer actions of olive oil may relate to the ability of its monounsaturated fatty acids and oleic acid to regulate carcinogens. In the context of the MD, the benefits associated with the consumption of several functional components may be intensified by certain forms of food preparation. In addition, the practice of more physical activity and the following of other lifestyle habits such as reduced alcohol intake and cessation of smoking contributes to overall improvement in health.[7]

II. CANCERS AND THEIR MODULATION BY DIETARY, ENVIRONMENTAL, OR LIFESTYLE FACTORS

A. Colorectal Cancer

Significant progress has been made over the last decade in identifying factors that modify risk of colorectal cancer (CRC. Large international variation in CRC incidence and mortality rates, and the prominent increases in the incidence of CRC in groups that migrated from low- to high-incidence areas provided important evidence that lifestyle factors influence the development of this malignancy. These observations formed the basis for various hypotheses of lifestyle factors in the etiology of CRC neoplasia, and together with other hypotheses continue to be evaluated.[6]

Epidemiological and experimental evidence that dietary intake is an important etiological factor in colorectal neoplasia is convincing. Study designs used to test the existing hypotheses include: ecological studies, where patterns of consumption and cancer incidence or mortality rates are compared among different populations; case-control (retrospective) studies, where reported past diet as recalled by individuals afflicted with cancer is compared against recall among those without the disease; and prospective (or cohort) studies, where diet is assessed among cancer-free individuals and correlated with subsequent cancer occurrence or mortality. The totality of the data suggests that the Western diet contributes to the causation of ~50% of CRC; however, precisely which specific nutrients, foods, or combination of these are related to the development of CRC is not well known.[3,6]

The role of meat in the etiology of CRC has been contentious. Although some studies have associated consumption of large amounts of red meat with possible increased risk to the distal portion of the large intestine, others did not. The totality of the epidemiologic and experimental evidence support the rational behavior of moderate eating of red meat, mixed with diet containing dairy products, carbohydrates, vegetables, and fruits will not result in increase in CRC risk.[7] The recent population-based Fukuoka case-control Japanese CRC study showed that consumption of red meat (beef/pork and processed meat), total fat, saturated fat, or n-6 polyunsaturated fatty acid (PUFA) showed no clear association with the overall or subsite-specific risk of CRC. There was an almost significant inverse association between n-3 PUFA and the risk of CRC. High intake of fish was found to decrease the risk, particularly for distal colon.[8] Another recent large population-based cohort in women in Norway did not support the hypothesis of a protective effect of fish on CRC risk. An increased risk was, however, found for high consumption of poached lean fish.[9]

In a recent study in Canada, the strongest positive associations between colon cancer risk and increasing total fat intake were observed for proximal colon cancer in men and for distal colon cancer in both men and women. Increased consumption of vegetables, fruit, and whole-grain products did not reduce the risk of colon cancer. A modest reduction in distal colon cancer risk was noted in women who consumed yellow-orange vegetables. Significant positive associations were observed between proximal colon cancer risk in men and consumption of red meat and dairy products, and between distal colon cancer risk in women and total intake of meat and processed meat. Strong associations between bacon intake and both subsites of colon cancer in women were found. When men were compared with women directly by subsite, the results did not show a corresponding association. A significantly reduced risk of distal colon cancer was noted in women only with increasing intake of dairy products and of milk. Among men and women taking vitamin and mineral supplements for more than 5 years, significant inverse associations with colon cancer were most pronounced among women with distal colon cancer. These findings suggest that dietary risk factors for proximal colon cancer may differ from those for distal colon cancer.[10] Discrepancy between findings from cohort and case-control studies regarding total energy intake and colon cancer risk was found, making it impossible to draw any firm conclusions between total caloric intake and risk of CRC.[6]

In a recent Scottish study that looked at the association between various dietary fats and CRC risk, total and trans-monounsaturated fatty acids and palmitic, stearic, and oleic acids were dose-dependently associated with CRC risk, but these effects did not persist after further energy adjustments. Significant dose-dependent reductions in risk were associated with increased consumption of ω-3 PUFA. These associations persisted after including energy with the nutrient-energy-adjusted term or total energy-adjusted fatty acid intake. The observed different effects of various types of fatty acids underlie the importance of type of fat in the etiology and prevention of CRC.[11]

High consumption of fruits and vegetables has been shown to be associated with a decreased risk of CRC. Results of most published studies have shown an inverse association between intake of vegetables and colon cancer, while data for fruit consumption are less compelling.[4,6,7] Mechanisms responsible for the protective effect of fruit and vegetables include inhibition of nitrosamine formation, provision of substrate for making antineoplastic agents, diluting and binding of carcinogens, alteration of hormone metabolism, antioxidant effects, and the induction of detoxification enzymes—such as glutathione S transferases, GSTs—by cruciferous vegetables that is mainly attributed to the degradation products of glucosinolates (e.g., isothiocyanates and indoles).[6] A recent study found an increased risk of CRC for very low intake of total fruits and vegetables by men. Among subgroups of vegetables, green leafy vegetables were associated with a lower risk of CRC for men. Intake of fruits was not related to risk of CRC in men or women.[12] A recent pooled analysis of 14 cohorts found that fruits and vegetables were not strongly associated with colon cancer risk overall, but may be associated with a lower risk of distal colon cancer, particularly among nondrinkers of alcohol and among low consumers of red meat,[13] suggesting that diets plentiful in fruits and vegetables remain important in the benefits attained for other outcomes, including CVD and some other cancers.

The hypothesis that high consumption of dietary fiber reduces the risk of developing CRC was proposed >3 decades ago when it was observed in the 1960s that rural Ugandans consuming a diet rich in dietary fiber had a low rate of CRC. Several plausible pathophysiological processes, including stool bulking with subsequent dilution of colonic luminal carcinogens and production of anticarcinogenic short-chain fatty acids have been proposed to account for the ecologic association.[7] Many epidemiologic studies have examined this hypothesis with mixed conclusions. Earlier case-control studies tended to show a protective association with dietary fibers, whereas initial prospective cohorts did not. Results of adenoma recurrence trials with fiber interventions were generally null. The inconsistencies of findings concerning this association were recently exacerbated by two recent reports from large prospective European studies that showed an inverse relation between dietary fiber intake and CRC risk.[14,15] These results were followed by the findings of pooled prospective cohort studies that showed either no association or, at most, an increased risk only in persons who consumed small amounts of dietary fiber.[16] The association with whole grain was stronger for rectal than for colon cancer. A recent large prospective cohort showed that total dietary intake was not associated with CRC risk, whereas whole-grain consumption was associated with a moderate reduced risk.[17] Therefore, the epidemiologic evidence of a beneficial effect of whole-grain consumption with CRC reduction in risk necessitates further evaluations.

The role of calcium or vitamin D in CRC has been investigated in a variety of studies including animal studies, international correlation studies, case-control and cohort studies, and intervention studies of adenoma recurrence, in addition to human intervention studies on the effect of calcium supplementation on cell proliferation. It has been hypothesized that calcium might reduce colon cancer risk by binding secondary bile acids and ionized fatty acids to form insoluble soaps in the lumen of the colon, thus reducing the proliferative stimulus of these compounds on colon mucosa. Calcium can also directly influence the proliferative activity of the colon mucosa.[18] While results of analytical epidemiological studies for the association between calcium and CRC risk have been inconsistent, data from large cohort studies showed weak, nonsignificant inverse associations with no evidence of dose–response relationship. A meta-analysis of published literature on dairy products that was carried until the year 2002 found an inverse association between CRC and milk intake for cohort but not case-control studies, and no clear association was found between cheese or yogurt intake and CRC risk because data with different intake cut points across studies were combined.[19]

A recent pooled analysis of 10 cohorts in five countries in North America and Europe that included 534,536 individuals of both genders, among whom 4992 developed CRC during 6–12 years of follow-up, using a food frequency questionnaire (FFQ) at baseline, showed that milk consumption was statistically associated with reduced risk for cancers of the distal colon and rectum, although results for most other dairy foods were suggestive of inverse associations. Calcium intake was also inversely associated with risk of CRC, with the inverse association being statistically significant among those in the highest vitamin D intake category, although the difference in associations across vitamin D intake levels was not statistically significant. Fermented food products (e.g., yogurt, cheese) did not show association with CRC risk.[20]

Few epidemiological data have been published on the association between vitamin D and CRC.[6] They tend to show some association between the two, especially in the presence of calcium, lending support to the multiplicative effect of these two nutrients in colorectal carcinogenesis.[21]

The health effects of brewed green tea, consumed mostly in Asia, are attributed to numerous polyphenolic compounds, which represent 30% of dried leaf extract. These compounds include flavonols, flavandiols, flavonoids, and phenolic acids; however, most of the polyphenols found in green tea are monomeric flavan-3-ols, better known as catechins, including: (+)-catechin (C), (-)- epicatechin (EC), (+)-gallocatechin (GC), (-)-epigallocatechin (EGC), (-)-epicatechin gallate (ECG) and (-)-apigallocatechin gallate (EGCG. Among the catechins in green tea, EGCG has received scrutiny because of anticancer properties; the others were less pharmacologically active.[22]

A recent prospective study of Chinese women aged 40 to 70 years showed a significant dose–response relationship for both the amount of green tea consumed and duration in years of its consumption on both colon and rectal cancers, especially for those who consumed tea regularly.[23]

Black tea, most of that which is consumed in Western countries, contains a different kind of polyphenols (e.g., theaflavins and thearubigens as a result of oxidation of polyphenols and tannins), whereas other components are as in green tea;

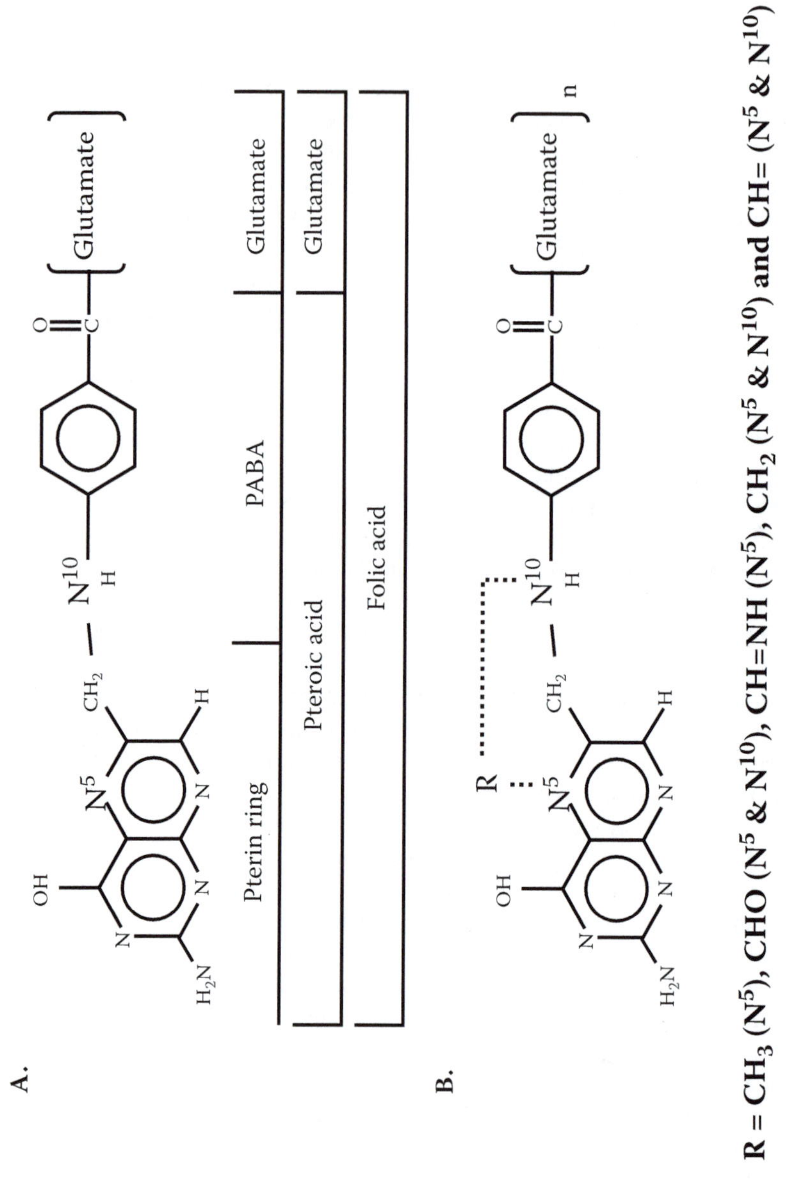

A.

B.

R = CH_3 (N^5), CHO (N^5 & N^{10}), CH=NH (N^5), CH_2 (N^5 & N^{10}) and CH= (N^5 & N^{10})

FIGURE 17.1 Chemical structure of folic acid (A) and folate (B.

these polyphenols seem to have chemopreventive properties, although studies carried in the 1970s and 80s suggested that black tea is mutagenic in *in vitro* assays and tannin-induced tumors in mouse, but not a rat model, when black tea was injected subcutaneously.[25] Although the totality of the evidence does not associate black tea consumption with CRC, the effect of smoking on CRC among tea consumers needs to be researched and clarified.[7]

Folate is a water-soluble B vitamin that is present abundantly in foods such as green leafy vegetables, asparagus, broccoli, Brussels sprouts, citrus fruit, legumes, dry cereals, whole grains, yeast, lima beans, livers and other organic meats (e.g., methyl group diets). Folic acid is the fully oxidized form of this vitamin (Figure 17.1). Except for the *de novo* synthesis by intestinal flora, mammals are unable to synthesize folate; therefore, the daily folate requirement must be obtained from dietary or supplemental sources. The Recommended Dietary Allowance (RDA) for both men and women in North America is 400 μg/day of dietary folate equivalents (DFEs). Folate deficiency appears to play an important role ion the pathogenesis of several disorders in humans including atherosclerosis, neural tube defects (NTD) and other congenital defects, adverse pregnancy outcomes, neuropsychiatric and cognitive disorders, and cancer.[26] Evidence for a protective effect of folate supplementation on NTD led the U.S. Public Health Service in 1992 to recommend that all women who are of reproductive age or capable of becoming pregnant to consume daily 400 μg of folic acid from supplements or fortified foods in conjunction with consumption of folate-rich foods. This recommendation was followed by the U.S. Food and Drug Administration to issue a regulation in 1996 requiring that all flour and uncooked cereal-grain products in the United States be fortified with folic acid (140 μg/100 g) by January 1998 (28) to provide on average 100 μg additional folic/day, with only a very small proportion of the population receiving >1 mg.[29] Higher supplemental levels of folic acid (1–5 mg/day) are routinely provided to certain subgroups of patients who are taking antifolate-based medications (methotrexate for rheumatoid arthritis, psoriasis, or Crohn's disease; sulfasalazine for ulcerative colitis) to minimize or prevent adverse effects relating to folate depletion; even higher supplemental levels in the range of 5–15 mg/day and sometimes up to 40–50 mg/day are given to patients with chronic renal failure on dialysis and renal transplant patients who are often hyperhomocysteinemic and are at high risk of developing premature atherosclerotic complications.[29]

The concept of a dual modulatory role of folate in carcinogenesis proposes that its deficiency enhances, whereas its supplementation reduces the risk of neoplastic transformation. Folate is an essential cofactor for the *de novo* biosynthesis of purines and thymidylate, and in this role folate plays an important role in DNA synthesis and replication. Consequently, folate deficiency in tissues with rapidly replicating cells results in ineffective DNA synthesis. In neoplastic cells where DNA replication and cell divisions are occurring at an accelerated rate, interruption of folate metabolism causes ineffective DNA synthesis, resulting in inhibition of tumor growth, which has been the basis for cancer chemotherapy using a number of antifolate agents (e.g., methotrexate and 5-flurouracil).[30] Furthermore, folate deficiency has been shown to induce regression and suppress progression of preexisting neoplasms in experimental models.[31] In contrast, folate deficiency in normal tissues appears to predispose them to neoplastic transformation and folate supplementation suppresses the development of tumors in normal tissue.[29] Epidemiologic studies collectively suggest an inverse association (in some case dose-dependent) between folate status (measured by either folate dietary/supplemental intake, or its blood levels) and the risk of several malignancies, including cancers of the colorectum, oropharynx, esophagus, stomach, pancreas, lungs, cervix, ovary, breast, neuroblastoma or leukemia.[30] Currently, it is unknown what effect folate deficiency and supplementation on the progression of early precursor or preneoplastic lesions of CRC (e.g., aberrant crypt foci, ACF) has on adenoma and to fully developed cancer. The mechanisms by which folate exerts dual modulatory effects on carcinogenesis, depending on the timing and dose of folate intervention, relate to its essential role in one carbon transfer reactions involved in DNA synthesis and biological methylation reactions.[29] Overall, inverse associations with CRC have been shown whether assessing diet or blood; studies of adenoma prevalence have also shown an association.[6,7]

Currently available evidence indicates that folate supplementation appears to be able to reverse preexisting genomic DNA hypomethylation and to increase the extent of genomic DNA methylation above the preexisting level.[32] Therefore, prevention or reversal of genomic DNA hypomethylation may be a mechanism by which folate supplementation suppresses neoplastic transformation in the colorectum, although it does not seem that genomic DA hypomethylation in the colorectum is a mechanism by which folate deficiency enhances colorectal carcinogenesis.[32] Because of lack of compelling evidence on the potential tumor-promoting effect, routine folic acid supplementation should not be recommended currently as a chemopreventive measure for CRC.

Additional evidence of a role for folate is that inherited variation in the activity of methylenetetrahydrofolate reductase (MTHFR), a critical enzyme in the production of the form of folate that supplies the methyl group for methionine synthesis, influence risk of colon cancer. In this gene-nutrient interaction pathway,[35] key nutrient and nonnutrient components are involved. Different endogenous forms of folate, 5-methyltetrahydrofolate and 5,10-methylenetetrahydrofolate are essential for DNA methylation and DNA synthesis, respectively. When levels of 5,10-methylene-tetrahydrofolate, which is required to convert deoxyuridylate to thymidylate, are low, misincorporation of uracil for thymidine may occur during DNA synthesis, possibly increasing spontaneous mutation rates, sensitivity to DNA-damaging agents, frequency of chromosomal aberrations, or errors in DNA replication. Folate deficiency is related to massive incorporation of uracil into DNA and to increased chromosomal breaks, and these abnormalities are reversed by folic acid supplementation.[36] When methionine intake is low, levels of S-adenosylmethionine decrease, which stimulates MTHFR to convert 5,10-methylenetetrahydrofolate to 5-methyltetrahydrofolate. Homocysteine is methylated by 5-methyltetrahydrofolate to form methionine. Low production of methionine may occur by insufficient folate levels, which can in turn result in a low supply of methyl groups for DNA methylation. DNA hypomethylation is among the earliest events observed in colon carcinogenesis;[32] however, it is unclear whether this process directly influences the carcinogenic process. Additional micronutrients involved in the DNA methylation process include vitamins B_6 and B_{12}. Furthermore, since alcohol is known to influence folate metabolism and methyl group availability,[6] its interaction with key micronutrients needs to be considered in this process.[37] Although folic acid is a key nutrient in CRC, much work is needed to identify specific key pathways of this process. Whether folate has a beneficial effect on CRC will be answered when the results of ongoing intervention trials are completed and reported.[38]

Diet alone is not an indicator of anyone's colorectal cancer risk. Other factors such as family history of colorectal or other cancers and age have an impact on whether a person will develop CRC. Lifestyle also contributes to one's CRC risk as well as to other health problems. For instance, persons with high cigarette use and alcohol consumption are more likely to have health problems including cancer and CVD. Those who are obese and those who have little or no physical activity are also at higher risk of health disorders, including cancer. A study that explored key lifestyle factors to prevent cancer using data from several other studies found that weekly vigorous exercise dropped the risk of colon cancer. A diet high in fiber foods and small amounts of meat also seemed to lower the risk of colon cancer.[39] A large number of epidemiological studies have investigated the association between physical activity and CRC, and the evidence for an inverse association was considered conclusive by the International Agency for Research in Cancer (IARC) in 2002.[40] A recent study also found that there is a risk for colonic polyps associated with high cholesterol levels.[41] However, another cohort that investigated the effects of occupational activity and leisure time activity on incident colon cancer risk in a Danish middle-aged population did not support the evidence of an inverse association between colon cancer risk and occupational activity or leisure time activity. In spite of this, avoiding a sedentary lifestyle by participating in different activities may reduce CRC risk.[42]

In a study that compared CRC in African Americans (AA) to Native Americans (NA), the higher CRC risk and mucosal proliferation rates observed in AA compared with NA were associated with higher dietary intakes of animal products and higher colonic populations of potentially toxic hydrogen and secondary bile-salt producing bacteria, giving support to the hypothesis that CRC risk is determined by interaction between the external (dietary) and internal (bacterial) environments.[43]

B. Breast Cancer

Breast cancer is the most commonly diagnosed cancer and the second most common cause of cancer mortality among women in the United States. Estimates indicate that there are at least 2.4 million women who are breast cancer survivors in America. Among these women, there is particular concern about the long-term risk of recurrence.[44] Changes in lifestyle habits such as diet have been proposed to modify risks. Results of observational epidemiologic studies on associations of dietary patterns high in fruits and vegetables, low in fat or both with risk of recurrence or survival are inconsistent. Although firm conclusions about the potential benefits of such dietary patterns from the results of those studies have not been established, a growing body of evidence is emerging from randomized clinical trials designed specifically to examine the effects of dietary interventions on breast cancer prognosis.[45]

Results of the Women's Healthy Eating and Living (WHEL) Study, a randomized multicenter controlled trial designed to assess whether an intensive dietary intervention aimed at increasing fruits to 3 servings/d, vegetables to 5 servings/d and fiber to 30 g/d, and decreasing fat intake to 15–20% of total calories would reduce the risk of recurrence, new primary invasive breast cancer, or mortality among survivors of early stage breast cancer. After an average follow-up period of 7.3 years, there were no differences in the risk of recurrence or incidence of a new primary breast cancer, or in the risk of overall mortality between the two groups. Similarly, there were no between-group prognostic differences according to baseline demographic characteristics, including body mass index, or clinical characteristics, including tumor stage and hormone receptor status, implying that a diet high in vegetables, fruits, and fibers, and low in fat did not reduce additional breast cancer events on mortality during the 7.3-year follow-up period. Furthermore, the intervention showed no benefit for women whose diet at baseline was low in fruits, vegetables, or fiber, or high in fat.[46]

Another randomized clinical trial, the Women's Intervention Nutrition Study (WINS), which enrolled 2437 women within 1 year of diagnosis of early stage breast cancer, designed specifically to assess whether a low-fat diet (15% of total calories) affects breast cancer recurrence or survival, gave results different from the WHEL study. Interim results showed a significant benefit on the hazard ratio or relapse-free survival after a median of 5 years of follow-up among women randomized to the low-fat dietary intervention group compared with the control group, which received minimal dietary guideline information.[47] Results of an exploratory analysis suggested that the beneficial effect of the low-fat intervention might be confined to women with estrogen and progesterone receptor-negative breast cancers. While there is debate regarding the differential effects of the low-fat intervention according to hormone receptor status and whether this difference could be explained by variation in the hazard rates for recurrences of hormone receptor-positive *versus* negative breast cancer according to length of follow-up,[84] a recent update and analysis of WINS data based on 8 years of follow-up demonstrated similar benefits in the low-fat diet group.[49] Available controversial evidence, however, based on large prospective cohorts[50–53] and meta-analysis[54] does not support the view that dietary fat decreases a woman's risk of developing cancer during postmenopausal years, although intake may be associated with higher risks of breast cancer for specific population subgroups such as menopausal hormone users or younger women.[40,55]

Exploratory analyses suggested a differential effect of the dietary intervention based on hormonal receptor status such that there was a stronger effect for dietary fat reduction on breast cancer recurrence in women with hormone receptor-negative cancers than in women with hormone receptor-positive cancers. When compared with estrogen receptor (ER)-negative status, a positive ER status was shown to be associated with a lower peak hazard of recurrence in the first 5 years, but a higher hazard of recurrence from years 5–12. This means that the ER-negative recurrences occur more frequently in early follow-up and ER-positive recurrences occur more frequently in later follow-ups. Because more recurrences are observed in ER-positive patients between 5 and 12 years, it seems possible that the differential effect of the dietary intervention on hormonal receptor status may be reduced after longer follow-up of these patients.[56] Therefore, evidence is insufficient to recommend for or against reduction in dietary fat to reduce risk of this cancer, although from a prevention perspective, interventions to control the amount of body fat (e.g., promotion of exercise and caloric restraint) are likely to have a greater impact on breast cancer incidence than a reduction in fat intake.

A key issue regarding conflicting results from the WHEL and WINS regarding the potential benefits of dietary modifications on long-term breast cancer prognosis is the difference in energy balance that was achieved between WINS and WHEL study participants. In WINS, over the 5-year follow-up, there was a continuous increase in the difference in self-reported total energy intake between the intervention and comparison groups. Consequently, women randomized to the low-fat intervention experienced significant weight loss, with a 6-lb (2.7 kg) weight difference between intervention and control women at 5 years.[47] Conversely, in the WHEL Study, self-reported total energy intake decreased to a comparable extent in both the intervention and comparison groups through 6 years of follow-up, and both groups experienced small weight gains (i.e., 0.6 and 0.4 kg, respectively).[57] It is unclear whether the difference in energy balance, as reflected by weight change, partly accounts for the beneficial effects of the intervention on survival observed in WINS and no intervention effects as observed in the WHEL Study. Taken together, these data support findings from observational studies suggesting that a high level of obesity, weight gain, or both after diagnosis is adversely associated with breast cancer disease-free survival and overall survival.[58]

Other related considerations raised by the results of the WHEL study include adherence to the intended dietary modification and validity of collected data. It is unclear whether the lack of adherence to the intervention goal for fat reduction explains any of the null findings of the study. The validity of some of the composites of the self-reported dietary data was also questioned because of inconsistencies in decreased caloric intake, without a corollary decrease in body weight.[45] Energy balance appears to play a crucial role in breast cancer. Being overweight is associated with a lower risk before menopause while increasing the risk of cancer after menopause. Regular exercise and avoidance of weight gain during adult life is beneficial to both overall health and prevention of postmenopausal breast cancer. For women in midlife or later who are already overweight, weight loss is desirable. Because of inconsistencies, it is not possible now to establish dietary recommendations for improving long-term prognosis for early stage breast cancer survivors.

It should be noted that bias in data reporting may be both random and nonrandom, and may be found with simpler as well as more advanced dietary instruments. A random bias will contribute to obscure relations between diet and breast cancer, whereas a systematic bias may obscure or aggravate such associations. Underreporting of nonprotein energy has been found to be substantial, particularly among those who are obese or have high dietary intakes. Such a nonrandom bias on the group level would tend to aggravate associations between dietary nonprotein diet and disease. Whether the net result of the random and nonrandom bias aggravates or obscures relations depends on the relative magnitude of the two.[59]

Adverse metabolic responses to high carbohydrate intake are at least in part mediated through insulin and insulin-like growth factors (IGF), which can in turn stimulate cancer growth.[38] These effects may theoretically be stronger in premenopausal women for whom nonestrogen growth factors may be more important, and in overweight women who may be insulin resistant and therefore more susceptible to the effects of rapidly absorbed carbohydrates. Women with type 2 diabetes who are chronically exposed to high insulin may have 10% to 20% higher risk of breast cancer. Carbohydrates and their quality as measured by glycemic index (GI) and glycemic load have been positively associated with breast cancer in some case-control studies. Yet, no overall association between carbohydrates or carbohydrate quality and breast cancer risk has been reported in prospective studies of adult diet.[61] Reported associations between carbohydrate quality and breast cancer according to tumor type, BMI, menopausal status, and physical activity need to be confirmed.

The association among carbohydrate and fiber intake and breast cancer has been less studied than the fat intake and breast cancer. A consistent inverse association between dietary fiber intake (from whole grains and raw vegetables) and breast cancer has been reported in case-control but not cohort studies.[62] Dietary fat promotes intestinal reabsorption of estrogens by enhancement of deconjugating enzyme activity, whereas intraluminal fiber retards the process. Further evidence appears in research comparing vegetarians with omnivores wherein urinary estrogen levels are higher in omnivores than vegetarians, and conversely fecal estrogens are higher in vegetarians than omnivores. Also, breast cancer incidence rates are lower in lifelong vegetarians than in omnivores.[63] In an intervention study that combined effects of dietary fat and fiber, no evidence supports the concept that a low-fat, high-fiber diet modifies serum hormone concentrations; reduction in available hormones in circulating blood would in turn reduce the risk of breast cancer.[64]

To date, a fairly consistent pattern of lower energy expenditure and higher hormone concentrations in AA girls and premenopausal women compared with non-Hispanic white girls and women has been shown, whereas data on energy expenditure in Hispanic whites and Asians have not been published. Given the secular trends in obesity and in ages at onset of puberty and menarche as well as ethnic group differences in energy expenditure, it is unknown whether energy expenditure is set *in utero*, and if so, it is not known how that programming influences prevention research. Identification of the intensity of physical activity to reduce breast cancer risk may require an assessment of a woman's nutritional status at birth.[65] Thus, fetal programming of reproductive function (indicated by responsiveness of steroid hormone levels to intensity of physical activity in the reproductive years), dietary intervention, energy expenditure and weight loss are factors to consider in a program aimed at cancer prevention.

Free serum estrogen E_2 levels vary over the menstrual cycle by level of physical activity in women who differ by body fatness or ponderal index at birth.[65] High rates of small for gestational age (SGA), i.e., <10% of gender-specific birth weight-for-gestation age, but greater chances of survival within weight-for-gestation groups and lower energy expenditure in AA than non-Hispanic white girls support the possibility that AA girls are born with a lower energy expenditure than non-Hispanic white girls. Similar data are not available for Hispanics and Asians in the United States. Recent data show that catch-up growth in the first 2 years of life among those born SGA influences age at puberty and menarche.[66] These issues raise the question of whether dietary interventions should be tailored for prevention by early life growth trajectories coupled with physical activity to enhance efficacy, or whether to refine selection of participants in future dietary trials, for example, to gene polymorphism for LDL-C in AAs that are suppressed with increasing dietary cholesterol intake to tailor prevention modalities.[67] The role of molecular markers during specific windows of life course such as the gene polymorphism in cytochrome P450 that vary by ethnic group and early pubertal development are currently being explored in a large study of young AA and Mexican American girls.[62] The challenge would be to figure a way to tailor interventions at puberty (and therefore greater cumulative life exposure to hormones) for various ethnic groups. At the same time, new tools are needed for dietary and physical activity assessment to forecast prevention and intervention modalities later in life as other windows for modification of hormonal influence on breast cancer risk arises. It is clear from the limited epidemiologic evidence that diet in early life may matter, most possibly due to increased mammary susceptibility to carcinogens.[61]

Alcohol consumption monotonically increases risk of breast cancer; each additional 10 g of alcohol (~1 drink) consumed daily corresponds to a 9% increase in breast cancer risk, and the risk increases with increasing categories of alcohol, as consumption of ≥30g/day of alcohol was significantly associated with a 43% increase in risk.[68] In an updated analysis of the National Health Service (NHS) with 5346 cases, alcohol intake as low as half a drink daily associated with a variety of alcoholic beverages and drinking patterns was significantly associated with breast cancer risk.[69] Estrogen levels increase significantly with consumption of one or two alcoholic drinks daily, suggesting a potential mechanism through which alcohol may increase the risk of breast cancer. Using data from 274,688 women participating in the European Prospective Investigation into Cancer and Nutrition (EPIC) supports previous findings that recent alcohol intake increases the risk of breast cancer.[70]

High intake of folic acid has consistently been shown to minimize the excess risk of breast cancer associated with regular alcohol consumption, especially for postmenopausal breast cancer cases.[71] Analyses of plasma folic acid levels confirm this mitigating effect, which is strongest in women who consume at least one drink daily.[72] The public health implications of the positive association between any alcohol consumption and breast cancer are complicated by the protective effect of moderate alcohol consumption on CVD and the overall reduction in total mortality. Women who consume alcohol regularly may benefit from a multivitamin containing folate to lessen their risk of breast cancer.[71]

The results of case-control studies on the effect of soy intake on breast cancer risk have been mixed. A recent meta-analysis of 12 case-control and six cohort studies showed a modest inverse association between high soy intake and breast cancer risk.[74] However, the inconsistencies among studies, coupled with the potentially adverse estrogenic effects of soy components[75] makes it now difficult to make overall recommendations regarding soy intake.

Although no significant association between a diet high in fruit and vegetables, whole grains and low-fat dairy products (prudent diet) or a diet high in refined grains, processed meat, high-fat dairy and desserts (Western diet) was observed in relation to overall risk of breast cancer,[76] a prudent diet containing fruits and vegetables in particular, may protect against ER-negative tumors after menopause, and among postmenopausal smokers a Western diet may increase breast cancer risk.[61] Neither fruit nor vegetable consumption in adulthood seems to protect against overall breast cancer. The Pooling Project analysis showed no effect of adult consumption of fruit and vegetables on breast cancer incidence.[77] This lack of association was recently confirmed in an EPIC cohort of 10 European countries.[78]

Dairy products were not associated with breast cancer incidence in the Pooling Project.[79] In a prospective analysis from the NHS, no association was seen among postmenopausal women, but was observed among premenopausal women who consumed dairy products once a day compared with women who consumed them less than three times a month.[80] Both calcium and vitamin D were inversely related to risk of postmenopausal breast cancer; the strong correlation between these nutrients precluded distinguishing their effect.[81] A large prospective study that evaluated the association between vitamin D intake and breast cancer risk in 34,321 postmenopausal women showed strong association with intake of >800 IU/day of vitamin D in the first 5 years after baseline dietary assessment.[82] In another prospective study, dietary calcium and other components of dairy products were inversely related to risk of postmenopausal breast cancer, especially among women with ER-positive tumors.[83]

Retrospective data seem to suggest that elevated serum carotenoids are associated with lower risk of breast cancer,[61] but prospective studies have not found significant overall associations among vitamins E and C, selenium, or coffee on breast cancer risk.[84]

Among the prospective epidemiologic studies conducted on gene–diet interactions and breast cancer incidence, today there is no association that is consistent, strong, and statistically significant, except for alcohol intake, overweight, and weight gain for postmenopausal breast cancer in women. The apparent lack of association between diet and breast cancer incidence may reflect a true absence of an association, or may be due to measurement error exceeding the variation in the diet studied, lack of sufficient follow-up, or focus on an age range of low susceptibility. The risk of breast cancer can be rationally reduced by avoidance of weight gain in adulthood and limiting alcohol consumption.[85]

Findings of significant differences in physical activity levels based on demographic characteristics suggest the importance of promoting physical activity, particularly among breast cancer survivors of ethnic minority or lower educational levels.[86] Beneficial health effects on breast cancer survival were seen following combination of a physically active lifestyle with high vegetable and fruit intake.[57] Data indicate that several aspects of physical activity reduce risk of breast cancer in a dose-dependent manner. Physical activity appears to be most important for women who are postmenopausal and have not recently been exposed to HRT. While lifetime activity is important, activity close to the time of diagnosis also appears to be important, suggesting that even if women have not previously been active, they might well benefit from increasing physical activity not only for cardiovascular fitness, but also to reduce risk of breast cancer. These associations appear to be important for both Hispanic/American Indians and non-Hispanic white women living in the southwestern United States and for women regardless of their body weight.[87] Increasing physical activity to 30–60 minutes per day may be a good recommendation for the general population.

C. Head and Neck Cancers

Head and Neck (H&N) cancers include cancers of the tongue oropharynx, floor of the mouth, hard/soft palate, buccal mucosa, gum, tonsil, tonsilar pillar, larynx, and oropharyngeal wall. Almost 40,000 cases and 200,000 deaths are attributed worldwide to oral and oropharyngeal cancers, with approximately 58% cases identified in the southern tier of Asia.[88] Indeed, oral cancer is quite high in Asia, with a general increase of about eightfold across central and east Asia. Fewer than 50% of cases may be expected to survive more than 5 years, with poorer survival expected for patients with regional or advanced disease, or for those who experience cancer recurrences after treatment.[89] Most H&N cancers are staged as regional disease, and localized therapy has limited effects on nearby tissue. This is consistent with the concept of a "field cancerization effect"[90] as genetic damage throughout the oropharyngeal cavity induced by tobacco and related products lead to a second lesion. Overall, 10–30% of patients will be diagnosed with a second primary tumor, perhaps exceeding that of cancer at any other body site, and about 4% of patients with H&N cancer who receive curative treatment will be diagnosed with a second primary each year.[91]

A prudent diet, that is low in calories, monounsaturated fats, or red/processed meat should be avoided, together with increased consumption of fruits, vegetables, and cereals rich in micronutrients and fibers in order to reduce the risks of H&N cancer.[92] In a study that evaluated the relation between laryngeal carcinoma in Uruguayan men and dietary patterns, drinking pattern was directly associated with risk of laryngeal carcinoma, western patterns displayed a significant increase in risk, whereas healthy patterns were protective. Moreover, most dietary patterns were associated with supraglottic cancer, supporting a possible etiological difference between supraglottic and glottic carcinomas.[93] In a prospective study that investigated the relation between H&N cancers and alcohol consumption in the NIH-AARP Diet and Health Study, drinking >three alcoholic beverages per day was associated with increased risk in men and women, but consumption of up to one drink per day may be associated with reduced risk relative to nondrinking.[94]

Cancers of the H&N impose a tremendous health burden, particularly among communities with high tobacco and alcohol, paan, or betel use. Observational epidemiology and basic research studies provide the framework necessary to develop a highly focused diet abundant in cruciferous vegetables rich in isothiocyanates and indoles (believed to increase carcinogen metabolism, induce apoptosis, and reduce the risk of developing a primary H&N tumor. These studies characterize investigated populations and permit comprehensive dietary assessment and other measurements relevant to disease progression. Moreover, buccal cells and tissues from the oral cavity are relatively simple to procure, and clinical outcomes such as a secondary primary may be combined with biochemical and cellular biomarker analyses to investigate the mechanisms of action systematically and within target tissue. This focused approach may reveal an acceptable and low cost option to reduce the risk of H&N cancer.[95]

D. Gastric Cancer

In 2002, gastric cancer was the second most frequent cause of cancer deaths worldwide and the fourth most common cancer, with an estimated 650,000 deaths and 880,000 new cases per year. Almost two-thirds of these new cases occurred in developing countries. In Japan, gastric cancer accounted for 51,000 deaths in 2004, or 16% of all cancer deaths, with a total of 13,000 new cases detected in 2000, or 19% of all incident cancers.[97] In the United States[98] and Europe,[99] gastric cancer used to be one of the most common cancers; however, mortality rates have fallen dramatically over the last 50 years in all Western countries without any specific intervention taken to eradicate the bacterium *Helicobacter pylori* infection known to be a risk factor for gastric cancer development, but not by itself a sufficient cause for its development,[100] and gastric cancer is now less common. This worldwide decline in incidence is likely attributed to the spread of refrigeration, the use of which would inversely correlate with salting and other salt-based methods of preservation such as curing and smoking, and with the overall volume of salt in the diet.[4]

Substantial evidence from ecological, case-control, and cohort studies strongly suggests that the risk may be increased with a high intake of various traditional salt-preserved foods and salt per se, and decreased with a high intake of fruits and vegetables, particularly fruits. However, it remains unclear which constituents in fruit and vegetables play a significant role in gastric cancer prevention,[101] among them vitamin C is a plausible candidate that is supported by a relatively large body of epidemiological evidence, and may protect against the progression against mucosal atrophy.[102] Consumption of green tea, rich in antioxidant polyphenols (catechins) such as EGCG, together with quitting smoking, is possibly associated with a decreased risk of gastric cancer,[103] although the protective effects have been for the most part identified in Japanese women, most of whom are nonsmokers.[101] A large prospective EPIC-EURGAST study of ~520,000 participants aged 35–70 years showed that a higher socioeconomic position was associated with a reduced risk of gastric adenocarcinoma, which was strongest for cardia cancer or intestinal histological subtype, suggesting different risk profiles according to educational levels. These effects appear to be explained only partially by established risk factors.[104]

E. Lung Cancer

Tobacco smoking was identified as the single most powerful cause of the lung cancer epidemic.[105] Associations between other factors and lung cancer risk were found, including workplace agents (e.g., asbestos, arsenic, chromium, nickel, and radon), environmental (positive smoking, indoor radon, heavy air pollution), lifestyle and behavioral (physical activity, diet), reproductive, genetic and epigenetic,[106] socioeconomic, and other factors.[107] While smoking is known to be closely associated with less healthful nutrition habits, the associations between dietary factors and lung cancer are likely to be very weak in comparison with smoking. A hospital-based case-control study in Prague, Czech Republic, involving 569 female lung cancer patients and 2120 control subjects that investigated the differences in the impact of diet and physical exercise on lung cancer risk in female nonsmokers versus smokers, found that diet and physical exercise are important factors contributing to variation in risk among women. Their importance seemed to vary in relation to status of smoking, the dominant factor in the etiology of lung cancer. A protective effect was observed among nonsmoking women frequently drinking black tea. Among smoking women, protective effects appeared for milk/dairy products, vegetables, apples, and physical exercise, while the inverse statistical association for wine was not significant. The observed interactions (effect modifications) of the impact of some dietary items upon lung cancer risk in women at different levels of the smoking habit deserve further investigation.[108]

In an EPIC study conducted between 1992 and 2000 on 478,590 individuals to investigate the association of fruit and vegetable consumption and lung cancer incidence, a significant inverse association between vegetable consumption and lung cancer incidence in smokers was ascertained.[109] A recent ongoing case-control study in Houston, Texas, of 1676 incident lung cancer cases and 1676 matched health controls, dietary zinc and copper intakes were associated with reduced risk of lung cancer.[110] Given the known limitations of case-control studies, these findings must be interpreted with caution and warrant further investigation.

A recent case-control in Galicia, Spain, with 295 cases and 322 controls, studied the association of meat and fish consumption with risk of lung cancer. While total meat consumption was found to be a protective factor for lung cancer, its frequency of consumption was very high among the participants. On the other hand, substantially lower consumption frequencies of fish would appear to increase risk of lung cancer regardless of the type of fish.[111] Because of these unexpected findings, results need to be reinvestigated in a prospect cohort setting.

F. Ovarian Cancer

Long known as the "silent killer," ovarian cancer, which is the second most common gynecological malignancy and the most deadly in the United States, could be recognized by a vigilant gynecologist in spite of its subtle syndromes. This year, 21,000 women are expected to be diagnosed with the cancer, and 15,000 will die.[112] In a cohort of 97,275 eligible women in the California Teacher Study who completed a baseline dietary assessment in 1995–1996 to study the relation between diet and risk of ovarian cancer, 280 women had developed invasive or borderline ovarian cancer by December 31, 2003. Intakes of isoflavones were associated with lower risk of ovarian cancer. On the other hand, intake of isothiocyanates or foods high in isothiocyanates was not associated with ovarian cancer risk, nor was intake of micronutrients, antioxidant vitamins, or other micronutrients. Although dietary consumption of isoflavones may be associated with decreased ovarian cancer risk, most dietary factors are unlikely to play a major role in ovarian cancer development.[113] However, a case-control study conducted in China during 1999–2000 on 254 cases and 652 age-matched controls to investigate whether the intake of α-carotene, β-carotene, β-cryptoxanthin, lutein, zeaxanthin, and lycopene is inversely associated with ovarian cancer risk, found that higher intake of these carotenoids can reduce the risk of epithelial ovarian cancer.[114]

A recent case-control study that investigated the relationship between ovarian cancer risk and calcium, lactose, vitamin D, and dairy products found no statistically significant inverse association between total calcium intake and ovarian cancer, but found an inverse association between dietary calcium intake and ovarian cancer. When considered alone, supplemental calcium was not associated with risk of ovarian cancer. This finding may reflect the fact that calcium from dietary sources is more bioavailable than calcium from supplements and therefore may have a stronger effect on ovarian carcinogenesis.[115] These results for dietary calcium are consistent with two case-control studies[116,117] and inconsistent with a prospective study[118] that found a weak but nonsignificant association. No statistically significant relations were found for consumption of specific dairy foods, lactose, or vitamin D with ovarian cancer risk. The possibility of a decreased risk of ovarian cancer for dietary calcium merits further evaluation.[115]

A Japan Collaborative Cohort (JACC) Study established in 1988–1990 that consisted of 46,465 men and 64,327 women observed until the end of 2003 found that high intakes of dried or salted fish and Chinese pickled/fermented cabbage were potential risk factors for ovarian cancer death. In contrast, however, a high intake of soy bean curd (tofu) might have preventive effects against the risk.[119] Recently, a prospective study of 40,000 postmenopausal women aged 50 to 79 on a low-fat diet (20% of calories) was found to reduce their chance of ovarian cancer by 40% (120) within the EPIC Study that investigated the relation of IGF-I and its major binding protein IGFBP-3. Measured in serum samples of 214 women who subsequently developed ovarian cancer and 388 matched controls, the study found there was no association between the circulating IGF-I or IGFBP-3 levels and the risk of ovarian cancer. However, there was an effect among women aged 55 or younger. Relations between IGFP-3 and ovarian cancer before age 55 were in the same direction as for IGF-I, but less strong and statistically not significant. In women aged over 55, there was no association between serum IGF-I or IGFBP-3 and ovarian cancer risk. These results suggest that the circulating levels of IGF-I may play a potentially important role in the development of ovarian cancer in women of a pre- or perimenopausal age.[121]

G. Endometrial Cancer

Endometrial cancer is the most common female gynecological cancer in the United States. Because obesity and unopposed estrogens are strong risk factors for endometrial cancer, and fat intake has been postulated to affect both risk factors, its role in the etiology of this disease has received some attention. The role of dietary fat and cholesterol on endometrial cancer risk was reviewed in1997; the evidence for an increased endometrial cancer risk was deemed "possible" for saturated/animal fat and "insufficient" total fat and cholesterol.[4]

Because dietary fat has been postulated to affect obesity and estrogen levels, two important risk factors for endometrial cancer, its association with this disease has received some attention. The current evidence for several dietary lipids in the peer-reviewed literature until December 2007 was reviewed recently in two cohorts and nine case-control studies in a meta-analysis. A case-control data suggested an increased risk for total, saturated, and animal fat. However, the limited available cohort data do not support the associations.[122] Additional data, particularly from prospective studies, are needed before conclusions can be drawn. A recent analysis from a population-based case-control study in Wisconsin including 240 cases and 2342 controls under 80 years old to evaluate the association of body mass index (BMI), weight gain, and weight cycling with endometrial cancer risk found that weight and lack of weight stability are associated with risk of endometrial cancer.[123] Within a recent cohort of 103,882 women ages 50 to 71 at baseline in 1995 to 1996, 677 cases of endometrial cancer were ascertained in the NIH-AARP Diet and Health Study. Results showed that both current adiposity and adult weight gain are associated with substantial increases in the risk of endometrial cancer, with relations particularly evident among never users of menopausal HRT.[124]

The role of dietary nutrients in the etiology of endometrial cancer was evaluated in a population-based case-control study of 1204 newly diagnosed endometrial cancer cases and 1212 age frequency-matched controls in Shanghai, China. Dietary macronutrients associated with endometrial cancer risk depend on their sources, with intake of animal origin nutrients being related to higher risk and intake of plant origin nutrients related to lower risk. Dietary fiber, retinol, β-carotene, vitamins C, E, and supplements were found to decrease endometrial cancer risk.[125]

The etiologic role of physical activity in endometrial cancer risk remains unclear, given the few epidemiologic studies that have been conducted. To investigate this relation more fully, an analysis was undertaken in the EPIC Study. During an average 6.6 years of follow-up, 689 incident endometrial cancer cases were identified from an analytic cohort within EPIC of 253,023 women. No clear associations between each type of activity and endometrial cancer risk were found for total study population combined. Associations were more evident in the stratified results, with premenopausal women who were active versus inactive experiencing significant risk. No effect modification by BMI, HRT, oral contraceptive use, or energy intake was found. No evidence of a protective effect of increased physical activity was reported for all women, but some support for a benefit among premenopausal women was found to be most pronounced for those performing household activities.[125]

H. Prostate Cancer

Prospective studies between prostate cancer risk and fruit and vegetable intake have been inconsistent, some showing either nonstatistically significant inverse association or no association, although there have been indications of a potential benefit of cruciferous vegetables.[127–129] None of the prospective studies reported statistically significant inverse associations with increasing intake of fruits. However, these studies were not conducted in populations uniformly screened with prostate-specific antigen (PSA) and only one included control for history of PSA.[129] Moreover, only a few of these cohorts represented large-scale v initiatives[126,129] (i.e., they ascertained ≥600 patients with prostate cancer), several had relatively crude assessment of diet, many did not consider specific fruit or vegetable subgroups, and one prospective study reported risk with respect to total fruit and vegetable intake in relation to organ-contained and extraprostatic cancer,[128] and one additional study reported disease-stratified findings for cruciferous vegetable intake.[129]

A recent study among participants in the screened arm of the Prostate, Lung, Colorectal and Ovarian (PLCO) Cancer Screening Trial, examined whether fruit and vegetable intake is associated with a reduced risk of prostate cancer among approximately 30,000 men, including more than 1300 patients with prostate cancer. This trial avoided the risk of differential screening, which can lead to bias.[130] Findings indicated that intakes of cruciferous and dark green vegetables, especially broccoli and cauliflower, were associated with a decreased risk of aggressive, particularly extraprostatic, prostate cancer. Aggressive prostate cancer is biologically virulent and associated with poor prognosis. Therefore, if the observed association is found to be causal, a possible means of reducing the burden of this disease may be primary prevention through increased consumption of broccoli, cauliflower, and possibly spinach.[131]

Neither flavonoids[132] nor regular multivitamin use[133] were associated with risk of early or localized prostate cancer, whereas supplemental vitamin E by itself was not protective against prostate cancer. Increasing consumption of γ-tocopherol from foods was associated with a reduced risk of clinically related disease.[134] A recent Finish cohort of 29,133 male smokers, aged 50 to 69 years old, among whom 1732 diagnosed with incident prostate cancer between 1985 and 2004 were used to study serum and dietary vitamin E in relation to prostate cancer.[135] The inverse serum α-tocopherol prostate cancer association was greater among those who were supplemented with either α-tocopherol or β-carotene during the trial. There were no associations between prostate cancer and the individual dietary tocopherols and tocotrienols. Thus, higher prediagnostic serum concentrations of α-tocopherol, but not dietary vitamin E, was associated with a lower risk of developing prostate cancer, particularly advanced prostate cancer.[135]

To evaluate the association of meat and dairy food consumption with the risk of developing prostate cancer in 1989, 3892 men 35+ years old, participated in the CLUE II Cohort study of Maryland's Washington County, named for the study slogan "Give us a 'clue' to cancer and heart disease." Results showed that overall, consumption of processed meat and pork, but not total meat or red meat, was associated with possible increased risk of total prostate cancer in this prospective study. Higher intake of dairy food, but not calcium, was positively associated with prostate cancer. Further investigation into the mechanism by which processed meat and dairy consumption might increase the risk of prostate cancer is suggested.[136]

It has been hypothesized that the fat content, especially saturated fat, might underlie the association between meat consumption and prostate cancer risk by influencing the production of sex steroid hormones.[4] However, the results of studies evaluating the association between cancer and fat intake have been inconsistent. Adjustments for intake of saturated fat did not attenuate the association of processed meat or pork with high-stage disease. In contrast to prior studies, no consistent associations between calcium intake and prostate cancer risk was observed in this cohort, although the level of calcium intake was lower than in studies that found a positive association.[136] Further research examining the possible higher risk of prostate cancer in men who consume large amounts of processed meat or pork products such as sausages, hot dogs, ham or lunch meat, or bacon is warranted.

To date, the strongest evidence regarding diet and prostate cancer relates to energy balance. Urologists aspiring to best clinical practice should encourage their patients to achieve a healthy body weight through regular exercise and a healthful plant-based diet rich in fruits, vegetables, and whole grains. Advocating functional foods or supplements explicitly for cancer control purposes would currently be premature.[137] Various measures of physical activity with prostate cancer risk among men in the American Society for Cancer Prevention Study II Nutrition Cohort, a large prospective study of U.S. adults enrolled in 1992/1993 as well as from a food frequency questionnaire (FFQ) completed as part of an earlier study in 1982 were examined. During the 9-year prospective follow-up, 5503 incident prostate cancer cases were identified among 72,174 men who were cancer-free at enrollment. Findings were inconsistent with most previous studies that found no association between recreational physical activity and overall prostate cancer risk, but suggest physical activity may be associated with reduced risk of aggressive prostate cancer.[138] A large EPIC nested case-control study found that serum IGF-I concentrations were not strongly associated with prostate cancer risk, although the results were comparable with small increase in risk, particularly for advanced-stage disease; no association for IGFBP-3 was found.[139]

I. Urinary Bladder Cancer

Approximately 357,000 new cases of urinary bladder cancer (UBC) occurred worldwide in 2002.[140] UBC is the seventh most common cancer worldwide in men (109.1 new cases per 100,000 person-years) and the 17th in women (2.5 per 100,000 person-years. These differences in incidence rates between genders have been attributed in part to differences in smoking habits. High incidence rates are observed in developing countries. The highest incidence rate in men was in Egypt (37.1 per 100,000 person-years. In women, the highest incidence rate was recorded in Zambia (13.8 per 100,000 person-years. A similar pattern is observed for mortality rates that tended to increase in men in the majority of European countries between 1960 and 1990, with a subsequent decline in many countries.[141] The difference between incidence and mortality rates suggest that UBC has a long progression period. In the United States, the 5-year relative survival rate ranges from 97% for those diagnosed with stage I to 22% for those with stage IV.[142] In Europe, the overall rate was 71%, varying widely across countries.[143]

Cigarette smoking and occupational exposure to aromatic amines are the main known causes of UBC. Phenacetin, chlornaphazine, and cyclophosphamide also increase UBC risk. Chronic infection by the helmenthic worm *Schistosoma haematobium* is a cause of squamous cell carcinoma. NAT2 show acetylator and GSTM1 null genotypes, alone and in interaction with tobacco, are associated with an increased risk. Consumption of vegetables and fresh fruits protects against this tumor.[144]

These risk factors have been mainly investigated in Caucasians and it is uncertain whether they play the same role in individuals of different ethnicity. Further research is needed to disentangle whether established risks or protective and susceptibility factors have a different effect on different UBC subgroups according to pathological or molecular characteristics. Similarly, an in-depth study of endogenous factors such as inflammation, oxidative stress, and hormonal status may help in identifying further causes of UBC as well as elucidating the reason for sex differences in incidence.[144] Genetic factors appear to play a role in this cancer, but whether they correspond to low penetrance cancer predisposing polymorphisms acting together or interacting with environmental factors is not certain.[145]

J. Other Cancers

1. Pancreatic Cancer

The relation between risk factor and pancreatic cancer has been studied in a large American Cancer Society Cancer Prevention Study II Nutrition Cohort to examine the associations between measures of adiposity, recreational physical activity, and pancreatic cancer risk. Information on current weight and weight at age 18, location of weight gain, and recreational physical activity were obtained at baseline in 1992 via FFQ for 145,627 men and women who were cancer free at enrollment. During the 7 years of follow-up, 242 incident pancreatic cancer cases were identified among these participants. This study, along with several recent studies, supports the hypothesis that obesity and central adiposity are associated with pancreatic cancer risk. No differences in pancreatic cancer incidence rates were found between men and women who were most active (>31.5 metabolic equivalent hours per week) at baseline compared with men and women who reported no recreational physical activity.[146]

2. Kidney Cancers

Kidney cancers account for almost 2% of all cancers worldwide, with 150,000 new cases and 78,000 deaths from the disease occurring annually.[147] The incidence of kidney cancer has increased significantly worldwide in both males and females. Between 1988 and 1992, the incidence of renal cancer among males per 100,000 person-year in the United States was 34.1,[148] in Finland 12.1, in Norway 9.0, and in Japan 6.5.[149] The incidence of renal cancer among females in the same time period in the United States was 5.7,[148] in Finland 6.7, Norway 5.0 and Japan 2.5.[149]

Several potential risk factors have been identified such as smoking, obesity, kidney diseases, hypertension, occupational factors, hormonal status, socioeconomic status, alcohol, coffee or tea intake.[150] The association of meat consumption as a potential risk for kidney cancer has been studied in several case-control studies, but the evidence has been inconsistent.[151] A recent meta-analysis of 13 case-control studies published between 1966 and 2006 showed that increased consumption of all meat, red meat, poultry, and processed meat is associated with an increased risk of renal cancer. Reduction of meat consumption is an important approach to decreasing the incidence of kidney cancer in the general population.[152] Another recent analysis of the role of diet in the high-risk population of central Europe among 1065 incident kidney cancer cases and 1509 controls in Russia, Romania, Poland, and the Czech Republic showing an increased risk associated with dairy products, preserved vegetables, and red meat, provides clues to the high rates of kidney cancer in this population.[153] On the other hand, prospectively examined associations between intakes of fruits, vegetables, vitamins A, C and E, and carotenoids and risk of renal cell cancer in women and men in 88,759 women in the Nurses' Health Study from 1980–2000 and 47,828 men in the Health Professional Follow-up Study from 1986 to 2000 in which dietary intake was assessed every 2–4 years, found that fruit and vegetable consumption may reduce the risk of renal cell cancer in men.[154]

3. Skin Cancer

In the United States, 5 million cases of skin cancers, basal cell carcinoma (BCC) and squamous cell carcinoma (SCC) occur each year.[155] Incidence rates are generally increasing in white populations worldwide,[156] so that the costs of treatment of BCC and SCC tumors exceed the cost of treatment of all other cancers and place a disproportionate burden on healthcare costs.[157] Excessive sun exposure causes skin cancer by mutagenic, immunosuppressive, and oxidative stress-inducing mechanisms.[158] Animal studies show that diet, specifically the intake of lutein, vitamins E, C and selenium, or a combination of these and other antioxidants can protect against oxidative damage in the skin by directly quenching reactive oxygen species and scavenging free radicals.[159] In addition, dietary n-3 fatty acids can dramatically reduce the plasma coetaneous proinflammatory and immunosuppressive prostaglandin E synthasase type 2 (PGE_2) concentration in mice, whereas dietary n-fatty acids increase PGE_2.[160] Dietary n-3 fatty acids also can greatly reduce the inflammatory response and enhance the delayed-type hypersensitivity immune response after UV light exposure in mice when compared with an equivalent dietary amount of n-6 fatty acids.[160]

Evidence in humans regarding the association between dietary intake and the risk of developing BCC and SCC tumors suggests a positive relation between fat intake and skin cancers but an inconsistent relation with other nutrients.[161] Consumption of green leafy vegetables and unmodified dairy products can each influence the cumulative incidence of SCC after adjustment for sun exposure in persons with a history of skin cancer.[162]

A recent investigation of the association between empirically determined dietary pattern and the risk of BCC and SCC in which data collected in a prospective community-based study in Nambour, Australia in 1360 adults aged 25–75 years between 1992 and 2002, with adjustments for the sun-exposure histories of participants and other established risk factors for these cancers was undertaken to investigate the association between dietary patterns and BCC and SCC. A dietary pattern characterized by high meat and fat intakes increases SCC tumor risk, particularly in persons with a skin cancer history, but there was no association between the dietary patterns and BCC tumors.[163]

A case-control study reported protective effects of vegetables, fish, and legumes on the risk of BCC and SCC combined.[164] In a population-based case-control study, an inverse association was found between the consumption of hot black tea and SCC risk. Therefore, given the involvement of oxidative damage in skin carcinogenesis,[159] the Australian study adds to the evidence that the consumption of leafy green vegetables that contain antioxidants and a variety of vitamins, minerals, and other bioactive substances such as polyphenols may underlie the protective effect of the vegetable and fruit dietary pattern in persons who are susceptible to skin cancer.[165]

No association was found between dietary patterns and BCC tumor risk in persons with or without a prior history of skin cancer; this lack of an association may reflect the distinctly different pathogenesis of BCC and SCC tumors. In a randomized, double-blind, controlled trial, the role of retinol in preventing SCC, but not BCC, was found.[166] In a nested case-control study, no association was found between BCC and carotenoids (except lutein), vitamin E, or selenium, as measured by either serum biomarkers or dietary intake.[167]

Cutaneous malignant melanoma (CMM) is related to pigmentary traits, history of sun exposure and sunburns, and number of melanocytic naevi. Limited and inconsistent information is available on the association between the risk of CMM and dietary factors. A case control Italian study carried out between 1992 and 1994 on 542 CCM cases and 538 controls showed no appreciable association between CMM risk and selected food items, including fish, meat, vegetables, fruit, dairy products, whole-meal bread, alcohol, coffee, and tea. Consumption of tea appeared to have a protective effect on CMM risk.[168] Another population case-control Italian study found that excess energy-adjusted intake of linoleic acid and a lower consumption of soluble carbohydrates may increase melanoma risk.[169] Another case-control study in the United States that used 502 CCM cases and 565 controls concluded that foods rich in vitamin D and carotenoids and low in alcohol may be associated with a reduction in risk for melanoma.[170] The above analysis on the relation between CMM and diet should be repeated in larger prospective studies. The relationship between cancer and environmental and dietary factors is presented in Table 17.1.

III. MOLECULAR MECHANISMS AND TARGETS

A. DNA Repair Pathways

At the fundamental level, cancer is a genetic disease in which the initial mechanism leading to carcinogenesis involves damage to DNA. The genome is continuously subject to damage from both exogenous agents and endogenous processes (e.g., UV component of sunlight and ingested genotoxic chemicals, products of cellular metabolism including reactive oxygen species (ROS) such as hydroxyl radicals and hydrogen peroxide, and spontaneous chemical degradation of bases in DNA including deamination of cysteine, adenine, and 5-methylcytosine. In addition, copying errors in the form of misrepaired bases and small insertion or deletion loops may result from slippage of DNA polymerase during replication of repetitive sequences. The telomeric ends of chromosomes shorten by ~100 base pair per cell division, leading eventually to chromosomal instability and replicative senescence.[171] Moreover, the epigenetic making of DNA (DNA methylation) alters in response to exposure to a wide range of agents, including dietary compounds, leading to changes in gene expression.[32]

TABLE 17.1

The Relationship Between Cancer and Environmental Factors, Physical Activity, and Obesity

Cancer	Evidence	Factors Associated with Decreased Risk	Factors Associated with Increased Risk
CRC	Convincing Probable	Physical activity	Processed/overcooked red meat, alcohol intake Obesity, central adiposity, exposure to tobacco products earlier in life
Premenopausal breast	Convincing	Breast feeding, physical activity	Alcohol intake
	Probable		Attained height
Postmenopausal breast	Convincing	Breast feeding, physical activity	Overweight/obesity, alcohol intake
	Probable		Attained height
H&N	Convincing		Alcohol intake
	Probable		
Gastric	Probable	Allium-containing vegetables	Preserved salty foods, grilled meat
Lung	Convincing	Fruits, physical activity, non–smoking	Smoking
	Probable		Alcohol intake
Ovarian	Probable	Low fat diet taken late in life Birth control pills for women of childbearing age Isoflavones & carotenoids	Dried or salted fish & Chinese pickled/fermented cabbage
Endometrial	Convincing	Physical activity	Overweight/obesity, central adiposity, menopausal estrogen therapy
	Probable		Saturated/animal fat
Prostate	Probable		Milk and dairy foods
Bladder	Convincing Probable		Cigarette smoking, occupational exposure Inflammation, oxidative stress, hormonal status, tysanomas in Caucasians
Pancreatic	Probable		Obesity, central adiposity
Kidney	Probable	Fruit and vegetable consumption	Meat consumption
SCC/BSC	Convincing		UV exposure from sunlight
Skin	Probable	Vitamin D, tea and carotenoids with CMM	High meat and fat with SCC
Liver	Convincing		Aflatoxin contaminated foods, alcohol
Gallbladder	Probable		Central adiposity

The repair phenomenon becomes functionally important only if the damage is not detected and resolved in a timely and effective manner by repair systems. In mammals, there are five highly conserved DNA repair pathways encoded by ~150 genes, which appear to have arisen early in evolution[172] and include:

- Direct reversal (DR), which operates via proteins acting directly on a damaged base with DNA to correct its structure without removing the damaged nucleotide as in case of the protein methylguanine-methyltransferaser (MGMT), which removes alkyl groups from the O^6–position of guanine. Failure to remove each alkyl group results in a G→A transition mutation following replication. MGMT transfers the alkyl group from guanine to a cysteine residue within the enzyme to restore the damaged guanine.
- Base-excision repair (BER), which repairs DNA damage such as oxidation caused by ROS, deamination, and hydroxylation arising from cellular metabolism and spontaneous depurination. BER occurs at ~10^4 events per human cell per day. The most frequent lesions repaired by BER are apurinic/apyrimidinic (AP) sites where the base is missing from the DNA backbone by either a short-patch repair where a single nucleotide is inserted into the AP site by DNA polymerase β and sealed by a DNA ligase, or long-patch repair in which an additional 2–13 nucleotides are removed and the gap is repaired by polymerase β and sealed by a ligase.
- Nucleotide excision repair (NER), which removes lesions causing structural distortion of the DNA helix such as pyrimidine dimers produced by UV exposure, and hydrocarbon DNA adducts such as those derived from food and smoking, including 2-amino-1-methyl-6-phenylimidazo[4,5-b]pyridine (PhIP) sand benxzo[a]pyrene diol epoxide (BPDE. Two types of NER exist: (i) global genomic repair (GGR), which surveys the genome for DNA distortions, and (ii) transcription-coupled repair (TCR), which focuses on damage that blocks elongating RNA polymerases. These two pathways differ only in the way the DNA damage is detected.
- Repair of double strand breaks, which are the most dangerous lesions in term of cytotoxicity and mutagenicity. It is carried out by homologous recombination (HR) and nonhomologous end joining (NHE).
- DNA mismatch repair (MMR), which is responsible primarily for detecting and repairing copying mistakes made during replication in order to provide a 100-fold increase in the fidelity of replication. Additionally, alkyl adducts and oxidatively damaged bases are also repaired by MMR, which involves 26 genes and their encoded proteins that act in three stages to remove and repair damage by their encoded proteins. It should be realized that inside the cell, DNA defects are detected and repaired in the context of chromatin.[172]

It is also instructive to realize that ~1% of a cell's DNA is found within the mitochondria (mtDNA), which appears to be more vulnerable to sustained damage than is naked DNA because it is more directly exposed to oxidative damage from the respiratory chain within the organelle, is not protected by histones, and has a less developed repair machinery. There is evidence only for the presence of DR and BER activity in mtDNA, which may explain the observation of sustained age-related accumulation of mitochondrial mutations in apparently normal human tissue.[172]

About 70% of CpG dinucleotides in the human genome are methylated at position 5 on the cytosine ring. Methylation patterns are heritable from one cell generation to the next by the enzyme DNMT1. However, mistakes are made in this process and the policing of DNA methylation marks is several orders of magnitude poorer than that of the primary DNA sequence.[172]

B. Nutritional Modulation of DNA Repair

The strongest evidence for an effect of a nutrient on DNA repair is an observational study that found NER to be 18% lower in adults with the lowest compared with the highest tertile of folate intake.[173] One of the earliest *in vivo* studies showed that an abnormally high rate of DNA repair in children with Down syndrome was made normal by zinc supplementation.[174] On the other hand, all the studies in which healthy volunteers were supplemented with individual nutrients were without effect on DNA repair, and most of them employed peripheral blood lymphocytes (PBL). A recent intervention study in healthy adults given 1.2 mg folic acid/d for 12 weeks found no evidence for BER, and the volunteers in the lowest quartile of folate status distribution at baseline had lower BER after supplementation.[175] Nevertheless, positive effects on DNA repair were reported in studies in which healthy adults were supplemented with a reduced form of coenzyme Q_{10},[176] or in those consuming an extra 1–3 kiwifruits per day,[177] or in volunteers randomized to a supplement of 200g cooked, minced carrots per day.[178] However, in the latter study, supplementation with another whole food (tinned mandarin oranges) or with amounts of α- and β-carotene equivalent to those in the carrots had no detectable effect on DNA repair.[178]

A study that investigated a tissue other than PBL used a Comet assay in rectal mucosal cells and in PBL from alcoholics and control subjects. In contrast with findings for PBL, a repair of endonuclease III-specific lesions by rectal cells was undetectable.[179] Obviously, more work is needed to discern whether individual tissues show differential capacity for DNA repair and whether such repair can be enhanced by nutritional intervention.[172]

C. Epigenetic Mechanisms

Evidence is accumulating to demonstrate that a variety of bioactive food components as well as energy consumption can influence DNA methyltransferases, methylcytosine guanine dinucleotide-binding proteins, histone-modifying enzymes, and chromatin remodeling factors. One of the most important mechanisms by which mutation could influence DNA repair is through methylation of the promoter region of repair genes leading to gene silencing.[32]

With the exception of folate, which may alter DNA methylation via its role as a methyl donor, the mechanisms of action of most dietary factors with respect to DNA methylation are poorly understood. An exception is the dietary phenol EGCG, which, at relatively low concentrations, inhibited DNMT1 by fitting into its catalytic pocket.[180] When cancer cells were treated *in vitro* by EGCG, demethylation of the previously hypermethylated promoters ensued and reexpression of the silenced genes that induced the DNA repair genes MGMT and MLH1.[180] Other dietary constituents such as the short-chain fatty acid butyrate and the phytochemicals diallyl sulphide and sulphoraphane act as inhibitors of histone deacetylase, thereby regulating gene expression.[181] It remains to be seen whether this is a mechanism through which nutritional factors can upregulate DNA repair.[172]

D. Apoptosis

Apoptosis, or cellular suicide, is one of the most potent defenses against cancer, since this process eliminates potential deleterious mutated cells. Many dietary cancer-preventive compounds, including selenium, EGCG, phenylethyl isothiocyannate, retinoic acid, sulforaphane, curcumin, apigenin, quercetin, and resveratrol inhibit apoptosis.[182] Distinct from the apoptotic events in the normal physiological process, which are mediated mainly by the interaction between death receptors and their relevant ligands, many bioactive dietary components appear to induce apoptosis through mitochondrial-mediated pathway. Dietary compounds generally induce oxidative stress, which downregulates antiapoptotic molecules such as Bcl-2 or Bcl-x and upregulates proapoptotic molecules such as Bax or Bak.[183] The imbalance between antiapoptotic and proapoptotic proteins elicits the release of cytochrome c from the mitochondrial membrane, which forms a complex with caspase-9 with the subsequent activation of caspases-3, -6 and -7. The activated caspases degrade important intracellular proteins, leading to the morphological changes and the phenotype of apoptotic cells.[184] To enhance this mitochondria-mediated apoptosis, dietary components also activate proapoptotic c-Jun N-terminal kinase (JNK) and inhibit antiapoptotic nuclear factor $_{k}$B (NF-$_{k}$B) signaling pathways.[183] Thus, the cytotoxic effects of dietary components on the cells can be monitored by measuring their effects on mitochondria, caspases and other apoptosis-related proteins.[185]

E. Inflammation and Immunity

Inflammation represents a physiological response to invading microorganisms, trauma, chemical irritation or foreign tissues. Although acute inflammation is usually beneficial, chronic inflammation is often detrimental to the host. Epidemiologic data show an association between chronic inflammatory conditions and subsequent malignant transformation in the inflamed tissue.[186] Evidence indicates that there are multiple mechanisms linking inflammation to cancer and that there are multiple targets for cancer prevention by bioactive dietary components. At the molecular level, free radicals and aldehydes produced during chronic inflammation can induce gene mutations and posttranslational modifications of key cancer-related proteins. In response to an inflammatory insult, proinflammatory cytokines such as tumor necrosis factor-α (TNF-α), Interleukin-1 (IL-1), IL-6, IL-12 and γ-interferon are synthesized and secreted resulting in an elevation in reactive oxygen and nitrogen species. This process is followed by the secretion of anti-inflammatory cytokines (e.g., IL-4, IL-10 and TGF-β) to reduce the accumulation of reactive species. The binding of pro-inflammatory cytokines to their receptors triggers many signaling pathways including the mitogen-activated protein kinase (MAPK) pathway, which can activate two redox-sensitive transcription factors, namely NF-$_k$B and the c-Jun part of activating protein-1 (AP-1). These transcription factors activate the expression of a wide variety of genes including inducible nitric oxide synthase (iNOS) and cyclooxygenase-2 (COX-2). These enzymes, in turn, directly influence reactive oxygen species (ROS) and eicosanoid levels.[185]

Chronic inflammation results in increased DNA damage, cellular proliferation, the disruption of DNA repair pathways, inhibition of apoptosis, and the promotion of angiogenesis and invasion,[186] all of which are important during the cancer process. Several of these mechanisms are amenable to influence by dietary constituents. Evidence exists that selected dietary components, including conjugated lenoleic acid, long chain ω-3 fatty acids such as those in fish oil, butyrate, EGCG, curcumin, resveratrol, genistein, luteolin, quercetin, and vitamins A and D, may influence the inflammatory process at various sites.[185]

F. Angiogenesis

Angiogenesis, the development of new blood vessels from endothelial cells, is a crucial process in tumor pathogenesis as it sustains malignant cells with nutrients and oxygen. During angiogenesis, endothelial cells are stimulated by various growth factors such as vascular endothelial growth factor (VEGF) and fibroblast growth factor (FGF), and are attracted to the site where the new blood supply is needed by inflammatory cytokines and chemokines.[187] Chemotactic migration along this gradient is, however, possible only through the degradation of extracellular matrix components.[188] This is accomplished *via* matrix metalloproteinases (MMPs).[188] Preventing the expansion of new blood vessel networks results in reduced tumor size and metastasis and is another mechanism whereby dietary components inhibit tumor growth. Dietary components that inhibit angiogenesis include PUFA and polyphenols such as EGCG, resveratrol, curcumin, and genistein.[185]

IV. Conclusions and Research Needs

In 1991 was estimated that tobacco use and poor diet accounted for about one third of cancer deaths in the United States. When combined with alcohol consumption, certain infectious diseases, and environmental and occupational carcinogens, about 75–80% of cancer deaths could in principle be prevented; diet (or nutrition) could be responsible for up to 30% of cancer deaths—at least as much as tobacco use.[3] Decades later and with much more evidence from large studies, we are still unsure which dietary factors affect cancer. For example, we are not still sure of the relation between consumption of fruits and vegetables and cancer incidence, the contribution of excess body weight to cancer development and death, between eating red meat and cancer, and whether fiber has a protective effect.

IARC estimated in 2002 that overweight and obesity (a BMI of 30 k/m^2 or greater) may be responsible for about 10% of breast and CRC cancer cases, and between 25% and 40% of kidney, esophageal, and endometrial cancers. With obesity, there are still many unanswered questions such as the magnitude to which obesity may contribute to the risk of cancer and other adverse health effects, whether a few extra pounds constitutes a cancer risk, and the appropriate way to measure all of these effects. In 2003, using data from the 900,000 Americans in the Cancer Prevention Study II, the risk of cancer death associated with excess weight and obesity was estimated to account for up to 20% of all cancer deaths in U.S. women and 14% for men. Cancer death rates were 52% higher in obese men than in normal-weight men, and the death rate for obese women was 62% higher than their normal-weight counterparts. It would seem that about 90,000 cancer deaths could be prevented if Americans maintained a healthy weight.[189] In 2005, obesity was reported to be associated with ~112,000 excess deaths and of them, more than 82,000 occurred in people with a BMI of 35 or higher.[190] However, it was also reported that being overweight (a BMI of between 25 and 30) was actually protective and associated with 86,000 fewer deaths relative to the normal weight (BMI between 18.5 and 25. Because of these uncertainties, research is needed to delineate the connection between cancer risk and different factors acting in different time frame that contribute to death from the various cancers.

Current dogma suggests that the positive correlation between obesity and cancer is driven by white adipose tissue that accompanies obesity, possibly through excess secretion of adipokines. Recent studies in fatless A-Zip/F1 mice, which have undetectable adipokine levels but display accelerated tumor formation, suggest that adipokines are not required for the enhanced tumor development. The A-Zip/F-1 mice are also diabetic and display elevated circulating levels of other factors frequently associated with obesity (insulin, IGF-1, and proinflammatory cytokines) and activation of several signaling pathways associated with carcinogenesis. Therefore, the risk factors underlying the obesity–cancer link need to be revisited. It is postulated that pathways associated with insulin resistance and inflammation, rather than adipocyte-derived factors, may represent key prevention and therapeutic targets for disrupting the obesity–cancer link.[191]

A multicenter prospective study carried out in 23 centers from 10 European countries (EPIC Study), including 519,978 subjects (366,521 women and 153,457 men), most aged 35–70 years, found that of the main food groups in major cancers, consumption of fruit was negatively associated with cancer of the lung, but not with prostate or breast cancer. Consumption of vegetables, mainly onion and garlic, reduced the risk of intestinal stomach cancer but was not associated with cancer of the lung, prostate, or breast. Consumption of red and processed meat was positively associated with CRC and with non-cardia stomach cancer in those infected by *H. pylori*. Fish intake was negatively associated with colorectal cancer risk. High alcohol intake increased the risk of breast cancer.[192]

More recently, it was shown that it is not a single dietary compound in the food that is responsible for increased risk, but a contribution of these dietary compounds interacting together (enhancing or negating the effect of other food components) that matter. Evidence suggests that bioactive food components can typically influence more than one process. It is essential to have a better understanding of how the response relates to exposure and credentialing which process is involved in bringing about a change in tumor incidence or tumor behavior. Credentialing is being defined as a determination of which cellular process(es) and which bioactive food components are most important for bringing about a phenotypic change. Additional attention is needed to determine the critical intake of dietary components, their duration, and when they should be provided to optimize the desired physiological response. Further research is also needed on the molecular targets for bioactive components and whether genetic and epigenetic events dictate the direction and magnitude of the response.[185]

Higher intake of a Western dietary pattern characterized by high intakes of meat, fat, refined grains, and sugary desserts, as compared to a prudent diet characterized by high intakes of fruits, vegetables, poultry, and fish, may be associated with a higher risk of recurrence and mortality among patients with stage III colon cancer treated with surgery and adjuvant chemotherapy. Further studies are needed to delineate which components of such a diet show the strongest association.[193]

In view of the substantial improvements in early detection and treatment, even more patients can expect to live 5 years after diagnosis. With improvements in longevity, the late-occurring adverse effects of cancer and its treatment are becoming increasingly apparent. Healthy lifestyle behaviors that encompass regular exercise, weight control, healthy nutrition, and some complementary practices, e.g., support groups and imagery, have the potential to greatly reduce cancer-treatment-associated morbidity and mortality in cancer survivors and can enhance the quality of life.[2]

Many dietary bioactive compounds, mostly phytochemicals, have been found to decrease the risk of carcinogenesis. Modulating the metabolism and disposition pathways of carcinogenesis represents one of the major mechanisms by which dietary compounds prevent carcinogenesis. The expression of phase I enzymes, which presumably mostly activates carcinogens, is mainly regulated by xenobiotics sensing nuclear receptors such as Ahr, CAR, PXR, and RXR. On the other hand, Phase II enzymes catalyze the conjugations of carcinogens and generally are transcriptionally controlled by the Nrf2/ARE signaling pathways, which regulate the expression of many detoxifying enzymes, and are a major target of dietary compounds. The final excretion of carcinogens and their metabolites is mediated by phase III transporters, which share many regulatory mechanisms with phase I/II enzymes. The expression of metabolizing enzymes and transporters is often coordinately regulated. Besides transcriptional regulation, the activities of phase I/II enzymes and phase III transporters could be directly activated or inhibited by dietary compounds. Furthermore, genetic polymorphisms have profound effects on the individual response to dietary compounds.[35]

Dietary bioactive food components that interact with the immune response have considerable potential to reduce the risk of cancer. Reduction of chronic inflammation or its downstream consequences may represent a key mechanism that can be reduced through targeting signal transduction or through antioxidant effects. Major classes of macronutrients provide numerous examples including amino acids such as glutamine or arginine, lipids such as ω-3 PUFA, DHA or EPA, or novel carbohydrates such as various sources of β-glucans. Vitamins such as C and E are commonly used as antioxidants, while zinc and selenium are minerals with a wide spectrum of impact on the immune system. Some of the most potent immunomodulators are phytochemicals such as polyphenols, EGCG, curcumin, or isothiocyanates. There is accumulating evidence for cancer prevention by probiotics and these may also activate the immune response.[194] Genomic approaches are becoming increasingly important in characterizing potential mechanisms of cancer prevention, optimizing the rational selection of dietary bioactive food components, or identifying humans with differing requirements for cancer protection, and more research should be directed to understand mechanistic interactions between these dietary components and cancer.

Early life nutrition has the potential to change chromatin structure, to alter gene expression and consequently the phenotype, and to modulate health throughout the life course.[172] Whether later interventions can reverse adverse epigenetic markings is unknown and more research is needed on that.

REFERENCES

1. Parkin, P. M., Bray, F., Ferlay, J., and Pisani, P., Global cancer statistics, 2002. *CA Cancer J. Clin.* 55, 74–108, 2005.
2. Jones, L. W. and Demark-Wahnefried, W., Diet, exercise and complementary therapies after primary treatment for cancer. *Lancet Oncol.* 7, 1017–1026, 2006.
3. Doll, R. and Peto, P., The causes of cancer: quantitative estimates of avoidable risks of cancer in the United States today. *J. Natl. Cancer Inst.* 66, 1191–1308, 1981.
4. World Cancer Research Fund, Food, Nutrition and the Prevention of Cancer: A Global Perspective. American Institute for Cancer Research, Washington, DC, 1997.
5. Popkin, B. M., Understanding global nutrition dynamics as a step towards controlling cancer incidence. *Nature Rev. Cancer* 7, 61–67, 2007.
6. Martínez, M. E., Primary prevention of colorectal cancer: Lifestyle, nutrition, exercise: recent results. *Cancer Res.* 166, 177–211, 2005.
7. Ortega, R. M., Importance of functional foods in the Mediterranean diet. *Publ. Health Nutr.* 9, 1136–1140, 2006.
8. Engese, D., Andersen, V., Hjartåker A., and Lund, E., Meat, fish and fat intake in relation to subsite-specific risk of colorectal cancer: the Fukuoka Colorectal Cancer Study. *Cancer Sci.* 98, 590–597, 2007.
9. Engest, D., Andersen, V., Hjartåker, A., and Lund, E., Consumption of fish and risk of colon cancer in the Norwegian women and cancer (NOWAC) study. *Br. J. Nutr*, 98, 576–582, 2007.
10. Hu, J., Morrison, H., Mery, L. MesMeules, M., et al. and Macleod, M., Diet and vitamin or mineral supplementation and risk of colon cancer by subsite in Canada. *Eur. J. Cancer Prevent.* 16, 275–291, 2007.
11. Theodoratou, E., McNeill, G., Cetnarskyj, R., Tenesa, A, Barnetson, R., et al., Dietary fatty acid and colorectal cancer in case-control study. *Am. J. Epidemiol.* 166, 181–195, 2007.
12. Park, Y., Subar, A. F., Kipnis, V., Thompson, F. E., Mouw, T, et al., Fruit and vegetable intakes and risk of colorectal cancer in the NIH-AARP Diet and Health Study. *Am. J. Epidemiol.* 166, 170–180, 2007.
13. Koushik, A., Hunter, D. J., Spiegelman, D., Beeson, W. L., van den Brandt, P. A., et al., Fruits, vegetables, and colon cancer risk in a pooled analysis of 14 cohort studies. *J. Natl. Cancer Inst.* 99, 1471–1483, 2007.
14. Bingham, S. A., Day, N. E., Luben, R., Ferrari, P., Slimani, N., et al., Dietary fiber in food and protection against colorectal cancer in the European Prospective Investigation into Cancer and Nutrition (EPIC): An observational study. *Lancet* 361, 1496–1501, 2003.

15. Peters, U., Sinha, R., Chatterjee, N., Subar, A. F., Ziegler, R. G., et al., Dietary fibre and colorectal adenoma in a colorectal cancer early detection programme. *Lancet* 361, 1491–1495, 2003.
16. Park, Y., Hunter, D. J., Spiegelman, D, Bergkvist, L., Berrino, F., et al., Dietary fiber intake and risk of colorectal cancer: A pooled analysis of prospective cohort studies. *JAMA* 294, 2849–2857, 2005.
17. Schatzkin, A., Mouw, T., Park, Y., Subar, A. F., Kipnis, V., et al., Dietary fiber and whole-grain consumption in relation to colorectal cancer in the NIH-AARP Diet and Health Study. *Am. J. Clin. Nutr.* 85, 1353–1360, 2007.
18. Lipkin, M. and Newmark, H., Effect of added dietary calcium on colonic epithelial cell proliferation in subjects at high risk for familial colonic cancer. *N. Engl. J. Med.* 313, 1381–1384, 1985.
19. Norat, T. and Riboli, E., Dietary products and colorectal cancer: A review of possible mechanisms and epidemiological evidence. *Eur. J. Clin. Nutr.* 57, 1–17, 2003.
20. Cho, E., Smith-Werner, S. A., Spiegelman, D., Beeson, W. L., van den Brandt, P. A., et al., Dietary foods, calcium and colorectal cancer: A pooled analysis of 10 cohort studies. *J. Natl. Cancer Inst.* 96, 1015–1022, 2004.
21. Jacobs, E. T., Martínez, M. E., and Alberts, D. S., Research and public health implications of the intricate relationship between calcium and vitamin D in the prevention of colorectal neoplasia. *Natl. Cancer Inst.* 95, 1736–1737.
22. Kumar, N., Shibata, D., Helm, J., Coppola, D., and Malafa, M., Green tea polyphenols in the prevention of colon cancer. *Front. Biosci.* 12, 2309–2315, 2007.
23. Yang, G., Shu, X. O., Li, H., Chow, W. H., Ji, B. T., et al., Prospective cohort study of green tea consumption and colorectal cancer risk in women. *Cancer Epidemiol. Biomark. Prevent.* 16, 1219–1223, 2007.
24. Hoc, T., Chen, C. W., Wanasundera, U. N., and Shahidi, F., in *Natural Antioxidant: Chemistry, Health Effects, and Applications*, Shahidi, F., Ed., American Oil Chemical Society, Champaign, IL, 1997, 213.
25. Kapadin, G. J., Paul, B. D., Chung, E. D., Ghosh, B., and Pradhan, S. N., Carcinogenicity of *Camellia sinesis* (tea) and some tannin-containing folk medicinal herbs administered subcutaneously in rats. *J. Natl. Cancer Inst.* 57, 207–209, 1976.
26. Kim, Y. I., Will mandatory folic acid fortification prevent or promote cancer? *Am. J. Clin. Nutr.* 80, 1123–1128, 2004.
27. Bailey, L. B., Rampersaud, G. C., and Kauwell, G. P., Folic acid supplements and fortification affect the risk for neural tube defects, vascular disease and cancer: Evolving science. *J. Nutr.* 133, 1961S–1968S, 2003.
28. Food and Drug Administration, Food standards: Amendment of standards of identity for enriched grain products to require addition of folic acid. Final rule, 21 CFR Parts 136, 137 and 139. *Fed. Regist.* 61, 878108807, 1996.
29. Kim, Y. I., Folate and colorectal cancer: An evidence-based critical review. *Molec. Nutr. Food Res.* 51, 267–292, 2007.
30. Choi, S. W. and Mason, J. B., Folate status: Effects on pathways of colorectal carcinogenesis. *J. Nutr.* 132, 2413S–2418S, 2002.
31. Bills, N. D., Hinrichs, S. H., Morgan, R., and Clifford, A. J., Delayed tumor onset in transgenic mice fed a low-folate diet. *J. Natl. Cancer Inst.* 84, 332–337, 1992.
32. Ahmed, F. E., Colorectal cancer epigenetics: The role of environmental factors and the search for molecular biomarkers. *J. Env. Sci. Health* C25, 101–154, 2007.
33. Kim, Y. I., Nutritional epigenetics: Impact of folate deficiency on DNA methylation and colon cancer susceptibility. *J. Nutr.* 135, 2703–2709, 2005.
34. Ma, J., Stampfer, M. J., Giovannucci, E., Artigas, C., Hunter, D. J., et al., Methylenetetrahydrofolate reductase polymorphism, dietary interactions and risk of colorectal cancer. *Cancer Res.* 57, 1098–1102, 1997.

35. Ahmed, F. E., Gene–gene, gene–environment & multiple interactions in colorectal cancer. *J. Environ. Sci. Health* C24, 1–101, 2006.
36. Blount, B. C., Mack, M. M., Wehr, C. M., MacGregor, J. T., Hiatt, R. A., et al., Folate deficiency causes uracil misincorporation into human DNA and chromosome breakage: Implications for cancer and neuronal damage. *Proc. Natl Acad. Sci. USA* 94, 3290–3295, 1997.
37. Kim, D. O., The interactive effect of methyl-group diet and polymorphism of methylenetetrahydrofolate reductase on the risk of colorectal cancer. *Mutat. Res.* 622, 14–18, 2007.
38. Ahmed, F. E., Effect of diet, lifestyle, and other environmental/chemopreventive factors on colorectal cancer development, and assessment of the risks. *J. Environ. Sci. Health* C22, 1–57 (2004.
39. Doyle, V. C., Nutrition and colorectal cancer risk: A literature review. *Gastroenterol. Nurs.* 30, 178– 182, 2007.
40. International Agency for Research on Cancer, *Handbook of Cancer Prevention: Weight Control and Physical Activity*. IARC Press, Lyon, France, 2002.
41. Jeejeebhoy, K., Lifestyle factors key to staving off colon cancer. *Med. Post* 41, 21–29, 2005.
42. Johnsen, N. F., Christensen, J., Thomsen, B. L., Olsen, A., Loft, S., et al., Physical activity and risk of colon cancer in a cohort of Danish middle aged men and women. *Eur. J. Epidemiol.* 21, 877–884, 2006.
43. O'Keefe, S. J., Chung, D., Mahmoud, N., Sepulveda, A. R., Manafe, M., et al., Why do African Americans get more colon cancer than Native Americans? *J. Nutr.* 137, 175S–182S, 2007.
44. Ries, A. G., Melbert, D., Krapcho, M., Mariotto, A., Miller, B. A., et al., Eds., SEER Cancer Statistics Review, 1975–2004. National Cancer Institute, Bethesda, MD. http://seer.cancer.gov/csr/1975_2004/.
45. Gapstur, S. M. and Khan, S., Fat, fruits, vegetables, and breast cancer survivorship. *JAMA* 298, 335–336, 2007.
46. Pierce, J. P., Natarajan, L, Caan, B. J., Parker, B. A., Greenberg, E. R., et al., Influence of a diet very high in vegetables, fruit and fiber and low fat on prognosis following treatment for breast cancer: The Women's Healthy Eating and Living (WHEL) randomized trial. *JAMA* 298, 289–298, 2007.
47. Chlebowski, R. T., Blackburn, G. L., Thomson, C. A., Nixon, D. W., Shapiro, A., et al., Dietary fat reduction and breast cancer outcome: Interim efficacy results from the Women's Intervention Study. *J. Natl. Cancer Inst.* 98, 1767–1776, 2006.
48. Kurt, M. and Altundag, K., Dietary fat reduction and breast cancer outcome: Interim efficacy results from the Women's intervention Nutrition Study. *J. Natl. Cancer Inst.* 99, 899–901, 2007.
49. Chlebowski, R. T., Blackburn, G. L., and Elashoff, R., Mature analysis from the Women's intervention Nutrition Study (WINS) evaluating dietary fat reduction and breast cancer outcome. *Breast Cancer Res. Treat.* 100 (Suppl 1), S16, 2006.
50. Hunter, D. J., Spiegelman, D., Adami, H. O., Beeson, L., and van den Brandt, P. A., et al., Cohort studies of fat intake and the risk of breast cancer—a pooled analysis. *N. Engl. J. Med.* 334, 356–361, 1996.
51. Smith-Warner, S. A., Spiegelman, D., Adami, H. O., Beeson, L., et al., Types of dietary fat and breast cancer: A pooled analysis of cohort studies. *Int. J. Cancer* 92, 767–774, 2001.
52. Thiébaut, A. C. M., Kipnis, V., Chang, S. C., Subar, A. F., Thompson, F. E., et al., Dietary fat and postmenopusal invasive breast cancer in the National Institute of Health–AARP Diet and Health Study Cohort. *J. Natl. Cancer Inst.* 99, 451–462, 2007.
53. Prentice, R. L., Caan, B., Chlebowski, R. T., Patterson, R., Kuller, L. H., et al., Low-fat dietary pattern and risk of invasive breast cancer. *JAMA* 295, 629–642, 2006.

54. Boys, N. F., Stone, J., Vogt, K. N., Connelly, B. S., Martin, L. J., and Minkin, S., Dietary fat and breast cancer risk revisited: A meta-analysis of the published literature. *Br. J. Cancer* 89, 1672–1685, 2003.
55. van den Brandt, P. A., Spiegelman, D., Yaun, S. S., Adami, H. O., Beeson, L., et al., Pooled analysis of prospective cohort studies on height, weight and breast cancer risk. *Am. J. Epidemiol.* 152, 514–527, 2000.
56. Saphner, T., Tormey, D. C., and Gray, R., Annual hazard rates of recurrence for breast cancer after primary therapy. *J. Clin. Oncol.* 14, 2738–2746, 1996.
57. Pierce, J. P., Stefanick, M. L., Flatt, S. W., Natarajan, L., Sternfeld, B., et al., Greater survival after breast cancer in physically active women with high vegetable-fruit intake regardless of obesity. *J. Clin. Oncol.* 25, 2345–2351, 2007.
58. Goodwin, P. J., Energy balance and cancer prognosis, breast cancer, in *Cancer Prevention and Management Through Exercise and Weight Control*, McTeran, A., Ed., Taylor & Francis, Boca Raton, FL, 2006.
59. Heitmann, B. L. and Frederiksen, P., Imprecise methods may both obscure and aggravate a relation between fat and breast cancer. *Eur. J. Clin. Nutr.* 61, 925–927, 2007.
60. Wolf, I., Sadetzki, S., Catane, R., Karaski, A., and Kaufman, B., Diabetes mellitus and breast cancer. *Lancet Oncol.* 6, 103–111, 2005.
61. Linos, E., Holmes, M. D., and Willett, W. C., Diet and breast cancer. *Curr. Oncol Rep.* 9, 31–41, 2007.
62. Key, T. J., Allen, N. E., Spencer, E. A., and Travis, R. C., Nutrition and breast cancer. *Breast* 12, 412–416, 2003.
63. Dos Santos Silva, I., Mangtani, P., McCormack, V., Bhakta, D., Sevak, L., and McMichael, A. J., Lifelong vegetarianism and risk of breast cancer: A population-based case-control study among South Asian migrant women living in England. *Int. J. Cancer* 99, 238–244, 2002.
64. Forman, M. R., Changes in dietary fat and fiber and serum hormone concentrations: Nutritional strategies for breast cancer prevention over the life course. *J. Nutr.* 137, 170S–174S, 2007.
65. Jasienska, G., Thune, I., and Ellison, P. T., Fatness at birth predicts adult susceptibility to ovarian suppression: An empirical test of the predictive adaptive response hypothesis. *Proc. Natl Acad. Sci. USA* 103, 12759–12762, 2006.
66. Ibanez, L. and de Zegher, F., Puberty and prenatal growth. *Mol. Cell. Endocrinol.* 254–255, 22–25, 2006.
67. Topol, E. J., Cholesterol, racial variation and targeted medicines. *Nature Med.* 11, 122–123, 2005.
68. Zhang, S. M., Lee, I. M., Manson, J., Cook, N. R., Willett, W. C., and Buring, J. E., Alcohol consumption and breast cancer risk in the Women's Health Study. *Am. J. Epidemiol.* 165, 667–676, 2007.
69. Chen, W. Y., Willett, W. C., and Rossner, G. A., Moderate alcohol consumption and breast cancer risk. *J. Clin. Oncol. Proc. ASCO* 23, 515, 2005.
70. Tjonneland, A., Christensen, J., Olsen, A., Stripp, C., Thomsen, B. L., et al., Alcohol intake and breast cancer risk: The European Prospective Investigation into Cancer and Nutrition (EPIC. *Cancer Causes Cont.* 18, 361–373, 2007.
71. Ericson, U. M., Sonestedt, E., Gullberg, B., Olsson, H., and Wirfalt, E., High folate intake is associated with lower breast cancer incidence in postmenopausal women in the Malmo Diet and Cancer cohort. *Am. J. Clin. Nutr.* 86, 434–443, 2007.
72. Zhang, S. M., Willett, W. C., Selhub, J., Hunter, D. J., and Giovannucci, E. L., Plasma folate, vitamin B6, vitamin B12, homocysteine, and risk of breast cancer. *J. Natl. Cancer Inst.* 95, 373–380, 2003.

73. Fuchs, C. S., Stampfer, M. J., Colditz, G. A., Giovannuci, E. L., Manson, J. E., et al., Alcohol consumption and mortality among women. *N. Engl. J. Med.* 332, 1245–1250, 1995.
74. Trock, B. J., Hilakivi-Clarke, L. and Clarke, R., Meta-analysis of soy intake and breast cancer risk. *J. Natl. Cancer Inst.* 98, 459–471, 2006.
75. Hargreaves, D. F., Potten, C. S., Harding, C., Shaw, L. E., Morton, M. S., et al., Two-week dietary soy supplementation has an estrogenic effect on normal premenopausal breast. *J. Clin. Endocrin. Metab.* 84, 4017–4024, 1999.
76. Adebamowo, C. A., Hu, F. B., Cho, E., Spiegelman, D., Holmes, M. D., et al., Dietary patterns and the risk of breast cancer. *Ann. Epidemiol.* 15, 789–795, 2005.
77. Smith-Warner, S. A., Spiegelman, D., Yaun, S. S., Adami, H. O., Beeson, W. L., et al., Intake of fruits and vegetables and risk of breast cancer: A pooled analysis of cohort studies. *JAMA* 285, 769–776, 2001.
78. van Gils, C. H., Peeters, P. H., Buene-de-Mesquita, H. B., Boschaizen, H. C., Lahmann, P. H., et al., Consumption of vegetables and fruits and risks of breast cancer. *JAMA* 293, 183–193, 2005.
79. Missmer, S. A., Smith-Warner, S. A., Spiegelman, D., Yaun, S. S., Adami, H. O., et al., Meat and dairy food consumption and breast cancer: A pooled analysis of cohort studies. *Int. J. Epidemiol.* 31, 78–85, 2002.
80. Shin, M. H., Holmes, M. D., Hankinson, S. E., Wu, K., Colditz, G. A., and Willett, W. C., Intake of dairy products, calcium, and vitamin D and risk of breast cancer. *J. Natl. Cancer Inst.* 94, 1301–1311, 2002.
81. Lin, J., Manson, J. E., Lee, I. M., Cook, N. R., Buring, J. E., and Zhang, S. M., Intakes of calcium and vitamin D and breast cancer risk in women. *Arch. Intern. Med.* 167, 1050–1059, 2007.
82. Robien, K., Cutler, G. J., and Lazovich, D., Vitamin D intake and breast cancer risk in postmenopausal women: The Iowa Women's Health Study. *Curr. Cancer Control* 18, 775–782, 2007.
83. McCullough, M. L., Rodriguez, C., Diver, W. R., Fegelson, H. S., Stevens, V. L., Thun, M. J., and Calle, E. E., Dairy, calcium, and vitamin D intake and postmenopausal breast cancer risk in the Cancer Prevention Study II Nutrition Cohort. *Cancer Epidemiol. Biomark. Prev.* 14, 2898–2904, 2005.
84. Holmes, M. D. and Willett, W. C., Does diet affect breast cancer risk? *Breast Cancer Res.* 6, 170–178, 2004.
85. Michels, K. B., Mohllajee, A. P., Roset-Bahmanyar, E., Beehler, G. P., and Moyich, K. B., Diet and breast cancer: A review of the prospective observational studies. *Cancer* 109, 2712–2749, 2007.
86. Hong, S., Bardwell, W. A., Natarajan, L., Flatt, S. W., Rock, C. L., et al., Correlates of physical activity levels in breast cancer survivors participating in the Women's Health Eating and Living (WHEL) Study. *Breast Cancer Res. Treat.* 101, 225–232, 2007.
87. Slattery, M. L., Edwards, S., Murtaugh, M. A., Sweeney, C., Herrick, J., et al., Physical activity and breast cancer risk among women in Southwestern United States. *Ann. Epidemiol.* 17, 342–353, 2007.
88. Nair, U., Bartsch, H., and Nair, J., Alert for an epidemic of oral cancer due to use of the betel quid substitutes gutkha and pan masala: A review of agents and causative mechanisms. *Mutagenesis* 19, 251–262, 2004.
89. Jemal, A., Siegel, R., Ward, E., Murray, T, Xu, J., Smigal, C., and Thun, M. J., Cancer statistics 2006. *CA Cancer J. Clin.* 56, 106–130, 2006.
90. Lippman, S. M. and Hong, W. K., Molecular markers of the risk of oral cancer. *N. Engl. J. Med.* 344, 1323–1326, 2001.

91. Khuri, F. R., Kim, E. S., Lee, J. J., Winn, R. J., Benner, S. E., et al., The impact of smoking status, disease stage, and index tumor site on second primary tumor incidence and tumor recurrence in the head and neck retinoid chemoprevention trial. *Cancer Epidemiol. Biomark. Prev.* 10, 823–829, 2001.
92. Taghavi, N. and Yazdi, I., Type of food and risk of oral cancer. *Arch. Iranian Med.* 10, 227–232, 2007.
93. De Stefani, E., Boffetta, P., Ronco, A. L., Deneo-Pellegrini, H., Acosta, G., and Mendilaharsu, M., Dietary patterns and risk of laryngeal cancer: An exploratory factor analysis in Uruguayan men. *Int. J. Cancer* 121, 1086–1091, 2007.
94. Freedman, N. D., Schatzkin, A., Leitzmann, M. F., Hollenbeck, A. R., and Abnet, C. C., Alcohol and head and neck cancer risk in a prospective study. *Br. J. Cancer* 96, 1469–1474, 2007.
95. Fowke, J. H., Head and neck cancer: A case for inhibition by isothiocyanates and indoles from cruciferous vegetables. *Eur. J. Cancer Prevent.* 16, 348–356, 2007.
96. International Agency for Research on Cancer, *World Cancer Report*. Stewart, B. W. and Kleihues, P., Eds., IAC Press, Lyon, France, 2003.
97. Marugame, T., Kamo, K., Katanoda, K., Ajiki, W., and Sobue, T., Cancer and incidence rates in Japan in 2000: Estimates based on data from 11 population-based cancer registries. *Jpn J. Clin. Oncol.* 36, 668–675, 2006.
98. National Cancer Institute, Cancer rates and risks: Cancer mortality in the United States, 1950–1991. Changing pattern for major cancers. http://seer.cancer.gov/publications/raterisk/index.html/.
99. La Vecchia, C., Franceschi, S., and Levi, F., Epidemiological research on cancer with a focus on Europe. *Eur. J. Cancer Prev.* 12, 5–14, 2003.
100. Makola, D., Peura, D. A., and Crowe, S. E., *Helicobacter pylori* infection and related gastrointestinal diseases. *J. Clin. Gastroenterol.* 410, 548–558, 2007.
101. Tsugane, S. and Sasazuki, D., Diet and the risk of gastric cancer: Review of epidemiological devidence. *Gastric Cancer* 10, 75–83, 2007.
102. Sasazuki, S., Sasaki, S., Tsubono, Y., Okubo, S., Hayashi, M., et al., The effect of 5-year vitamin C supplementation on serum pepsinogen level and Helicobacter pylori infection. *Cancer Sci.* 94, 378–382, 2003.
103. Freedman, N. D., Abnet, C. C., Leitzmann, M. F., Mouw, T., Subar, A. F., et al., A prospective study of tobacco, alcohol, and the risk of esophageal and gastric cancer subtypes. *Am. J. Epidemiol.* 165, 1424–1433, 2007.
104. Nagel, G., Linseisen, J., Boshuizen, H. C., Pera, G., Del Giudice, G., et al., Socioeconomic position and the risk of gastric and esophageal cancer in the European Prospective Investigation into Cancer and Nutrition (EPIC–EURGAST. *Int. J. Epidemiol.* 36, 66–76, 2007.
105. International Agency for Research on Cancer, *Monographs on the Evaluation of Carcinogenic Risks to Humans*, Vol 83, *Tobacco smoke and involuntary smoking*, IARC Press, Lyon, France, 2004.
106. Shields, P. G., Molecular epidemiology and smoking and lung cancer. *Oncogene* 21, 6870–6876, 2002.
107. Ekberg-Aronsson, M., Nilsson, P. M., Nilsson, J. A., Pehrsson, K., and Lofdahl, C. G., Socio-economic status and lung cancer risk including histologic subtyping—a longitudinal study. *Lung Cancer* 51, 21–29, 2006.
108. Kubik, A., Zatloukal, P., Tomasek, L., Pauk, N., Havel, L., Dolezal, J., and Plesko, I., Interactions between smoking and other exposures associated with lung cancer risk in women: Diet and physical activity. *Neoplasma* 54, 83–88, 2007.

109. Linseisen, J., Rohrmann, S., Miller, A. B., Bueno-de-Mesquita, H. B., Buchner, F. L., et al., Fruit and vegetable consumption and lung cancer risk: Updated information from the European Prospective Investigation into Cancer and Nutrition (EPIC). *Int. J. Cancer* 121, 1103–1114, 2007.
110. Mahabir, S., Spitz, M. R., Barrera, S. L., Beaver, S. H., Etzekl, C., and Forman, M. R., Dietary zinc, copper and selenium, and risk of lung cancer. *Int. J. Cancer* 120, 1108–1115, 2007.
111. Dosil-Síaz, O., Ruano-Ravina, A., Gestal-Otero, J. J. and Barros-Dios, J. M., Meat and fish consumption and risk of lung cancer: A case-control study in Galicia, Spain. *Cancer Lett.* 252, 115–122, 2007.
112. Twombly, R. Cancer killer may be "silent" no more. *J. Natl. Cancer Inst.* 99, 1359–1362, 2007.
113. Chang, E. T., Lee, V. S., Canchola, A. J., Clarke, C. A., Purdie, D. M., et al., Diet and risk of ovarian cancer in the California Teachers Study Cohort. *Am. J. Epidemiol.* 165, 802–813, 2007.
114. Zhang, M., Holman, C. D., and Binns, C. W., Intake of specific carotenoids and the risk of epithelial ovarian cancer. *Br. J. Nutr.* 98, 187–193, 2007.
115. Koralek, D. O., Bertone-Johnson, E. R., Leitzmann, M. F., Sturgeon, S. R., Lacer, J. V. Jr., Schairer, C., and Schatzkin, A., Relationship between calcium, lactose, vitamin D, and dairy products and ovarian cancer. *Nutr. Cancer* 56, 22–390, 2007.
116. Goodman, M. T., Wu, A. H., Tung, K. H., McDuffie, K., Kolonel, L. N., et al., Association of dairy producvts, lactose, and calcium with the risk of ovarian cancer. *Am. J. Epidemiol.* 156, 148–157, 2002.
117. Bidoli, E., La Vecchia, C., Taslamini, R., Negri, E., Parpinel, M., et al., Micronutrients and ovarian cancer: A case-control study in Italy. *Ann. Oncol.* 12, 1589–1593, 2001.
118. Kushi, L. H., Mink, P. J., Folsom, A. R., Anderson, K. E., Zheng, W., et al., Prospective study of diet and ovarian cancer. *Am. J. Epidemiol.* 149, 21–31, 1999.
119. Sakauchi, F., Khan, M. M., Mori, M., Kubo, T. and Fujino, Y., et al., Dietary habits and risk of ovarian cancer death in a large-scale cohort study (JACC) in Japan. *Nutr. Cancer* 57, 138–145, 2007.
120. Kiani, F., Knutsen, S., Singh, P., Ursin, G., and Fraser, G., Dietary risk factors for ovarian cancer: The Adventist Health Study. *Cancer Causes Cont.* 17, 137–146, 2006.
121. Peeters, P. H., Lukanova, A., Allen, N., Berrino, F., Key, T., et al., Serum IGF-I, its major binding protein (IGFP-3) and epithelial ovarian cancer risk: The European Prospective Investigation into Cancer and Nutrition (EPIC). *Endocrine–Rel. Cancer* 14, 81–90, 2007.
122. Bandera, E. V., Kushl, L. H., Moore, D. F., Gifkins, D. M., and McCullough, M. L., Dietary lipids and endometrial cancer: The current epidemiologic evidence. *Cancer Causes Cont.* 18, 687–703, 2007.
123. Trentham-Dietz, A., Nichols, H. B., Hampton, J. M., and Newcomb, P. A., Weight change and risk of endometrial cancer. *Int. J. Epidemiol.* 35, 151–158, 2006.
124. Chang, S. C., Lacey, J. V., Brinton, L. A., Hartage, P., Adams, K., et al., Lifetime weight history and endometrial cancer risk by type of menopausal hormone in the NIH-AARP diet and health study. *Cancer Epidemiol. Biomark. Prev.* 16, 723–730, 2007.
125. Xu, W. H., Dai, Q., Xiang, Y. B., Zhao, G. M., Ruan, Z. X., Cheng, J. R., et al., Nutritional factors in relation to endometrial cancer: A report from a population-based case-control study in Shanghai, China. *Int. J. Cancer* 120, 1776–1781, 2007.
126. Friedenreich, C., Cust, A., Lahmann, P. H., Steindorf, K., Boutron-Ruault, M. C., et al., Physical activity and risk of endometrial cancer: The European prospective investigation into cancer and nutrition. *Int. J. Cancer* 121, 347–355, 2007.

127. Schuurman, A. G., Goldbohm, R. A., Dorant, E., and van den Brandt, P. A., Vegetable and fruit consumption and prostate cancer risk: A cohort study in The Netherlands. *Cancer Epidemiol. Biomark. Prev.* 7, 673–680, 1998.
128. Stram, D. O., Hankin, J. H., Wilkens, L. R., Park, S., Henderson, B. E., et al., Prostate cancer incidence and intake of fruits, vegetables and related micronutrients: The multiethnic cohort study (USA). *Cancer Causes Cont.* 17, 1193–1207, 2006.
129. Giovannucci, E., Rimm, E. B., Liu, Y., Stampfer, M. J., and Willett, W. C., A prospective study of cruciferous vegetables and prostate cancer. *Cancer Epidemiol. Biomark. Prev.* 12, 1403–1409, 2003.
130. Kristal, A. R. and Stanford, J. L., Cruciferous vegetables and prostate cancer risk: Confounding by PSA screening. *Cancer Epidemiol. Biomark. Prev.* 13, 265–273, 2004.
131. Kirsh, V. A., Peters, U., Mayne, S. T., Subar, A. F., Chatterjee, N., et al., Prospective study of fruit and vegetable intake and risk of prostate cancer. *J. Natl Cancer Inst.* 99, 1200–1209, 2007.
132. Bosetti, C., Bravi, F., Talamini, R., Parpinel, M., Gnagnarella, P., et al., Flavonoids and prostate cancer risk: A study in Italy. *Nutrition Cancer* 56, 123–127, 2006.
133. Lawson, K. A., Wright, M. E., Subur, A., Mouw, T., Hollenbeck, A., Schatzkin, A., and Leitzmann, M. F., Multivitamin use and risk of prostate cancer in the National Institute of Health-AARP Diet and Health Study. *J. Natl. Cancer Inst.* 99, 751–764, 2007.
134. Wright, M. E., Weinstein, S. J., Lawson, K. A., Albanes, D., Subar, A. F., et al, Supplemental and dietary vitamin E intakes and risk of prostate cancer in a large prospective study. *Cancer Epidemiol. Biomark. Prev.* 16, 1128–1135, 2007.
135. Weinstein, S. J., Wright, M. E., Lawson, K. A., Snyder, K., Mannisto, S., et al., Serum and dietary vitamin E in relation to prostate cancer risk. *Cancer Epidemiol. Biomark. Prev.* 16, 1253–1259, 2007.
136. Rohrmann, S., Platz, E. A., Kavanaugh, C. J., Thuita, L., Hoffman, S. C., and Helzlsouer, K. J., Meat and dairy consumption and subsequent risk of possible cancer in a U. S. Cohort study. *Cancer Causes Cont.* 18, 41–48, 2007.
137. Demark-Wahenfried, W. and Moyad, M. M., Dietary intervention in the management of prostate cancer. *Curr. Opin. Urol.* 17, 168–174–2007.
138. Patel, A. V., Rodriguez, C., Jacobs, E. J., Solomon, L., Thun, M. J., and Calle, E. E., Recreational physical activity and risk of prostate cancer in a large cohort of U. S. men. *Cancer Epidemiol. Biomark. Prev.* 14, 275–279, 2005.
139. Allen, N. E., Key, T. J., Appleby, P. N., Travis, R. C., Roddam, A. W., Rinaldi, S., et al., Serum insulin-like growth factor (IGF)-I and IGF-binding protein-3 concentrations and prostate cancer risk: Results from the European Prospective Investigation into Cancer and Nutrition. *Cancer Epidemiol. Biomark. Prev.* 16, 1121–1127, 2007.
140. Farlay, J., Bray, F., Pisani, P., and Parkin, D. M., *GLOBOCAN 2002: Cancer incidence, mortality and prevalence worldwide*, version 1.0. IARC CancerBase No. 5. IARC Press, Lyon, France, 2004.
141. Levi, F., Lucchini, F., Negri, E., Boyle, P., and La Vecchia, C., Cancer mortality in Europe, 1995–1999, and an overview of trends since 1960. *Int. J. Cancer* 110, 155–169, 2004.
142. Gloeckler-Ries, L. A., Reichman, M. E., Lewis, D. R., Hankey, B. F., and Edwards, B. K., Cancer survival and incidence from the Surveillance, Epidemiology, and End Results (SEER) program. *Oncologist* 8, 541–552, 2003.
143. Sant, M., Aareleid, T., Berrino, F., Bielska-Lasota, M., Carli, P. M., et al., EUROCARE-3: survival of cancer patients diagnosed 1990–1994—results and commentary. *Ann. Oncology* 14, v61–v118, 2003.
144. Murta-Nascimento, C., Schmitz-Dräger, B. J., Zeegers, M. P., Steineck, G., Kogevinas, M., et al., Epidemiology of urinary bladder cancer: From tumor development to patient's death. *World J. Urol.* 25, 285–295, 2007.

145. Murta-Nascimento, C., Silverman, D. T., Kogevinas, M., Garcia-Closas, M., Rothman, N., et al, Risk of bladder cancer associated with family history of cancer: Do low-penetrance polymorphisms account for the increase in risk? *Cancer Epidemiol. Biomark. Prev.* 16, 1595–1600, 2007.
146. Patel, A. V., Rodriguez, C., Bernstein, L., Chao, A., Thun, M. J., and Calle, E. E., Obesity, recreational physical activity, and risk of pancreatic cancer in a large U. S. Cohort. *Cancer Epidemiol. Biomark. Prev.* 14, 459–466, 2005.
147. Parkin, D. M., Pisani, P., and Ferlay, J., Global cancer statistics. *CA Cancer J. Clin.* 49, 33–64, 1999.
148. Ries, L. A. E. M. and Kosary, C. L., SEER Cancer Statistics Review, 1973–1997. National Cancer Institute, Bethesda, MS, 2000.
149. Mathew, A., Devesa, S. S., Fraumeni, J. F. Jr., and Chow, W. H., Global increases in kidney cancer incidence, 1973–1992. *Eur. J. Cancer Prev.* 11, 171–178, 2002.
150. Dhote, R., Pellicer-Coeuret, M., Thiounn, N., Debre, B., and Vidal-Trecan, G., Risk factors for adult renal cell carcinoma: A systematic review and implications for prevention. *BJU Int.* 86, 20–27, 2000.
151. Tavani, A., La Vecchia, C., Gallus, S., Lagiou, P, Trichopoulos, D., et al., Red meat intake and cancer risk: A study in Italy. *Int. J. Cancer* 86, 425–428, 2000.
152. Faramawi, M., Johnson, E., Fry, M. W., Sall, M., and Yi, Z., Consumption of different types of meat and the risk of renal cancer: Meta-analysis of case-control studies. *Cancer Causes Cont.* 18, 125–133, 2007.
153. Hsu, C. C., Chow, W. H., Boffetta, P., Moore, L., Zaridze, D., et al., Dietary risk factors for kidney cancer in Eastern and Central Europe. *Am. J. Epidemiol.* 166, 62–70, 2007.
154. Lee, J. E., Giovannucci, E., Smith-Warner, S. A., Spiegelman, D., Willett, W. C., and Curhan, G. C., Intakes of fruits, vegetables, vitamins A, C and E, and carotenoids and risk of renal cell cancer. *Cancer Epidemiol. Biomark. Prev.* 15, 1204–1211, 2006.
155. American Cancer Society, Cancer facts and Figures 2005. ACS, Atlanta, GA, 2005.
156. Christenson, L. J., Borrowman, T. A., Vachon, C. M., Tollefson, M. M., Otley, C. C., Weaver, A. L., and Roenigh, R. K., Incidence of basal cell and squamous cell carcinoma in a population younger than 40 years. *JAMA* 294, 681–690, 2005.
157. Joseph, A. K., Mark, T. L., and Mueller, C., The period prevalence and costs of treating nonmelanoma skin cancers in patients over 65 years of age covered by Medicare. *Dermatol. Surg.* 27, 955–959, 2001.
158. Ahmed, F. E. and Setlow, R. B., Different rate limiting steps in excision repair of ultraviolet- and N-acetoxy-2-acetylaminofluorene damaged DNA in normal human fibroblasts. *Proc. Natl Acad. Sci. the United States* 74, 1548–1552, 1977.
159. Sies, H. and Stahl, W., Nutritional protection against skin damage from sunlight. *Ann. Rev. Nutr.* 24, 173–200, 2004.
160. Black, H. S. and Rhodes, L. E., The potential of omega-3 fatty acids in the prevention of non-melanoma skin cancer. *Cancer Detect. Prev.* 30, 224–232, 2006.
161. McNaughton, S., Marks, G., and Green, A., Role of dietary factors in the development of basal cell and squamous cell cancer of the skin. *Cancer Epidemiol. Biomark. Prev.* 14, 1596–1607, 2005.
162. Hughes, M. C., Van der Pols, J. C., Marks, G. C., and Green, A. C., Food intake and risk of squamous cell carcinoma of the skin in a community: The Nambour Skin Cancer Cohort Study. *Int. J. Cancer* 119, 1953–1960, 2006.
163. Ibiebele, T. I., van der Pols, J. C., Hughes, M. C., Marks, G. C., Williams, G. M., and Green, A. C., Dietary pattern in association with squamous cell carcinoma of the skin: A prospective study. *Am. J. Clin. Nutr.* 85, 1401–1408, 2007.
164. Kune, G. A., Banneman, S., Field, B., Watson, L. F., Cleland, H., Merenstein, D., and Viletta, L., Diet, alcohol, smoking, serum beta-carotene and vitamin A in male nonmelanocytic skin cancer patients and controls. *Nutr. Cancer* 18, 237–244, 1992.

165. Hakim, I. A., Harris, R. B., and Ritenbaugh, C., Fat intake and risk of squamous cell carcinoma of the skin. *Nutr. Cancer* 36, 155–162, 2000.
166. Moon, T. E., Levine, N., Cartmel, B., Bangert, J. L., Rodney, S., et al., Effect of retinol in preventing squamous cell skin cancer in moderate-risk subjects: A randomized, double-blind, controlled trial. Southwest Skin Cancer Prevention Study Group. *Cancer Epidemiol. Biomark. Prev.* 6, 949–956, 1997.
167. McNaughton, S., Marks, G., Gaffney, P., Williams, G., and Green, A., Antioxidant and basal cell carcinoma of the skin: A nested case-control study. *Cancer Causes Control* 16, 609–618, 2005.
168. Naldi, L., Gallus, S., Tavani, A., Imberti, G. L. and La Vecchia, C., Risk of melanoma and vitamin A, coffee and alcohol: A case-control study from Italy. *Eur. J. Cancer Prev.* 13, 503–508, 2004.
169. Vincenti, M., Pellacani, G., Malagoli, C., Bassissi, S., Sieri, S., et al., A population-based case-control study of diet and melanoma risk in northern Itlay. *Public Health Nutr.* 8, 1307–1314, 2005.
170. Millen, A. E., Tucker, M. A., Hartge, P., Halpren, A., and Elder, A., Diet and melanoma in a case-control study. *Cancer Epidemiol. Biomark. Prev.* 13, 1042–1051, 2004.
171. Hoeijmakers, J. H. J., Genome maintenance mechanism for preventing cancer. *Nature* 411, 366–374, 2001.
172. Mathers, J. C., Coxhead, J. M., and Tyson, J., Nutrition and DNA repair—Potential molecular mechanisms of action. *Curr. Cancer Drug Targets* 7, 325–334, 2007.
173. Wei, Q., Shen, H., Wang, L. E., Duphorne, C. M., Pillow, P. C., et al., Association between low dietary folate intake and suboptimal cellular DNA repair capacity. *Cancer Epidemiol. Biomark. Prev.* 12, 963–969, 2003.
174. Chirricolo, M., Musa, A. R., Monti, D., Zannotti, M., and Franceschi, C., Enhanced DNA repair in lymphocytes of Down syndrome patients: The influence of zinc nutritional supplementation. *Mutat. Res.* 295, *105–111*, 1993.
175. Basten, G. P., Duthie, S. J., Pirie, L., Vaughn, N., Hill, M. H., and Powers, H. J., Sensitivity of markers of DNA stability and DNA repair activity to folate supplementation in healthy volunteers. *Br. J. Cancer* 94, 1942–1947, 2006.
176. Tomasetti, M., Alleva, R., Borghi, B., and Collins A. R., *In vivo* supplementation with coenzyme Q_{10} enhances the recovery of human lymphocytes from oxidative DNA damage. *FASEB J.* 15, 1425–1427, 2001.
177. Collins, A. R., Harrington, V., Drew, J., and Melvin, R., Nutritional modulation of DNA repair in human intervention study. *Carcinogenesis* 24, 511–515, 2003.
178. Astley, S. B., Elliott, R. M., Archer, D. B., and Southon, S., Evidence that dietary supplementation with carotenoids and carotenoid-rich foods modulates the DNA damage: Repair balance in human lymphocytes. *Br. J. Nutr.* 91, 63–72, 2004.
179. Pool-Zobel, B. L., Domacher, I., Lambertz, R., Knoll, M., and Seitz, H. K., Genetic damage and repair in human rectal cells for biomonitoring: Sex differences, effects of alcohol exposure and susceptibilities in comparison to peripheral blood lymphocytes. *Mutat. Res.* 551, 127–134, 2004.
180. Fang, M. Z., Wang, Y., Ai, N., Hou, Z., Sun, Y., Lu, H., et al., Tea polyphenol (-) –epigallocatechin-3-gallate inhibits DNA methyltransferase and reactivates methylation-silenced genes in cancer cell lines. *Cancer Res.* 63, 7563–7570, 2003.
181. Dashwood, R. H., Myzak, M. C., and Ho, E., Dietary HDHC inhibitors: Time to rethink weak ligands in cancer chemotherapy. *Carcinogenesis* 27, 344–349, 2006.
182. Martin, K. R., Targeting apoptosis with dietary bioactive agents. *Exp. Biol. Med.* 231, 117–129, 2006.
183. Chen, C. and Kong, A. N., Dietary cancer-chemopreventive compounds: From signaling and gene expression to pharmacological effects. *Trends Pharmacol. Sci.* 26, 318–326, 2005.

184. Thornberry, N. A. and Lazebnik, Y., Caspases: enemies within. *Science* 281, 1312–1316, 1998.
185. Davis, C. D. Nutritional interactions: Credentialing of molecular targets for cancer prevention. *Exp. Biol. Med.* 232, 176–183, 2007.
186. Hofseth, L. J. and Ying, L., Identifying and diffusing weapons of mass inflammation in carcinogenesis. *Biochim. Biophys. Acta.* 1765, 74–84, 2006.
187. Albini, A., Tosetti, F., Benelli, R., and Noonan, D. M., Tumor inflammatory angiogenesis and its chemoprevention. *Cancer Res.* 65, 10637–10641, 2005.
188. Li, M., Yamamoto, H., Adachi, Y., Maruyama, Y., and Shinomura, Y., Role of matrix metalloproteinase-7 (matrilysin) in human cancer invasion, apoptosis, growth, and angiogenesis. *Exp. Biol. Med.* 231, 20–27, 2006.
189. Twombly, R., The big fat question: What is the role of excess weight in cancer risk, mortality? *J. Natl. Cancer Inst.* 97, 1110–1112, 2005.
190. Mark, D. H., Deaths attributable to obesity. *JAMA* 293, 1918–1919, 2005.
191. Hursting, S. D., Nunez, N. P., Varticovski, L., and Vinson, C., The obesity cancer link: Lessons learned from a fatless mouse. *Cancer Res.* 67, 2391–2393, 2007.
192. Gonzalez, C. A. and Riboli, E., Diet and cancer prevention: Where we are, where we are going. *Nutr. Cancer* 56, 225–231, 2006.
193. Meyerhardt, J. A., Niedzwiecki, D., Hollis, D., Saltz, L. B., Hu, F. B., et al., Association of dietary patterns with cancer recurrence and survival in patients with stage III colon cancer. *JAMA* 98, 754–764, 2007.
194. Ferguson, L. R. and Philpott, M., Cancer prevention by dietary active components that target the immune response. *Curr. Cancer Drug Targets* 7, 459–464, 2007.

Appendix A

Recommended Dietary Allowances (RDAs) and Adequate Intakes (AIs) of Carbohydrates, Fiber, Fat, Protein, and Water for Adults, 31–70y

	Men		Women[a]	
Nutrient	**31–50y**	**51–70y**	**31–50y**	**51–70y**
Carbohydrates (g/d)	**130**	**130**	**130**	**130**
Total fiber (g/d	38*	30*	25*	21*
n-6 PUFAs (g/d)	17*	14*	12*	11*
n-3 PUFAs (g/d)	1.6*	1.6*	1.1*	1.1*
Protein (g/d)[b]	**56**	**56**	**46**	**46**
Total water (L/d)	3.7*	3.7*	2.7*	2.7*
From foods (L/d)	0.7*	0.7*	0.5*	0.5*
From beverages L/d)	3.0*	3.0*	2.2*	2.2*

Note: Recommended Dietary Allowances (RDAs) are in bold type and Adequate Intakes (AIs) in ordinary type followed by an asterisk (*). RDAs and AIs can both be used as goals for individual intake.

[a] Nonpregnant, nonlactating.

[b] Or 0.8 g/kg body weight/d.

Adapted from: Institute of Medicine, National Academy of Sciences, Dietary Reference Intakes publications.[18,26]

Appendix B

Recommended Dietary Allowances (RDAs) and Adequate Intakes (AIs) of Vitamins for Adults, 31–70y

	Men		Women[a]	
Nutrient	**31–50y**	**51–70y**	**31–50y**	**51–70y**
Vitamin A (μg/d)[b]	**900**	**900**	**700**	**700**
Vitamin C (mg/d)	**90**	**90**	**75**	**75**
Vitamin D (μg/d)[c,d]	5*	10*	5*	10*
Vitamin E (mg/d)[e]	**15**	**15**	**15**	**15**
Vitamin K (μg/d)	120*	120*	90*	90*
Thiamin (mg/d)	**1.2**	**1.2**	**1.1**	**1.1**
Riboflavin (mg/d)	**1.3**	**1.3**	**1.1**	**1.1**
Niacin (mg/d)[f]	**16**	**16**	**14**	**14**
Vitamin B_6 (mg/d)	**1.3**	**1.7**	**1.3**	**1.5**
Folate (μg/d)[g]	**400**	**400**	**400**	**400**
Vitamin B_{12} (μg/d)	**2.4**	**2.4**[h]	**2.4**	**2.4**[h]
Pantothenic Acid (mg/d)	5*	5*	5*	5*
Biotin (μg/d)	30*	30*	30*	30*
Choline (mg/d)[i]	550*	550*	425*	425*

Note: Recommended Dietary Allowances (RDAs) are in bold type and Adequate Intakes (AIs) in ordinary type followed by an asterisk (*). RDAs and AIs can both be used as goals for individual intake.

[a] Nonpregnant, nonlactating.

[b] As retinol activity equivalents (RAEs). 1 RAE = 1 μg retinol, 12 μg ß-carotene, 24 μg α-carotene, or 24 μg ß-cryptoxanthin. To calculate RAEs from REs of provitamin A carotenoids in foods, divide the REs by 2. For preformed vitamin A in foods or supplements and for provitamin A carotenoids in supplements, 1 RE = 1 RAE.

[c] Calciferol. 1μg calciferol = 40 IU vitamin D.

[d] In the absence of adequate exposure to sunlight.

[e] As α-tocopherol. α-tocopherol includes RRR-α-tocopherol, the only form of α-tocopherol that occurs naturally in foods, and the 2R-stereoisomeric forms of α-tocopherol (RRR-, RSR-, RRS-, and RSS-α-tocopherol) that occur in fortified foods and supplements. It does not include the 2S-stereoisomeric forms of α-tocopherol (SRR-, SSR-, SRS-, and SSS- α-tocopherol), also found in fortified foods and supplements.

[f] As niacin equivalents (NE). 1 mg of niacin = 60 mg of tryptophan.

[g] As dietary folate equivalents (DFE). 1 DFE = 1 μg food folate = 0.6 μg of folic acid from fortified food or as a supplement consumed with food = 0.5 μg of a supplement taken on an empty stomach.

[h] Because 10 to 30% of older people may malabsorb food-bound B_{12}, it is advisable for those older than 50 years to meet their RDA mainly by consuming foods fortified with B_{12} or a supplement containing B_{12}.

[i] Although AIs have been set for choline, there are few data to assess whether a dietary supply of choline is needed at all stages of the life cycle, and it may be that the choline requirement can be met by endogenous synthesis at some of these stages.

Adapted from: Institute of Medicine, National Academy of Sciences, Dietary Reference Intakes publications.[16,29–31]

Appendix C

Recommended Dietary Allowances (RDAs) and Adequate Intakes (AIs) of Minerals for Adults, 31–70y

	Men		Women[a]	
Nutrient	**31–50y**	**51–70y**	**31–50y**	**51–70y**
Calcium (mg/d)	1,000*	1,200*	1,000*	1,200*
Chromium (μg/d)	35*	30*	25*	20*
Chloride (g/d)[b]	2.3*	2.0*	2.3*	2.0*
Copper (μg/d)	**900**	**900**	**900**	**900**
Fluoride (mg/d)	4*	4*	3*	3*
Iodine (μg/d)	**150**	**150**	**150**	**150**
Iron (mg/d)	**8**	**8**	**18**	**8**
Magnesium (mg/d)	**420**	**420**	**320**	**320**
Manganese (mg/d)	2.3*	2.3*	1.8*	1.8*
Molybdenum (μg/d)	**45**	**45**	**45**	**45**
Phosphorus (mg/d)	**700**	**700**	**700**	**700**
Potassium (g/d)	4.7*	4.7*	4.7*	4.7*
Selenium (μg/d)	**55**	**55**	**55**	**55**
Sodium (g/d)	1.5*	1.3*	1.5*	1.3*
Zinc (mg/d)	**11**	**11**	**8**	**8**

Note: Recommended Dietary Allowances (RDAs) are in bold type and Adequate Intakes (AIs) in ordinary type followed by an asterisk (*). RDAs and AIs may both be used as goals for individual intake.

[a] Nonpregnant, nonlactating.

[b] The AI for chloride is set at a level equivalent on a molar basis to that of sodium.

Adapted from: Institute of Medicine, National Academy of Sciences, Dietary Reference Intakes publications.[16,26,30,31]

Appendix D

Tolerable Upper Intake Levels (ULs) of Vitamins for Adults[a], 31–70y

Vitamin	UL	Vitamin	UL
Vitamin A (μg/d)[b]	3,000	Vitamin B_6 (mg/d)	100
Vitamin C (mg/d)	2,000	Folate (μg/d)[c]	1,000
Vitamin D (μg/d)	50	Vitamin B_{12}	ND[d]
Vitamin E (mg/d)[c,e]	1,000	Pantothenic Acid	ND
Vitamin K	ND	Biotin	ND
Thiamin	ND	Choline (g/d)	3.5
Riboflavin	ND	Carotenoids[f]	ND
Naicin (mg/d)[c]	35		

Note: Tolerable upper intake levels (ULs) are the maximum levels of daily nutrient intakes that are likely to pose no risk of adverse effects. Unless otherwise specified, the UL represents total intake from food, water, and supplements.

[a] Men and nonpregnant, nonlactating women.

[b] As preformed vitamin A only.

[c] The ULs for vitamin E, niacin, and folate apply to synthetic forms obtained from supplements, fortified foods, or a combination of the two.

[d] ND = Not determinable due to lack of data of adverse effects in this age group and concern with regard to lack of ability to handle excess amounts. Source of intake should be from food only to prevent high levels of intake.

[e] As α-tocopherol; applies to any form of supplements α-tocopherol.

[f] β-Carotene supplements are advised only to serve as a provitamin A source for individuals at risk of vitamin A deficiency.

Adapted from: Institute of Medicine, National Academy of Sciences, Dietary Reference Intakes publications.[16,29–31]

Appendix E

Tolerable Upper Intake Levels (ULs) of Minerals for Adults[a], 31–70y

Mineral	UL	Mineral	UL
Arsenic[b]	ND[c]	Manganese (mg/d)	11
Boron (mg/d)	20	Molybdenum (μg/d)	2,000
Calcium (g/d)	2.5	Nickel (mg/d)	1.0
Chloride (g/d)	3.6	Phosphorus (g/d)	4
Chromium	ND	Potassium[d]	ND
Copper (μg/d)	10,000	Selenium (μg/d)	400
Fluoride (mg/d)	10	Silicon[e]	ND
Iodine (μg/d)	1,100	Sodium (g/d)	2.3
Iron (mg/d)	45	Vanadium (mg/d)[f]	1.8
Magnesium (mg/d)[g]	350	Zinc (mg/d)	40

Note: Tolerable upper intake levels (ULs) are the maximum levels of daily nutrient intakes that are likely to pose no risk of adverse effects. Unless otherwise specified, the UL represents total intake from food, water, and supplements.

[a] Men and nonpregnant, nonlactating women.

[b] Although the UL was not determined for arsenic, there is no justification for adding arsenic to food or supplements.

[c] ND = Not determinable due to lack of data of adverse effects in this age group and concern with regard to lack of ability to handle excess amounts. Source of intake should be from food only to prevent high levels of intake.

[d] Caution is warranted given concerns about adverse effects when consuming excess amounts of potassium from potassium supplements while on drug therapy or in the presence of undiagnosed chronic disease.

[e] Although silicon has not been shown to cause adverse effects in humans, there is no justification for adding silicon to supplements.

[f] Although vanadium in food has not been shown to cause adverse effects in human, there is no justification for adding vanadium to food and vanadium supplements should be used with caution.

Adapted from: Institute of Medicine, National Academy of Sciences, Dietary Reference Intakes publications.[16,26,30,31]

Appendix F

Recommended Dietary Intakes (RDIs) and Adequate Intakes (AIs) of Dietary Fiber, Fat, Protein, and Water for Adults, 31–70y, living in Australia and New Zealanda

	Men		Women[a]	
Nutrient	**31–50y**	**51–70y**	**31–50y**	**51–70y**
Dietary fiber (g/d)	30*	30*	25*	25*
n-6 PUFAs (g/d)	13*	13*	8*	8*
n-3 PUFAs (g/d)	1.3	1.3	0.8	0.8
DHA/EPA/DPA (mg/d)[c]	160**	160**	90**	90**
Protein (g/d)	**64**	**64**	**46**	**46**
Total water (L/d)	3.4*	3.4*	2.8	2.8*
From fluids (L/d)	2.6*	2.6*	2.1*	21*

Note: Recommended Dietary Intakes (RDIs) are in bold type and Adequate Intakes (AIs) in ordinary type followed by an asterisk (*). RDIs and AIs may both be used as goals for individual intake.

[a] An UL has not been established from these nutrients with one exception. The UL for DHA/EPA/DPA[c] is 3,000 mg/d.

[b] Nonpregnant, nonlactating.

[c] Docosahexaenoic acid/eicosapentaenoic acid/docosapentaenoic acid.

Adapted from: National Health and Medical Research Council, Commonwealth of Australia and New Zealand Government, Nutrient Reference Values for Australia and New Zealand. Available at: http://www.nrv.gov.au. Accessed January 25, 2008.[19]

Appendix G

Recommended Dietary Intakes (RDIs) and Adequate Intakes (AIs) of Vitamins for Adults, 31–70y, living in Australia and New Zealand

	Men		Women[a]	
Nutrient	**31–50y**	**51–70y**	**31–50y**	**51–70y**
Vitamin A (μg/d)[b]	**900**	**900**	**700**	**700**
Vitamin C (mg/d)	**45**	**45**	**45**	**45**
Vitamin D (μg/d)[c]	5*	10*	5*	10*
Vitamin E (mg/d)[d]	10*	10*	7*	7*
Vitamin K (μg/d)	70*	70*	60*	60*
Thiamin (mg/d)	**1.2**	**1.2**	**1.1**	**1.1**
Riboflavin (mg/d)	**1.3**	**1.3**	**1.1**	**1.1**
Niacin (mg/d)[e]	**16**	**16**	**14**	**14**
Vitamin B_6 (mg/d)	**1.3**	**1.7**	**1.3**	**1.5**
Folate (μg/d)[f]	**400**	**400**	**400**	**400**
Vitamin B_{12} (μg/d)	**2.4**	**2.4**[g]	**2.4**	**2.4**[g]
Pantothenic Acid (mg/d)	6*	6*	4	4*
Biotin (μg/d)	30*	30*	25*	15*
Choline (mg/d)	550*	550*	425*	425*

Note: Recommended Dietary Intakes (RDIs) are in bold type and Adequate Intakes (AIs) in ordinary type followed by an asterisk (*). RDIs and AIs may both be used as goals for individual intake.

[a] Nonpregnant, nonlactating.

[b] As retinol equivalents (REs).

[c] 1 μg cholecalciferol = 0.2 μg 25(OH)D. 1 IU = 0.025 μg cholecalciferol or 0.005 μg 25(OH)D.

[d] As α-tocopherol equivalents.

[e] As niacin equivalents (NE).

[f] As dietary folate equivalents. 1 μg DFE = 1 μg food folate or 0.5 μg folate acid on an empty stomach or 0.6 μg folic acid with meals or as fortified foods.

[g] The natural vitamin B_{12} in foods may be less bioavailable to the substantial number of older adults who have atrophic gastritis with low stomach acid secretion. People with this condition may require higher intakes of vitamin B_{12}-rich foods, vitamin B_{12}-fortified foods or supplements.

Adapted from: National Health and Medical Research Council, Commonwealth of Australia and New Zealand Government, Nutrient Reference Values for Australia and New Zealand. Available at http://www.nrv.gov.au. Accessed January 25, 2008.[19]

Appendix H

Recommended Dietary Intakes (RDIs) and Adequate Intakes (AIs) of Minerals for Adults, 31–70y, living in Australia and New Zealand

	Men		Women[a]	
Nutrient	**31–50y**	**51–70y**	**31–50y**	**51–70y**
Calcium (mg/d)	**1,000**	**1,000**	**1,000**	**1,300**
Chromium (μg/d)	35*	35*	25*	25*
Copper (μg/d)	1700*	1700*	1200*	1200*
Fluoride (mg/d)	4*	4*	3*	3*
Iodine (μg/d)	**150**	**150**	**150**	**150**
Iron (mg/d)	**8**	**8**	**18**	**8**
Magnesium (mg/d)	**420**	**420**	**320**	**320**
Manganese (mg/d)	5.5*	5.5*	5.0*	5.0*
Molybdenum (μg/d)	**45**	**45**	**45**	**45**
Phosphorus (mg/d)	**1000**	**1000**	**1000**	**1000**
Potassium (g/d)	3.8*	3.8*	2.8*	2.8*
Selenium (μg/d)	**70**	**70**	**60**	**60**
Sodium (g/d)[b]	0.46-0.92*	0.46-0.92*	0.46-0.92*	0.46-0.92*
Zinc (mg/d)	**14**	**14**	**8**	**8**

Note: Recommended Dietary Intakes (RDIs) are in bold type and Adequate Intakes (AIs) in ordinary type followed by an asterisk (*). RDIs and AIs may both be used as goals for individual intake.

[a] Nonpregnant, nonlactating.

[b] This AI may not apply to highly active people who lose large amounts of sweat on a daily basis.

Adapted from: National Health and Medical Research Council, Commonwealth of Australia and New Zealand Government, Nutrient Reference Values for Australia and New Zealand. Available at: http://www.nrv.gov.au. Accessed January 25, 2008.[19]

Appendix I

Upper Levels of Intake (ULs) of Vitamins for Adults[a], 31–70y, living in Australia and New Zealand

Vitamin	UL	Vitamin	UL
Vitamin A (μg/d)	3,000	Vitamin B_6 (mg/d)	50
Vitamin C (mg/d)	NP[bc]	Folate (μg/d)[d]	1,000
Vitamin D (mg/d)	80	Vitamin B_{12}	NP
Vitamin E (mg/d)	300	Pantothenic Acid	NP
Vitamin K	NP	Biotin	NP
Thiamin	NP	Choline (g/d)	3.5
Riboflavin	NP	β-Carotene	NP[e]
Naicin (mg/d)	35/900[f]		

Note: Upper levels of intake (ULs) are the highest average daily nutrient intake levels likely to pose no adverse health effects to almost all individuals in the general population. As intake increases above the UL, the potential risk of adverse effects increases.

[a] Men and nonpregnant, nonlactating women.

[b] NP = Not possible to set.

[c] It is not possible to establish an UL for vitamin C, but 1,000 mg/d is a prudent limit.

[d] As folic acid.

[e] The UL for β-carotene cannot be established for supplemental use and does not need to be established for food use.

[f] 35 mg as nicotinic acid/900 mg as nicotinamide.

Adapted from: National Health and Medical Research Council, Commonwealth of Australia and New Zealand Government, Nutrient Reference Values for Australia and New Zealand. Available at: http://www.nrv.gov.au. Accessed January 25, 2008.[19]

Appendix J

Upper Levels of Intake (ULs) of Minerals for Adults[a], 31–70y, living in Australia and New Zealand

Mineral	UL	Mineral	UL
Calcium (g/d)	2.5	Molybdenum (μg/d)	2,000
Chromium	NP[b]	Nickel (mg/d)	1.0
Copper (μg/d)	10,000	Phosphorus (g/d)	4
Fluoride (mg/d)	10	Potassium	NP[c]
Iodine (μg/d)	1,100	Selenium (μg/d)	400
Iron (mg/d)	45	Sodium (g/d)	2.3
Magnesium (mg/d)	350[d]	Zinc (mg/d)	40
Manganese (mg/d)	NP[e]		

Note: Upper Levels of Intake are the highest levels of continuing daily nutrient intake likely to pose no adverse health effects in almost all individuals.

[a] Men and nonpregnant, nonlactating women.

[b] NP = Not possible to set.

[c] No UL has been set for potassium from dietary sources. High potassium intakes can cause gastrointestinal discomfort and stress that may include ulceration and perforation. Arrhythmia can also arise from the resulting hypercalcemia. Caution is warranted given concerns about adverse effects when consuming excess amounts of potassium from potassium supplements while on drug therapy or in the presence of undiagnosed chronic disease.

[d] As a supplement.

[e] Manganese intake beyond that normally present in food and beverages could represent a health risk, but there are insufficient data to set an UL.

Adapted from: National Health and Medical Research Council, Commonwealth of Australia and New Zealand Government. Nutrient Reference Values for Australia and New Zealand. Available at http://www.nrv.gov.au. Accessed January 25, 2008.[19]

Appendix K

World Health Organization's Recommended Nutrient Intakes of Vitamins for Adults, 19–65y

	Men	Women	
Nutrient	**19-65y**	**19-50y**[a]	**51-65y**[b]
Vitamin A (μg RE[c]/d)	600	500	500
Vitamin C (mg/d)	45	45	45
Vitamin D (μg/d)	5-10[d]	5	10
Vitamin E (mg-α-TE[e]/d)	10.0	7.5	7.5
Vitamin K (μg/d)	65	55	55
Thiamin (mg/d)	1.2	1.1	1.1
Riboflavin (mg/d)	1.3	1.1	1.1
Niacin (mg NE[f]/d)	16	14	14
Vitamin B_6 (mg/d)	1.3-1.7[g]	1.3	1.5
Folate (μg DFE[h]/d)	400	400	400
Vitamin B_{12} (μg/d)	2.4	2.4	2.4
Pantothenic Acid (mg/d)	5.0	5.0	5.0
Biotin (μg/d)	30	30	30

[a] Premenopausal.
[b] Menopausal.
[c] Retinol equivalent.
[d] 5 μg/d for those 19-50y; 10 μg/d for those 51-65y.
[e] α-Tocopherol equivalent.
[f] Niacin equivalent.
[g] 1.3 mg/d for those 19-50y; 1.7 mg/d for those 51-65y.
[h] Dietary folate equivalent.

Adapted from: World Health Organization, *Vitamin and Mineral Requirements in Human Nutrition,* 2nd Ed. 2004.[32]

Appendix L

World Health Organization's Recommended Nutrient Intakes of Minerals for Adults, 19–65y

	Men	Women	
Nutrient	**19-65y**	**19-50y[a]**	**51-65y[b]**
Calcium (mg/d)	1000	1000	1300
Iron (mg/d)[c]			
15% Bioavailability	9.1	19.6	7.5
12% Bioavailability	11.4	24.5	9.4
10% Bioavailability	13.7	29.4	11.3
5% Bioavailability	27.4	58.8	22.6
Iodine (µg/d)	150	150	150
Selenium (µg/d)	34	26	26
Magnesium (mg/d)	260	220	220
Zinc (mg/d)[d]			
High bioavailability	4.2	3.0	3.0
Moderate bioavailability	7.0	4.9	4.9
Low bioavailability	14.0	9.8	9.8

[a] Premenopausal.

[b] Menopausal.

[c] For those in developing countries 5% and 10% bioavailability values generally are used. For those consuming more Western-type diets, 12% and 15% would be appropriate, depending primarily on meat intake.

[d] High bioavailability = assumed 50% bioavailability (generally refined diets low in cereal fiber and phytic acid); medium bioavailability = assumed 30% bioavailability (generally mixed diets containing animal or fish protein); low bioavailability = assumed 15% bioavailability (generally diets high in unrefined, unfermented, and ungerminated cereal grain, high in phytic acid, and negligible animal protein).

Adapted from: World Health Organization, Vitamin and Mineral Requirements in Human Nutrition, 2nd Ed. 2004.[32]

Appendix M

Daily Values for Adults and Children 4 Years of Age and Older

Vitamin A—5000 IU	Sodium—2400 mg
Vitamin C—60 mg	Calcium—1000 mg
Vitamin D—400 IU	Iron—18 mg
Vitamin E —30 IU	Phosphorus—1000 mg
Vitamin K—80 μg	Iodine—150 μg
Thiamin—1.5 mg	Magnesium—400 mg
Riboflavin—1.7 mg	Zinc—15 mg
Niacin—20 mg	Selenium 70 μg
Vitamin B_6—2.0 mg	Copper—2.0 mg
Folate—400 μg	Manganese—2.0 mg
Vitamin B_{12}—6.0 μg	Chromium—120 μg
Biotin—300 μg	Molybdenum—75 μg
Pantothenic Acid—10 mg	Chloride—3400 mg

Adapted from: U.S. Food and Drug Administration, A Food Labeling Guide: Reference Values for Nutrition Labeling. Available at http://www.cfsan.fda.gov/~dms/flg-7a.html, editorial revisions June, 1999, accessed February 20, 2008.[35]

Appendix N

Basic Recommended and Personal Recommendations Expected to Reduce the Incidence of Cancer, According to the World Cancer Research Fund and American Institute for Cancer

Recommendation 1

Body Fatness: Be as lean as possible within the normal range of body weight

Personal Recommendations

Ensure that body weight through childhood and adolescent growth projects toward the lower end of the normal BMI range at age 21

Maintain body weight within the normal range from age 21

Avoid weight gain and increases in waist circumference throughout adulthood

Recommendation 2

Physical Activity: Be physically active as part of everyday life

Personal Recommendations

Be moderately physically active, equivalent to brisk walking, for at least 30 minutes every day

As fitness improves, aim for ≥60 minutes of moderate, or for ≥30 minutes of vigorous physical activity every day

Limit sedentary habits such as watching television

Recommendation 3

Foods and Drinks that Promote Weight Gain: Limit consumption of energy-dense foods. Avoid sugary drinks

Personal Recommendations

Consume energy-dense foods sparingly

Avoid sugary drinks

Consume "fast foods" sparingly, if at all

Recommendation 4

Plant Foods: Eat mostly foods of plant origin

Personal Recommendations

Eat at least 5 portions/servings (≥400 g or 14 oz) of a variety of non-starchy vegetables and of fruits every day

Eat relatively unprocessed cereals (grains) and/or pulses (legumes) with every meal

Limit refined starchy foods

People who consume starchy roots or tubers as staples also to ensure intake of sufficient non-starchy vegetables, fruits, and pulses (legumes)

Recommendation 5

Animal Foods: Limit intake of red meat and avoid processed meat

Personal Recommendation

People who eat red meat to consume <500 g (18 oz) a week, very little if any to be processed

Recommendation 6

Alcoholic Drinks: Limit alcoholic drinks

Personal Recommendation

If alcoholic drinks are consumed, limit consumption to ≤2 drinks a day for men and ≤1 drink a day for women

Recommendation 7

Preservation, Processing, Preparation: Limit consumption of salt. Avoid moldy cereals (grains) or pulses (legumes)

Personal Recommendations

Avoid salt-preserved, salted, or salty foods; preserve foods without using salt

Limit consumption of processed foods with added salt to ensure an intake <5 g (2.4 g sodium) a day

Do not eat moldy cereals (grains) or pulses (legumes)

Recommendation 8

Dietary Supplements: Aim to meet nutritional needs through diet alone

Personal Recommendation

Dietary supplements are not recommended for cancer prevention.

Adapted from: World Cancer Research Fund/American Institute for Cancer Research, *Food Nutrition, Physical Activity, and the Prevention of Cancer: A Global Perspective*, American Institute for Cancer Research, Washington, DC, 2007.[39]

Index

A

B

C

D

E

F

G

H

I

K

L